# Glial Neurobiology in Mental Illness

# Glial Neurobiology in Mental Illness

Editor: Jaxon Blakeley

AMERICAN
MEDICAL PUBLISHERS
www.americanmedicalpublishers.com

AMERICAN
MEDICAL PUBLISHERS
www.americanmedicalpublishers.com

**Cataloging-in-Publication Data**

Glial neurobiology in mental illness / edited by Jaxon Blakeley.
p. cm.
Includes bibliographical references and index.
ISBN 979-8-88740-134-8
1. Mental illness. 2. Neuroglia. 3. Neurobiology. 4. Mental health. 5. Neuropsychology.
6. Neuropsychiatry. I. Blakeley, Jaxon.
RC454.4 .G55 2023
616.89--dc23



American Medical Publishers,
41 Flatbush Avenue,
1st Floor, New York,
NY 11217, USA

ISBN 979-8-88740-134-8 (Hardback)

# Contents

# Preface

The world is advancing at a fast pace like never before. Therefore, the need is to keep up with the latest developments. This book was an idea that came to fruition when the specialists in the area realized the need to coordinate together and document essential themes in the subject. That's when I was requested to be the editor. Editing this book has been an honour as it brings together diverse authors researching on different streams of the field. The book collates essential materials contributed by veterans in the area which can be utilized by students and researchers alike.

Mental illness refers to a mental or behavioral pattern which causes significant interference with the functioning of a person. The behavioral patterns can be remitting, relapsing or persistent, and can occur in isolated episodes. Glial cells are important for proper functioning of neurons and dysfunction in glial cells can result in various mental illnesses, like psychiatric disorders, autism, glioblastoma and multiple sclerosis. They do not produce electrical impulses and are found in the peripheral nervous system and the central nervous system. They help homeostasis, produce myelin in the peripheral nervous system, while providing protection and support to the neurons. Glial cells comprise ependymal cells, oligodendrocytes, microglia and astrocytes in the central nervous system. They are made up of satellite cells and schwann cells in the peripheral nervous system. This book strives to provide a fair idea about glial neurobiology in mental illness and to help develop a better understanding of the latest advances in their clinical management. Those with an interest in this field would find it helpful.

Each chapter is a sole-standing publication that reflects each author's interpretation. Thus, the book displays a multi-facetted picture of our current understanding of application, resources and aspects of the field. I would like to thank the contributors of this book and my family for their endless support.

**Editor**

# 1

# Serum S100B Protein is Specifically Related to White Matter Changes in Schizophrenia

*Berko Milleit[1,2]*, Stefan Smesny[1], Matthias Rothermundt[3,4], Christoph Preul[5], Matthias L. Schroeter[6], Christof von Eiff[7]†, Gerald Ponath[3,8], Christine Milleit[1,9], Heinrich Sauer[1] and Christian Gaser[1,5]*

[1] Department of Psychiatry, Jena University Hospital, Jena, Germany, [2] St. Joseph-Krankenhaus, Dessau-Roßlau, Germany, [3] Department of Psychiatry, University of Muenster, Muenster, Germany, [4] Department of Psychiatry, St. Rochus Hospital, Telgte, Germany, [5] Department of Neurology, Jena University Hospital, Jena, Germany, [6] Max Planck Institute for Human Cognitive and Brain Sciences and Clinic for Cognitive Neurology, Leipzig, Germany, [7] Institute of Medical Microbiology, University of Muenster, Muenster, Germany, [8] Department of Neurology, School of Medicine, Yale University, New Haven, CT, USA, [9] Department of Psychiatry, Sophien- und Hufeland-Klinikum, Weimar, Germany

***Correspondence:**
Berko Milleit
berko.milleit@yahoo.de

**†Present Address:**
Christof von Eiff,
Pfizer Pharma GmbH, Berlin, Germany

**Background:** Schizophrenia can be conceptualized as a form of dysconnectivity between brain regions. To investigate the neurobiological foundation of dysconnectivity, one approach is to analyze white matter structures, such as the pathology of fiber tracks. S100B is considered a marker protein for glial cells, in particular oligodendrocytes and astroglia, that passes the blood brain barrier and is detectable in peripheral blood. Earlier Studies have consistently reported increased S100B levels in schizophrenia. In this study, we aim to investigate associations between S100B and structural white matter abnormalities.

**Methods:** We analyzed data of 17 unmedicated schizophrenic patients (first and recurrent episode) and 22 controls. We used voxel based morphometry (VBM) to detect group differences of white matter structures as obtained from T1-weighted MR-images and considered S100B serum levels as a regressor in an age-corrected interaction analysis.

**Results:** S100B was increased in both patient subgroups. Using VBM, we found clusters indicating significant differences of the association between S100B concentration and white matter. Involved anatomical structures are the posterior cingulate bundle and temporal white matter structures assigned to the superior longitudinal fasciculus.

**Conclusions:** S100B-associated alterations of white matter are shown to be existent already at time of first manifestation of psychosis and are distinct from findings in recurrent episode patients. This suggests involvement of S100B in an ongoing and dynamic process associated with structural brain changes in schizophrenia. However, it remains elusive whether increased S100B serum concentrations in psychotic patients represent a protective response to a continuous pathogenic process or if elevated S100B levels are actively involved in promoting structural brain damage.

**Keywords: schizophrenia, S100B, white matter, voxel based morphometry, VBM, first episode psychosis**

## INTRODUCTION

Structural abnormalities in the brains of schizophrenic patients have been frequently reported using post mortem (Harrison, 1999) and *in vivo* magnetic resonance imaging (MRI) techniques (Pearlson and Marsh, 1999; Wright et al., 2000; Gupta et al., 2015). Schizophrenia has been shown to be associated with ventricular enlargement and slightly decreased overall brain volume. Regional volume abnormalities were mainly localized in limbic structures and the temporal lobe (Bogerts et al., 1990; Wright et al., 2000). Neuroanatomical findings include decreased presynaptic and dendritic markers consistent with reduced neuron size and increased neuron density (Pakkenberg, 1993; Harrison, 1999). These findings and results from neuropsychological and neuroimaging studies of function have led to the notion of a disturbance of connectivity between brain regions (Andreasen et al., 1998; Lipska and Weinberger, 2002).

Consequently, abnormalities in interconnecting white matter (WM) structures have attracted interest (Davis et al., 2003). While investigations of global white matter volume have been inconclusive, local changes in white matter have been demonstrated in prefrontal cortex, temporo-parietal and parieto-occipital regions, splenium, cingulum, and posterior capsule, supporting the hypothesis of abnormal connectivity in schizophrenia (Davis et al., 2003; Kubicki et al., 2007; Ellison-Wright et al., 2008). However, the pathophysiological processes underlying structural abnormalities, their time dimension, and the relation to symptomatology and outcome are still to a large extent ambiguous. Structural abnormalities of the brain parenchyma like white matter myelin disturbance, deterioration of the neuropil, loss of synaptic connectivity, and functional impairment of oligodendrocytes have been proposed to contribute to the etiology of schizophrenia (Selemon and Goldman-Rakic, 1999; Davis et al., 2003; Katsel et al., 2011; Streitbuerger et al., 2012; Hercher et al., 2014).

S100B is a small acidic $Ca^{2+}$-binding protein that is found in high abundance within the central nervous system (CNS). It is secreted by astrocytes and oligodendrocytes, and is also expressed in ependyma and neurons (Donato, 2001; Eldik and Wainwright, 2003; Schroeter et al., 2013). A post mortem histological study in human brain tissue showed that S100B immunostained cells in cortical regions have astrocytic morphology while most S100B positive cells located in white matter regions resembled oligodendrocytes (Steiner et al., 2007).

As a rather small protein with a molecular weight of 21kDa in its biologically active homodimeric form, S100B passes the blood brain barrier, and thus is detectable as a brain derived protein in peripheral blood (Reiber, 2001). Measurements of S100B in serum have been proven to valuably reflect the S100B concentration in cerebrospinal fluid (CSF) in healthy individuals as well as in patients with various neurological diseases (Reiber, 2001). In schizophrenic patients, increased S100B serum concentration is a repeatedly reported finding (Aleksovska et al., 2014).

Though many effects of S100B have been explored, the pathophysiologic role of elevated S100B levels in schizophrenia is not yet clarified. S100B is implicated in a number of $Ca^{2+}$-dependent regulation processes, including phosphorylation, enzyme activity, cell metabolism, and signaling pathways (Donato, 2001; Rothermundt et al., 2004a). Extracellular effects of S100B depend on its local concentration. While nanomolar concentrations have been demonstrated to be neuroprotective and neurotrophic, micromolar concentrations have been shown to have neurotoxic effects and to induce apoptosis (Eldik and Wainwright, 2003; Gonçalves et al., 2008). Hence, S100B elevation can be considered to be a secondary attempt to protect nervous tissue, e.g., against glutamate induced stress (Ahlemeyer et al., 2000). Contrariwise, pathologic overproduction of S100B could also induce neuroinflammatory responses and thus make S100B a brain damaging agent itself (Eldik and Wainwright, 2003).

This study aims to ascertain whether there are associations between S100B elevation as a possible marker for glial function or dysfunction and local structural white matter changes in brains of schizophrenic patients. We utilized a voxel based morphometry (VBM) approach, since it is an established automated and thereby user-independent method well suited to detect local structural differences in the whole brain without prior definition of regions of interest by analysing *in vivo* magnetic resonance images (MRI; Ashburner and Friston, 2000; Honea et al., 2005). Building on prior knowledge from previous neuroimaging studies, interaction analyses, and histological post mortem studies, we hypothesized that an interaction between S100B and WM can be found in interconnecting fronto-temporal white matter structures (Steiner et al., 2008; Streitbuerger et al., 2012; Schroeter et al., 2013) and other repeatedly reported white matter structures within the frontal and temporal lobe as well as in cingulum bundle and corpus callosum (White et al., 2008).

## METHODS

### Subjects

We investigated 17 consecutively admitted patients from the inpatient unit of the Department of Psychiatry of the Jena University Hospital fulfilling DSM IV criteria for schizophrenia (all Caucasians, epidemiologic data in **Table 1**). Eleven patients suffered their first acute psychotic episode (FEP), of which 8 were drug-naïve and 3 free of neuroleptic medication for at least 5 days. Six patients had been psychotic for more than one time, thus suffering from a recurrent acute psychotic episode (REP). Of those, 2 patients were still naïve in terms of neuroleptic drugs; 4 were free of neuroleptic medication for at least 4 days. Diagnosis was made for each patient by two independent board-certified psychiatrists (St. S., H. S.) and confirmed by structured clinical interview. Patients were compared to 22 healthy volunteers (all Caucasian, epidemiological data given in **Table 1**). None of the healthy controls had a personal or family history of psychiatric disorder. Subjects with any acute or chronic inflammatory disease or recent treatment with non-steroidal or steroidal anti-inflammatory drugs were excluded from the study. For all subjects, blood samples were taken for S100B serum level analysis and high-resolution MRI was performed. The study was approved by the Research Ethics Committee of the Jena

**TABLE 1 | Epidemiological data and status of medication for each group.**

| | Control Group | First episode patients | Recurrent episode patients |
|---|---|---|---|
| Number (N) | 22 | 11 | 6 |
| Gender (male/female) | 9/13 | 5/6 | 1/5 |
| Age (years ± SD) | 34.73 (±10.30) | 30.53 (±9.95) | 42.00 (±9.28) |
| Drug-naïve (number) | | 8 | 2 |
| Drug-free (number, duration of drug-free period) | | 3 (5–14 days) | 4 (4 days–5 months) |
| Previous medication | | Risperidone | Risperidone, Olanzapine, Haloperidole |

University Hospital. All subjects gave written informed consent to participate in the study.

## Acquiring and Storage of Blood Samples

Venous blood (10 ml) was taken from an antecubital vein using a 19-gauge butterfly attached to a dry plastic syringe. Blood was allowed to clot for 30 min at room temperature. Serum was separated by centrifugation (10 min at 3000 rpm) within 2 h after collection and stored in 1 ml aliquots at −72°C. Mean duration of storage was 28.6 days (range: 12–56 days, SD: ±10.0 days). After thawing, sera were re-centrifuged and stirred carefully in order to avoid any inhomogeneities of the specimen.

## Analysis of S100B Protein Levels

S100B concentrations were determined by applying the LIAISON Sangtec 100 assay (AB Sangtec Medical, Bromma, Sweden), a quantitative automated luminometric immunoassay, according to the manufacturer's instructions. The assay's lower detection limit for S100B is 0.02 $\mu gl^{-1}$. The intra-assay (within-run) imprecision (CVs) is between 2.6 and 6.4 %, depending on concentration. The inter-assay variation (CVs) is between 2.2 and 10.7 %. Analytical recovery ranges between 91 and 100.

## Acquisition of Structural Data and Image Processing

High-resolution MRI was performed on a 1.5 T Philips Gyroscan ACSII system. We acquired 256 sagittal slices using a T1-weighted sequence (TR = 13 ms, TE = 5 ms, flip angle 25°) with isotropic voxel size of 1 × 1 × 1 $mm^3$. Data preprocessing and analysis was performed using SPM2 software (Statistical Parametric Mapping; Wellcome Department of Cognitive Neurology, London, UK).

For morphometric analysis of the data we used voxel-based morphometry (VBM). VBM is a fully automatic technique to computationally analyze of differences in local gray or white matter volume. This method involves the following steps: (i) spatial normalization of all images to a standardized anatomical space by removing differences in overall size, position, and global shape; (ii) extraction of gray and white matter from the normalized images; and (iii) analysis of differences in local gray and white matter volume across the whole brain (Ashburner and Friston, 2000). We applied an optimized method of VBM (Ashburner and Friston, 2000; Good et al., 2001) using the VBM2 Toolbox (http://dbm.neuro.uni-jena.de/vbm). The spatial normalization to the standard anatomical space was performed in a two-stage process. In the first step, we registered each image to the International Consortium for Brain Mapping (ICBM) template (Montreal Neurological Institute, Montreal, Canada), which approximates Talairach space. The normalized images of all subjects were averaged and smoothed with a 8 mm full-width at half-maximum (FWHM) Gaussian kernel; this averaged image was then used as a new template to reduce scanner- and population-specific bias. In the second normalization step, we locally deformed each image of our entire group to the new template using a non-linear spatial transformation. This accounts for the remaining shape differences between the images and the template and improves the overlap of corresponding anatomical structures. Finally, normalized images were corrected for non-uniformities in signal intensity and partitioned into gray and white matter, cerebrospinal fluid, and background using a modified mixture model cluster analysis. The resulting maps represent the local probability of belonging to a particular tissue type via voxel-wise values between 0 and 1. Because we applied spatial registration the same voxel location in each image should approximately correspond to the same brain structure. Using the probability values, we examined the relative concentration of one tissue type [i.e., the proportion of gray matter (GM) to other tissue types within a region]. We restricted the statistical analysis to areas with a minimum probability value of 0.1 to avoid possible edge effects around tissue borders. To remove unconnected non-brain voxels (e.g., rims between brain surface and meninges), we applied a series of morphological erosions and dilations to the segmented images (Good et al., 2001). Because these segmentations are often affected by noise we introduced spatial constraints based on neighboring voxels by using a Markov Random Field Model (Cuadra et al., 2005). The resulting white matter images were smoothed with a 12 mm FWHM Gaussian kernel.

## Statistical Analysis

Statistical analysis of S100B serum levels was performed using the software package SPSS 15 for Windows. For evaluation of group differences, univariate analysis of variance (ANOVA) was performed using S100B concentration as the dependent variable, GROUP as a between-subject factor, and GENDER and AGE as covariates. To further investigate group differences found to be significant in ANOVA, we performed multiple pairwise group comparisons using a two-tailed Student's $t$-test with significance defined as $p < 0.05$ (corresponding to $p < 0.0167$ Bonferroni adjusted alpha).

Groupwise comparison of white matter imaging data was performed using a general linear model implemented in the software package SPM2. To account for variance related to age effects (due to different mean age between the patient groups), we included age as a confounding variable into the model. For resulting statistics, we set the significance threshold at $p < 0.001$. Only clusters exceeding the expected number of voxels per cluster (according to the Gaussian Random Field theory) were considered.

Assessment of associations between S100B concentration and structural abnormalities was realized using a general linear model in SPM2 with S100B concentration defined as a regressor. To account for age-related effects, we included age as confounding variable into the model. For pairwise group comparison, this type of analysis equals an interaction model (Smesny et al., 2010) testing for different regression slopes of white matter density related to S100B concentration between the groups in each voxel (S100B concentration vs. group interaction). Because variance was expected to differ between samples, we applied a non-sphericity correction. Again, all statistical images were thresholded at $p < 0.001$ and only clusters exceeding the expected number of voxels per cluster were reported. To support the anatomical labeling of our findings, we used the Mori MRI Atlas of Human White Matter (Mori et al., 2005).

## RESULTS

### Sample Characteristics and S100B Serum Concentration

There was a difference in mean age between groups (**Table 1**). Group differences in mean age at the time of investigation originate from the natural age of onset and the course of the disease, leading to a consistently higher age in recurrent-episode patients ($t$-test: for FEP vs. REP: $p = 0.001$, for C vs. REP: $p = 0.006$, for C vs. FEP: $p = 0.271$). We took this into account by considering age as a covariate in all following analyses, thus assuring our findings are not due to effects of age. In terms of gender distribution, Fisher's exact test (gender by group) yielded $p = 0.280$ for C vs. FEP, $p = 0.059$ for C vs. REP, and $p = 0.055$ for FEP vs. REP, indicating that the gender distribution was not statistically significant. Also, univariate ANOVA and correlation analysis did not reveal any significant effect of GENDER or AGE on S100B serum concentration. Univariate ANOVA resulted in significant effects of GROUP on S100B levels ($F = 6.310$, $p < 0.005$; AGE and GENDER corrected model: $F = 4.011$, $p = 0.009$). The $t$-test results were congruent with previous findings that reported significantly higher S100B serum concentrations in both patient groups compared to controls (C vs. FEP: $p = 0.006$, C vs. REP: $p = 0.008$). No significant group differences were found between first and recurrent episode patients. Results and statistical information of S100B serum concentration analysis are presented in **Table 2**. A graphical presentation of the data is shown in **Figure 1**.

**TABLE 2 | Results and corresponding statistical information of S100B serum concentration analysis, specified in μg/ml.**

| | Control Group | First episode patients | Recurrent episode patients |
|---|---|---|---|
| Range | 0.01–0.10 | 0.03–0.13 | 0.05–0.12 |
| Mean ± SD | 0.057 ± 0.023 | 0.084 ± 0.028 | 0.089 ± 0.026 |
| Median | 0.06 | 0.08 | 0.09 |
| 95% confidence interval | 0.047–0.067 | 0.065–0.103 | 0.061–0.116 |

### VBM-Based Pairwise Group Comparison of Brain Imaging Data

By performing a VBM-Based group comparison of MRI data, we found local white matter structural differences between patients and controls as well as between both patient groups. A detailed listing of the results of this analysis is presented in **Table 3**.

When comparing healthy controls with patients suffering from their first psychotic episode (C vs. FEP), structural differences in white matter were located in the right medial orbital gyrus of the frontal lobe (diminished white matter in patients) and in white matter of the parietal lobe corresponding to the posterior cingulum bundle (increased white matter in patients). The VBM-based comparison of white matter between healthy controls and patients suffering from a recurrent psychotic episode (C vs. REP) yielded more and larger clusters denoting differences between these groups than between controls and first episode patients. The largest cluster indicating diminished white matter in recurrent episode patients was located in the medial area of the occipital lobe and was assigned to the inferior fronto-occipital fasciculus. Others were located in the cuneus, left frontal lobe, and frontal white matter assigned to the corticothalamic tract. Increased white matter in recurrent episode patients was found in the right superior temporal gyrus assigned to the inferior longitudinal fasciculus, and in the left cerebellum.

There were clusters indicating diminished white matter in first episode patients as compared to recurrent episode patients (FEP vs. REP). These were located in the left and right pontine area assigned to the corticospinal tract, the left occipital lobe, the left parahippocampal area, and the right frontal lobe.

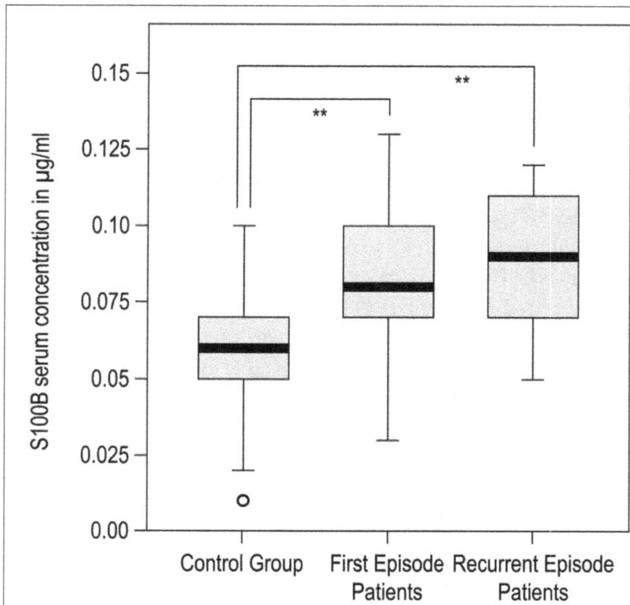


**FIGURE 1 | SPSS generated boxplot for results of S100B serum concentration analysis.** Black bar within box: median, gray box: 25–75% quartiles; small black bars: minimum to maximum; circles: outliners. Significant group differences are marked with **$p < 0.01$.

**TABLE 3 | Results of group comparison of white matter brain structure between controls and patient groups (VBM-based analysis).**

| Group comparison | Cluster size | *T*-value (voxel) | Anatomical region | Assigned white matter structure |
|---|---|---|---|---|
| C > FEP | 251 | 4.25 | Frontal lobe, medial orbital gyrus R | |
| C < FEP | 209 | 4.37 | Parietal lobe, region of gyrus Andrei Retzii L | Subcallosal white matter, Posterior cingulum bundle |
| C > REP | 3606* | 7.08 | Occipital lobe, median area L | Inferior fronto-occipital fasciculus |
| | 615 | 4.77 | Cuneus L/R | |
| | 194 | 4.03 | Frontal lateral white matter compartment R | Corona radiata, Corticothalamic tract |
| | 519 | 3.49 | Frontal lobe, F1 region L | |
| C < REP | 299 | 4.00 | Temporal lobe, superior temporal gyrus, Angular gyrus R | Inferior longitudinal fasciculus, Arcuate fasciculus |
| | 711 | 3.97 | Cerebellum L | |
| FEP > REP | 1033 | 5.40 | Occiptal lobe, median and basal parts L | Inferior fronto-occipital fasciculus |
| | 2064 | 4.82 | Middle and upper pontine area, lateral circumference, cerebellar peduncle L | Corticospinal tract |
| | 209 | 4.57 | Parahippocampal area T4/T5 L | Fornix |
| | 519 | 4.04 | Middle and upper pontine area, lateral circumference, cerebellar peduncle R | Corticospinal tract |
| | 265 | 3.78 | Frontal lobe, F1 region, middle part R | |
| FEP < REP | n.s. | n.s. | n.s. | n.s. |

*Between-group differences in white matter structure were found in reported clusters. Only clusters showing group differences at a significance level of $p < 0.001$ and exceeding the expected number of voxels per cluster according to the Gaussian Random Field theory are reported. *$p < 0.001$ (cluster-level, FWE corrected for multiple comparisons). Anatomic labeling, corresponding cluster size and T-value are shown for each cluster. The type of group comparison is indicated in the form A < / > B, where A > B indicates lower white matter in group B compared to A and vice versa. Lateralization is marked with L for left and R for right hemisphere. Anatomical names of white matter structures were assigned using Mori: MRI Atlas of Human White Matter (Mori et al., 2005). C, control; FEP, first episode patients; REP, recurrent episode patients. C, control; FEP, first episode patients; REP, recurrent episode patients.*

## Associations of S100B Serum Levels and White Matter Structure in Healthy Controls

We did not find statistically significant associations between S100B serum concentration and white matter brain structure in healthy controls.

## VBM-Based Pairwise Group Comparison of Associations between S100B Serum Levels and White Matter Brain Structure

We found differences in the association between local white matter structures and S100B concentration (denoted as *interaction* in the following text) between patients and controls as well as between both patient groups. A detailed listing of the results of this VBM-Based interaction analysis is presented in **Table 4**. **Figures 2–4** show localization and dimensions of each significant cluster listed in **Table 4** as an overlay onto the averaged T1-image of all subjects in axial and sagittal plane. Also shown are scatter plots and corresponding regression lines of S100B concentration vs. white matter values obtained from the 1st eigenvariate of the corresponding cluster.

Differences in the association between S100B and white matter between healthy controls and first episode patients (C vs. FEP) could be found in the left and right superior temporal gyrus assigned to the inferior longitudinal fasciculus (negative association in patients, illustrated in **Figure 2**: clusters 1, 2, and 3) and in the right postcentral dorsal white matter compartment assigned to the posterior cingulum bundle (steeper regression gradient in patients, **Figure 2**: cluster 4). In both cases, local white matter was diminished in patients.

In recurrent episode patients, there was a similar finding in the right postcentral white matter (posterior cingulum bundle, **Figure 3**: cluster 6). Also, there was a finding located in the superior temporal gyrus of the left temporal lobe (**Figure 3**: cluster 6), but the association between S100B and white matter was positive in recurrent episode patients and negative in first episode patients.

This type of interaction (negative association between S100B and white matter in first episode patients, positive association in recurrent episode patients) was also found in the direct comparison of both patient groups. With the chosen level of significance, a cluster in the right superior temporal gyrus could be identified (**Figure 3**: cluster 7). Additionally, a larger cluster (**Figure 3**: cluster 9, cluster-size 1289) could be detected in the right fronto-parietal white matter compartment, and was assigned to the superior longitudinal fasciculus. Other findings were located in the right temporal lobe and left postcentral region.

## VBM-Based Pairwise Group Comparison between S100B and Gray Matter

We followed a hypothesis driven approach and considered S100B as a protein associated with white matter (Schroeter et al., 2013). However, to complete the picture, we additionally calculated

**TABLE 4 | Results of pairwise group comparison of associations between S100B concentrations and white matter brain structure (VBM-based interaction analysis).**

| Interaction | Cluster Number | Cluster Size | *T*-Value (voxel) | Anatomical region | Assigned white matter structure |
|---|---|---|---|---|---|
| C > FEP | 1 | 175 | 3.80 | Temporal lobe, superior temporal gyrus L | Inferior longitudinal fasciculus<br>Arcuate fasciculus |
| | 2 | 880 | 5.13 | Temporal lobe, superior temporal gyrus R | Inferior longitudinal fasciculus<br>Arcuate fasciculus |
| | 3 | 400 | 4.17 | Dorsal parietal white matter compartment<br>Postcentral region R | Superior longitudinal fasciculus |
| C < FEP | 4 | 1214 | 5.55 | Parietal white matter compartment<br>Postcentral region R | Posterior cingulum bundle |
| C > REP | n.s. | n.s. | n.s. | n.s. | |
| C < REP | 5 | 818 | 4.28 | Temporal lobe, superior temporal gyrus<br>Angular gyrus L | Superior longitudinal fasciculus<br>Arcuate fasciculus |
| | 6 | 617 | 4.58 | Parietal white matter compartment<br>Postcentral region R | Posterior cingulum bundle |
| FEP > REP | n.s. | n.s. | n.s. | n.s. | |
| FEP < REP | 7 | 416 | 4.19 | Temporal lobe, superior temporal gyrus,<br>Insula R | Inferior longitudinal fasciculus |
| | 8 | 945 | 5.32 | Temporal lobe, T1/T2 region | Arcuate fasciculus |
| | 9 | 1289 | 4.84 | Fronto-parietal white matter compartment R | Superior longitudinal fasciculus |
| | 10 | 220 | 4.06 | Parietal lobe, Postcentral region | |

*Abbreviations, labeling and data structure as in* ***Table 3****. Interaction type is indicated in the form A < / > B, whereby A > B indicates a significantly steeper gradient of regression (association between S100B and white matter) of A as compared to B and vice versa. Clusters are numbered for easier identification in figures and discussion. C, control; FEP, first episode patients; REP, recurrent episode patients.*

results for gray matter in the same way as we did for white matter. It resulted in only 2 small clusters in the bordering region between gray and white matter—one next to the posterior cingulum bundle and one in the temporal lobe approximately corresponding to the neighborhood of the localization of cluster 2 in the white matter analysis but with much smaller extent (data not shown).

## DISCUSSION

This interaction analysis utilized a combined approach of voxel based brain morphometry and quantitative analysis of S100B serum concentration. It aimed to identify correlations between S100B concentration and white matter brain structure changes for schizophrenic patient groups at different stages of the disorder as compared to healthy controls. It also intended to show anatomic localizations of group differences. To minimize possible confounding effects, we ensured that all patients were free of antipsychotic medication at the time of investigation. Recurrent episode patients were significantly older at the time of investigation than controls and first episode patients. We took this into account by considering age as a nuisance variable in all VBM-based analyses and demonstrated that our findings were not due to age effects. Furthermore, investigation of patient subgroups (first episode and recurrent episode patients) allowed us to characterize patterns of S100B-associated structural brain abnormalities not only at the time of initial schizophrenic manifestation, but also at a recurrent episode stage.

### S100B Serum Concentration

S100B serum concentration was significantly increased in both patient groups when compared to healthy volunteers (**Table 2**, **Figure 1**), which constitutes a replication of findings in other first episode and chronic patient populations (Rothermundt et al., 2004a; Aleksovska et al., 2014). We did not find differences in S100B serum concentration between first and recurrent episode patients. When interpreting the latter result, one should bear in mind that, at the time of investigation, patients of both groups were unmedicated (or drug naïve) and had suffered an acute psychotic episode. Based on findings from other studies demonstrating that S100B decreases only in some patients when medicated (Rothermundt et al., 2001), or that it stays elevated even after 24 weeks of treatment in chronic patients (Rothermundt et al., 2004b), it is reasonable to assume that S100B elevation in schizophrenic patients is associated with pathophysiological processes inherent to psychotic episode in schizophrenia or, more likely, the disorder itself (Rothermundt et al., 2004a).

### VBM-Based Pairwise Group Comparison of Brain Imaging Data

In this section, we will discuss the results of the pairwise group comparison of white matter brain imaging data as presented in Section *VBM-Based Pairwise Group Comparison of Brain Imaging Data* and **Table 3**. While the main goal of this study was to identify possible interrelations between structural white matter changes and S100B concentration (see

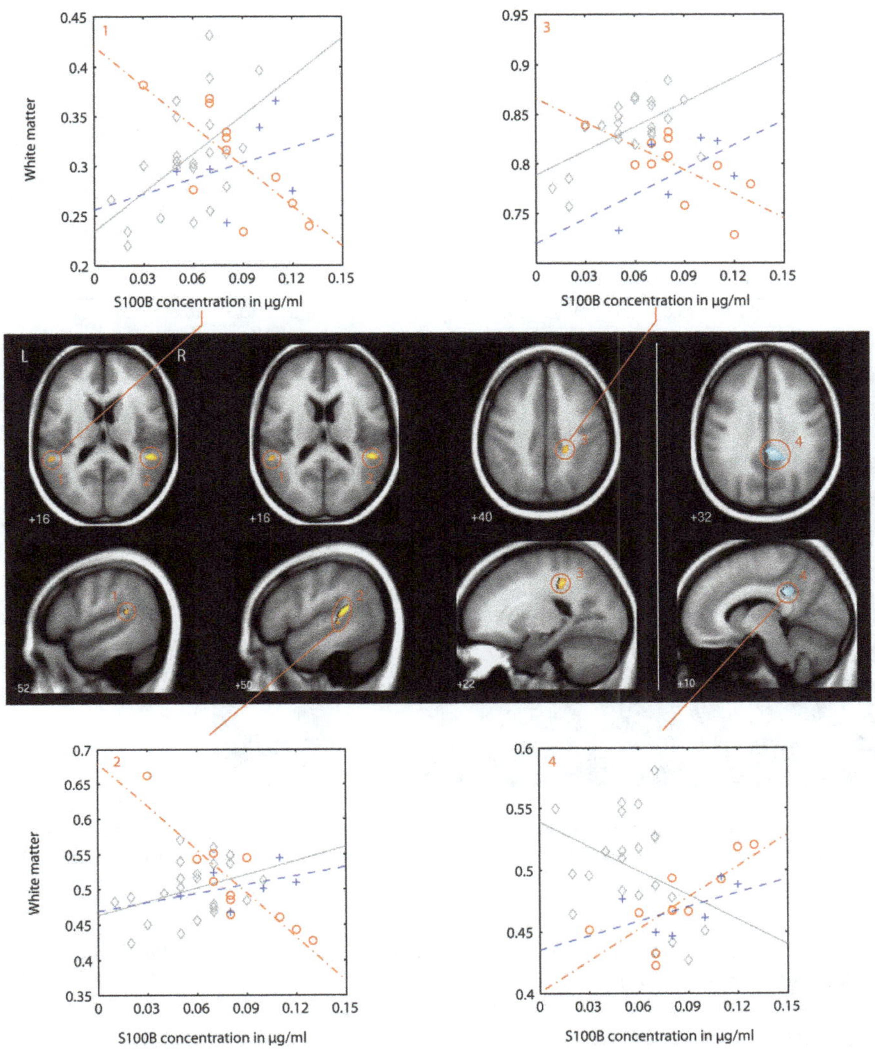


**FIGURE 2 | VBM-based pairwise group comparison of associations between S100B concentration and white matter brain structure (interaction analysis): controls (C) vs. first episode patients (FEP).** Clusters shown are significant as stated and numbered in **Table 4** and are shown as overlay to the T1 average image in axial and sagittal plane for each group comparison as indicated below anatomical images. The T1 averaged image was obtained from images of all participants of this study. Positive interaction (regression of group $A > B$) is indicated by red/yellow color, negative interaction ($A < B$) by blue color (colorbar with corresponding $T$-values shown in **Figure 3**). Numbering of clusters is as according to **Table 4**. Scatter plots showing S100B concentration against white matter values (obtained from 1st Eigenvariate of its corresponding cluster) and corresponding regression lines are demonstrated exemplarily for each found interaction pattern. Color coding in scatter plots: gray, C, controls; red, FEP, first episode patients; blue, REP, recurrent episode patients.

Sections *Associations of S100B Serum Levels and White Matter Structure in Healthy Controls* and *VBM-based Pairwise Group Comparison of Correlations between S100B Serum Levels and White Matter Brain Structure*), presentation and discussion of just the structural findings may be helpful for understanding and embedding results of the following interaction analysis into a broader neuroanatomical and pathophysiological context.

## First Episode Patients

We found differences in local white matter structures already present in the brains of first episode patients when compared to controls, even though most of these patients were drug-naïve. These differences were located in frontal regions (diminished WM) and parietal white matter structures (elevated WM) corresponding to the posterior part of the cingulum bundle.

Only few studies analyzing whole brain white matter structure in untreated first episode patients have been conducted so far (Kubicki et al., 2007; Kyriakopoulos and Frangou, 2009; Samartzis et al., 2014). Reductions of fractional anisotropy (FA) were found, among other regions, in the right parietal WM (Kyriakopoulos and Frangou, 2009). A recent DTI-based study revealed lower FA bilaterally in regions corresponding to the superior and inferior longitudinal fasciculus, the forceps major, the thalamic radiation, and the corpus callosum (Pérez-Iglesias et al., 2010). These and our findings strengthen the notion of disturbed white matter integrity being present already in very

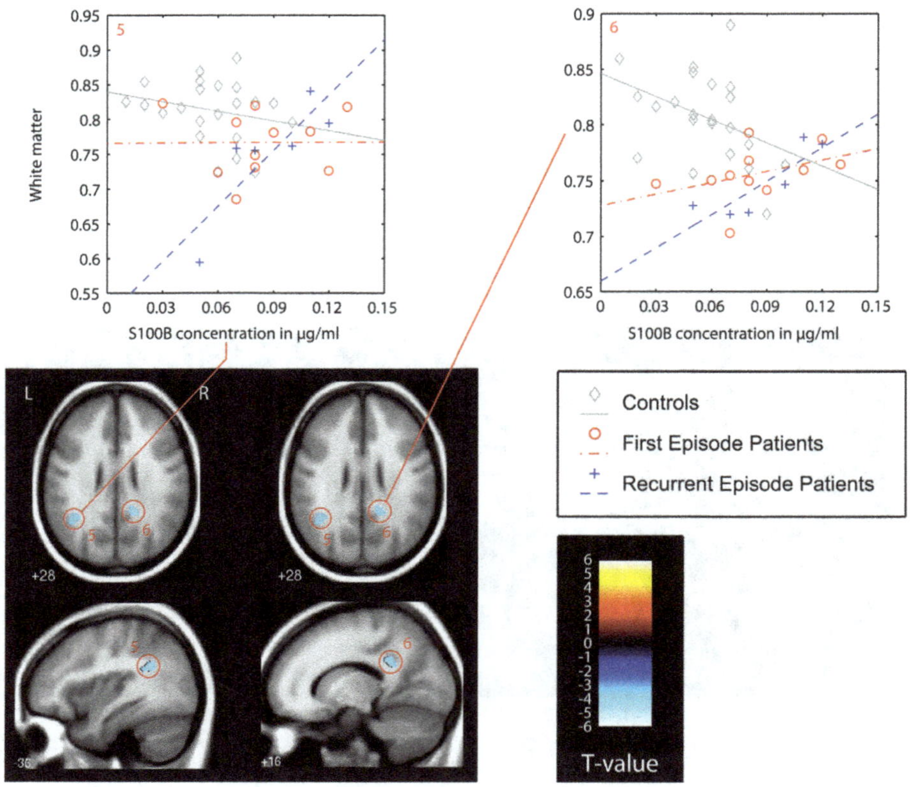


**FIGURE 3 | VBM-based interaction analysis: control group (C) vs. recurrent episode patients (REP).** Presentation as in **Figure 2**. In this figure also: color bar (*T*-values) and color/symbol coding for scatter plots in **Figures 2–4**: gray, C, controls; red, FEP, first episode patients; blue, REP, recurrent episode patients.

early stages of the disorder (Pantelis et al., 2005; Begré and Koenig, 2008; Kyriakopoulos and Frangou, 2009).

## Recurrent Episode Patients

In recurrent episode patients we found both, areas with diminished and increased local white matter (when compared to the control group). The largest cluster (3606 voxels) with the highest *T*-score (7.08) showing locally diminished WM was located in the left occipital lobe in the region corresponding to the inferior fronto-occipital fasciculus. Another area of diminished WM was located in the right frontal white matter corresponding to the corticothalamic tract. These results are in line with previous VBM-based studies (Suzuki et al., 2002), as well as DTI-based studies that describe abnormalities of those structures in terms of decreased FA or reduced track length (Kubicki et al., 2005; Mitelman et al., 2007; Ellison-Wright and Bullmore, 2009). Abnormalities of these WM structures provide evidence supporting the hypothesis of cerebral dysconnectivity in schizophrenia (Konrad and Winterer, 2008; Ellison-Wright and Bullmore, 2009).

Increased WM was found in the left cerebellum and the temporal white matter corresponding to the arcuate fasciculus, structures that have been repeatedly reported to be altered in schizophrenia as well (Douaud et al., 2007; Kubicki et al., 2007; Ellison-Wright and Bullmore, 2009). The possible meaning and relevance of temporal lobe findings are discussed in more detail in Section *VBM-based Pairwise Group Comparison of Correlations between S100B Serum Levels and White Matter Brain Structure.*

## First Episode vs. Recurrent Episode Patients

When comparing the first episode and recurrent episode patient groups, we found clusters indicating locally diminished white matter in the REP group but not in the FEP group. Although this was not a longitudinal study and these results must be interpreted cautiously, these findings may refer to an ongoing process of structural remodeling during the disease course. Such a process has been proposed in several previously published studies (DeLisi, 1999; Pantelis et al., 2003; Brans et al., 2008; Pol and Kahn, 2008).

In our sample, we found that the fornix and the inferior fronto-occipital fasciculus (see Section *Recurrent Episode Patients*) differ significantly between the FEP and REP groups. The fornix is one of the main pathways connecting the hippocampus with other brain regions and has repeatedly been shown to be altered in schizophrenia (Kubicki et al., 2005; Kuroki et al., 2006). It has also been associated with memory impairment (Nestor et al., 2007). Also, we found that the cerebellar peduncles and other structures corresponding to the corticospinal tract differ significantly between the patient groups. Structural changes of the cerebellar peduncles could contribute to some cognitive symptoms, since they are part of the frontal-thalamic-cerebellar

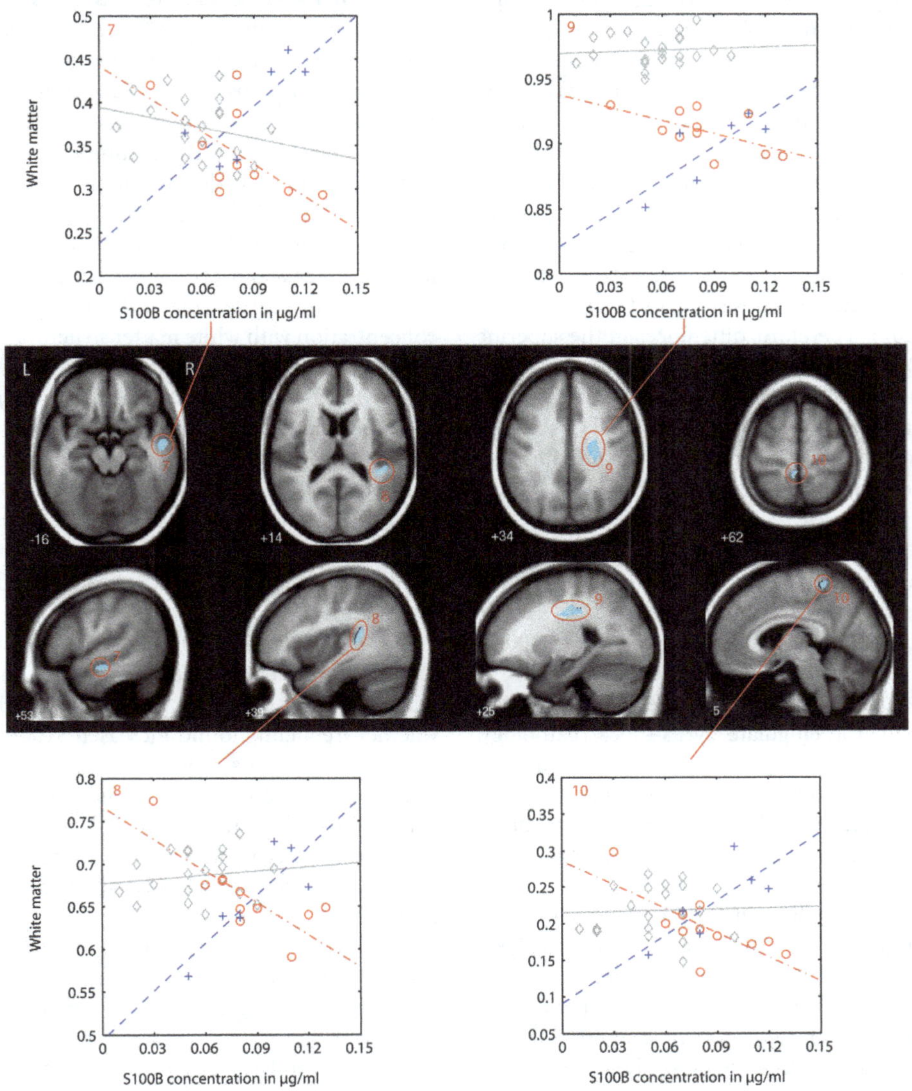


**FIGURE 4 | VBM-based interaction analysis: first episode patients (FEP) vs. recurrent episode patients (REP).** Presentation as in **Figure 2**. Color coding in scatter plots: gray, C, controls; red, FEP, first episode patients; blue, REP, recurrent episode patients.

circuitry that is thought to be disturbed in schizophrenic patients (Andreasen et al., 1998). The idea of a possible change in these structures over the course of the disease is supported by results of some DTI-based studies which reported reduced FA in early (Kyriakopoulos et al., 2008) and later disease stages (Okugawa et al., 2006), but not in chronic schizophrenic patients (Wang et al., 2003).

## VBM-based Pairwise Group Comparison of Correlations between S100B Serum Levels and White Matter Brain Structure

In the following, we will discuss the results of the VBM-based interaction analysis (for cluster numbering and anatomical localization, see **Table 4** and **Figures 2–4**) for all three group comparisons made (C vs. FEP, C vs. REP, and FEP vs. REP). This type of analysis was intended to test which local differences in structural imaging data between groups can be explained by differences of the chosen regressor S100B.

In first episode patients, S100B-associated differences to controls were located in the white matter of regions of the left and right superior temporal gyrus (STG), and in the postcentral region (clusters 1, 2, and 3). At these localizations, increased S100B concentrations were associated with diminished local white matter values (negative correlation). In the right cingulum bundle (cluster 4), first episode patients showed a positive correlation between S100B concentrations and white matter values.

Structural abnormalities of the temporal lobe rank among the most consistently reported morphometric findings in first episode patients (Bogerts et al., 1990; Pearlson and Marsh, 1999; Honea et al., 2005). As extensively discussed elsewhere, volume differences might follow from changes in neuropil and white matter (Selemon and Goldman-Rakic, 1999; Davis et al., 2003; Walterfang et al., 2005). Furthermore, white matter volume differences involving the inferior longitudinal fasciculus have been found in a subgroup of schizophrenic patients (Sigmundsson et al., 2001). Results from studies investigating white matter fiber tracts with more subtle *in vivo* methods, such as diffusion tensor imaging (DTI) or magnetization transfer imaging (MTI), strengthen the hypothesis that disturbed integrity of white matter structures is present in patients suffering from schizophrenic psychosis (Kubicki et al., 2005, 2007; Ashtari et al., 2007). Therefore, differences in the superior temporal gyrus (STG) are of special interest, as these structures include Heschl's gyrus and planum temporale. Disturbances in these structures and the inferior longitudinal fasciculus connecting Broca's and Wernicke's area may account for the pathophysiology of hearing voices (Dierks et al., 1999; Ashtari et al., 2007).

Alterations of the cingulum bundle have been consistently reported in previous studies investigating white matter abnormalities in schizophrenia (Sigmundsson et al., 2001; Kubicki et al., 2003, 2005; Shergill et al., 2007; Peters et al., 2008). As the cingulum bundle connects limbic structures—and is also known to interconnect the thalamus, prefrontal, parietal, and temporal lobes with the cingulate gyrus—local pathology of these structures already detectable in first episode patients might contribute to the hypothesis of dysconnection of the hippocampal/temporolimbic complex with the dorsolateral prefrontal cortex (Lipska and Weinberger, 2002; Mori et al., 2005).

While there was a joint finding in the posterior cingulum bundle of both patient groups, the striking result of our analysis was significant differences between both patient groups. These are localized in the right superior temporal gyrus (superior and inferior longitudinal fasciculus), right middle temporal lobe, in the postcentral region, and in a large region of the right fronto-temporal white matter that corresponds to the right superior longitudinal fasciculus. In all of these regions, first episode patients had a negative correlation of S100B concentration to white matter values while recurrent episode patients had a positive correlation (**Figure 4**).

There is a significant body of evidence for disturbed white matter configuration in temporal regions, including the STG, the insula (Ashtari et al., 2007; Mitelman et al., 2007; Shergill et al., 2007; Ellison-Wright and Bullmore, 2009), and the fronto-temporal white matter structures including the superior longitudinal fasciculus (Kubicki et al., 2005; Samartzis et al., 2014). A progression of structural temporal changes has been reported (Kasai et al., 2003a,b; Ellison-Wright et al., 2008) while another follow-up study did not find significant progression of structural changes in temporal regions (DeLisi and Hoff, 2005).

Although based on a cross-sectional analysis, our results suggest differences in the structural abnormalities of these regions between schizophrenic patients of earlier (FEP) and later (REP) stages in terms of a diverging correlation with S100B concentrations.

## Summary and Conclusions

There were significantly different correlations between S100B concentration and local white matter formations between both patient groups and healthy controls, as well as between first episode and recurrent episode patients. Structural white matter changes showing a different correlation with S100B between groups are located in brain regions that have been previously described extensively in the literature to be affected in schizophrenic patients. Also, these structures are integral parts in hypotheses about the physical foundation of neurocognitive symptoms in schizophrenia. A divergent association of S100B concentration with white matter structural changes could already be detected in the very early stage of the disorder (FEP). While there was a finding in the cingulum bundle that appears to be stable during the course of the disease, the correlation of S100B concentrations with white matter structural changes was found to be reversed between patient groups at different stages of disorder, especially in the white matter of the superior temporal gyrus corresponding to the inferior longitudinal fasciculus and fronto-temporal white matter corresponding to the superior longitudinal fasciculus.

We conclude that S100B is involved in an ongoing dynamic process associated with local structural changes in white brain matter of schizophrenic patients. Still, the question is open whether frequently found increased S100B serum concentration in psychotic patients at different stages of disorder is a secondary attempt of protection against an ongoing harmful process or if pathologically elevated S100B levels themselves can be held responsible for structural brain damage, either directly or as part of a biochemical network (Hanson and Gottesman, 2005; Monji et al., 2009).

Considering the range of measured S100B concentrations (**Table 2**), massive glial or neuronal destruction is unlikely to be the cause of S100B increase in schizophrenia (Rothermundt et al., 2004a).

A recent study by Streitbuerger et al. (2012) investigated the correlation between serum S100B levels and gray matter and white matter parameters with MRI (T1-weighted and diffusion tensor imaging) in healthy subjects. Here, S100B was specifically related to the diffusion tensor imaging parameters fractional anisotropy and radial diffusivity, the latest an indicator of myelin changes, in the corpus callosum, anterior forceps, and superior longitudinal fasciculus in female subjects. In contrast, there was no association between gray matter T1 data and S100B. Histological data confirmed a co-localization of S100B with oligodendrocyte markers in the human corpus callosum in this study. The authors showed additionally, that S100B was most abundantly expressed in the corpus callosum according to the whole genome Allen Human Brain Atlas. Based on these data, one might conclude that serum S100B represents a biomarker for white matter tracts and, consequently, oligodendroglia, which might have led to the association between white matter parameters and schizophrenia in our study, without relevant effects on gray matter.

Given the fact that S100B is involved in many different regulation processes and also linked to glutamatergic and cytokine systems (Ahlemeyer et al., 2000; Tramontina et al., 2006; Müller and Schwarz, 2007; Gonçalves et al., 2008), elevated S100B in schizophrenic psychosis could be an expression of other cross-linked and ongoing biochemical pathophysiological processes. Thus, the exact relation of S100B with structural changes remains open. On the other hand, S100B is a protein that exerts paracrine and autocrine effects on neurons and glia, and thus plays an important role in cell proliferation and differentiation, cellular energy metabolism, and cytoskeletal modification (Rothermundt et al., 2004a; Gonçalves et al., 2008). Hence, S100B might also be directly involved in processes leading to structural white matter changes in schizophrenia.

## Limitations of the Study

We included patients at different stages of the disorder to cover the entire course of the disease in a cross-sectional design. Cross-sectional studies have their limitations in the interpretation of the results when discussing questions about progression of structural changes. The sample sizes used in this study are considered to be moderate (Honea et al., 2005). However, an essential aspect of this study was to investigate unmedicated patients and also to compare first episode patients with patients at a later stage of the disease. Thus, the sample size was limited due to the small number of patients fulfilling these criteria.

All patients participating in this study were either neuroleptic-naïve or unmedicated. Due to practical and ethical reasons, of those who were unmedicated, some patients were off medication only for 4 respective 5 days, and some individuals had received haloperidole as previous medication. Considering the effects of antipsychotic medication on brain structure (Lieberman et al., 2005), it would have been desirable to have had a longer medication-free period before obtaining MRI data, so we cannot completely rule out a possible effect of medication on the results, especially in the REP group.

Patient groups differed in mean age. To ensure that found differences between these groups were not predominantly caused by effects of age, we included age as nuisance variable in all analyses. By this method a possible influence of age on the results can be diminished but not completely be ruled out.

A correlation ($r = 0.538$, $p < 0.001$) between S100B and body mass index (BMI) has been reported in healthy controls (Steiner et al., 2010a), though such correlation was not found in patients suffering from schizophrenia (Steiner et al., 2010b). However, S100B might have other sources than the brain, e.g., adipose tissue (Gonçalves et al., 2010) and it is recommendable to consider body mass index in future studies.

There was also an imbalance in the gender ratio. Differences in brain structure between men and women are at least in part a matter of overall size. While such size and shape differences are controlled by normalizing each image to the ICBM template (see *Section Acquisition of Structural Data and Image Processing*), a possible influence of gender on our results cannot completely be ruled out. Also, gender specific correlations between serum S100B and white matter parameters have been found in a previous study (Streitbuerger et al., 2012). Hence, we re-performed analyses with a reduced sample including female subjects only (data not shown). Although this lead to a considerable reduction of sample size, main effects were comparable (findings in cingulum bundle, temporal lobe findings).

For the statistical analysis, a stringent threshold of $p = 0.001$ was chosen to exclude false positives resulting from unaccounted confounding variables (Ashburner and Friston, 2000). Furthermore, having exclusively found significant changes in anatomical structures previously described to be altered in schizophrenia in a non-region-of-interest-approach, it is reasonable to assume that our results are valid.

We used VBM to find local differences in white matter values of T1 weighted MR images and assigned detected clusters to anatomical fiber structures according to an atlas of human brain white matter, presuming that localizations of clusters found in our analysis correspond to these structures. This method cannot show the fiber tracts themselves, including their directions and disruptions. To prove that these fiber tracts are indeed disrupted and that the disruptions are associated with S100B, future studies in this field should also utilize techniques such as DTI or MTI.

## AUTHOR CONTRIBUTIONS

BM performed data analyses with SPM and SPSS, wrote MATLAB scripts to plot graphs, made tables and figures, and conceptualized and wrote the article. SS had the original idea and made the concept of this interaction analysis. He also screened patients, made diagnoses and obtained MRI-data. MR, GP, CV did the measurement of S100B protein, wrote the methods part of S100B measurement, contributed to and revised the text of the manuscript, especially in the discussion regarding S100B protein. CP assigned the found clusters to anatomical white matter structures, did proof reading, and contributed to the discussion regarding neuroanatomical points. MS made major contributions to introduction and discussion and especially helped with connecting the results to findings of other studies in this field. CM did additional statistical analysis, made extensive literature research on the topic, maintained the literature database, wrote most of the introduction, and contributed to the logical structure of the manuscript. HS is the head of department. He provided all means to conduct the study, contributed to the original design, diagnosis of patients, obtaining of MRI-data, and to the text of the manuscript. CG is the senior author. He provided all knowledge and means to perform VBM analysis, wrote the VBM toolbox and scripts to make slice overlays. He provided intensive help in preparing and performing computer analyses, and wrote all MR-related parts of the manuscript.

## FUNDING

Stefan Smesny was supported by the German Research Foundation (DFG), grant Sm 68/1-1. Christian Gaser was supported by the German Federal Ministry of Education and Research (BMBF), grant 01EV0709.

## ACKNOWLEDGMENTS

The authors would like to thank the staff of the Department of Psychiatry of the Jena University Hospital for their extensive support to this study and the staff of the Department of Diagnostic and Interventional Radiology of the University of Jena for their support in obtaining the high-resolution MRI scans. Also, the authors would like to thank Rachel A. Yotter for proof-reading and helpful comments on the manuscript.

## REFERENCES

Ahlemeyer, B., Beier, H., Semkova, I., Schaper, C., and Krieglstein, J. (2000). S-100beta protects cultured neurons against glutamate- and staurosporine-induced damage and is involved in the antiapoptotic action of the 5 HT(1A)-receptor agonist, Bay x 3702. *Brain Res.* 858, 121–128. doi: 10.1016/S0006-8993(99)02438-5

Aleksovska, K., Leoncini, E., Bonassi, S., Cesario, A., Boccia, S., and Frustaci, A. (2014). Systematic review and meta-analysis of circulating S100B blood levels in schizophrenia. *PLoS ONE* 9:e106342. doi: 10.1371/journal.pone.0106342

Andreasen, N. C., Paradiso, S., and O'Leary, D. S. (1998). "Cognitive dysmetria" as an integrative theory of schizophrenia: a dysfunction in cortical-subcortical-cerebellar circuitry? *Schizophr. Bull.* 24, 203–218.

Ashburner, J., and Friston, K. J. (2000). Voxel-based morphometry–the methods. *Neuroimage* 11, 805–821. doi: 10.1006/nimg.2000.0582

Ashtari, M., Cottone, J., Ardekani, B. A., Cervellione, K., Szeszko, P. R., Wu, J., et al. (2007). Disruption of white matter integrity in the inferior longitudinal fasciculus in adolescents with schizophrenia as revealed by fiber tractography. *Arch. Gen. Psychiatry* 64, 1270–1280. doi: 10.1001/archpsyc.64.11.1270

Begré, S., and Koenig, T. (2008). Cerebral disconnectivity: an early event in schizophrenia. *Neuroscientist* 14, 19–45. doi: 10.1177/1073858406298391

Bogerts, B., Ashtari, M., Degreef, G., Alvir, J. M., Bilder, R. M., and Lieberman, J. A. (1990). Reduced temporal limbic structure volumes on magnetic resonance images in first episode schizophrenia. *Psychiatry Res.* 35, 1–13. doi: 10.1016/0925-4927(90)90004-P

Brans, R. G. H., van Haren, N. E. M., van Baal, G. C. M., Staal, W. G., Schnack, H. G., Kahn, R. S., et al. (2008). Longitudinal MRI study in schizophrenia patients and their healthy siblings. *Br. J. Psychiatry* 193, 422–423. doi: 10.1192/bjp.bp.107.041467

Cuadra, M. B., Cammoun, L., Butz, T., Cuisenaire, O., and Thiran, J. P. (2005). Comparison and validation of tissue modelization and statistical classification methods in T1-weighted MR brain images. *IEEE Trans. Med. Imaging* 24, 1548–1565. doi: 10.1109/TMI.2005.857652

Davis, K. L., Stewart, D. G., Friedman, J. I., Buchsbaum, M., Harvey, P. D., Hof, P. R., et al. (2003). White matter changes in schizophrenia: evidence for myelin-related dysfunction. *Arch. Gen. Psychiatry* 60, 443–456. doi: 10.1001/archpsyc.60.5.443

DeLisi, L. E. (1999). Regional brain volume change over the life-time course of schizophrenia. *J. Psychiatr. Res.* 33, 535–541. doi: 10.1016/S0022-3956(99)00028-X

DeLisi, L. E., and Hoff, A. L. (2005). Failure to find progressive temporal lobe volume decreases 10 years subsequent to a first episode of schizophrenia. *Psychiatry Res.* 138, 265–268. doi: 10.1016/j.pscychresns.2005.02.005

Dierks, T., Linden, D. E., Jandl, M., Formisano, E., Goebel, R., Lanfermann, H., et al. (1999). Activation of Heschl's gyrus during auditory hallucinations. *Neuron* 22, 615–621. doi: 10.1016/S0896-6273(00)80715-1

Donato, R. (2001). S100: a multigenic family of calcium-modulated proteins of the EF-hand type with intracellular and extracellular functional roles. *Int. J. Biochem. Cell Biol.* 33, 637–668. doi: 10.1016/S1357-2725(01)00046-2

Douaud, G., Smith, S., Jenkinson, M., Behrens, T., Johansen-Berg, H., Vickers, J., et al. (2007). Anatomically related grey and white matter abnormalities in adolescent-onset schizophrenia. *Brain* 130, 2375–2386. doi: 10.1093/brain/awm184

Eldik, L. J. V., and Wainwright, M. S. (2003). The Janus face of glial-derived S100B: beneficial and detrimental functions in the brain. *Restor. Neurol. Neurosci.* 21, 97–108.

Ellison-Wright, I., and Bullmore, E. (2009). Meta-analysis of diffusion tensor imaging studies in schizophrenia. *Schizophr. Res.* 108, 3–10. doi: 10.1016/j.schres.2008.11.021

Ellison-Wright, I., Glahn, D. C., Laird, A. R., Thelen, S. M., and Bullmore, E. (2008). The anatomy of first-episode and chronic schizophrenia: an anatomical likelihood estimation meta-analysis. *Am. J. Psychiatry* 165, 1015–1023. doi: 10.1176/appi.ajp.2008.07101562

Gonçalves, C. A., Leite, M. C., and Guerra, M. C. (2010). Adipocytes as an important source of serum S100B and possible roles of this protein in adipose tissue. *Cardiovasc. Psychiatry Neurol.* 2010, 790431. doi: 10.1155/2010/790431

Gonçalves, C. A., Leite, M. C., and Nardin, P. (2008). Biological and methodological features of the measurement of S100B, a putative marker of brain injury. *Clin. Biochem.* 41, 755–763. doi: 10.1016/j.clinbiochem.2008.04.003

Good, C. D., Johnsrude, I. S., Ashburner, J., Henson, R. N., Friston, K. J., and Frackowiak, R. S. (2001). A voxel-based morphometric study of ageing in 465 normal adult human brains. *Neuroimage* 14, 21–36. doi: 10.1006/nimg.2001.0786

Gupta, C. N., Calhoun, V. D., Rachakonda, S., Chen, J., Patel, V., Liu, J., et al. (2015). Patterns of gray matter abnormalities in schizophrenia based on an international mega-analysis. *Schizophr. Bull.* 41, 1133–1142. doi: 10.1093/schbul/sbu177

Hanson, D. R., and Gottesman, I. I. (2005). Theories of schizophrenia: a genetic-inflammatory-vascular synthesis. *BMC Med. Genet.* 6:7. doi: 10.1186/1471-2350-6-7

Harrison, P. J. (1999). The neuropathology of schizophrenia. A critical review of the data and their interpretation. *Brain* 122(Pt 4), 593–624. doi: 10.1093/brain/122.4.593

Hercher, C., Chopra, V., and Beasley, C. L. (2014). Evidence for morphological alterations in prefrontal white matter glia in schizophrenia and bipolar disorder. *J. Psychiatry Neurosci.* 39, 376–385. doi: 10.1503/jpn.130277

Honea, R., Crow, T. J., Passingham, D., and Mackay, C. E. (2005). Regional deficits in brain volume in schizophrenia: a meta-analysis of voxel-based morphometry studies. *Am. J. Psychiatry* 162, 2233–2245. doi: 10.1176/appi.ajp.162.12.2233

Kasai, K., Shenton, M. E., Salisbury, D. F., Hirayasu, Y., Lee, C. U., Ciszewski, A. A., et al. (2003b). Progressive decrease of left superior temporal gyrus gray matter volume in patients with first-episode schizophrenia. *Am. J. Psychiatry* 160, 156–164. doi: 10.1176/appi.ajp.160.1.156

Kasai, K., Shenton, M. E., Salisbury, D. F., Hirayasu, Y., Onitsuka, T., Spencer, M. H., et al. (2003a). Progressive decrease of left Heschl gyrus and planum temporale gray matter volume in first-episode schizophrenia: a longitudinal magnetic resonance imaging study. *Arch. Gen. Psychiatry* 60, 766–775. doi: 10.1001/archpsyc.60.8.766

Katsel, P., Byne, W., Roussos, P., Tan, W., Siever, L., and Haroutunian, V. (2011). Astrocyte and glutamate markers in the superficial, deep, and white matter layers of the anterior cingulate gyrus in schizophrenia. *Neuropsychopharmacology* 36, 1171–1177. doi: 10.1038/npp.2010.252

Konrad, A., and Winterer, G. (2008). Disturbed structural connectivity in schizophrenia primary factor in pathology or epiphenomenon? *Schizophr. Bull.* 34, 72–92. doi: 10.1093/schbul/sbm034

Kubicki, M., McCarley, R., Westin, C. F., Park, H. J., Maier, S., Kikinis, R., et al. (2007). A review of diffusion tensor imaging studies in schizophrenia. *J. Psychiatr. Res.* 41, 15–30. doi: 10.1016/j.jpsychires.2005.05.005

Kubicki, M., Park, H., Westin, C. F., Nestor, P. G., Mulkern, R. V., Maier, S. E., et al. (2005). DTI and MTR abnormalities in schizophrenia: analysis of white matter integrity. *Neuroimage* 26, 1109–1118. doi: 10.1016/j.neuroimage.2005.03.026

Kubicki, M., Westin, C. F., Nestor, P. G., Wible, C. G., Frumin, M., Maier, S. E., et al. (2003). Cingulate fasciculus integrity disruption in schizophrenia: a magnetic resonance diffusion tensor imaging study. *Biol. Psychiatry* 54, 1171–1180. doi: 10.1016/S0006-3223(03)00419-0

Kuroki, N., Kubicki, M., Nestor, P. G., Salisbury, D. F., Park, H. J., Levitt, J. J., et al. (2006). Fornix integrity and hippocampal volume in male schizophrenic patients. *Biol. Psychiatry* 60, 22–31. doi: 10.1016/j.biopsych.2005.09.021

Kyriakopoulos, M., and Frangou, S. (2009). Recent diffusion tensor imaging findings in early stages of schizophrenia. *Curr. Opin. Psychiatry* 22, 168–176. doi: 10.1097/YCO.0b013e328325aa23

Kyriakopoulos, M., Vyas, N. S., Barker, G. J., Chitnis, X. A., and Frangou, S. (2008). A diffusion tensor imaging study of white matter in early-onset schizophrenia. *Biol. Psychiatry* 63, 519–523. doi: 10.1016/j.biopsych.2007.05.021

Lieberman, J. A., Tollefson, G. D., Charles, C., Zipursky, R., Sharma, T., Kahn, R. S., et al. (2005). Antipsychotic drug effects on brain morphology in first-episode psychosis. *Arch. Gen. Psychiatry* 62, 361–370. doi: 10.1001/archpsyc.62.4.361

Lipska, B., and Weinberger, D. (2002). A neurodevelopmental model of schizophrenia: neonatal disconnection of the hippocampus. *Neurotox. Res.* 4, 469–475. doi: 10.1080/1029842021000022089

Mitelman, S. A., Torosjan, Y., Newmark, R. E., Schneiderman, J. S., Chu, K. W., Brickman, A. M., et al. (2007). Internal capsule, corpus callosum and long associative fibers in good and poor outcome schizophrenia: a diffusion tensor imaging survey. *Schizophr. Res.* 92, 211–224. doi: 10.1016/j.schres.2006.12.029

Monji, A., Kato, T., and Kanba, S. (2009). Cytokines and schizophrenia: Microglia hypothesis of schizophrenia. *Psychiatry Clin. Neurosci.* 63, 257–265. doi: 10.1111/j.1440-1819.2009.01945.x

Mori, S., Wakana, S., Nagae-Poetscher, L. M., and van Zijl, P. C. M. (2005). *MRI Atlas of Human White Matter.* Amsterdam: Elsevier.

Müller, N., and Schwarz, M. J. (2007). The immunological basis of glutamatergic disturbance in schizophrenia: towards an integrated view. *J. Neural. Transm. Suppl.* 72, 269–280. doi: 10.1007/978-3-211-73574-9_33

Nestor, P. G., Kubicki, M., Kuroki, N., Gurrera, R. J., Niznikiewicz, M., Shenton, M. E., et al. (2007). Episodic memory and neuroimaging of hippocampus and fornix in chronic schizophrenia. *Psychiatry Res.* 155, 21–28. doi: 10.1016/j.pscychresns.2006.12.020

Okugawa, G., Nobuhara, K., Minami, T., Takase, K., Sugimoto, T., Saito, Y., et al. (2006). Neural disorganization in the superior cerebellar peduncle and cognitive abnormality in patients with schizophrenia: a diffusion tensor imaging study. *Prog. Neuropsychopharmacol. Biol. Psychiatry* 30, 1408–1412. doi: 10.1016/j.pnpbp.2006.05.014

Pakkenberg, B. (1993). Total nerve cell number in neocortex in chronic schizophrenics and controls estimated using optical disectors. *Biol. Psychiatry* 34, 768–772. doi: 10.1016/0006-3223(93)90065-L

Pantelis, C., Velakoulis, D., McGorry, P. D., Wood, S. J., Suckling, J., Phillips, L. J., et al. (2003). Neuroanatomical abnormalities before and after onset of psychosis: a cross-sectional and longitudinal MRI comparison. *Lancet* 361, 281–288. doi: 10.1016/S0140-6736(03)12323-9

Pantelis, C., Yücel, M., Wood, S. J., Velakoulis, D., Sun, D., Berger, G., et al. (2005). Structural brain imaging evidence for multiple pathological processes at different stages of brain development in schizophrenia. *Schizophr. Bull.* 31, 672–696. doi: 10.1093/schbul/sbi034

Pearlson, G. D., and Marsh, L. (1999). Structural brain imaging in schizophrenia: a selective review. *Biol. Psychiatry* 46, 627–649. doi: 10.1016/S0006-3223(99)00071-2

Pérez-Iglesias, R., Tordesillas-Gutiérrez, D., Barker, G. J., McGuire, P. K., Roiz-Santiañez, R., Mata, I., et al. (2010). White matter defects in first episode psychosis patients: a voxelwise analysis of diffusion tensor imaging. *Neuroimage* 49, 199–204. doi: 10.1016/j.neuroimage.2009.07.016

Peters, B. D., de Haan, L., Dekker, N., Blaas, J., Becker, H. E., Dingemans, P. M., et al. (2008). White matter fibertracking in first-episode schizophrenia, schizoaffective patients and subjects at ultra-high risk of psychosis. *Neuropsychobiology* 58, 19–28. doi: 10.1159/000154476

Pol, H. E. H., and Kahn, R. S. (2008). What happens after the first episode? A review of progressive brain changes in chronically ill patients with schizophrenia. *Schizophr. Bull.* 34, 354–366. doi: 10:1093/schbul/sbm168

Reiber, H. (2001). Dynamics of brain-derived proteins in cerebrospinal fluid. *Clin. Chim. Acta* 310, 173–186. doi: 10.1016/S0009-8981(01)00573-3

Rothermundt, M., Missler, U., Arolt, V., Peters, M., Leadbeater, J., Wiesmann, M., et al. (2001). Increased S100B blood levels in unmedicated and treated schizophrenic patients are correlated with negative symptomatology. *Mol. Psychiatry* 6, 445–449. doi: 10.1038/sj.mp.4000889

Rothermundt, M., Ponath, G., and Arolt, V. (2004a). S100B in schizophrenic psychosis. *Int. Rev. Neurobiol.* 59, 445–470. doi: 10.1016/S0074-7742(04)59017-7

Rothermundt, M., Ponath, G., Glaser, T., Hetzel, G., and Arolt, V. (2004b). S100B serum levels and long-term improvement of negative symptoms in patients with schizophrenia. *Neuropsychopharmacology* 29, 1004–1011. doi: 10.1038/sj.npp.1300403

Samartzis, L., Dima, D., Fusar-Poli, P., and Kyriakopoulos, M. (2014). White matter alterations in early stages of schizophrenia: a systematic review of diffusion tensor imaging studies. *J. Neuroimaging* 24, 101–110. doi: 10.1111/j.1552-6569.2012.00779.x

Schroeter, M. L., Sacher, J., Steiner, J., Schoenknecht, P., and Mueller, K. (2013). Serum S100B represents a new biomarker for mood disorders. *Curr. Drug Targets* 14, 1237–1248. doi: 10.2174/138945011131499 90014

Selemon, L. D., and Goldman-Rakic, P. S. (1999). The reduced neuropil hypothesis: a circuit based model of schizophrenia. *Biol. Psychiatry* 45, 17–25. doi: 10.1016/S0006-3223(98)00281-9

Shergill, S. S., Kanaan, R. A., Chitnis, X. A., O'daly, O., Jones, D. K., Frangou, S., et al. (2007). A diffusion tensor imaging study of fasciculi in schizophrenia. *Am. J. Psychiatry* 164, 467–473. doi: 10.1176/appi.ajp.164.3.467

Sigmundsson, T., Suckling, J., Maier, M., Williams, S., Bullmore, E., Greenwood, K., et al. (2001). Structural abnormalities in frontal, temporal, and limbic regions and interconnecting white matter tracts in schizophrenic patients with prominent negative symptoms. *Am. J. Psychiatry* 158, 234–243. doi: 10.1176/appi.ajp.158.2.234

Smesny, S., Milleit, B., Nenadic, I., Preul, C., Kinder, D., Lasch, J., et al. (2010). Phospholipase A2 activity is associated with structural brain changes in schizophrenia. *Neuroimage* 52, 1314–1327. doi: 10.1016/j.neuroimage.2010.05.009

Steiner, J., Bernstein, H. G., Bielau, H., Berndt, A., Brisch, R., Mawrin, C., et al. (2007). Evidence for a wide extra-astrocytic distribution of S100B in human brain. *BMC Neurosci.* 8:2. doi: 10.1186/1471-2202-8-2

Steiner, J., Bernstein, H. G., Bielau, H., Farkas, N., Winter, J., Dobrowolny, H., et al. (2008). S100B-immunopositive glia is elevated in paranoid as compared to residual schizophrenia: a morphometric study. *J. Psychiatr. Res.* 42, 868–876. doi: 10.1016/j.jpsychires.2007.10.001

Steiner, J., Schiltz, K., Walter, M., Wunderlich, M. T., Keilhoff, G., Brisch, R., et al. (2010a). S100B serum levels are closely correlated with body mass index: an important caveat in neuropsychiatric research. *Psychoneuroendocrinology* 35, 321–324. doi: 10.1016/j.psyneuen.2009.07.012

Steiner, J., Walter, M., Guest, P., Myint, A. M., Schiltz, K., Panteli, B., et al. (2010b). Elevated S100B levels in schizophrenia are associated with insulin resistance. *Mol. Psychiatry* 15, 3–4. doi: 10.1038/mp.2009.87

Streitbuerger, D. P., Arelin, K., Kratzsch, J., Thiery, J., Steiner, J., Villringer, A., et al. (2012). Validating serum S100B and neuron-specific enolase as biomarkers for the human brain - a combined serum, gene expression and MRI study. *PLoS ONE* 7:e43284. doi: 10.1371/journal.pone.0043284

Suzuki, M., Nohara, S., Hagino, H., Kurokawa, K., Yotsutsuji, T., Kawasaki, Y., et al. (2002). Regional changes in brain gray and white matter in patients with schizophrenia demonstrated with voxel-based analysis of MRI. *Schizophr. Res.* 55, 41–54. doi: 10.1016/S0920-9964(01)00224-9

Tramontina, F., Tramontina, A. C., Souza, D. F., Leite, M. C., Gottfried, C., Souza, D. O., et al. (2006). Glutamate uptake is stimulated by extracellular S100B in hippocampal astrocytes. *Cell. Mol. Neurobiol.* 26, 81–86. doi: 10.1007/s10571-006-9099-8

Walterfang, M., Wood, S. J., Velakoulis, D., Copolov, D., and Pantelis, C. (2005). Diseases of white matter and schizophrenia-like psychosis. *Aust. N.Z. J. Psychiatry* 39, 746–756. doi: 10.1080/j.1440-1614.2005.01678.x

Wang, F., Sun, Z., Du, X., Wang, X., Cong, Z., Zhang, H., et al. (2003). A diffusion tensor imaging study of middle and superior cerebellar peduncle in male patients with schizophrenia. *Neurosci. Lett.* 348, 135–138. doi: 10.1016/S0304-3940(03)00589-5

White, T., Nelson, M., and Lim, K. O. (2008). Diffusion tensor imaging in psychiatric disorders. *Top. Magn. Reson. Imaging* 19, 97–109. doi: 10.1097/RMR.0b013e3181809f1e

Wright, I. C., Rabe-Hesketh, S., Woodruff, P. W., David, A. S., Murray, R. M., and Bullmore, E. T. (2000). Meta-analysis of regional brain volumes in schizophrenia. *Am. J. Psychiatry* 157, 16–25. doi: 10.1176/ajp.157.1.16

2

# Introducing Directly Induced Microglia-Like (iMG) Cells from Fresh Human Monocytes: A Novel Translational Research Tool for Psychiatric Disorders

*Masahiro Ohgidani[1], Takahiro A. Kato[1,2]* and Shigenobu Kanba[1]*

*[1] Department of Neuropsychiatry, Graduate School of Medical Sciences, Kyushu University, Fukuoka, Japan, [2] Brain Research Unit, Innovation Center for Medical Redox Navigation, Kyushu University, Fukuoka, Japan*

***Correspondence:**
*Takahiro A. Kato,
Department of Neuropsychiatry,
Graduate School of Medical
Sciences, Kyushu University and
Brain Research Unit, Innovation
Center for Medical Redox Navigation,
Kyushu University, 3-1-1 Maidashi
Higashi-ku, Fukuoka 812-8582,
Japan
takahiro@npsych.med.kyushu-u.ac.jp*

Microglia, glial cells with immunological functions, have been implicated in various neurological diseases and psychiatric disorders in rodent studies, and human postmortem and PET studies. However, the deeper molecular implications of living human microglia have not been clarified. Here, we introduce a novel translational research approach focusing on human microglia. We have recently developed a new technique for creating induced microglia-like (iMG) cells from human peripheral blood. Two cytokines, GM-CSF and IL-34, converted human monocytes into the iMG cells within 14 days, which show various microglial characterizations; expressing markers, forming a ramified morphology, and phagocytic activity with various cytokine releases. We have already confirmed the applicability of this technique by analyzing iMG cells from a patient of Nasu-Hakola disease (NHD; Ohgidani et al., 2014). We herein show possible applications of the iMG cells in translational research. We believe that this iMG technique will open the door to explore various unknown dynamic aspects of human microglia in psychiatric disorders. This also opens new routes for psychopharmacological approach such as drug efficacy screening and personalized medicine.

**Keywords: microglia, regenerative medicine, translational research, psychiatric disorders, schizophrenia, mood disorders, GM-CSF, IL-34**

Recently, the roles of microglia, immune cells in the brain, have been highlighted not only by neuroscientists but also by a variety of clinical researchers, especially in the field of neurology and psychiatry (Hughes, 2012). The pathophysiology of microglia has been suggested in various neuronal diseases and psychiatric disorders by human postmortem and positron emission tomography (PET) studies (Steiner et al., 2008; van Berckel et al., 2008; Takano et al., 2010; Gupta et al., 2014). Furthermore, microglial modulation has been proposed as an intervention in brain diseases including psychiatric disorders by recent clinical trials using minocycline, an antibiotic with microglial inhibitory effects (Miyaoka et al., 2008; Levkovitz et al., 2010; Chaudhry et al., 2012; Hayakawa et al., 2014). It has also been suggested that minocycline acts to modulate social interactions not only in psychiatric patients but also in healthy volunteers (Kato et al., 2012; Watabe et al., 2012, 2013). On the other hand, various psychotropic drugs have been revealed to

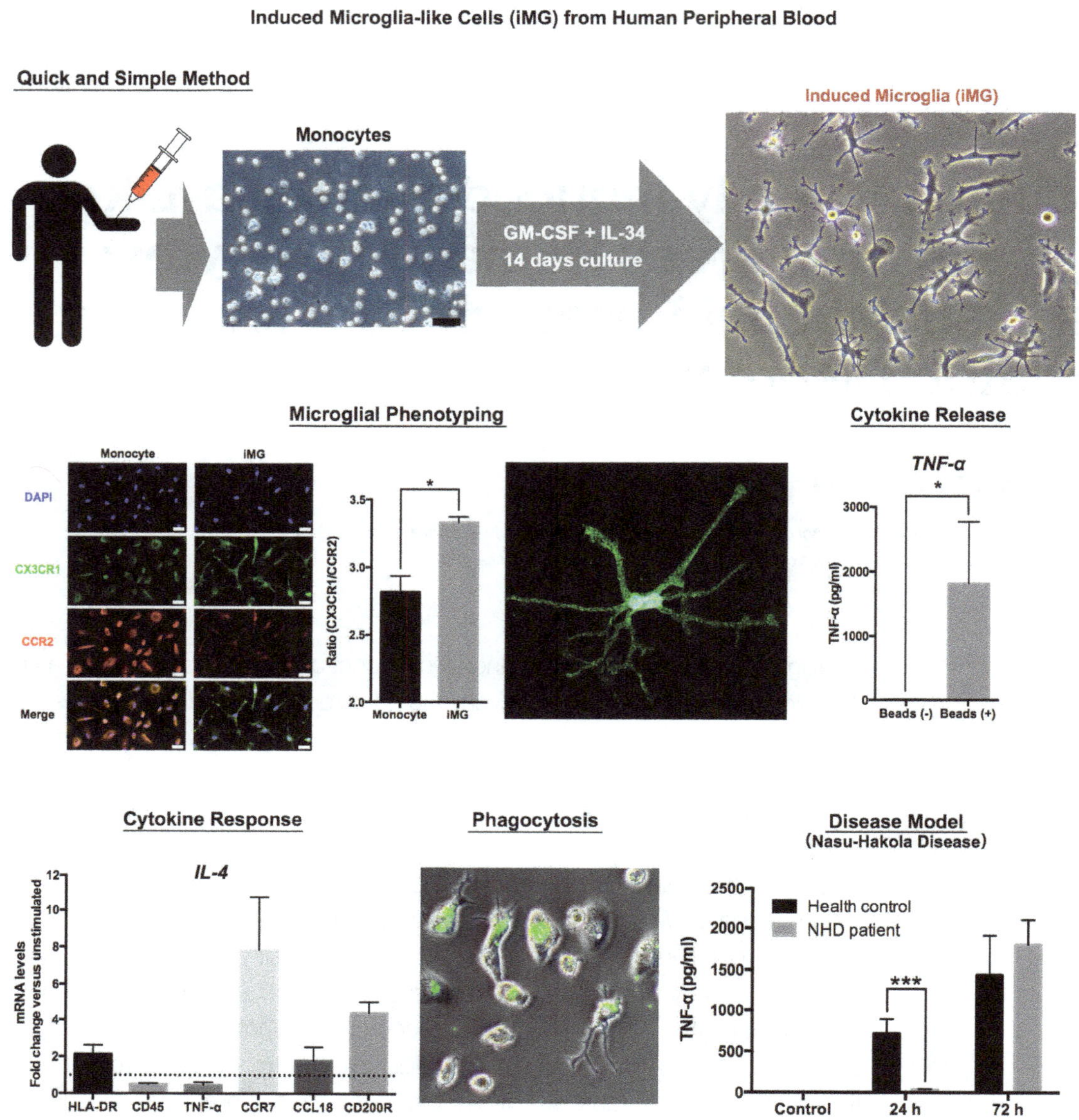


**FIGURE 1 | Induced Microglia-like Cells (iMG) from Human Peripheral Blood.**

inhibit microglial over-activation in *in vitro* experiments using rodent cells (Kato et al., 2007, 2008, 2011a,b; Bian et al., 2008; Seki et al., 2013).

The above reports have strongly suggested that maladaptive microglial activation may play a crucial role in various brain disorders (Block et al., 2007; Hanisch and Kettenmann, 2007; Kato et al., 2013). However, the deeper dynamic molecular actions of living human microglia in real patients have not been well clarified due to technical and ethical issues (such as difficulties involved in human brain biopsies). Until now, almost all human microglia research has been conducted using the postmortem brain or PET. These approaches have revealed important roles for activated microglia in psychiatric patients such as schizophrenia and autism (Steiner et al., 2008; van Berckel et al., 2008; Takano et al., 2010; Suzuki et al., 2013; Gupta et al., 2014). However, using these methods, it is difficult to ascertain the molecular pathological mechanisms such as the signaling pathway and gene expression pattern. On the other hand, animal (rodent) studies with cytological and histological analysis can reveal the various deeper dynamic actions of microglia at molecular levels (Nimmerjahn et al., 2005; Wake et al., 2009; Kettenmann et al., 2011). In fact, microglial activation has been shown in a variety of cytological and histological analyses using rodent models of brain diseases (Wu et al., 2002; Yoshiyama et al., 2007). Molecular biological analysis using rodent primary cultures and cell strains has been the standard method until now (Kato et al., 2007, 2008, 2011a,b; Bian et al., 2008; Seki et al., 2013; Mizoguchi et al., 2014a,b). In fact, rodent studies have been very vital in microglial research, however the question remains- how much does human pathology reflect in rodents? Can schizophrenia model mice have delusions and/or hallucinations? Even though a variety of rodent models of psychiatric disorders exist, it is extremely hard to validate deeper psychopathologies in rodents.

Thus, human studies using living brain cells derived from psychiatric patients have been warranted to evaluate the interactions of microglial activities and deeper psychopathology including psychiatric symptoms. A novel term "cellular model" has emerged in addition to "animal model" in the research of various physical diseases. The technology to obtain human neuronal cells from non-brain tissues (e.g., skin) by novel reproductive techniques such as induced pluripotent stem (iPS) cells (Takahashi et al., 2007) and directly induced neuronal (iN) cells (Pang et al., 2011; Liu et al., 2013) has emerged, and these tools have just recently been applied to psychiatric research (Kim, 2010; Brennand et al., 2011; Wen et al., 2014). Further, iPS technology can produce glial cells such as astrocytes (Juopperi et al., 2012) and progenitor of oligodendrocytes (Wang et al., 2013). However, to our knowledge, there exist no reports on the production of microglia by iPS technology. Very recently, we have developed a novel technique to create induced microglia-like cells (iMG) from human peripheral blood (Ohgidani et al., 2014).

The brain is mostly composed of ectomorphic cells such as neurons, astrocytes and oligodendrocytes. Microglia is the only mesomorphic cell in the brain (Kettenmann et al., 2011). Therefore, we tried to induce microglia-like cells from peripheral monocytes, which have the same origin as mesomorphic cells. To determine what cytokines can induce iMG cells from human peripheral monocytes, we tested the effects of cytokines. Surprisingly, the cocktail of both granulocyte-macrophage colony-stimulating factor (GM-CSF) and interleukin (IL) −34 successfully induced small soma bodies bearing numerous branched collaterals, which expressed the specific morphology of ramified microglia-small soma with extensive radial ramifications. The iMG cells express the essential characteristics of human microglia such as surface markers and drug responses, phagocytosis and cytokine production (**Figure 1**).

We first utilized the iMG cells as a "cellular disease model" focusing on one of the most famous primary microglia-oriented diseases, the Nasu-Hakola disease (NHD; Hakola, 1972; Nasu et al., 1973). NHD is a very rare autosomal recessive disease, and the responsible two genes, which are expressed in microglia in the brain, are DNAX-activation protein of 12 kDA (DAP12) and triggering receptor expressed on myeloid cells 2 (TREM2; Paloneva et al., 2000, 2002). The deeper pathophysiological roles of microglia have not been well understood. Thus, we investigated the pathophysiology of NHD using the iMG technique. In agreement with genetic diagnosis, the iMG cells from a NHD patient (141delG in DAP12 gene) showed significantly lower expression of DAP12 than those from a healthy control (HC). Interestingly, the response of producing pro-inflammatory cytokines (TNF-α and IL-6) was delayed in the iMG cells from the NHD patient as compared to those from HC. Furthermore, we have also confirmed the delayed cytokine productions in the NHD model of iMG cells which was prepared by siRNA (Ohgidani et al., 2014). These novel findings may help to understand the hitherto unknown pathophysiological aspects of NHD.

In this way, we believe that the iMG technique will enable the clarification of novel pathophysiological dysfunctions of human microglia as a translational research tool in various brain diseases including psychiatric disorders. We believe that the iMG technique will enable the exploration and development of psychiatric research especially to the following areas;

## Multidimensional Correlation Analysis with Clinical Data, Brain Imaging Data and iMG

By combining clinical data, brain imaging data, and the iMG data from the same patient will be able to clarify the dynamic interaction between a specific psychopathology and a specific microglial activation (**Figure 2-(1)**). For example, the aberration of TREM, which is expressed in microglia, has recently been observed in psychiatric disorders such as bipolar disorder (Weigelt et al., 2011) and Alzheimer's disease (Jonsson et al., 2013). Analyzing the TREM aberration of iMG cells from psychiatric patients can help to clarify the main role of TREM in psychopathology, which in turn may assist in the psychiatric evaluation of diagnosis and severity.

## Drug Evaluation and Personalized Medicine

We previously reported the neuroprotective effects of psychotropic drugs via suppressing microglial activation using rodent microglial cells (Kato et al., 2007, 2008, 2011a,b; Bian et al., 2008; Seki et al., 2013). The iMG technique may help to predict drug responses before treating patients. Drug efficacy screening using iMG cells can predict which drug will

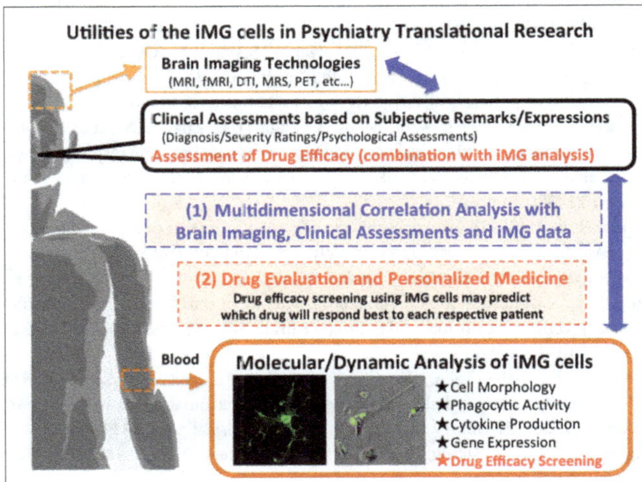


**FIGURE 2 | Utilities of the iMG cells in Psychiatry Translational Research.**

respond best to each respective patient, and the technique may be applied as a companion diagnostic tool, which has raised expectations for the application of "order-made" medicine with a reduction in side effects and a shortening of treatment period (**Figure 2-(2)**).

## Conclusion

We introduced a novel translational research approach focusing on human microglia-like cells using the iMG technique. Before reaching a conclusion, we need to mention a recent considerable discussion regarding functional differences between yolk sac derived microglia and monocyte derived microglia (Ginhoux et al., 2010; Katsumoto et al., 2014). We should keep it in our mind that the iMG cells are originated from monocytes, which may be different from the functions of yolk sac derived microglia. In addition, because IL-34 is a tissue-restricted ligand of CSF1R and this cytokine is associated with the development of other types of monocyte-derived cells such as Langerhans cells and possibly dendritic cells (Wang et al., 2012), which should also be considered. Despite these propositions, we believe that the iMG technique, at least to some extent, can analyze human microglial pathology in a living state, which had been impossible until recently. We hope that this translational method will open the door to explore various unknown dynamic aspects of human microglia in brain diseases, especially psychiatric disorders. This opens new routes for not only understanding the psychopathological mechanism of psychiatric disorders but also psychopharmacological approach such as drug efficacy screening and personalized medicine.

## Acknowledgments

This work was supported in part by the Japanese Ministry of Education, Culture, Sports, Science, and Technology KAKENHI (Grant-in-Aid 26713039 for Young Scientists (A) to TAK, Grant-in-Aid 26860933 for Young Scientists (B) to MO, and Grant-in-Aid 25117011 for Scientific Research on Innovative Areas [Glia assembly] to SK); Japan Agency for Medical Research and Development (AMED)-The Japanese Ministry of Health, Labour and Welfare (H27 - Seishin-Syogai Taisaku-Jigyo to SK); Takeda Science Foundation (to TAK); and SENSHIN Medical Research Foundation (to TAK, MO, and SK).

## References

Bian, Q., Kato, T., Monji, A., Hashioka, S., Mizoguchi, Y., Horikawa, H., et al. (2008). The effect of atypical antipsychotics, perospirone, ziprasidone and quetiapine on microglial activation induced by interferon-gamma. *Prog. Neuropsychopharmacol. Biol. Psychiatry* 32, 42–48. doi: 10.1016/j.pnpbp.2007.06.031

Block, M. L., Zecca, L., and Hong, J. S. (2007). Microglia-mediated neurotoxicity: uncovering the molecular mechanisms. *Nat. Rev. Neurosci.* 8, 57–69. doi: 10.1038/nrn2038

Brennand, K. J., Simone, A., Jou, J., Gelboin-Burkhart, C., Tran, N., Sangar, S., et al. (2011). Modelling schizophrenia using human induced pluripotent stem cells. *Nature* 473, 221–225. doi: 10.1038/nature09915

Chaudhry, I. B., Hallak, J., Husain, N., Minhas, F., Stirling, J., Richardson, P., et al. (2012). Minocycline benefits negative symptoms in early schizophrenia: a randomised double-blind placebo-controlled clinical trial in patients on standard treatment. *J. Psychopharmacol.* 26, 1185–1193. doi: 10.1177/0269881112444941

Ginhoux, F., Greter, M., Leboeuf, M., Nandi, S., See, P., Gokhan, S., et al. (2010). Fate mapping analysis reveals that adult microglia derive from primitive macrophages. *Science* 330, 841–845. doi: 10.1126/science.1194637

Gupta, S., Ellis, S. E., Ashar, F. N., Moes, A., Bader, J. S., Zhan, J. N., et al. (2014). Transcriptome analysis reveals dysregulation of innate immune response genes and neuronal activity-dependent genes in autism. *Nat. Commun.* 5:5748. doi: 10.1038/ncomms6748

Hakola, H. P. A. (1972). Neuropsychiatric and genetic aspects of a new hereditary disease characterized by progressive dementia and lipomembranous polycystic osteodysplasia. *Acta Psychiat. Scand. Suppl.* 232, 1–173.

Hanisch, U. K., and Kettenmann, H. (2007). Microglia: active sensor and versatile effector cells in the normal and pathologic brain. *Nat. Neurosci.* 10, 1387–1394. doi: 10.1038/nn1997

Hayakawa, K., Kato, T. A., Kohjiro, M., Monji, A., and Kanba, S. (2014). Minocycline, a microglial inhibitor, diminishes terminal patients' delirium? *Am. J. Geriatr. Psychiatry* 22, 314–315. doi: 10.1016/j.jagp.2013.11.003

Hughes, V. (2012). Microglia: the constant gardeners. *Nature* 485, 570–572. doi: 10.1038/485570a

Jonsson, T., Stefansson, H., Steinberg, S., Jonsdottir, I., Jonsson, P. V., Snaedal, J., et al. (2013). Variant of TREM2 associated with the risk of Alzheimer's disease. *N. Engl. J. Med.* 368, 107–116. doi: 10.1056/NEJMoa1211103

Juopperi, T. A., Kim, W. R., Chiang, C. H., Yu, H. M., Margolis, R. L., Ross, C. A., et al. (2012). Astrocytes generated from patient induced pluripotent stem cells recapitulate features of Huntington's disease patient cells. *Mol. Brain* 5:17. doi: 10.1186/1756-6606-5-17

Kato, T., Mizoguchi, Y., Monji, A., Horikawa, H., Suzuki, S. O., Seki, Y., et al. (2008). Inhibitory effects of aripiprazole on interferon-gamma-induced microglial activation via intracellular Ca2+ regulation *in vitro*. *J. Neurochem.* 106, 815–825. doi: 10.1111/j.1471-4159.2008.05435.x

Kato, T., Monji, A., Hashioka, S., and Kanba, S. (2007). Risperidone significantly inhibits interferon-gamma-induced microglial activation *in vitro*. *Schizophr. Res.* 92, 108–115. doi: 10.1016/j.schres.2007.01.019

Kato, T. A., Monji, A., Mizoguchi, Y., Hashioka, S., Horikawa, H., Seki, Y., et al. (2011a). Anti-inflammatory properties of antipsychotics via microglia modulations: are antipsychotics a 'fire extinguisher' in the brain of schizophrenia? *Mini Rev. Med. Chem.* 11, 565–574. doi: 10.2174/138955711795906941

Kato, T. A., Monji, A., Yasukawa, K., Mizoguchi, Y., Horikawa, H., Seki, Y., et al. (2011b). Aripiprazole inhibits superoxide generation from phorbol-myristate-acetate (PMA)-stimulated microglia *in vitro*: implication for antioxidative psychotropic actions via microglia. *Schizophr. Res.* 129, 172–182. doi: 10.1016/j.schres.2011.03.019

Kato, T. A., Watabe, M., Tsuboi, S., Ishikawa, K., Hashiya, K., Monji, A., et al. (2012). Minocycline modulates human social decision-making: possible impact of microglia on personality-oriented social behaviors. *PLoS One* 7:e40461. doi: 10.1371/journal.pone.0040461

Kato, T. A., Yamauchi, Y., Horikawa, H., Monji, A., Mizoguchi, Y., Seki, Y., et al. (2013). Neurotransmitters, psychotropic drugs and microglia: clinical implications for psychiatry. *Curr. Med. Chem.* 20, 331–344. doi: 10.2174/0929867311320030003

Katsumoto, A., Lu, H., Miranda, A. S., and Ransohoff, R. M. (2014). Ontogeny and functions of central nervous system macrophages. *J. Immunol.* 193, 2615–2621. doi: 10.4049/jimmunol.1400716

Kettenmann, H., Hanisch, U. K., Noda, M., and Verkhratsky, A. (2011). Physiology of microglia. *Physiol. Rev.* 91, 461–553. doi: 10.1152/physrev.00011.2010

Kim, K. S. (2010). Induced pluripotent stem (iPS) cells and their future in psychiatry. *Neuropsychopharmacology* 35, 346–348. doi: 10.1038/npp.2009.108

Levkovitz, Y., Mendlovich, S., Riwkes, S., Braw, Y., Levkovitch-Verbin, H., Gal, G., et al. (2010). A double-blind, randomized study of minocycline for the treatment of negative and cognitive symptoms in early-phase schizophrenia. *J. Clin. Psychiatry* 71, 138–149. doi: 10.4088/JCP.08m04666yel

Liu, M. L., Zang, T., Zou, Y. H., Chang, J. C., Gibson, J. R., Huber, K. M., et al. (2013). Small molecules enable neurogenin 2 to efficiently convert human fibroblasts into cholinergic neurons. *Nat. Commun.* 4:2183. doi: 10.1038/ncomms3183

Miyaoka, T., Yasukawa, R., Yasuda, H., Hayashida, M., Inagaki, T., and Horiguchi, J. (2008). Minocycline as adjunctive therapy for schizophrenia: an open-label study. *Clin. Neuropharmacol.* 31, 287–292. doi: 10.1097/WNF.0b013e3181593d45

Mizoguchi, Y., Kato, T. A., Horikawa, H., and Monji, A. (2014a). Microglial intracellular Ca2+ signaling as a target of antipsychotic actions for the treatment of schizophrenia. *Front. Cell. Neurosci.* 8:370. doi: 10.3389/fncel.2014.00370

Mizoguchi, Y., Kato, T. A., Seki, Y., Ohgidani, M., Sagata, N., Horikawa, H., et al. (2014b). Brain-derived neurotrophic factor (BDNF) induces sustained intracellular Ca2+ elevation through the up-regulation of surface transient receptor potential 3 (TRPC3) channels in rodent microglia. *J. Biol. Chem.* 289, 18549–18555. doi: 10.1074/jbc.M114.555334

Nasu, T., Tsukahar, Y., and Terayama, K. (1973). A lipid metabolic disease-"membranous lipodystrophy"-an autopsy case demonstrating numerous peculiar membrane-structures composed of compound lipid in bone and bone marrow and various adipose tissues. *Acta Pathol. Jpn.* 23, 539–558. doi: 10.1111/j.1440-1827.1973.tb01223.x

Nimmerjahn, A., Kirchhoff, F., and Helmchen, F. (2005). Resting microglial cells are highly dynamic surveillants of brain parenchyma *in vivo*. *Science* 308, 1314–1318. doi: 10.1126/science.1110647

Ohgidani, M., Kato, T. A., Setoyama, D., Sagata, N., Hashimoto, R., Shigenobu, K., et al. (2014). Direct induction of ramified microglia-like cells from human monocytes: dynamic microglial dysfunction in Nasu-Hakola disease. *Sci. Rep.* 4:4957. doi: 10.1038/srep04957

Paloneva, J., Kestilä, M., Wu, J., Salminen, A., Bohling, T., Ruotsalainen, V., et al. (2000). Loss-of-function mutations in TYROBP (DAP12) result in a presenile dementia with bone cysts. *Nat. Genet.* 25, 357–361. doi: 10.1038/77153

Paloneva, J., Manninen, T., Christman, G., Hovanes, K., Mandelin, J., Adolfsson, R., et al. (2002). Mutations in two genes encoding different subunits of a receptor signaling complex result in an identical disease phenotype. *Am. J. Hum. Genet.* 71, 656–662. doi: 10.1086/342259

Pang, Z. P. P., Yang, N., Vierbuchen, T., Ostermeier, A., Fuentes, D. R., Yang, T. Q., et al. (2011). Induction of human neuronal cells by defined transcription factors. *Nature* 476, 220–223. doi: 10.1038/nature10202

Seki, Y., Kato, T. A., Monji, A., Mizoguchi, Y., Horikawa, H., Sato-Kasai, M., et al. (2013). Pretreatment of aripiprazole and minocycline, but not haloperidol, suppresses oligodendrocyte damage from interferon-gamma-stimulated microglia in co-culture model. *Schizophr. Res.* 151, 20–28. doi: 10.1016/j.schres.2013.09.011

Steiner, J., Bielau, H., Brisch, R., Danos, P., Ullrich, O., Mawrin, C., et al. (2008). Immunological aspects in the neurobiology of suicide: elevated microglial density in schizophrenia and depression is associated with suicide. *J. Psychiatr. Res.* 42, 151–157. doi: 10.1016/j.jpsychires.2006.10.013

Suzuki, K., Sugihara, G., Ouchi, Y., Nakamura, K., Futatsubashi, M., Takebayashi, K., et al. (2013). Microglial activation in young adults with autism spectrum disorder. *JAMA Psychiatry* 70, 49–58. doi: 10.1001/jamapsychiatry.2013.272

Takahashi, K., Tanabe, K., Ohnuki, M., Narita, M., Ichisaka, T., Tomoda, K., et al. (2007). Induction of pluripotent stem cells from adult human fibroblasts by defined factors. *Cell* 131, 861–872. doi: 10.1016/j.cell.2007.11.019

Takano, A., Arakawa, R., Ito H., Tateno, A., Takahashi, H., Matsumoto, R., et al. (2010). Peripheral benzodiazepine receptors in patients with chronic schizophrenia: a PET study with [C-11]DAA1106. *Int. J. Neuropsychopharmacol.* 13, 943–950. doi: 10.1017/s1461145710000313

van Berckel, B. N., Bossong, M. G., Boellaard, R., Kloet, R., Schuitemaker, A., Caspers, E., et al. (2008). Microglia activation in recent-onset schizophrenia: a quantitative (R)-[C-11]PK11195 positron emission tomography study. *Biol. Psychiatry* 64, 820–822. doi: 10.1016/j.biopsych.2008.04.025

Wake, H., Moorhouse, A. J., Jinno, S., Kohsaka, S., and Nabekura, J. (2009). Resting microglia directly monitor the functional state of synapses *in vivo* and determine the fate of ischemic terminals. *J. Neurosci.* 29, 3974–3980. doi: 10.1523/JNEUROSCI.4363-08.2009

Wang, S., Bates, J., Li, X. J., Schanz, S., Chandler-Militello, D., Levine, C., et al. (2013). Human iPSC-derived oligodendrocyte progenitor cells can myelinate and rescue a mouse model of congenital hypomyelination. *Cell Stem Cell* 12, 252–264. doi: 10.1016/j.stem.2012.12.002

Wang, Y., Szretter, K. J., Vermi, W., Gilfillan, S., Rossini, C., Cella, M., et al. (2012). IL-34 is a tissue-restricted ligand of CSF1R required for the development of Langerhans cells and microglia. *Nat. Immunol.* 13, 753–760. doi: 10.1038/ni.2360

Watabe, M., Kato, T. A., Monji, A., Horikawa, H., and Kanba, S. (2012). Does minocycline, an antibiotic with inhibitory effects on microglial activation, sharpen a sense of trust in social interaction? *Psychopharmacology (Berl)* 220, 551–557. doi: 10.1007/s00213-011-2509-8

Watabe, M., Kato, T. A., Tsuboi, S., Ishikawa, K., Hashiya, K., Monji, A., et al. (2013). Minocycline, a microglial inhibitor, reduces 'honey trap' risk in human economic exchange. *Sci. Rep.* 3:1685. doi: 10.1038/srep01685

Weigelt, K., Carvalho, L. A., Drexhage, R. C., Wijkhuijs, A., de Wit, H., van Beveren, N. J. M., et al. (2011). TREM-1 and DAP12 expression in monocytes of patients with severe psychiatric disorders. EGR3, ATF3 and PU.1 as important transcription factors. *Brain Behav. Immun.* 25, 1162–1169. doi: 10.1016/j.bbi.2011.03.006

Wen, Z. X., Nguyen, H. N., Guo, Z. Y., Lalli, M. A., Wang, X. Y., Su, Y. J., et al. (2014). Synaptic dysregulation in a human iPS cell model of mental disorders. *Nature* 515, 414–418. doi: 10.1038/nature13716

Wu, D. C., Jackson-Lewis, V., Vila, M., Tieu, K., Teismann, P., Vadseth, C., et al. (2002). Blockade of microglial activation is neuroprotective in the 1-methyl-4-phenyl-1,2,3,6-tetrahydropyridine mouse model of Parkinson disease. *J. Neurosci.* 22, 1763–1771.

Yoshiyama, Y., Higuchi, M., Zhang, B., Huang, S. M., Iwata, N., Saido, T. C., et al. (2007). Synapse loss and microglial activation precede tangles in a P301S tauopathy mouse model. *Neuron* 53, 337–351. doi: 10.1016/j.neuron.2007.01.010

# 3

# Maternal Immune Activation Evoked by Polyinosinic: Polycytidylic Acid does not Evoke Microglial Cell Activation in the Embryo

*Silke Smolders[1,2†], Sophie M. T. Smolders[1,3,4,5†], Nina Swinnen[1], Annette Gärtner[2], Jean-Michel Rigo[1†], Pascal Legendre[3,4,5†] and Bert Brône[1*†]*

*[1] BIOMED – Hasselt University, Hasselt, Belgium, [2] Laboratory of Neuronal Differentiation, VIB Center for the Biology of Disease, Leuven and Center for Human Genetics, KU Leuven, Leuven, Belgium, [3] INSERM, UMR S 1130, Université Pierre et Marie Curie, Paris, France, [4] CNRS, UMR 8246, Université Pierre et Marie Curie, Paris, France, [5] UM 119 NPS, Université Pierre et Marie Curie, Paris, France*

***Correspondence:**
*Bert Brône,
BIOMED – Hasselt University,
Martelarenlaan 42, 3500 Hasselt,
Belgium
bert.brone@uhasselt.be*

*† These authors have contributed equally to this work.*

Several studies have indicated that inflammation during pregnancy increases the risk for the development of neuropsychiatric disorders in the offspring. Morphological brain abnormalities combined with deviations in the inflammatory status of the brain can be observed in patients of both autism and schizophrenia. It was shown that acute infection can induce changes in maternal cytokine levels which in turn are suggested to affect fetal brain development and increase the risk on the development of neuropsychiatric disorders in the offspring. Animal models of maternal immune activation reproduce the etiology of neurodevelopmental disorders such as schizophrenia and autism. In this study the poly (I:C) model was used to mimic viral immune activation in pregnant mice in order to assess the activation status of fetal microglia in these developmental disorders. Because microglia are the resident immune cells of the brain they were expected to be activated due to the inflammatory stimulus. Microglial cell density and activation level in the fetal cortex and hippocampus were determined. Despite the presence of a systemic inflammation in the pregnant mice, there was no significant difference in fetal microglial cell density or immunohistochemically determined activation level between the control and inflammation group. These data indicate that activation of the fetal microglial cells is not likely to be responsible for the inflammation induced deficits in the offspring in this model.

**Keywords: neuropsychiatric disorders, maternal immune activation, microglia, embryo, cortex**

## Introduction

Schizophrenia and autism are neurodevelopmental disorders that can arise early during postnatal life. Although genetic deficits are important risk factors, perturbations of local environment, especially during pregnancy, are suspected to play a central role in the occurrence of these neurodevelopmental disorders. Maternal immune activation (MIA) during pregnancy is considered as a risk factor for schizophrenia and autism in the offspring (Brown, 2012). To study the mechanisms behind this association several animal models were developed in which pregnant rodents were infected with the influenza virus, polyinosinic:polycytidylic acid [poly (I:C)] or lipopolysaccharide (LPS) (Patterson, 2009). These models confirmed that prenatal infection leading to MIA can lead to behavioral and neurological disorders in the offspring (Shi et al., 2003; Meyer et al., 2006; Fortier et al., 2007; Lowe et al., 2008; Harvey and Boksa, 2012; Giovanoli et al., 2013; Squarzoni et al., 2014). During MIA evoked by poly (I:C), an elevated maternal serum cytokine, interleukin-6 (IL-6), was found to be critical for the development of these neurological deficits in the offspring (Samuelsson et al., 2006; Smith et al., 2007). Differences in behavioral abnormalities observed in the offspring at adult age are critically dependent on the time of maternal poly (I:C) challenge, being related to differences in cytokine responses in the fetal brain shortly after the induction of MIA (Meyer et al., 2006, 2008). However, the source of the cytokine response in the fetal brain remains a matter of debate as it can originate from maternal, placental and/or embryonic tissue. An endogenous increase in fetal brain cytokine production was demonstrated using mRNA analysis of the cytokine expression level upon maternal poly (I:C) challenge during the late gestation stage in mice (17 embryonic days, E17; Meyer et al., 2006). This was not observed when maternal poly (I:C) challenge was performed at mid gestation stage (E9; Meyer et al., 2006), a developmental age at which immature microglia, the resident immune cells of the brain, have not yet invaded the fetal central nervous system (CNS; Ginhoux et al., 2010; Rigato et al., 2011; Swinnen et al., 2013).

Microglia colonize the brain early during embryonic development (E11.5 in the mouse embryo; Ginhoux et al., 2010; Rigato et al., 2011; Swinnen et al., 2013) and are known to control several developmental processes in the brain at perinatal developmental stages (Cunningham et al., 2013; Squarzoni et al., 2014; Michell-Robinson et al., 2015). First, embryonic microglia have been shown to be involved in angiogenesis through close contact with vessel sprouts and endothelial tip cells and the secretion of soluble factors that stimulate angiogenesis during development (Fantin et al., 2010; Rymo et al., 2011). Secondly, during CNS development microglial cells clear cellular debris and induce programmed cell death in developing neurons via the production of superoxide ions (Marin-Teva et al., 2004; Wakselman et al., 2008) and tumor necrosis factor (TNF)-α (Sedel et al., 2004). Thirdly, several studies have pointed toward an important role for microglia in synaptic remodeling and synapse elimination (Tremblay et al., 2010; Paolicelli et al., 2011; Schafer et al., 2012; Zhan et al., 2014). Finally, microglial cells can also influence the development and differentiation of neural cells. Microglia-conditioned media can influence embryonic precursor migration and differentiation in primary cultures (Aarum et al., 2003; Jonakait et al., 2011). In addition, microglial cells can regulate cortical precursor proliferation and astrogenesis (Nakanishi et al., 2007). Primary culture experiments on embryonic precursor cultures showed that microglial cells are important for precursor proliferation and astrogenesis. In microglia-depleted cultures and cultures from PU.1 knock out embryos proliferation and astrogenesis were decreased. Addition of microglia to these cultures restored both processes and an abnormal increase in microglial cell numbers resulted in increased astrogenesis (Antony et al., 2011). Deactivation of embryonic microglia with tetracyclines or elimination via the macrophages suicide technique led to an increase in neural precursor cells, while microglial activation had the opposite effect (Cunningham et al., 2013).

Maternal immune activation induces an imbalance in cytokines levels, of which maternal IL-6 has been shown to be a critical mediator in inducing the effects of MIA on brain development and behavioral changes (Smith et al., 2007). IL-6 is known to induce activation of adult microglial cells; leading to the production of pro-inflammatory factors, such as nitric oxide, reactive oxygen species, proteolytic enzymes, and TNF-α by microglial cell cultures (Krady et al., 2008), microglial proliferation (*in vitro*; Streit et al., 2000) and infiltration (*in vivo*; Lacroix et al., 2002) or the upregulation of microglial CX3CR1, making them more sensitive to fractalkine signaling (Lee et al., 2010). An imbalance in cytokine levels caused by MIA might thus be able to activate embryonic microglia, even at early developmental stages, and alter their normal functions. This can trigger a cascade of events that could lead to developmental defects observed in the offspring of LPS or poly (I:C) treated pregnant mice. Indeed, MIA evoked by LPS injection evoked microglia activation and enhanced phagocytosis of neural precursors by microglia at prenatal stages in rats (Cunningham et al., 2013). However, the question remains whether an endogenous increase in fetal brain cytokine production in response to maternal poly (I:C) challenge is of microglial origin. Accordingly it remains unclear whether poly (I:C)-induced MIA results in the activation of embryonic microglia during fetal development.

To determine to what extent MIA evoked by poly (I:C) can alter cortex invasion by microglia and/or change embryonic microglial cell activation state, we evoked MIA using a single (at E11.5) or a double injection (at E11.5 and E15.5) of poly (I:C) (Meyer et al., 2006; Shi et al., 2009). This developmental time window is an important time point for cortex invasion by immature microglia as their cell density dramatically increases during this period (Swinnen et al., 2013). We show that poly (I:C)-induced MIA does not affect microglial density and activation level during embryonic development suggesting that pathological activation of embryonic microglial cells at the onset of their colonization processes cannot explain neurological deficits observed at postnatal stages in offspring after poly (I:C)-induced MIA.

## Materials and Methods

### Animals

All experiments were conducted in accordance with the European Community guiding principles on the care and use of animals and with the approval of the Ethical Committee on Animal Research of Hasselt University. Mice were maintained in the animal facility of the Hasselt University in accordance with the guidelines of the Belgian Law and the European Council Directive. To visualize microglia in the embryonic cortex the transgenic CX3CR1-eGFP knock-in mice (Jung et al., 2000) were used. The heterozygous CX3CR1-eGFP embryos used in this study were obtained by crossing wild type C57BL/6 females with homozygous CX3CR1-eGFP +/+ male mice (obtained from the European Mouse Mutant Archive - EMMA with the approval of Jung et al., 2000). The day of conception was designated as embryonic day 0.5 (E0.5).

## Maternal Immune Activation

At day E11.5 (single injection) or at E11.5 and E15.5 (double injection) mice received i.p. a dose of poly (I:C) (20 mg/kg; Polyinosinic–polycytidylic acid potassium salt; Sigma–Aldrich, Bornem, Belgium) or vehicle (saline). Five hours after injection the maternal blood was collected, the serum was aliquoted and stored at −80°C until the IL-6 assay was performed (Shi et al., 2003; Smith et al., 2007). The maternal IL-6 concentrations were determined using the Mouse IL-6 ELISA Kit from Thermo Scientific (Rockford, IL, USA), following the manufacturer's instructions. The analysis was conducted using a FLUOstar OPTIMA plate reader (BMG Labtech, Ortenberg, Germany).

## Fluorescent Immunostaining of Embryonic Brains

Pregnant mice were sacrificed and embryonic tissue processed as described before (Swinnen et al., 2013). The heads of E11.5 and E12.5 embryos were fixed in 4% paraformaldehyde for 3 h at 4°C and 5 h for E17.5 embryos. After fixation, the embryonic heads were cryoprotected overnight in phosphate-buffered saline (PBS) + 30% sucrose, frozen in optimal cutting temperature compound (Tissue-Tek) and stored at −80°C until sectioned. Ten micrometer-thick coronal tissue sections were cut on a Leica CM1900 uv cryostat, mounted on Superfrost Plus glasses and stored at −20°C until staining.

To check whether embryonic microglia can be directly activated by poly (I:C), IL-6 or LPS, 300-μm thick coronal brain slices (E15.5) were cultured for 24 h with either saline, poly (I:C) (50 μg/ml), IL-6 (10 ng/ml), or LPS (1 μg/ml). To this end, pregnant mothers were euthanized at E15.5. Embryonic brains were isolated in ice-cold PBS-glucose (pH 7.4; 25 mM), embedded in 3% low melting agarose (Fisher Scientific) and sliced coronally at a thickness of 300 μm using a Microm HM650V Vibrating Blade Microtome. Slices were mounted on MilliCell organotypic inserts (Millipore) and maintained in semi-hydrous conditions at 37°C and 5% $CO_2$ for 24 h. The media consisted of Neurobasal medium supplemented with 2 mM L-glutamine, B27 supplement, N2 supplement, and 0.5% penicillin–streptomycin (all from Invitrogen) with either saline, poly (I:C) (50 μg/ml), IL-6 (10 ng/ml) or LPS (1 μg/ml) added. Afterward slices were fixed for 1 h in 4% PFA and cryoprotected overnight in PBS + 30% sucrose, frozen in optimal cutting temperature compound (Tissue-Tek) and stored at −80°C until sectioned. Ten micrometer-thick coronal tissue sections were cut on a Leica CM1900 uv cryostat, mounted on Superfrost Plus glasses and stored at −20°C until staining.

In order to determine the activation state of the microglia, we used antibodies against interleukin (IL)-1β, inducible nitric oxide synthase (iNOS) and Mac-2/Galectin-3 (Rigato et al., 2011; Cunningham et al., 2013). All primary antibodies and working solutions are listed in **Table 1**.

**TABLE 1 | Overview of the antibodies used for immunostainings and flow cytometry experiments.**

| Antibody | Company | Reference | Dilution |
|---|---|---|---|
| **Immunohistochemistry** | | | |
| Anti-IL1β (rabbit polycl.) | Abcam | ab9722 | 1:100 |
| Anti-iNOS (rabbit polycl.) | Abcam | ab15323 | 1:250 |
| Anti-Mac-2 (rat monocl.) | American type culture collection | TIB-166 | 1:250 |
| **Flow cytometry** | | | |
| Anti-IL1β PE (rat monocl.) | LifeSpan BioSciences | LS-C184791 | 1:300 |
| Anti-iNOS PE-Cy7 (rat monocl.) | eBioscience | 25-5920 | 1:300 |
| Anti-Mac-2 PE (rat monocl.) | eBioscience | 12-5301 | 1:300 |

## Isolation of Microglia and Flow Cytometry Experiments

Brains were isolated from CX3CR1-eGFP E17.5 embryos from mothers subjected to a single saline or poly (I:C) injection on E11.5, or a double poly (I:C) injection on E11.5 and E15.5. All steps occurred at 4°C or on ice, unless stated otherwise, to avoid microglia activation. Meninges were removed, the cortical area identical to the immunohistochemical analysis was dissected out and incubated during 30 min at 30°C in DMEM/F-12(1:1) + GlutaMAX (Life Technologies) containing 48 U/ml Papain from papaya latex (Sigma). Papain containing supernatants was discarded and the tissue was mechanically disrupted in medium through fast pipetting using a 1 ml pipet. Afterward, the homogenate was centrifuged at 400*g* during 5 min, resuspended in 40% isotonic Percoll (GE Healthcare) and centrifuged at 700*g* during 10 min without break. The pellet was resuspended in PBS and filtered through a 35 μm cell strainer. Cell suspensions were fixed and permeablized in Cytofix/Cytoperm buffer (BD Cytofix/Cytoperm$^{TM}$ Plus Fixation/Permeabilization Kit, BD Biosciences) during 20 min on ice, washed and incubated on ice for 30 min in Perm/Wash buffer with a mix of fluorochrome-conjugated rat anti-mouse antibodies: iNOS-PE-Cy7 (clone CXNFT, eBioscience), Mac-2-PE (clone eBioM3/38, eBioscience) and, IL1β-PE (clone 11n92, LifeSpan BioSciences) (**Table 1**). The following isotype controls were used: Rat IgG2aκ PE-Cy7, Rat IgG2aκ PE and Rat IgG2b PE (all from eBioscience). After washes, cells were resuspended in FACS buffer (PBS, 2% FCS, sodium azide), acquired in a FACS Aria II and analyzed with FACS Diva 6.1.3 software (BD Biosciences). Isotype-marker overlay graphs were created in FlowJo 10.0.8 Software. Inside the singlet population, the eGFP positive microglia (1000–12000 cells per experiment) were gated (**Figure 5A**), and within this population, the percentage of Mac-2, iNOS, and IL1β positive microglia was analyzed. Isotype controls were used to gate the positive cell population (**Figure 5B**). Per group, embryos were derived from one to three different mothers (saline, single poly (I:C), double poly(I:C)). BV-2 cells (Supplementary Data) were used as positive controls for the different antibodies (Supplementary Figure S1).

## Analysis and Statistics

Quantitative analysis of microglial cells was performed on images of coronal embryonic brain sections. We focused our analysis on the cerebral cortex area located dorsally to the lateral ganglionic eminences (LGE) and medial ganglionic eminences (MGE), containing the frontal and pariental cortex on E11.5 and E12.5, and the somatosensory and motor cortex at E17.5. This region of the cortex is well characterized on the functional and cellular level and the two GE structures are the major sources of cortical interneurons during embryonic neurogenesis (Tan et al., 1998; Anderson et al., 2001). For the quantifications of the hippocampal area at E17.5 only the dorsal hippocampus was included in the analysis.

Images were taken with a Nikon Eclipse 80i microscope and a Nikon digital sight camera DS-2MBWc [10x Nikon plan objective (numerical aperture (NA) of 0.25) and a 20x Plan Fluor objective (NA of 0.5)]. Images (1600 × 1200) were analyzed with ImageJ 1.45e software (NIH, USA; http://rsb.info.nih.gov/ij/). Only eGFP-positive cell bodies were taken into account for the measurements. Density analysis was performed by counting the number of eGFP positive cell bodies per $mm^2$ (Swinnen et al., 2013). For analysis of activation state we calculated the percentage of the eGFP positive cells that were also showing immunoreactivity for the activation marker. All values are expressed as mean ± SEM. The number of sections used is indicated as *n*, the number of embryos or blood samples as *N*; # sections/# embryos is thus designated in the text as *n/N*. Statistical significance was assessed by non-parametric Mann–Whitney test or Kruskal–Wallis test, *P*-values smaller than 0.05 were considered significant.

## Results

An increase in IL-6 level in the maternal blood is a crucial factor in the development of MIA-induced deficits and changes observed in the offspring (Smith et al., 2007). To control that the poly (I:C) injection procedure we used evoked an increase in IL-6 level in the maternal blood, we analyzed the IL-6 level in the maternal serum samples 5 hours after injection of either saline or poly (I:C). We found a significant increase ($P < 0.0001$; Mann–Whitney test) in the level of IL-6 in the sera of female mice primed with poly (I:C) (1876 ± 389.2 pg/ml, $N = 22$) when compared to those injected with saline (14.8 ± 3.3 pg/ml, $N = 26$), thus indicating that the mice in the poly (I:C) group effectively suffered from a systemic immune response.

In response to brain injury, microglia proliferate and shift to beneficial or detrimental activation states depending on the local environment. When activated, microglial cells adopt a phagocytic phenotype in order to clear dying cells (Kettenmann et al., 2011). In pathological conditions, such as in the mouse model of LPS-induced MIA, phagocytosis of neuronal precursor cells by microglia was also increased, which resulted in a decrease in the size of the precursor cell pool in the cerebral cortex (Cunningham et al., 2013). It must also be noted that microglial disturbances were also observed in patients suffering from autistic or schizophrenic disorders. Microglial activation has been observed in the brains of autistic (Vargas et al., 2005; Morgan et al., 2010) and schizophrenic patients (Radewicz et al., 2000; Wierzba-Bobrowicz et al., 2005; Monji et al., 2013). Recent studies also indicated that there is an increase in microglial density in different brain regions in the adult poly (I:C) MIA offspring (Juckel et al., 2011; Ratnayake et al., 2012).

To determine if poly (I:C)-evoked MIA alters the embryonic microglial cell colonization process in the fetal brain we compared cell density after single injection of poly (I:C), double injection of poly (I:C) or saline treatments, in the cortex at E11.5, E12.5 and at E17.5 (single injection) or at E17.5 (double injections) and in the hippocampal area at E17.5 (single and double injections). At all ages tested we did not find any significant difference in microglia cell density (Mann–Whitney test; $P > 0.05$, for detailed *P*-values see **Table 2**) in the cortex or in the hippocampus after a single or after double injections (**Figure 1**; **Table 2**), thus suggesting that poly (I:C)-evoked MIA does not alter early invasion of the cortex and the hippocampus by microglial cells in the embryo.

To determine if MIA induced a change in microglial activation level after a single poly (I:C) injection (E11.5), we performed an immunostaining for three different activation markers: Mac-2/Galectin-3, iNOS and IL1β at E11.5 and E17.5. Mac-2/Galectin-3 is a marker of microglial phagocytic activation state (Dumic et al., 2006; Rotshenker, 2009) while iNOS and IL1β are markers of a cytotoxic activation state (Cunningham et al., 2013). At E11.5 none of the microglia located in the cortex was immmunopositive for Mac-2 staining both after saline injection

**TABLE 2 | Microglial cell density in the cortex and hippocampal area of embryos derived from the control group and the group that was subjected to maternal inflammation at E11.5 or at E11.5 and E15.5.**

| Brain structure | Cortex | | | Hippocampus |
|---|---|---|---|---|
| **Embryonic age** | **E11.5** | **E12.5** | **E17.5** | **E17.5** |
| **Single injection at E11.5** | | | | |
| Saline | 48.6 ± 8.8 | 34.9 ± 2.8 | 59.6 ± 5.8 | 122.5 ± 4.9 |
| Poly (I:C) | 32.2 ± 5.7 | 37.8 ± 2.9 | 56.5 ± 4.3 | 111.6 ± 5.7 |
| *P* value | 0.191 | 0.375 | 0.573 | 0.435 |
| **Brain structure** | **Cortex** | | | **Hippocampus** |
| **Embryonic age** | **E17.5** | | | **E17.5** |
| **Double injection at E11.5 and E15.5** | | | | |
| Saline | 59.8 ± 3.1 | | | 95.3 ± 4.8 |
| Poly (I:C) | 57.8 ± 2.2 | | | 91.0 ± 5.7 |
| *P* value | 0.931 | | | 0.699 |

*Values are mean ± SEM of the number of microglial cells per $mm^2$, Mann–Whitney test was used for statistical analysis. When injected at E11.5 the numbers of embryonic brains in the saline and poly (I:C) group were, respectively: E11.5 = 4/5; E12.5 = 12/7; E17.5 cortex = 6/8; E17.5 hippocampus = 5/8. When injected at E11.5 and E15.5 numbers of embryonic brains in the saline and poly (I:C) group were, respectively: E17.5 cortex = 5/6; E17.5 hippocampus = 6/6.*

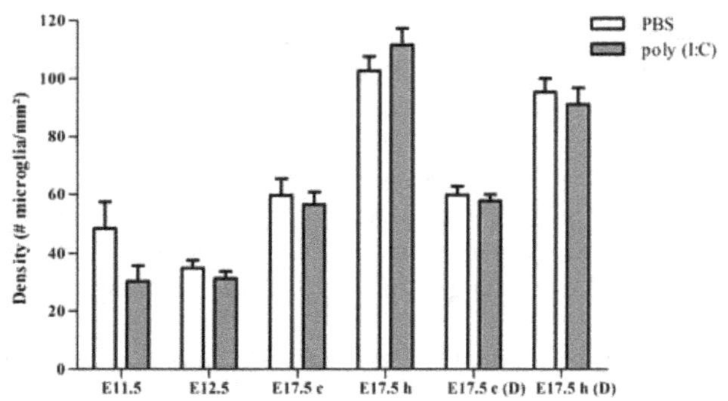


**FIGURE 1 | Embryonic microglial cell density is not increased after single and double injection of poly (I:C).** Microglial cell density in the cortex and hippocampal area was not affected after poly (I:C)-induced MIA. Values are mean ± SEM of the number of microglial cells per mm$^2$, Mann–Whitney test was used for statistical analysis. When injected at E11.5 the numbers of embryonic brains in the saline and poly (I:C) group were, respectively: E11.5 = 4/5; E12.5 = 12/7; E17.5 cortex = 6/8; E17.5 hippocampus = 5/8. When injected at E11.5 and E15.5 numbers of embryonic brains in the saline and poly (I:C) group were, respectively: E17.5 cortex = 5/6; E17.5 hippocampus = 6/6. c, cortex; h, hippocampal area; D, double injection.

($n/N$ = 14/3) and after poly (I:C) challenge ($n/N$ = 18/3; **Figure 2B1,B2**). At E17.5, 2.5 ± 0.5% ($n/N$ = 38/4) of the microglia in the cortex (**Figure 2A1,A2**) and 3.2 ± 0.7% ($n/N$ = 27/4) of the microglia in the hippocampal area expressed Mac-2 after saline injection. We did not find any significant difference (Kruskal–Wallis test; $P$ = 0.448) after poly (I:C) challenge. After poly (I:C) challenge, 1.9 ± 0.7% ($n/N$ = 23/4) of the microglia in the cortex and 2.5 ± 1% ($n/N$ = 15/4) of microglia in hippocampal area expressed Mac-2 (**Figures 2C1,C2,D1,D2**). We next investigated the expression of IL1β and iNOS (Cunningham et al., 2013) to determine if embryonic microglia can adopt a cytotoxic activation state after a single injection of poly (I:C). Induction of MIA by a single injection of poly (I:C) did not result in a significant increase in the percentage of microglia expressing IL1β either at E11.5 and E17.5 (Kruskal–Wallis test; $P$ = 0.136). In control conditions, 0 ± 0% ($n/N$ = 6/3) and 2.2 ± 1% ($n/N$ = 15/4) of microglia located in the cortex expressed IL1β at E11.5 and E17.5 (**Figure 3A1,A2**), respectively, while 3.1 ± 1.3% ($n/N$ = 17/4) expressed IL1β in the hippocampal area (E17.5). After poly (I:C) challenge, 3.3 ± 3.3% ($n/N$ = 10/3) and 3.5 ± 1% ($n/N$ = 19/4) of microglia located in the cortex expressed IL1β at E11.5 (**Figure 3B1,B2**) and at E17.5 (**Figure 3C1,C2**), respectively, while 7.2 ± 2.6% ($n/N$ = 17/4) expressed IL1β in the hippocampal area (E17.5; **Figure 3D1,D2**). We found similar results when analyzing iNOS expression at E11.5 and E17.5 in the cortex and in the hippocampal area (E17.5). Cortical iNOS expression in control conditions [E11.5: 8.3 ± 5.7%, $n/N$ = 10/3; E17.5: 2.0 ± 1.1%, $n/N$ = 15/4 (**Figure 4A1,A2**)] was not significantly different when compared to the poly (I:C) condition [E11.5: 0 ± 0%, $n/N$ = 8/3 (**Figure 4B1,B2**); E17.5: 1.9 ± 1.1%, $n/N$ = 12/4 (**Figure 4C1,C2**; Kruskal–Wallis test; $P$ = 0.471)]. In the hippocampal area, 1.5 ± 1.0% of microglia ($n/N$ = 14/4) express iNOS in control conditions while 0 ± 0%, of microglia ($n/N$ = 10/4) express iNOS after poly (I:C) challenge (**Figure 4D1,D2**, being not significantly different (Kruskal–Wallis test; $P$ = 0.471)).

This lack of change in embryonic microglia activation state after a single poly (I:C) injection could possibly lead only to a "primed" microglial state. Indeed, two injections of LPS were necessary in rat to elicit MIA induced microglia dysfunction during phagocytosis of cortical neural precursor cells (Cunningham et al., 2013), suggesting that the microglial phenotype could become only fully altered after the second inflammatory challenge. To determine if this is also the case for poly (I:C) we reanalyzed microglial density and activation level after a repeated injection of poly (I:C). Consequently, the mothers suffered from a double immune stimulation (on E11.5 as well as on E15.5). Despite the presence of a maternal immune response after both injections, there was no significant increase in microglial cell density (Mann–Whitney test; $P > 0.05$, for detailed $P$-values see **Table 2**) (**Figure 1**; **Table 2**). Microglial activation states were analyzed at E17.5 as described above. We did not find any significant difference (Kruskal–Wallis test; Mac-2, $P$ = 0.139; IL1β, $P$ = 0.945; iNOS, $P$ = 0.093) in the percentage of microglia expressing Mac-2, IL1β, or iNOS between control conditions and after double injections of poly (I:C). After double injections of poly (I:C) the percentage of microglia immunoreactive for Mac-2 antibody was 0 ± 0% ($n/N$ = 29/6) in the cortex (**Figure 2E1,E2**) and 2.0 ± 0.7% ($n/N$ = 22/6) in the hippocampal area (**Figure 2F1,F2**). In the cortex (**Figure 3E1,E2**) and hippocampal area (**Figure 3F1,F2**) 1.4 ± 0.7% ($n/N$ = 34/6) and 1.4 ± 1.0% ($n/N$ = 25/6) of the microglial cells showed immunoreactivity for the IL1β antibody, while 1.8 ± 0.7% ($n/N$ = 34/6) and 0 ± 0% ($n/N$ = 23/6) of the microglia were positive for iNOS in the cortex (**Figure 4E1,E2**) and hippocampal area (**Figure 4F1,F2**), respectively. These results indicate that even double injections of poly (I:C) did not evoke microglia activation in the embryo.

In addition to the immunohistochemical stainings, the presence of the activation markers on microglial cells at E17.5 was investigated by flow cytometry. The gating strategy and positive controls are shown in **Figures 5A,B** and Supplementary Figure S1. The results of the flow cytometric quantifications were similar to those obtained by immunohistochemistry. There was no significant difference in the proportion of microglial cells that were positive for Mac-2 after single poly (I:C) injection (16.8 ± 0.0%; N = 10) or double poly (I:C) injection (27.0 ± 4.6%; $N$ = 10) when compared to the control group (15.5 ± 4.3; $N$ = 5; **Figure 5C**, left; Kruskal–Wallis test, $P$ = 0.161). The proportion of microglial cells that were positive for IL1β in the control group (14.2 ± 3.1%; $N$ = 10) was not significantly different (**Figure 5C**, middle; Kruskal–Wallis test, $P$ = 0.093) to the percentage of microglia that was positive for IL1β after a single (22.3 ± 3.9%; $N$ = 8) or double poly (I:C) injection (16.0 ± 2.1%; $N$ = 6). The percentage of microglial cells positive for iNOS in the control group was 9.1 ± 2.8% ($N$ = 5). There was no significant effect (**Figure 5C**, right; Kruskal–Wallis test, $P$ = 0.816) of a single poly (I:C) (7.1 ± 1.5%; $N$ = 10) or double poly (I:C) challenge (9.9 ± 2.7%; $N$ = 10) on the percentage of microglia expressing this marker.

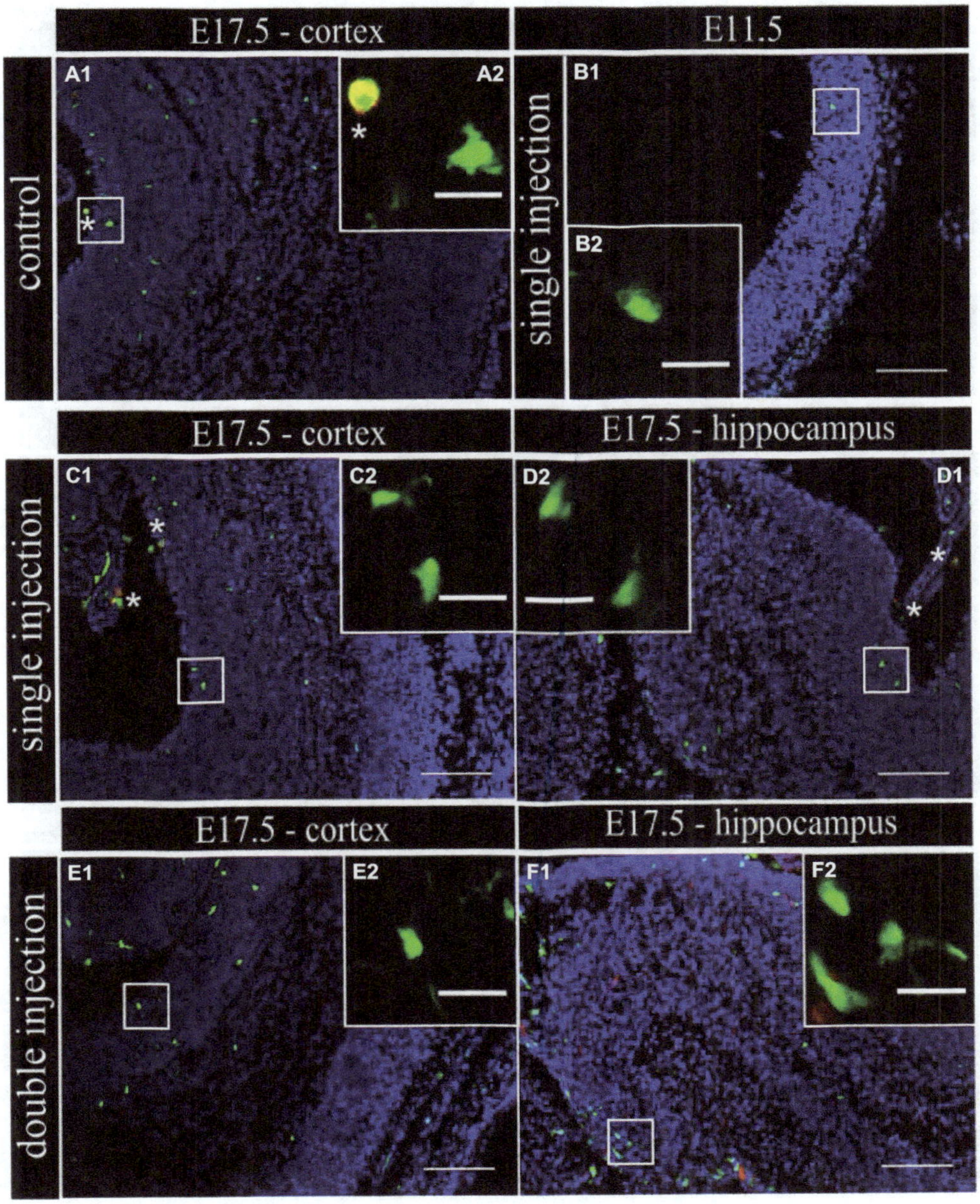


**FIGURE 2 | Embryonic microglial cell population is poorly immunoreactive to the Mac-2/Galectin-3 antibody after single and double injection of poly (I:C). (A–F1)** Coronal sections of embryonic brains, with cell nucleus staining in blue (DAPI) and microglial (CX3CR1-eGFP) cells in green. Immunohistochemical staining using a Mac-2 antibody (red) showed that at E17.5 almost no microglial cells in the cortex were immunoreactive for Mac-2 **(A2)** after injection with saline. At E11.5 **(B2)** and E17.5 **(C2,E2)** in the cortex and E17.5 hippocampal area **(D2,F2)** there was no increased percentage of microglial cells expressing the activation marker after poly (I:C) challenge compared to control. White square indicates the location of the cells in the tissue showed in the inset; * indicates a Mac-2 positive eGFP cell. Examples of one control brain area and poly (I:C) group only as they were not significantly different. Scale bar = 100 μm and for insets = 20 μm.

The absence of activation marker expression by microglia after poly (I:C) challenge raised the question whether fetal microglia can be directly activated by a poly (I:C) challenge as suspected for LPS (Cunningham et al., 2013) and IL-6 (Smith et al., 2007). To address this issue we analyzed the activation state of microglia in acute embryonic brain slices (E15.5) after exposure to IL-6, poly (I:C) or LPS. The percentage of microglial cells expressing Mac-2/Galectin-3, iNOS, and IL1β were analyzed 24 h after immune challenge of the slices (**Figure 6D**). **Figure 6** insets show examples of microglial cells that did (**Figures 6A–C2**) or did not show immunoreactivity (**Figures 6A–C3**) for the activation markers tested (Mac-2, IL1β, and iNOS). In control conditions 31 ± 5.9%, ($n/N$ = 23/4) of microglia were immunoreactive for Mac-2 antibody. This percentage was significantly higher (Kruskal–Wallis test; $P < 0.0001$) than that observed *in vivo* indicating that an *in vitro* environment promotes microglia

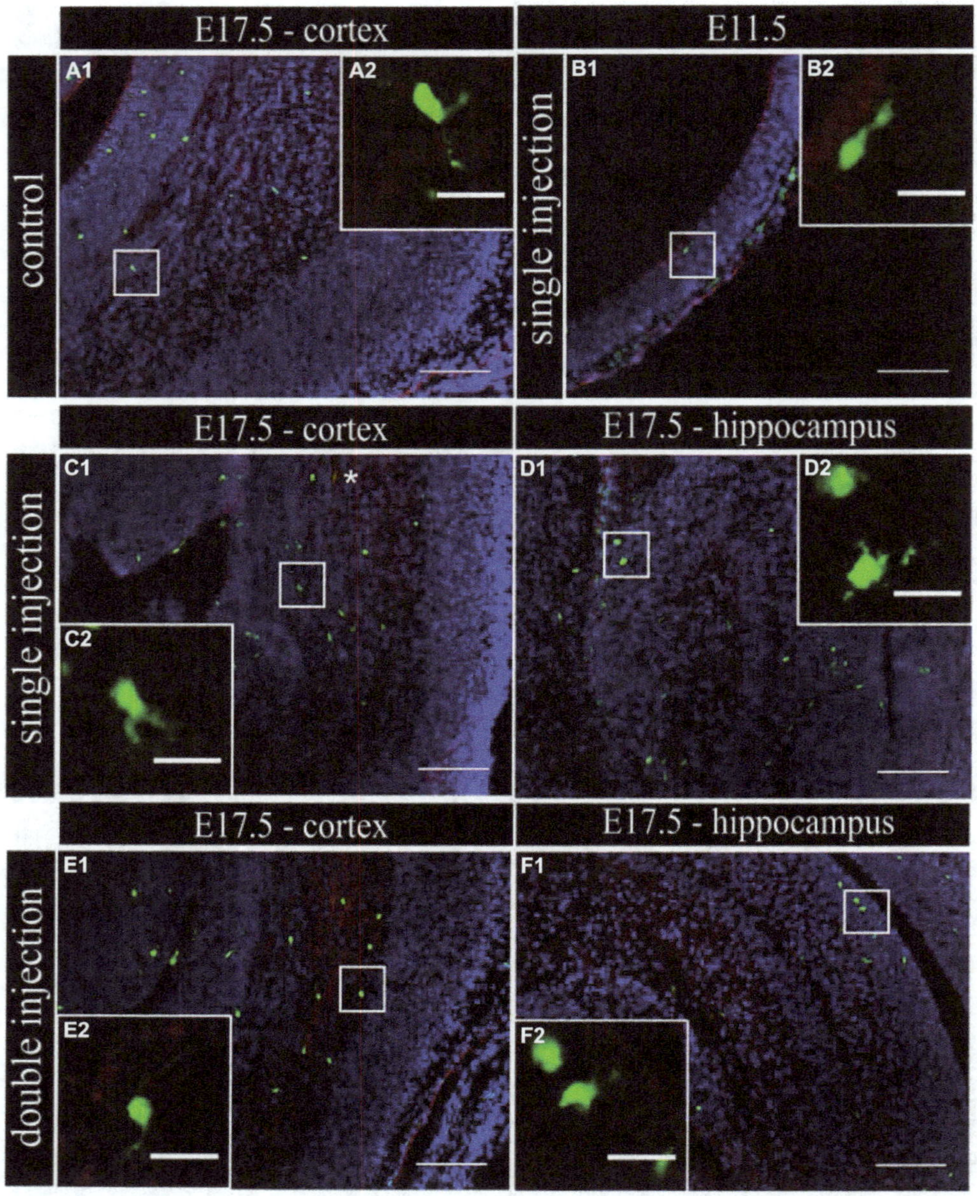


**FIGURE 3 | Embryonic microglia show no increased expression of IL1β after single and double injection of poly (I:C). (A–F1)** Coronal sections of embryonic brains, with cell nucleus staining in blue (DAPI) and microglial (CX3CR1-eGFP) cells in green. Immunohistochemical staining using an IL1β antibody (red) showed that at E17.5 almost no microglial cells in the cortex were immunoreactive for IL1β **(A2)** after injection with saline. At E11.5 **(B2)** and E17.5 **(C2,E2)** in the cortex and E17.5 hippocampal area **(D2,F2)** there was no increased percentage of microglial cells expressing the activation marker after poly (I:C) challenge compared to control. White square indicates the location of the cells in the tissue showed in the inset; * indicates an IL1β positive eGFP cell. Examples of one control brain area and poly (I:C) group only as they were not significantly different. Scale bar = 100 μm and for insets = 20 μm.

phagocytic activation state. However, there was no significant effect (Kruskal–Wallis test; $P = 0.274$) of IL-6, poly (I:C) or LPS treatment on the percentage of microglia being immunoreactive to Mac-2 antibody (**Figure 6D**), being 34 ± 5.5% ($n/N = 22/4$) after IL-6 exposure, 32 ± 6.7%, ($n/N = 18/5$) after poly (I:C) exposure and 47 ± 7.5% ($n/N = 21/5$) after LPS exposure (**Figure 6D**). As observed for Mac-2, the percentage of IL1β immunoreactive microglia was significantly higher than in *in vivo* conditions [in control conditions 52 ± 6.8%, ($n/N = 27/4$; Kruskal–Wallis test; $P < 0.0001$)] and for iNOS a trend to a higher percentage was observed under control conditions [in control conditions 18 ± 5.7%, ($n/N = 23/4$; Kruskal–Wallis test; $P = 0.091$)]. As shown in **Figure 6D** treatment with IL-6 or poly (I:C) did not significantly change the percentage of microglia immunoreactive for IL1β or iNOS antibodies. When looking at IL1β immunoreactivity, 36 ± 7.2% ($n/N = 16/4$) of the microglia was positive after IL-6 exposure and 54 ± 7.5%, ($n/N = 19/5$) after poly (I:C) exposure (**Figure 6D**). For iNOS they were

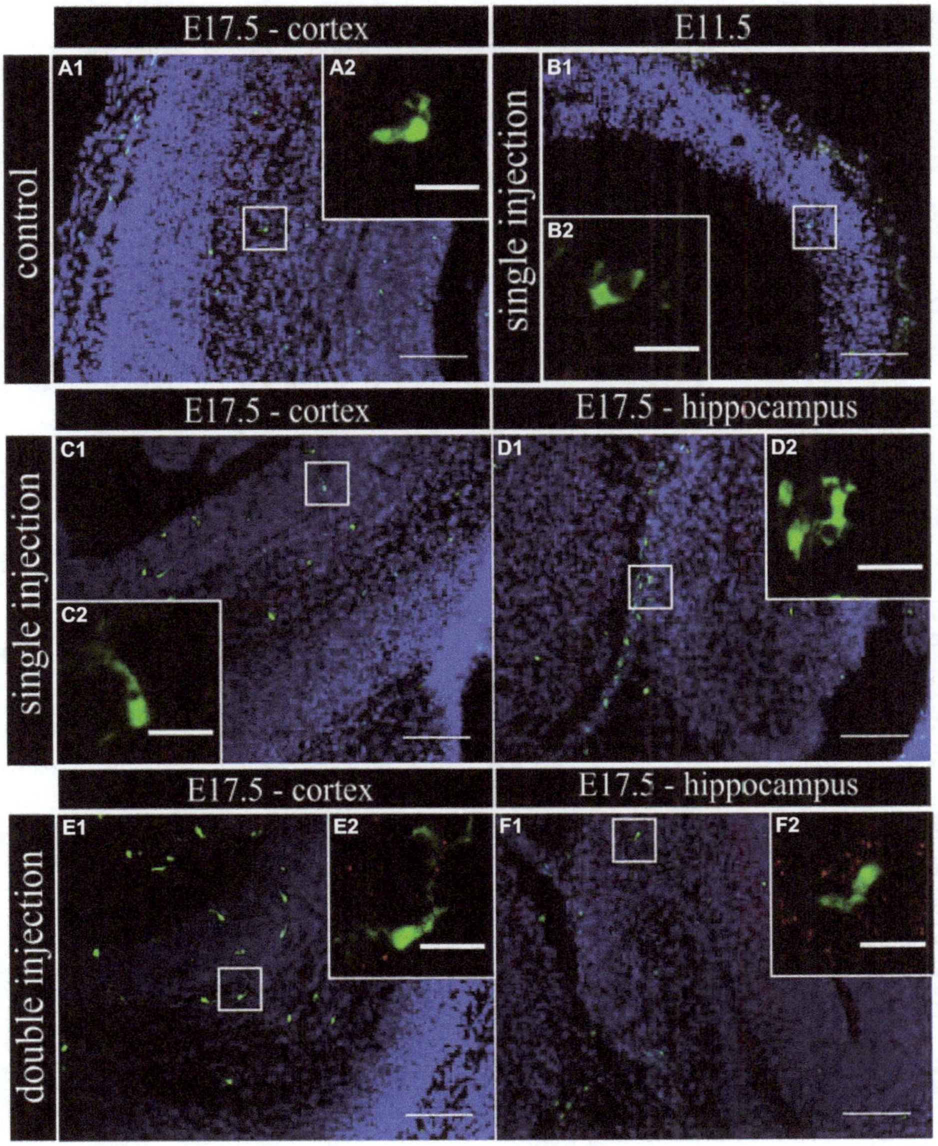


**FIGURE 4 | Embryonic microglia cell population is poorly immunoreactive to the iNOS antibody after single and double injection of poly (I:C). (A–F1)** Coronal sections of embryonic brains, with cell nucleus staining in blue (DAPI) and microglial (CX3CR1-eGFP) cells in green. Immunohistochemical staining using an iNOS antibody (red) showed that at E17.5 almost no microglial cells in the cortex were immunoreactive for iNOS **(A2)** after injection with saline. At E11.5 **(B2)** and E17.5 **(C2,E2)** in the cortex and E17.5 hippocampal area **(D2,F2)** there was no increased percentage of microglial cells expressing the activation marker after poly (I:C) challenge compared to control. White square indicates the location of the cells in the tissue showed in the inset. Examples of one control brain area and poly (I:C) group only as they were not significantly different. Scale bar = 100 μm and for insets = 20 μm.

30 ± 6.5% (*n/N* = 19/4) after IL-6 exposure and 25 ± 3.9%, (*n/N* = 25/5) after poly (I:C) exposure (**Figure 6D**). However, we found that LPS, contrary to IL-6 or poly (I:C), can directly activate microglia to a detrimental activation state. Indeed LPS exposure significantly increased the percentage of microglia immunoreactive for IL1β (Kruskal-Wallis test; $P = 0.025$) or iNOS antibodies (Kruskal-Wallis test; $P = 0.025$). In the presence of LPS 66 ± 5.5 (*n/N* = 22/5) and 42 ± 7.1% (*n/N* = 21/5) of microglia were immunoreactive for IL1β antibody or iNOS antibody, respectively.

## Discussion

Maternal immune activation-induced behavioral and neurological alterations observed in the offspring at juvenile and adult stages in animals are supposed to be correlated with the etiology of neuropsychiatric disorders in humans. Our study in mice demonstrates, for the first time, that MIA evoked by single or double poly (I:C) injections does not change microglia density and their activation state in the embryo *in vivo*. This suggests that the behavioral and neurological alterations in the

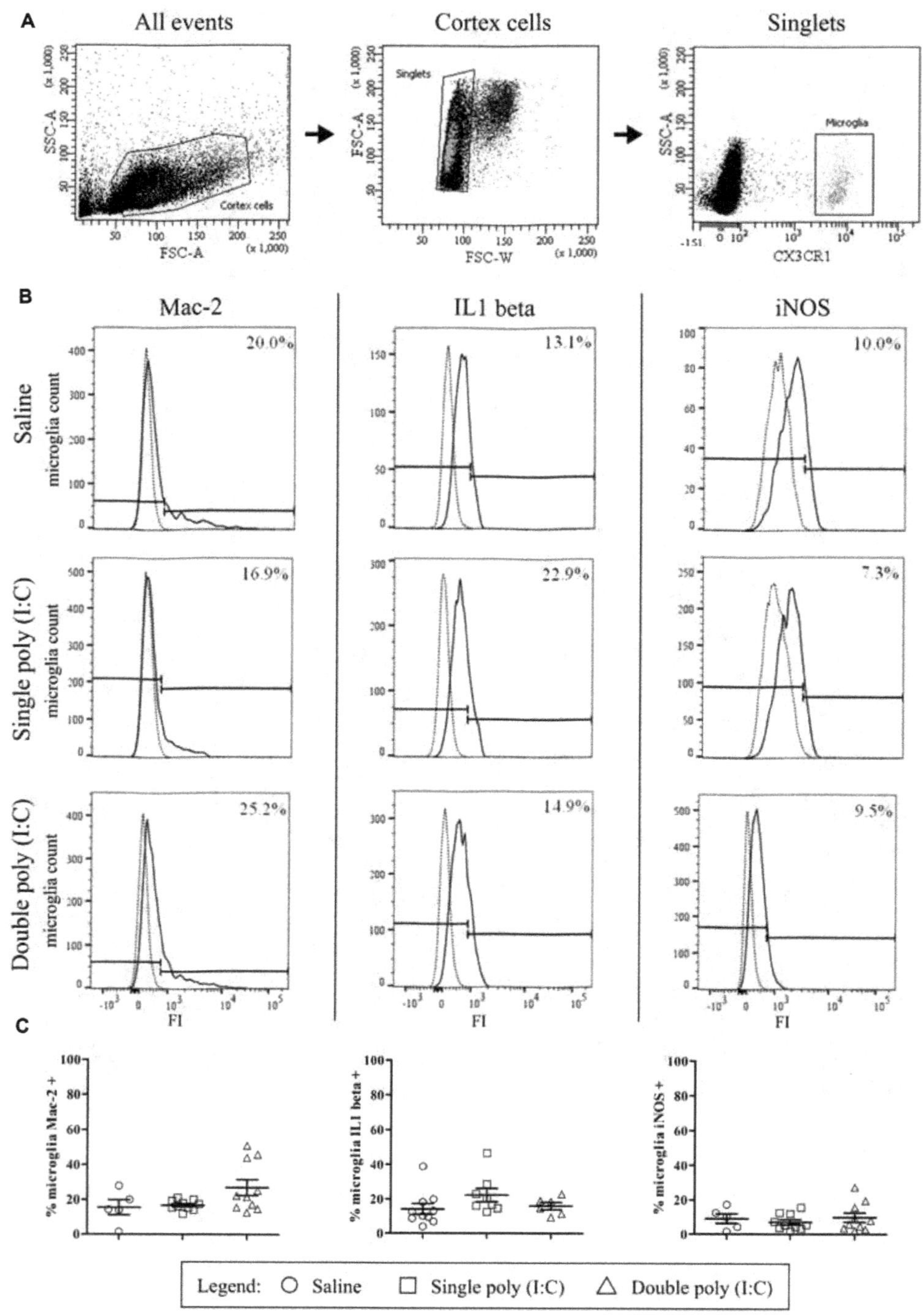


**FIGURE 5 | Flow cytometry reveals that embryonic microglial cells show a poor expression of activation markers Mac-2, IL1β and iNOS. (A)** Gating strategies for the microglial cells. In the whole embryonic cortex cell suspension, a gate was created on the non-debris population (left). Inside this population, single cells were selected (middle) and within this population, the microglial cells were gated based on CX3CR1-eGFP intensity (right). SSC, Side scatter; FSC, Forward scatter. **(B)** Gating strategies for positive Mac-2, iNOS and IL1β populations. Microglial cell count of representative samples is shown for Mac-2 (left), IL1β (middle) and iNOS (right; full lines) for embryos derived from saline, single poly (I:C) and double poly (I:C) injected mothers. Gates for positive populations were drawn based on the isotype fluorescence intensity (dotted lines). FI, fluorescence intensity. **(C)** Left panels: at E17.5 only a small percentage of microglial cells shows reactivity for Mac-2. There is no significant effect of poly (I:C) injection on this percentage. Number of embryos tested: Saline $N = 5$; single poly (I:C) $N = 10$ and double poly (I:C) $N = 10$. Middle panels: in control conditions, less than 15% of the microglial cells is positive for IL1β. There is no significant effect of poly (I:C) injection on this proportion. Number of embryos tested: Saline $N = 10$; single poly (I:C) $N = 8$ and double poly (I:C) $N = 6$. Right panels: at E17.5 less than 10% of the microglial cells is positive for iNOS. Poly (I:C) challenge has no significant effect on this percentage. Number of embryos tested: saline $N = 5$; single poly (I:C) $N = 10$ and double poly (I:C) $N = 10$.

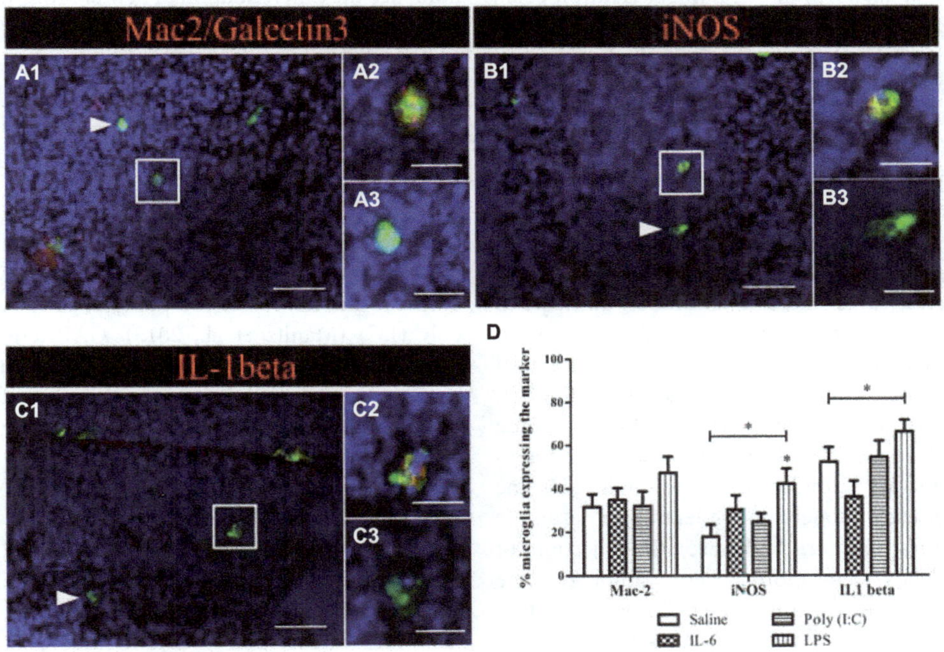


**FIGURE 6 | Microglial activation in acute brain slices.** Example of activation marker stainings on acute slices treated with LPS. **(A)** Immunohistochemical staining for Mac-2/Galectin-3 (red), nuclei were visualized with DAPI (blue; **A1**). Microglia (green) positive (**A1** white square, **A2**) for Mac-2/Galectin-3 (red) and microglia that do not express the marker (white triangle, **A3**) were present in the slice. **(B)** Immunohistochemical staining for iNOS (red), nuclei were visualized with DAPI (blue; **B1**). Microglial cells that were positive (white square **B1,B2**) and negative (white triangle **B1,B3**) for iNOS (red) were observed in the slice after LPS treatment. **(C)** Immunohistochemical staining for IL1β (red), nuclei were visualized with DAPI (blue; **C1**). Microglial cells that were positive (white square **C1,C2**) and negative (white triangle **C1,C3**) for IL1β (red) were observed in the slice after LPS treatment. Examples of the different immunostainings were taken from slices treated for 24 h with 1 μg/ml LPS. Scale bar = 50 μm and for inserts = 20 μm. White squares indicate the microglia positive for the marker and shown in higher magnification **(A–C2)**, white triangles indicate microglia negative for the marker and shown in higher magnification **(A–C3)**. **(D)** Quantification of the expression of three activation markers (Mac-2, iNOS, and IL1β) by microglia in E15.5 brain slices cultured for 24 h with IL-6 (10 ng/ml), poly (I:C) (50 μg/ml), or LPS (1 μg/ml). Kruskal–Wallis test was used for statistical analysis. Number of treated slices in control and IL-6 group $N = 4$; LPS and poly (I:C) group $N = 5$. Number of cryosections for Mac-2/iNOS/IL1β in: saline group $n = 23/23/27$; IL-6 group $n = 22/19/16$; poly (I:C) group $n = 18/25/19$; LPS group $n = 21/21/22$ (all derived from three different embryos). $^{*}p < 0.05$).

offspring cannot be related to the alteration of the activation state of embryonic microglial cells. Our *in vitro* studies indicated that microglia cannot be directly activated by poly (I:C) or IL-6 exposure, contrary to the activation observed upon LPS application.

Several observations suggest that the different infectious triggers induce differences in activation of embryonic microglia. The cytokine IL-6 can cross the placenta barrier *in vivo* when maternal inflammation was induced during mid-gestation (Kohmura et al., 2000; Ashdown et al., 2006; Dahlgren et al., 2006), but it is not clear whether poly (I:C) as well can cross the placenta (Brown and Patterson, 2011). LPS is shown to cross the placenta barrier *in vivo* when maternal inflammation was induced during early gestation (Cai et al., 2000; Kohmura et al., 2000), but this was not the case when LPS was injected at late gestation (Ashdown et al., 2006). Although extrapolation of these results to a poly (I:C) challenge would suggest that embryonic microglia are directly or indirectly activated in response to poly (I:C)-induced MIA at mid gestation, we could not find any evidence for microglia activation in this study. Previously, microglia dysfunction observed after poly (I:C)-induced MIA was only reported in offspring at postnatal and adult age (Juckel et al., 2011; Manitz et al., 2012). In that way it is of interest to compare in parallel the effect of MIA induced by different infectious agents on the embryonic microglia. Studies using single or repeated LPS challenge showed that this leads to microglial activation: in the fetal sheep brain, microglial cell numbers increased as well as the number of activated/amoeboid cells (Mallard et al., 2003; Hutton et al., 2008; Kuypers et al., 2013); in the rat embryo the percentage of microglia expressing iNOS and IL1β was increased (Cunningham et al., 2013) and postnatally a changed immunoreactivity by microglial cells was still observed (Cai et al., 2000); and in mice Iba-1 reactivity was increased during late embryonic and early postnatal stages (Le Belle et al., 2014). In conclusion, the time of injection and the nature of the infectious trigger determine whether an activation of the embryonic microglia does or does not participate to developmental neurological defects observed in MIA offspring (Garay et al., 2012). In addition the microglial response might be species dependent. However, a thorough comparison of the effect of MIA in different species is difficult to make for several reasons. For example, some studies use the mRNA and/or protein expression level of different cytokines as read-out (Garay et al., 2012) while others use immunohistochemistry (Cunningham et al., 2013; Giovanoli et al., 2013) or cell number (Hutton et al., 2008; Manitz et al., 2012) to investigate microglial cell activation after MIA. In addition, the effect of MIA is studied on several different postnatal and adult time points.

Microglial activation in postnatal to adult brains has been found to correlate to neurodevelopmental diseases. An active neuroinflammatory process, with microglial cell activation, was described in the brains of autistic patients (Vargas et al., 2005; Morgan et al., 2010) and of schizophrenic patients (Radewicz et al., 2000; Wierzba-Bobrowicz et al., 2005; Monji et al., 2013). However, it remains unclear if microglia activation participates to neuronal disorders or reflects a normal microglia response to neural dysfunctions. Our results show that poly (I:C)-induced MIA does not lead to activation of embryonic microglia. Yet, they cannot exclude that the embryonic microglial cells become primed, which could result in a more vigorous response to a subsequent inflammatory stimulation in the adult. In some neurodegenerative disease models in rodents (for example Alzheimer's, Parkinson's, and prion disease) the injection of LPS or poly (I:C) leads to a more severe pathology. The combined exposure of a prenatal immune challenge [poly (I:C) at E9] and peripubertal stress (from P30 to 40) resulted in the development of sensorimotor gating deficiencies and led to increased dopamine levels in the adult hippocampus (Giovanoli et al., 2013). At peripubertal age, the combination of both stressors resulted in altered neuroimmune responses, presented as increased microglial cell number and elevated levels of IL1β and TNFα in the hippocampus and prefrontal cortex (Giovanoli et al., 2013). These latter changes were transient, as they were not longer present in the adult. Finally, low doses of poly (I:C) worsened the deficits in pre-pulse inhibition and latent inhibition in 16 week-old mice with mutations in a schizophrenia susceptibility gene but had no effect in wild-type animals, thus indicating that genetic and environmental factors can interact to worsen the schizophrenia-related behavior (Lipina et al., 2013).

MIA induces not only a cytokine response in the maternal unit but also alters several cytokine levels in the placenta and in the fetus (Patterson et al., 2008; Pratt et al., 2013). Under normal conditions cytokines are present in the placental unit where they play an important role in controlling the tissue homeostasis and balance of the different T-cell types present in this structure. In addition, toll-like receptors (TLR), such as TLR-2 and 4, are expressed on human chorionic villi (Jonakait, 2007). Maternal injection with IL-6 is known lead to endocrine changes in the placenta (Hsiao and Patterson, 2011) and injection of a high dose of LPS results in placental inflammation (Girard et al., 2010) and induction of pro-inflammatory cytokines in the amniotic fluid (Gayle et al., 2004). In addition, a direct injection of LPS into the uteroplacental circulation leads to a reaction in the embryonic brain, suggesting the placental unit can contribute to perinatal brain damage through the induction of an inflammatory reaction as a response to infection during pregnancy (Hutton et al., 2008). This complicates elucidating the site where the cytokines act upon to potentially alter brain development since they can act directly on neural progenitors and neurons (Bauer et al., 2007; Deverman and Patterson, 2009). For example, IL-6 and LIF can influence the differentiation of neural progenitor cells (Nakanishi et al., 2007).

These data, in combination with the lack of microglial activation in our MIA study suggests that the acute maternal inflammation induced by poly (I:C) could affect other systems or cell types during embryonic stages. These MIA-induced early abnormalities might result in an altered CNS environment in the offspring that in turn affects the microglial cells at later developmental stages. This hypothesis is supported by the observed changes in neurotransmitter systems in the adult offspring and not in the pre-pubertal period after challenge with poly (I:C) (Manitz et al., 2012). GABAergic gene expression, like GABA receptor subunits and vesicular transporters, can be altered in the adult prefrontal cortex after MIA (Richetto et al., 2013). In addition, serotonin and glutamate signaling was altered (Holloway et al., 2013). These changes were not present at pre-pubertal ages. It is also important to note that, although microglia do not invade the CNS of mouse embryo at E9 (Rigato et al., 2011; Swinnen et al., 2013), poly (I:C) challenge at this gestation stage resulted in the suppression of spatial exploration in the adult (Meyer et al., 2006). This reinforces the idea that embryonic microglia dysfunction, if any, is unlikely to be the main mechanism inducing developmental disorders featuring pathological behavior. Accordingly, poly (I:C) challenge at E9 did not evoke any increase in cytokine mRNA level in the fetal brain (Meyer et al., 2006). Poly (I:C) might induce developmental deficits via direct action on neuronal development. However, our results cannot exclude that poly (I:C) evokes an embryonic microglia priming resulting in an exaggerated response of microglia to homeostatic disturbances at postnatal stages and subsequently makes neuronal dysfunction worse.

## Conclusion

Our findings show that a single and double injection of poly (I:C) is not sufficient to induce changes in fetal microglia activation phenotype during mid or late embryonic development. In addition they suggest a different response of the embryonic brain to MIA depending on the challenge procedure used.

## Author Contributions

Induction of MIA, IL-6 ELISA assays, immunohistochemical stainings, and quantifications were done by SS, SMTS, and NS. Guidance of the study, writing, and correction of the manuscript was performed by all authors.

## Acknowledgments

We want to thank Dorien Deluyker for assistance in blood sampling and Prof. Niels Hellings, Nele Claes, Tess DHaeze, and Marjan Vanheusden for advise concerning the flow cytometry experiments. Financial support for this research was granted by the Impulse financing tUL (transnationale Universiteit Limburg), the UHasselt, the Research Foundation of Flanders (FWO GOA0513), the Association Française contre les myopathies (AFM grant n° 18564) and the Interuniversity Attraction Poles Programme - Belgian State - Belgian Science Policy (IAP-P6/31 and P7/10).

## References

Aarum, J., Sandberg, K., Haeberlein, S. L., and Persson, M. A. (2003). Migration and differentiation of neural precursor cells can be directed by microglia. *Proc. Natl. Acad. Sci. U.S.A.* 100, 15983–15988. doi: 10.1073/pnas.2237050100

Anderson, S. A., Marin, O., Horn, C., Jennings, K., and Rubenstein, J. L. (2001). Distinct cortical migrations from the medial and lateral ganglionic eminences. *Development* 128, 353–363.

Antony, J. M., Paquin, A., Nutt, S. L., Kaplan, D. R., and Miller, F. D. (2011). Endogenous microglia regulate development of embryonic cortical precursor cells. *J. Neurosci. Res.* 89, 286–298. doi: 10.1002/jnr.22533

Ashdown, H., Dumont, Y., Ng, M., Poole, S., Boksa, P., and Luheshi, G. N. (2006). The role of cytokines in mediating effects of prenatal infection on the fetus: implications for schizophrenia. *Mol. Psychiatry* 11, 47–55. doi: 10.1038/sj.mp.4001748

Bauer, S., Kerr, B. J., and Patterson, P. H. (2007). The neuropoietic cytokine family in development, plasticity, disease and injury. *Nat. Rev. Neurosci.* 8, 221–232. doi: 10.1038/nrn2054

Brown, A. S. (2012). Epidemiologic studies of exposure to prenatal infection and risk of schizophrenia and autism. *Dev. Neurobiol.* 72, 1272–1276. doi: 10.1002/dneu.22024

Brown, A. S., and Patterson, P. H. (2011). *The Origins of Schizophrenia*. Columbia: Columbia University Press.

Cai, Z., Pan, Z. L., Pang, Y., Evans, O. B., and Rhodes, P. G. (2000). Cytokine induction in fetal rat brains and brain injury in neonatal rats after maternal lipopolysaccharide administration. *Pediatr. Res.* 47, 64–72. doi: 10.1203/00006450-200001000-00013

Cunningham, C. L., Martinez-Cerdeno, V., and Noctor, S. C. (2013). Microglia regulate the number of neural precursor cells in the developing cerebral cortex. *J. Neurosci.* 33, 4216–4233. doi: 10.1523/JNEUROSCI.3441-12.2013

Dahlgren, J., Samuelsson, A. M., Jansson, T., and Holmang, A. (2006). Interleukin-6 in the maternal circulation reaches the rat fetus in mid-gestation. *Pediatr. Res.* 60, 147–151. doi: 10.1203/01.pdr.0000230026.74139.18

Deverman, B. E., and Patterson, P. H. (2009). Cytokines and CNS development. *Neuron* 64, 61–78. doi: 10.1016/j.neuron.2009.09.002

Dumic, J., Dabelic, S., and Flogel, M. (2006). Galectin-3: an open-ended story. *Biochim. Biophys. Acta* 1760, 616–635. doi: 10.1016/j.bbagen.2005.12.020

Fantin, A., Vieira, J. M., Gestri, G., Denti, L., Schwarz, Q., Prykhozhij, S., et al. (2010). Tissue macrophages act as cellular chaperones for vascular anastomosis downstream of VEGF-mediated endothelial tip cell induction. *Blood* 116, 829–840. doi: 10.1182/blood-2009-12-257832

Fortier, M. E., Luheshi, G. N., and Boksa, P. (2007). Effects of prenatal infection on prepulse inhibition in the rat depend on the nature of the infectious agent and the stage of pregnancy. *Behav. Brain Res.* 181, 270–277. doi: 10.1016/j.bbr.2007.04.016

Garay, P. A., Hsiao, E. Y., Patterson, P. H., and Mcallister, A. K. (2012). Maternal immune activation causes age- and region-specific changes in brain cytokines in offspring throughout development. *Brain Behav. Immun.* 31, 54–68. doi: 10.1016/j.bbi.2012.07.008

Gayle, D. A., Beloosesky, R., Desai, M., Amidi, F., Nunez, S. E., and Ross, M. G. (2004). Maternal LPS induces cytokines in the amniotic fluid and corticotropin releasing hormone in the fetal rat brain. *Am. J. Physiol. Regul. Integr. Comp. Physiol.* 286, R1024–R1029. doi: 10.1152/ajpregu.00664.2003

Ginhoux, F., Greter, M., Leboeuf, M., Nandi, S., See, P., Gokhan, S., et al. (2010). Fate mapping analysis reveals that adult microglia derive from primitive macrophages. *Science* 330, 841–845. doi: 10.1126/science.1194637

Giovanoli, S., Engler, H., Engler, A., Richetto, J., Voget, M., Willi, R., et al. (2013). Stress in puberty unmasks latent neuropathological consequences of prenatal immune activation in mice. *Science* 339, 1095–1099. doi: 10.1126/science.1228261

Girard, S., Tremblay, L., Lepage, M., and Sebire, G. (2010). IL-1 receptor antagonist protects against placental and neurodevelopmental defects induced by maternal inflammation. *J. Immunol.* 184, 3997–4005. doi: 10.4049/jimmunol.0903349

Harvey, L., and Boksa, P. (2012). A stereological comparison of GAD67 and reelin expression in the hippocampal stratum oriens of offspring from two mouse models of maternal inflammation during pregnancy. *Neuropharmacology* 62, 1767–1776. doi: 10.1016/j.neuropharm.2011.11.022

Holloway, T., Moreno, J. L., Umali, A., Rayannavar, V., Hodes, G. E., Russo, S. J., et al. (2013). Prenatal stress induces schizophrenia-like alterations of serotonin 2A and metabotropic glutamate 2 receptors in the adult offspring: role of maternal immune system. *J. Neurosci.* 33, 1088–1098. doi: 10.1523/JNEUROSCI.2331-12.2013

Hsiao, E. Y., and Patterson, P. H. (2011). Activation of the maternal immune system induces endocrine changes in the placenta via IL-6. *Brain Behav. Immun.* 25, 604–615. doi: 10.1016/j.bbi.2010.12.017

Hutton, L. C., Castillo-Melendez, M., Smythe, G. A., and Walker, D. W. (2008). Microglial activation, macrophage infiltration, and evidence of cell death in the fetal brain after uteroplacental administration of lipopolysaccharide in sheep in late gestation. *Am. J. Obstet. Gynecol.* 198, 117.e1–e11. doi: 10.1016/j.ajog.2007.06.035

Jonakait, G. M. (2007). The effects of maternal inflammation on neuronal development: possible mechanisms. *Int. J. Dev. Neurosci.* 25, 415–425. doi: 10.1016/j.ijdevneu.2007.08.017

Jonakait, G. M., Pratt, L., Acevedo, G., and Ni, L. (2011). Microglial regulation of cholinergic differentiation in the basal forebrain. *Dev. Neurobiol.* 72, 857–864. doi: 10.1002/dneu.20969

Juckel, G., Manitz, M. P., Brune, M., Friebe, A., Heneka, M. T., and Wolf, R. J. (2011). Microglial activation in a neuroinflammational animal model of schizophrenia–a pilot study. *Schizophr. Res.* 131, 96–100. doi: 10.1016/j.schres.2011.06.018

Jung, S., Aliberti, J., Graemmel, P., Sunshine, M. J., Kreutzberg, G. W., Sher, A., et al. (2000). Analysis of fractalkine receptor CX(3)CR1 function by targeted deletion and green fluorescent protein reporter gene insertion. *Mol. Cell. Biol.* 20, 4106–4114. doi: 10.1128/MCB.20.11.4106-4114.2000

Kettenmann, H., Hanisch, U. K., Noda, M., and Verkhratsky, A. (2011). Physiology of microglia. *Physiol. Rev.* 91, 461–553. doi: 10.1152/physrev.00011.2010

Kohmura, Y., Kirikae, T., Kirikae, F., Nakano, M., and Sato, I. (2000). Lipopolysaccharide (LPS)-induced intra-uterine fetal death (IUFD) in mice is principally due to maternal cause but not fetal sensitivity to LPS. *Microbiol. Immunol.* 44, 897–904. doi: 10.1111/j.1348-0421.2000.tb02581.x

Krady, J. K., Lin, H. W., Liberto, C. M., Basu, A., Kremlev, S. G., and Levison, S. W. (2008). Ciliary neurotrophic factor and interleukin-6 differentially activate microglia. *J. Neurosci. Res.* 86, 1538–1547. doi: 10.1002/jnr.21620

Kuypers, E., Jellema, R. K., Ophelders, D. R., Dudink, J., Nikiforou, M., Wolfs, T. G., et al. (2013). Effects of intra-amniotic lipopolysaccharide and maternal betamethasone on brain inflammation in fetal sheep. *PLoS ONE* 8:e81644. doi: 10.1371/journal.pone.0081644

Lacroix, S., Chang, L., Rose-John, S., and Tuszynski, M. H. (2002). Delivery of hyper-interleukin-6 to the injured spinal cord increases neutrophil and macrophage infiltration and inhibits axonal growth. *J. Comp. Neurol.* 454, 213–228. doi: 10.1002/cne.10407

Le Belle, J. E., Sperry, J., Ngo, A., Ghochani, Y., Laks, D. R., Lopez-Aranda, M., et al. (2014). Maternal inflammation contributes to brain overgrowth and autism-associated behaviors through altered redox signaling in stem and progenitor cells. *Stem Cell Rep.* 3, 725–734. doi: 10.1016/j.stemcr.2014.09.004

Lee, K. M., Jeon, S. M., and Cho, H. J. (2010). Interleukin-6 induces microglial CX3CR1 expression in the spinal cord after peripheral nerve injury through the activation of p38 MAPK. *Eur. J. Pain* 14, 682. e1–e12. doi: 10.1016/j.ejpain.2009.10.017

Lipina, T. V., Zai, C., Hlousek, D., Roder, J. C., and Wong, A. H. (2013). Maternal immune activation during gestation interacts with Disc1 point mutation to exacerbate schizophrenia-related behaviors in mice. *J. Neurosci.* 33, 7654–7666. doi: 10.1523/JNEUROSCI.0091-13.2013

Lowe, G. C., Luheshi, G. N., and Williams, S. (2008). Maternal infection and fever during late gestation are associated with altered synaptic transmission in the hippocampus of juvenile offspring rats. *Am. J. Physiol. Regul. Integr. Comp. Physiol.* 295, R1563–R1571. doi: 10.1152/ajpregu.90350.2008

Mallard, C., Welin, A. K., Peebles, D., Hagberg, H., and Kjellmer, I. (2003). White matter injury following systemic endotoxemia or asphyxia in the fetal sheep. *Neurochem. Res.* 28, 215–223. doi: 10.1023/A:1022368915400

Manitz, M. P., Esslinger, M., Wachholz, S., Plumper, J., Friebe, A., Juckel, G., et al. (2012). The role of microglia during life span in neuropsychiatric disease - an animal study. *Schizophr. Res.* 143, 221–222. doi: 10.1016/j.schres.2012.10.028

Marin-Teva, J. L., Dusart, I., Colin, C., Gervais, A., Van Rooijen, N., and Mallat, M. (2004). Microglia promote the death of developing Purkinje cells. *Neuron* 41, 535–547. doi: 10.1016/S0896-6273(04)00069-8

Meyer, U., Murray, P. J., Urwyler, A., Yee, B. K., Schedlowski, M., and Feldon, J. (2008). Adult behavioral and pharmacological dysfunctions following disruption of the fetal brain balance between pro-inflammatory and IL-10-mediated anti-inflammatory signaling. *Mol. Psychiatry* 13, 208–221. doi: 10.1038/sj.mp.4002042

Meyer, U., Nyffeler, M., Engler, A., Urwyler, A., Schedlowski, M., Knuesel, I., et al. (2006). The time of prenatal immune challenge determines the specificity of inflammation-mediated brain and behavioral pathology. *J. Neurosci.* 26, 4752–4762. doi: 10.1523/JNEUROSCI.0099-06.2006

Michell-Robinson, M. A., Touil, H., Healy, L. M., Owen, D. R., Durafourt, B. A., Bar-Or, A., et al. (2015). Roles of microglia in brain development, tissue maintenance and repair. *Brain* 138, 1138–1159. doi: 10.1093/brain/awv066

Monji, A., Kato, T. A., Mizoguchi, Y., Horikawa, H., Seki, Y., Kasai, M., et al. (2013). Neuroinflammation in schizophrenia especially focused on the role of microglia. *Prog. Neuropsychopharmacol. Biol. Psychiatry* 42, 115–121. doi: 10.1016/j.pnpbp.2011.12.002

Morgan, J. T., Chana, G., Pardo, C. A., Achim, C., Semendeferi, K., Buckwalter, J., et al. (2010). Microglial activation and increased microglial density observed in the dorsolateral prefrontal cortex in autism. *Biol. Psychiatry* 68, 368–376. doi: 10.1016/j.biopsych.2010.05.024

Nakanishi, M., Niidome, T., Matsuda, S., Akaike, A., Kihara, T., and Sugimoto, H. (2007). Microglia-derived interleukin-6 and leukaemia inhibitory factor promote astrocytic differentiation of neural stem/progenitor cells. *Eur. J. Neurosci.* 25, 649–658. doi: 10.1111/j.1460-9568.2007.05309.x

Paolicelli, R. C., Bolasco, G., Pagani, F., Maggi, L., Scianni, M., Panzanelli, P., et al. (2011). Synaptic pruning by microglia is necessary for normal brain development. *Science* 333, 1456–1458. doi: 10.1126/science.1202529

Patterson, P., Xu, W., Smith, S., Devarman, B. (2008). "Maternal immune activation, cytokines and autism," in *Autism*, ed. A. W. Zimmerman (Totowa, NJ: Humana Press). doi: 10.1007/978-1-60327-489-0_13

Patterson, P. H. (2009). Immune involvement in schizophrenia and autism: etiology, pathology and animal models. *Behav. Brain Res.* 204, 313–321. doi: 10.1016/j.bbr.2008.12.016

Pratt, L., Ni, L., Ponzio, N. M., and Jonakait, G. M. (2013). Maternal inflammation promotes fetal microglial activation and increased cholinergic expression in the fetal basal forebrain: role of interleukin-6. *Pediatr. Res.* 74, 393–401. doi: 10.1038/pr.2013.126

Radewicz, K., Garey, L. J., Gentleman, S. M., and Reynolds, R. (2000). Increase in HLA-DR immunoreactive microglia in frontal and temporal cortex of chronic schizophrenics. *J. Neuropathol. Exp. Neurol.* 59, 137–150.

Ratnayake, U., Quinn, T. A., Castillo-Melendez, M., Dickinson, H., and Walker, D. W. (2012). Behaviour and hippocampus-specific changes in spiny mouse neonates after treatment of the mother with the viral-mimetic Poly I:C at mid-pregnancy. *Brain Behav. Immun.* 26, 1288–1299. doi: 10.1016/j.bbi.2012.08.011

Richetto, J., Calabrese, F., Riva, M. A., and Meyer, U. (2013). Prenatal immune activation induces maturation-dependent alterations in the prefrontal GABAergic transcriptome. *Schizophr. Bull.* 40, 351–361. doi: 10.1093/schbul/sbs195

Rigato, C., Buckinx, R., Le-Corronc, H., Rigo, J. M., and Legendre, P. (2011). Pattern of invasion of the embryonic mouse spinal cord by microglial cells at the time of the onset of functional neuronal networks. *Glia* 59, 675–695. doi: 10.1002/glia.21140

Rotshenker, S. (2009). The role of Galectin-3/MAC-2 in the activation of the innate-immune function of phagocytosis in microglia in injury and disease. *J. Mol. Neurosci.* 39, 99–103. doi: 10.1007/s12031-009-9186-7

Rymo, S. F., Gerhardt, H., Wolfhagen Sand, F., Lang, R., Uv, A., and Betsholtz, C. (2011). A two-way communication between microglial cells and angiogenic sprouts regulates angiogenesis in aortic ring cultures. *PLoS ONE* 6:e15846. doi: 10.1371/journal.pone.0015846

Samuelsson, A. M., Jennische, E., Hansson, H. A., and Holmang, A. (2006). Prenatal exposure to interleukin-6 results in inflammatory neurodegeneration in hippocampus with NMDA/GABA(A) dysregulation and impaired spatial learning. *Am. J. Physiol. Regul. Integr. Comp. Physiol.* 290, R1345–R1356. doi: 10.1152/ajpregu.00268.2005

Schafer, D. P., Lehrman, E. K., Kautzman, A. G., Koyama, R., Mardinly, A. R., Yamasaki, R., et al. (2012). Microglia sculpt postnatal neural circuits in an activity and complement-dependent manner. *Neuron* 74, 691–705. doi: 10.1016/j.neuron.2012.03.026

Sedel, F., Bechade, C., Vyas, S., and Triller, A. (2004). Macrophage-derived tumor necrosis factor alpha, an early developmental signal for motoneuron death. *J. Neurosci.* 24, 2236–2246. doi: 10.1523/JNEUROSCI.4464-03.2004

Shi, L., Fatemi, S. H., Sidwell, R. W., and Patterson, P. H. (2003). Maternal influenza infection causes marked behavioral and pharmacological changes in the offspring. *J. Neurosci.* 23, 297–302.

Shi, L., Smith, S. E., Malkova, N., Tse, D., Su, Y., and Patterson, P. H. (2009). Activation of the maternal immune system alters cerebellar development in the offspring. *Brain Behav. Immun.* 23, 116–123. doi: 10.1016/j.bbi.2008.07.012

Smith, S. E., Li, J., Garbett, K., Mirnics, K., and Patterson, P. H. (2007). Maternal immune activation alters fetal brain development through interleukin-6. *J. Neurosci.* 27, 10695–10702. doi: 10.1523/JNEUROSCI.2178-07.2007

Squarzoni, P., Oller, G., Hoeffel, G., Pont-Lezica, L., Rostaing, P., Low, D., et al. (2014). Microglia modulate wiring of the embryonic forebrain. *Cell Rep.* 8, 1271–1279. doi: 10.1016/j.celrep.2014.07.042

Streit, W. J., Hurley, S. D., Mcgraw, T. S., and Semple-Rowland, S. L. (2000). Comparative evaluation of cytokine profiles and reactive gliosis supports a critical role for interleukin-6 in neuron-glia signaling during regeneration. *J. Neurosci. Res.* 61, 10–20. doi: 10.1002/1097-4547(20000701)61:1<10::AID-JNR2>3.0.CO;2-E

Swinnen, N., Smolders, S., Avila, A., Notelaers, K., Paesen, R., Ameloot, M., et al. (2013). Complex invasion pattern of the cerebral cortex bymicroglial cells during development of the mouse embryo. *Glia* 61, 150–163. doi: 10.1002/glia.22421

Tan, S. S., Kalloniatis, M., Sturm, K., Tam, P. P., Reese, B. E., and Faulkner-Jones, B. (1998). Separate progenitors for radial and tangential cell dispersion during development of the cerebral neocortex. *Neuron* 21, 295–304. doi: 10.1016/S0896-6273(00)80539-5

Tremblay, M. E., Lowery, R. L., and Majewska, A. K. (2010). Microglial interactions with synapses are modulated by visual experience. *PLoS Biol.* 8:e1000527. doi: 10.1371/journal.pbio.1000527

Vargas, D. L., Nascimbene, C., Krishnan, C., Zimmerman, A. W., and Pardo, C. A. (2005). Neuroglial activation and neuroinflammation in the brain of patients with autism. *Ann. Neurol.* 57, 67–81. doi: 10.1002/ana.20315

Wakselman, S., Bechade, C., Roumier, A., Bernard, D., Triller, A., and Bessis, A. (2008). Developmental neuronal death in hippocampus requires the microglial CD11b integrin and DAP12 immunoreceptor. *J. Neurosci.* 28, 8138–8143. doi: 10.1523/JNEUROSCI.1006-08.2008

Wierzba-Bobrowicz, T., Lewandowska, E., Lechowicz, W., Stepien, T., and Pasennik, E. (2005). Quantitative analysis of activated microglia, ramified and damage of processes in the frontal and temporal lobes of chronic schizophrenics. *Folia Neuropathol.* 43, 81–89.

Zhan, Y., Paolicelli, R. C., Sforazzini, F., Weinhard, L., Bolasco, G., Pagani, F., et al. (2014). Deficient neuron-microglia signaling results in impaired functional brain connectivity and social behavior. *Nat. Neurosci.* 17, 400–406. doi: 10.1038/nn.3641

4

# Oligodendrocyte and Interneuron Density in Hippocampal Subfields in Schizophrenia and Association of Oligodendrocyte Number with Cognitive Deficits

*Peter Falkai*[1†], *Johann Steiner*[2†], *Berend Malchow*[1], *Jawid Shariati*[3], *Andreas Knaus*[3], *Hans-Gert Bernstein*[2], *Thomas Schneider-Axmann*[1], *Theo Kraus*[4], *Alkomiet Hasan*[1], *Bernhard Bogerts*[2] and *Andrea Schmitt*[1,5]*

[1] Department of Psychiatry and Psychotherapy, Ludwig Maximilians-University Munich, Munich, Germany, [2] Department of Psychiatry and Psychotherapy, University of Magdeburg, Magdeburg, Germany, [3] Department of Psychiatry and Psychotherapy, University of Göttingen, Göttingen, Germany, [4] Center for Neuropathology and Prion Research (ZNP), Ludwig Maximilians-University Munich, Munich, Germany, [5] Laboratory of Neuroscience (LIM27), Institute of Psychiatry, University of São Paulo, São Paulo, Brazil

***Correspondence:***
*Andrea Schmitt*
*andrea.schmitt@med.uni-muenchen.de*

*† These authors have contributed equally to this work.*

In schizophrenia, previous stereological post-mortem investigations of anterior, posterior, and total hippocampal subfields showed no alterations in total neuron number but did show decreased oligodendrocyte numbers in CA4, an area that corresponds to the polymorph layer of the dentate gyrus (DG). However, these investigations identified oligodendrocytes only on the basis of morphological criteria in Nissl staining and did not assess alterations of interneurons with immunohistochemical markers. Moreover, the association of findings in the posterior hippocampus with cognitive deficits remains unknown. On the basis of the available clinical records, we compared patients with definite and possible cognitive dysfunction; nine patients had evidence in their records of either definite ($n$ = 4) or possible ($n$ = 5) cognitive dysfunction. Additionally, we assessed the density of two oligodendrocyte subpopulations immunostained by the oligodendrocyte transcription factors Olig1 and Olig2 and of interneurons immunolabeled by parvalbumin. We investigated posterior hippocampal subregions in the post-mortem brains of the same schizophrenia patients (SZ; $n$ = 10) and healthy controls ($n$ = 10) we examined in our previously published stereological studies. Our stereological studies found that patients with definite cognitive deficits had decreased total/Nissl-stained oligodendrocyte numbers in the left ($p$ = 0.014) and right ($p$ = 0.050) CA4, left CA2/3 ($p$ = 0.050), left CA1 ($p$ = 0.027), and left ($p$ = 0.050) and right ($p$ = 0.014) subiculum of the anterior part of the hippocampus compared to patients with possible cognitive deficits. In the present study, we found no significant influence of definite cognitive deficits in the posterior part of the hippocampus, whereas in the entire hippocampus SZ with definite cognitive deficits showed decreased oligodendrocyte numbers in the left ($p$ = 0.050) and right ($p$ = 0.050) DG and left CA2/3 ($p$ = 0.050). We did not find significant differences in Olig1-, Olig2-, or parvalbumin-positive cell density between SZ and controls in any of the subregions of the posterior hippocampus.

Based on the results from our stereological study we hypothesize that a decreased number of oligodendrocytes in the anterior and entire hippocampus may be involved in cognitive deficits by impairing the connectivity of this structure in schizophrenia. In the posterior hippocampus, we could not replicate previously reported findings of decreased interneurons from the entire hippocampus.

**Keywords: schizophrenia, hippocampus, oligodendrocytes, interneurons, cognition, immunohistochemistry, post-mortem**

## INTRODUCTION

Schizophrenia has an unfavorable outcome in more than half of all patients and is linked to social and vocational disability (an der Heiden and Häfner, 2011). This unfavorable outcome is mainly due to negative symptoms, including cognitive dysfunction. While positive symptoms can be treated well by antipsychotics when given according to current guidelines (Hasan et al., 2012), effective treatment options for negative symptoms are still lacking. In this context, a recent meta-analysis revealed that cognitive dysfunction and residual negative symptoms are widely resistant to any known treatment (Fusar-Poli et al., 2015). Another meta-analysis, however, showed that antipsychotics have at least a moderate effect on cognitive impairments in schizophrenia (Desamericq et al., 2014). Cognitive impairments in schizophrenia involve deficits in episodic and working memory, for example, as well as in attention, processing speed, and problem solving (Nuechterlein et al., 2004; Falkai et al., 2011).

A cognitive cluster representing diminished verbal memory is related to decreased volume of the hippocampus (Geisler et al., 2015). Interestingly, in schizophrenia these verbal memory deficits have been found to be correlated with a loss of hippocampal volume, especially on the left side (Hasan et al., 2014). Recent examination of structural magnetic resonance imaging-based alterations in hippocampal subfields revealed decreased volumes of the cornu ammonis (CA) CA4/dentate gyrus (DG), CA2/3, and subiculum in schizophrenia patients (SZ) compared to healthy controls (Haukvik et al., 2015), but underlying alterations on the cellular level and their relationship to cognitive deficits remain unknown.

Recently, our group investigated the cytoarchitecture of the posterior, anterior, and entire hippocampus in post-mortem schizophrenia brains by evaluating neuronal, oligodendrocyte, and astrocyte numbers with design-based stereological estimation. In the posterior area, we found a significant reduction of oligodendrocyte numbers in the left and right CA4 regions (Schmitt et al., 2009). In the anterior part, we found a decreased number of oligodendrocytes in the left CA4, fewer neurons in the left DG, and smaller volumes of both the left CA4 and DG in SZ compared to healthy controls. In the entire hippocampus, both decreased oligodendrocyte numbers in the left CA4 and reduced volume remained significant (Falkai et al., 2016). In the Nissl-stained brain sections, however, we identified oligodendrocytes on the basis of morphological criteria only and did not distinguish between pyramidal neurons and interneurons. This approach may be relevant to our results, because in a stereological study, somatostatin-stained interneurons have been reported to be reduced in CA4, CA2/3, and CA1 and parvalbumin-stained interneurons in CA4 and CA1, although the total number of neurons was unchanged (Konradi et al., 2011). Moreover, the clinical consequence of our findings and the involvement of a deficit of premature or mature oligodendrocytes remains unknown. Oligodendrocytes are involved in myelination and ensure proper connectivity in neuronal networks. In SZ, deficits in myelination and brain connectivity have been found (Cassoli et al., 2015; Saia-Cereda et al., 2015), which are hypothesized to be related to symptoms of the disease and cognitive deficits (Mitterauer, 2011). In fact, in diffusion tensor imaging (DTI) studies verbal memory has been reported to be associated with decreased left-side dominant fractional anisotropy in the hippocampus and fornix of SZ (Lim et al., 2006; Nestor et al., 2007).

The aim of the present study was to address the question whether the findings of this study and those of our previous stereological studies in the anterior, posterior, and entire hippocampus (Schmitt et al., 2009; Falkai et al., 2016) can be connected to simple measures of cognitive dysfunction in this illness. Furthermore, we investigated whether the density of more premature oligodendrocytes, stained by the oligodendrocyte transcription factors Olig1, or of more mature oligodendrocytes stained by Olig2 respectively, or of parvalbumin-positive interneurons is altered in the posterior part of the hippocampus in the same post-mortem schizophrenia brains as previously investigated by design-based stereology in histologically stained sections (Schmitt et al., 2009; Falkai et al., 2016).

## MATERIALS AND METHODS

### Participant Characteristics

Post-mortem brains were obtained from the Düsseldorf Brain Collection (Bogerts et al., 1990) and the use of post-mortem material has been approved by the Ethics Committee of University of Magdeburg. Patients fulfilled ICD-9 criteria for schizophrenia and had been treated with typical antipsychotics for most of their illness. Exclusion criteria were alcohol or drug abuse and other neuropsychiatric disorders. We investigated the same sample as in our previously published stereological study of the posterior hippocampus in schizophrenia (Schmitt et al., 2009). Briefly, we assessed 10 patients with schizophrenia (mean [SD] age 55.1 [7.7] years; five males, five females;

**TABLE 1 | Characteristics of healthy controls and schizophrenia patients (SZ) and healthy controls investigated in the present study of the posterior hippocampus.**

| **Schizophrenia patients** | | | | | | | |
|---|---|---|---|---|---|---|---|
| No. | S | A | D | C | CPE | Cause of death | Last neuroleptic treatment |
| P3 | M | 48 | 18 | 2 | 3500 | Cardiac failure | Haloperidol, Haldoperidol Decanoate, Zuclopenthixol |
| P9 | M | 65 | 26 | 1 | 540 | Pulmonary insufficiency | Haloperidol, Fluphenazine |
| P10 | M | 46 | 18 | 1 | 250 | Pulmonary embolism | Clozapine, Levomepromazine |
| P14 | M | 51 | 28 | 2 | 350 | Ileus | Perphenazine, Promethazine |
| P20 | M | 47 | 23 | 2 | 640 | Cardiac arrest | Fluphenazine, Benperidol, Levomepromazine |
| P7 | F | 66 | 30 | 1 | 800 | Myocardial infarction | Benperidole, Fluphenazine |
| P12 | F | 53 | 20 | 2 | 2495 | Myocardial infarction | Perphenazine, Pericyazine |
| P13 | F | 60 | 16 | 1 | 0 | Pneumonia | Fluphenazine |
| P18 | F | 63 | 23 | 1 | 988 | Suicide | Haloperidol |
| P23 | F | 52 | 28 | n.a. | n.a. | Suicide by drowning | n.a. |
| **Healthy controls** | | | | | | | |
| N29 | M | 47 | | | | Coronary thrombosis | |
| N20 | M | 64 | | | | Aneurysm rupture | |
| N3 | M | 56 | | | | Pancreatitis | |
| N10 | M | 50 | | | | Myocardial infarction | |
| N23 | M | 38 | | | | Myocardial infarction | |
| N34 | F | 64 | | | | Peritonitis | |
| N22 | F | 47 | | | | Renal failure | |
| N27 | F | 50 | | | | Aneurysm rupture | |
| N21 | F | 52 | | | | Ovarial carcinoma | |
| N19 | F | 33 | | | | Coronary thrombosis | |

*S = Gender (M = male, F = female), A = age at death (years), D = duration of disease, C = Cognitive deficits: 1 = possible cognitive deficits, 2 = definite cognitive deficits, CPE = dose of neuroleptics (mg/day) in chlorpromazine equivalents, n.a.= no data available.*

mean [SD] post-mortem interval [PMI] 42.0 [17.2] h; mean [SD] disease duration: 23.0 [4.9] years) and 10 age- and gender-matched healthy controls without a history of a neuropsychiatric disorder, alcohol or drug abuse, dementia, neurological illness, trauma, or chronic terminal disease (mean [SD] age 50.2 [10.1] years; 5 males, 5 females; mean [SD] PMI 36.8 [20.3] h; **Table 1**). The mean daily dose of neuroleptic treatment during the last 90 days had been documented and calculated in chlorpromazine equivalents (CPE; Rey et al., 1989). Brains were uniformly fixed in toto in 10% phosphate buffered paraformaldehyde for about 7 months (pH 7.0, $t$ = 15–20°C). Then, the frontal and occipital parts of the brain were separated from the middle part, which was located between the lateral geniculate nucleus and the splenium of the corpus callosum, i.e., containing the anterior and posterior hippocampus. From this middle part, 20 μm coronal sections containing both hemispheres were cut on a Polycut S Leica microtome. The thickness of each section was determined by focusing through the section and subtracting the z-axis coordinate of the lower from that of the upper surface by the microcator, part of the Olympus microscope. The mean (SD) section thickness after histological procedure was 18.7 (1.1) μm.

Within the hippocampus, we analyzed two sections per brain, taken from the posterior part of the hippocampal formation, which spanned from the lateral geniculate nucleus to the level of the splenium of the corpus callosum. The subregions to be investigated separately were the CA1, CA2/3, and CA4 (deep polymorph layer of the DG), and subiculum. CA2 and CA3 were lumped together as described in the literature because these small regions are difficult to separate at the microscopic level (Schmitt et al., 2009).

## Immunohistochemistry

Immunohistochemical staining was prepared as described previously (Mosebach et al., 2013). Briefly, sections were deparaffinized, and antigen demasking was performed by boiling the sections for 4 min in 10 mM citrate buffer (pH 6.0). Sections were then preincubated with 1.5% $H_2O_2$ for 10 min to block endogenous peroxidase activity. Non-specific binding sites were blocked with 10% normal goat serum for 60 min and washings with Phosphate buffered saline (PBS) buffer. Monoclonal mouse anti-Olig1 antibody (R&D Systems, Abingdon, UK, dilution 1:50) or rabbit anti-Olig2 antibody (Millipore/Merck Darmstadt, Germany, dilution 1:150) was applied for 72 h at 4°C for immunostaining of Olig1- or Olig2-positive oligodendrocytes, respectively. Then, the streptavidin-biotin technique was used to incubate sections with a biotinylated anti-mouse (GE Healthcare, Freiburg, Germany, dilution 1:100) or anti-rabbit (DakoCyomation, Glostrup, Denmark, dilution: 1:100) antibody, respectively. Chromogen 3,3'-diaminobenzidine (DAB) and ammonium nickel sulfate were used to visualize the reaction product. Parvalbumin-positive interneurons were immunolabeled under the same conditions with a monoclonal antibody to the protein (Sigma, Taufkirchen, Germany; dilution 1:500) and an anti-mouse peroxidase secondary antibody (Biozol, Germany, dilution 1:50; Bernstein et al., 2007).

## Evaluation of Olig1-, Olig2- and Parvalbumin-Stained Sections

A rater blinded to diagnosis analyzed the regions of interest in both hemispheres at 400× magnification by using a stereological workstation consisting of a modified light microscope (BX50;

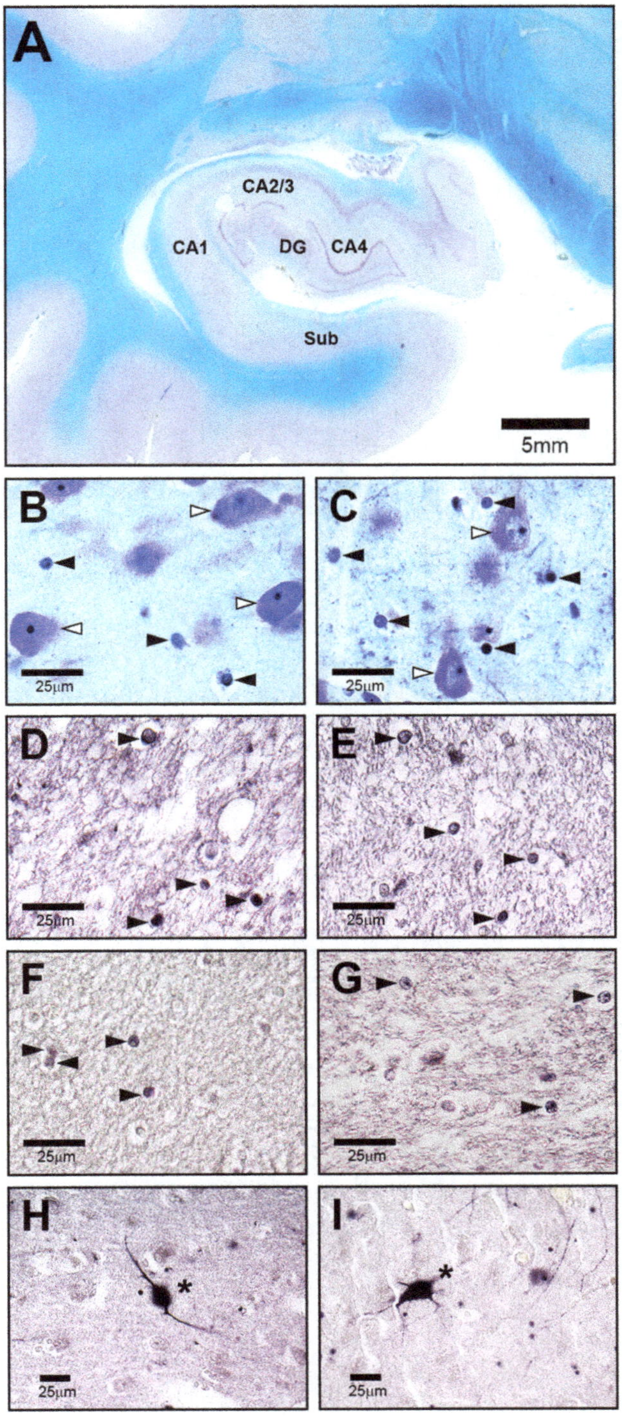


**FIGURE 1 | Representative high-power photomicrographs of 20 µm-thick coronal sections from a schizophrenia patient (SZ) (C,E,G,I) and a healthy control (A,B,D,F,H). (A)** Overview of subregions including cornu ammonis (CA) 1, 2–3, 4, dentate gyrus (DG) and subiculum (Sub) in a Nissl and myelin stained section. The following sections show CA4. **(B,C)** White arrowheads indicate neurons, black arrowheads point to oligodendrocytes. **(D,E)** Olig1 immunostained stained section with black arrowheads showing oligodendrocytes. **(F,G)** Olig2 immunolabeled section with black arrowheads showing oligodendrocytes. **(H,I)** Parvalbumin stained section with asterisks pointing to immunopositive neurons.

Olympus, Tokyo, Japan), Olympus Uplan Apo objectives (1.5×, 20×, 50×, 100× oil), motorized specimen stage for automatic sampling, electronic microcator, CCD color video camera, PC with frame grabber board, stereology software (Stereoinvestigator, MBF Bioscience Williston, VT, USA), and 17" monitor. Boundaries of hippocampal subfields were traced on video images displayed on the computer screen, and volumes were calculated in both sections. The numerical cell density of Olig1-, Olig2-, and parvalbumin-stained cells (**Figure 1**) was measured in the subregions by using the optional dissector and expressed as cells/mm$^3$. Because the actual mean (SD) thickness of the sections was 18.7 (1.1) µm, two well-defined optical planes within the sections were used (distance 16 µm between the upper and lower guard zones), and all stained cells that came into focus while passing from the upper to the lower optical plane (plane of the dissector) were counted. The individual volume shrinkage factors (VSF) were calculated from the measured linear shrinkage factor (LSF) with the following formula: VSF = (LSF) (Mosebach et al., 2013). The intra-class correlation coefficients for intra-rater reliability were 0.81 for Olig1, 0.95 for Olig2, and 0.83 for the parvalbumin-stained cells.

## Evaluation of Cognitive Deficits in Schizophrenia Patients (SZ)

In our correlation analysis, we used results from Nissl-stained serial section of the anterior and posterior part of the hippocampus (Schmitt et al., 2009; Falkai et al., 2016). We searched for a surrogate marker of cognitive dysfunction in the group of SZ. Therefore, an independent psychiatrist (J. Steiner) who was blind to the histological results evaluated the medical records and used a three-point semi-quantitative scale to rate patients' level of cognitive deficits (0 = no cognitive deficits, 1 = possible cognitive deficits, 2 = definite cognitive deficits). The rater searched for descriptions of deficits in the domains of attention, verbal learning, working memory, and executive functions and for indications of a decrease in cognitive performance or increase in residual symptoms over time. Patients who clearly had any of these symptoms were defined as having definite cognitive deficits; and those with marginal or borderline symptoms, possible cognitive deficits. Nine patients had either definite ($n = 4$) or possible ($n = 5$) deficits (**Table 1**); no records were available for one patient. It was not possible to formalize this kind of classification by scales (Ortakov et al., 1999).

## Statistical Analysis

The significance level was $\alpha = 0.05$, and all tests were two-tailed. Statistical analyses were performed with IBM SPSS statistics 22.

In the first analysis, outcome measures were densities from immunohistochemical Olig1, Olig2, and parvalbumin stainings in the hippocampal subfields CA1, CA2/3, CA4, and the subiculum. The independent factor was diagnostic group (SZ, controls). Because Levene's test detected significant variance inhomogeneities between the groups, we used non-parametric Mann-Whitney U tests to analyze diagnostic group differences.

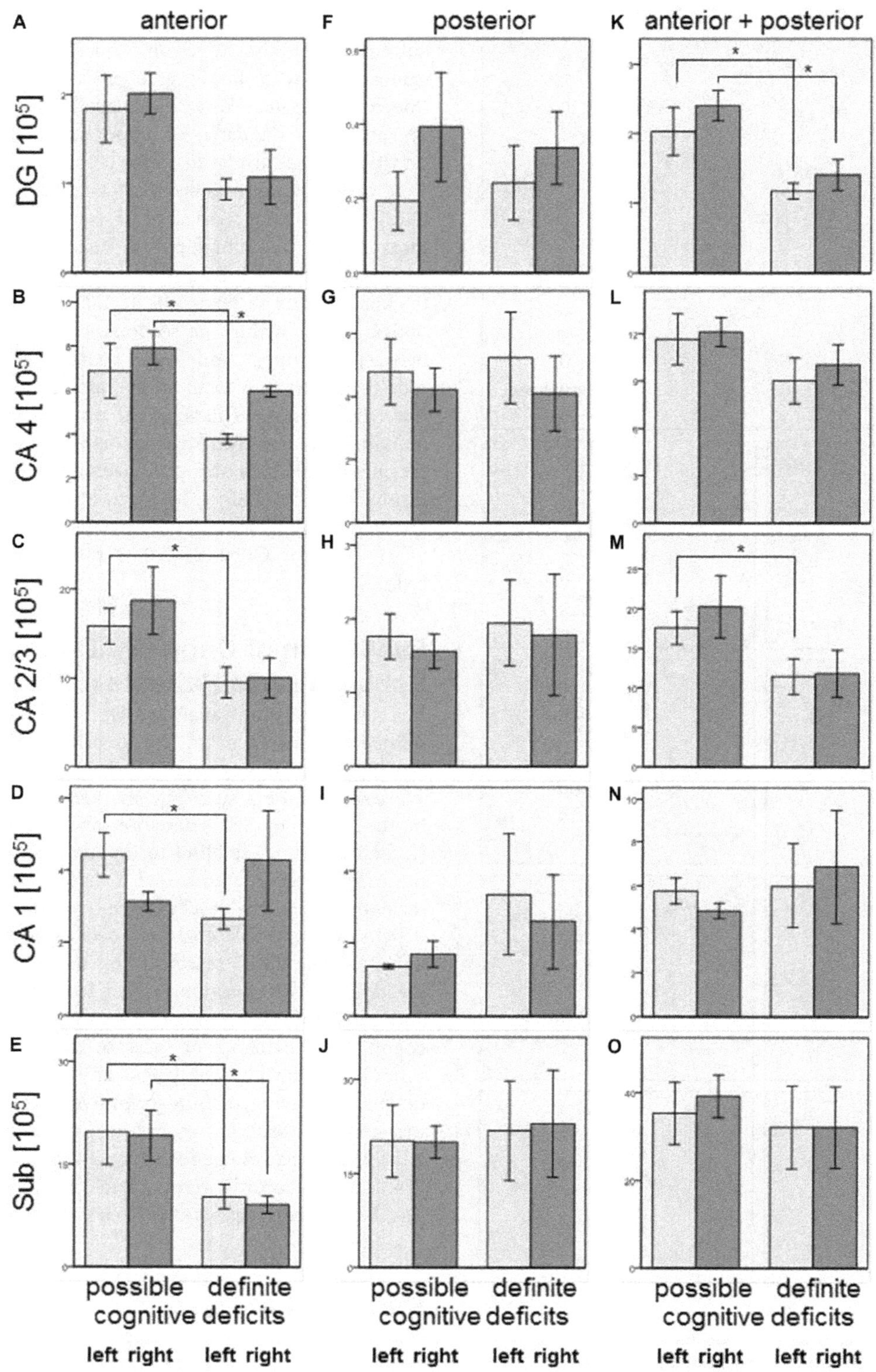


**FIGURE 2 | Left column (A–E): Number of oligodendrocytes [$\times 10^5$] in SZ with definite and possible cognitive deficits in anterior hippocampus: DG (DG, (A)), CA4 (B), CA2/3 (C), CA1 (D), and subiculum (Sub, (E)).** Columns represent mean oligodendrocyte number, and bars represent standard error of the mean. Light gray columns: left hemisphere; dark gray columns: right hemisphere. Decreased oligodendrocyte number in SZ with definite cognitive deficits were observed in CA4 (left and right), CA2/3 (left), CA1 (left), and subiculum (left and right). Middle column **(F–J)**: Number of oligodendrocytes [$\times 10^5$] in SZ with definite and possible cognitive deficits in posterior hippocampus: DG **(F)**, CA4 **(G)**, CA2/3 **(H)**, CA1 **(I)**, and Sub **(J)**. Columns represent mean oligodendrocyte number,

(*Continued*)

**FIGURE 2 | Continued**
and bars represent standard error of the mean. Light gray columns: left hemisphere; dark gray columns: right hemisphere. No significant differences were found between patients with definite and possible cognitive deficits. Right column **(K–O)**: Number of oligodendrocytes [$\times 10^5$] in SZ with definite and possible cognitive deficits in entire (anterior + posterior) hippocampus: DG, **(K)**, CA4 **(L)**, CA2/3 **(M)**, CA1 **(N)**, and Sub **(O)**. Columns represent mean oligodendrocyte number, and bars represent standard error of the mean. Light gray columns: left hemisphere; dark gray columns: right hemisphere. Decreased oligodendrocyte numbers in SZ with definite cognitive deficits were observed in DG (left and right) and CA2/3 (left). $^*p < 0.05$.

Cell densities were correlated with age at death, PMI, dose of neuroleptic treatment in CPE and disease duration by means of Spearman correlations for the total sample and separately for SZ and controls.

In addition to densities of oligodendrocytes and interneurons, outcome measures of the second analysis were the number of oligodendrocytes and neurons, estimated stereologically, and the structure volumes in the subfields (CA1, CA2/3, CA4, DG, and subiculum) of the anterior, posterior, and entire hippocampus of SZ, as published in Falkai et al. (2016). The independent factor was cognitive deficits (definite or possible). Means, standard deviations, and standard errors of the mean were calculated for all outcome measures for left and right hemispheres separately. We applied Levene's test of variance homogeneity to compare the two groups with different degrees of cognitive deficits. Because this test found significant variance inhomogeneities for several variables, patients with definite and possible deficits were compared with non-parametric Mann-Whitney U tests.

For this explorative study with small group sizes, especially as regards the analysis of the influence of cognitive deficits on cell numbers or densities within the group of SZ, the results are presented without error probability correction. If a Bonferroni adjustment of the type I error probability had been applied, no significant differences would remain between SZ and controls. However, if the error probability was adjusted the power of detecting existing mean differences would be too low.

## RESULTS

### Impact of Cognitive Deficits on Total Oligodendrocyte Numbers (Nissl Staining)

Our simple classification of cognitive deficits indicated that patients with a definite cognitive dysfunction had a more pronounced reduction of oligodendrocyte total cell numbers (combined staining with cresyl violet (Nissl) and myelin (luxol fast blue), Schmitt et al., 2009; Falkai et al., 2016) than patients with only a possible cognitive deficit. In the anterior hippocampus, SZ patients with definite cognitive deficits showed significantly lower numbers of oligodendrocytes in the left CA1 (−40%, $p$ = 0.027), left CA2/3 (−40%, $p$ = 0.050), left (−45%, $p$ = 0.014) and right (−25%, $p$ = 0.050) CA4, and left (−48%, $p$ = 0.050) and right (−52%, $p$ = 0.014) subiculum. In the posterior part of the hippocampus, definite cognitive deficits appeared to have no significant influence, while in the entire hippocampus SZ patients with definite cognitive deficits showed decreased oligodendrocyte numbers in the left (−42%, $p$ = 0.050) and right (−41%, $p$ = 0.050) DG and left CA2/3 (−35%, $p$ = 0.050; **Figure 2**). In patients with definite cognitive dysfunction, the number of neurons was not significantly lower in the DG of the anterior, posterior, or entire hippocampus (**Figure 3**). However, it has to be noted that patients with definite cognitive deficits had received a higher daily dose of neuroleptics during the last 90 days expressed in CPE compared to patients with only a possible cognitive deficit (1906 ± 1333 vs. 388 ± 302 mg/day, $p$ = 0.032).

### Densities of Olig1-, Olig2- and Parvalbumin-Positive Cells

We did not find significant differences between SZ and controls in any of the subregions of the posterior hippocampus in the number of Olig1-, Olig2-, or parvalbumin-positive cells. However, in the SZ we found trends towards a decrease in Olig1-positive oligodendrocytes in the right CA2/3 (−57%, $p$ = 0.070), right CA4 (−54%, $p$ = 0.096), and right subiculum (−39%, $p$ = 0.082). The SZ and controls showed no significant differences with respect to the mean densities of Olig2-positive oligodendrocytes in the investigated subregions of the posterior part of the hippocampus, but the density of parvalbumin-stained interneurons was increased in the left CA1 region in the SZ (+124%, $p$ = 0.033) and showed a trend towards an increase in the right CA4 (+175%, $p$ = 0.067; see **Figure 4**).

In the total sample of SZ and healthy controls, females showed higher Olig1 cell densities than males in the left (+138%, $p$ = 0.009) and right (+126%, $p$ = 0.005) CA1, left CA2/3 (+201%, $p$ = 0.008), and left CA4 (+47%, $p$ = 0.026) subregions. With respect to Olig2-stained cells, females had increased cell densities in the left (+54%, $p$ = 0.011) and right (+52%, $p$ = 0.004) CA1, left (+61%, $p$ = 0.007) and right (+69%, $p$ = 0.006) CA2/3, and left subiculum (+33%, $p$ = 0.007). Furthermore, females had an increased density of parvalbumin-positive interneurons compared to males in the left (+192%, $p$ = 0.016) and right (+92%, $p$ = 0.032) CA2/3, and left subiculum (+169%, $p$ = 0.033; see **Figure 5**).

In healthy controls, age correlated negatively with the density of Olig1-positive cells in the left CA2/3 (rho = −0.743, $p$ = 0.035) and right CA4 (rho = −0.671, $p$ = 0.034), whereas in SZ no significant correlations between age and cell densities were observed. In controls, the PMI correlated with oligodendrocyte density (Olig1, CA1 right: rho = 0.715, $p$ = 0.020, CA2/3 left: rho = 0.749, $p$ = 0.033), but not with Olig2 or interneuron density. No significant correlations of Olig1-, Olig2- or interneuron densities with disease duration were observed. The Olig2 density correlated with CPE in the right subiculum (rho = 0.833, $p$ = 0.010), but no other correlations with dose of neuroleptic treatment had been found (**Figure 6**).

Furthermore, the densities of Olig1-, Olig2-, and parvalbumin-stained cells did not differ between patients

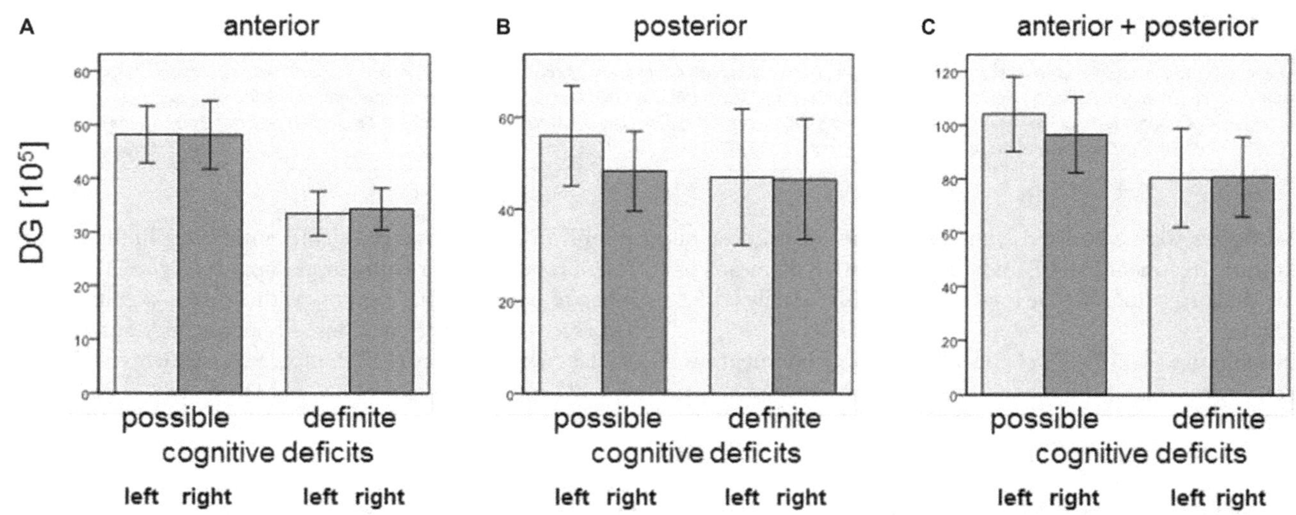


**FIGURE 3 | Number of neurons [$\times 10^5$] in (A) anterior, (B) posterior, and (C) entire DG in SZ patients with definite and possible cognitive deficits.** Columns represent means, and bars represent standard error of the mean.

with definite and possible cognitive deficits in any of these areas of the posterior hippocampus.

## DISCUSSION

Our recent design-based stereology investigation of the posterior part of the hippocampus in post-mortem schizophrenia brains revealed a significant bilateral reduction of oligodendrocytes in the left and right CA4 regions (Schmitt et al., 2009). In a subsequent study, we evaluated the anterior part of the hippocampus in the same cases and calculated results for the entire hippocampus. This study replicated the reduction of oligodendrocyte numbers, but only for the left CA4 region in schizophrenia (Falkai et al., 2016). Noteworthy is that no other histological components, including neurons and astroglia, showed alterations in the anterior or posterior portion of the hippocampus in schizophrenia, which is in contrast to the reduction of interneurons in schizophrenia found in a stereological study of the hippocampus and published also in reviews (Konradi et al., 2011; Heckers and Konradi, 2015). However, the study by Konradi et al. (2011) provided stereological data. Also, our evaluation of cell densities may have more methodological bias based on effects of tissue shrinkage which is caused by fixation or staining procedures.

To connect the reduction of oligodendrocytes with clinical outcome, we used the available case notes to subdivide the SZ into those with definite or possible cognitive dysfunction. Nine of the 10 patients showed either definite or possible deficits. Of interest is that on the basis of our stereological data we found a relation between definite cognitive dysfunction and reduced oligodendrocytes in several subregions of the anterior and entire hippocampus, which might point to a central role of oligodendrocytes in cognitive dysfunction in schizophrenia. Oligodendrocytes are important in myelination and are an integral part of the connectome, which allows brain regions to communicate with each other efficiently and quickly (Cassoli et al., 2015). Therefore, we hypothesize that a reduction in oligodendrocytes in the hippocampus might well be an underlying psycho-architectural substrate of cognitive dysfunction in schizophrenia. The fornix, which comprises the white matter tract of the hippocampus, shows decreased fractional anisotropy in first-episode and chronic SZ (Rametti et al., 2009; Abdul-Rahman et al., 2011; Kunimatsu et al., 2012; Fitzsimmons et al., 2014), and these alterations in the fornix correlate with impairment in declarative-episodic memory (Kuroki et al., 2006; Lim et al., 2006). Moreover, oligodendrocyte-related gene variants are related to white matter tract integrity and cognitive performance in SZ and healthy controls (Voineskos et al., 2013). Our results and those findings from magnetic resonance imaging studies support the hypothesis of structural and functional disconnectivity in a hippocampal-medial prefrontal network, leading to profound cognitive deficits in schizophrenia (Hutcheson et al., 2015).

Because in our stereological studies (Schmitt et al., 2009; Falkai et al., 2016), Nissl staining allows oligodendrocytes to be distinguished only morphologically from interneurons, we used Olig1, Olig2, and parvalbumin to stain sections adjacent to those in the same brains previously evaluated by design-based stereology. In accordance with our findings of unchanged neuron numbers in the Nissl-staining stereological study, we found no difference between schizophrenia and healthy controls in the density of a subgroup of 20% of interneurons stained by parvalbumin in the posterior part of the hippocampus (Freund and Buzsaki, 1996). This is in contrast to previously reported reductions of the total number of parvalbumin-positive interneurons in CA4 and CA1 and the density of parvalbumin-stained interneurons in CA2 (Benes et al., 1998; Knable et al., 2004) or all subfields (Zhang and Reynolds, 2002). However, these studies have conflicting results with respect to the affected subregions, and they did not separate

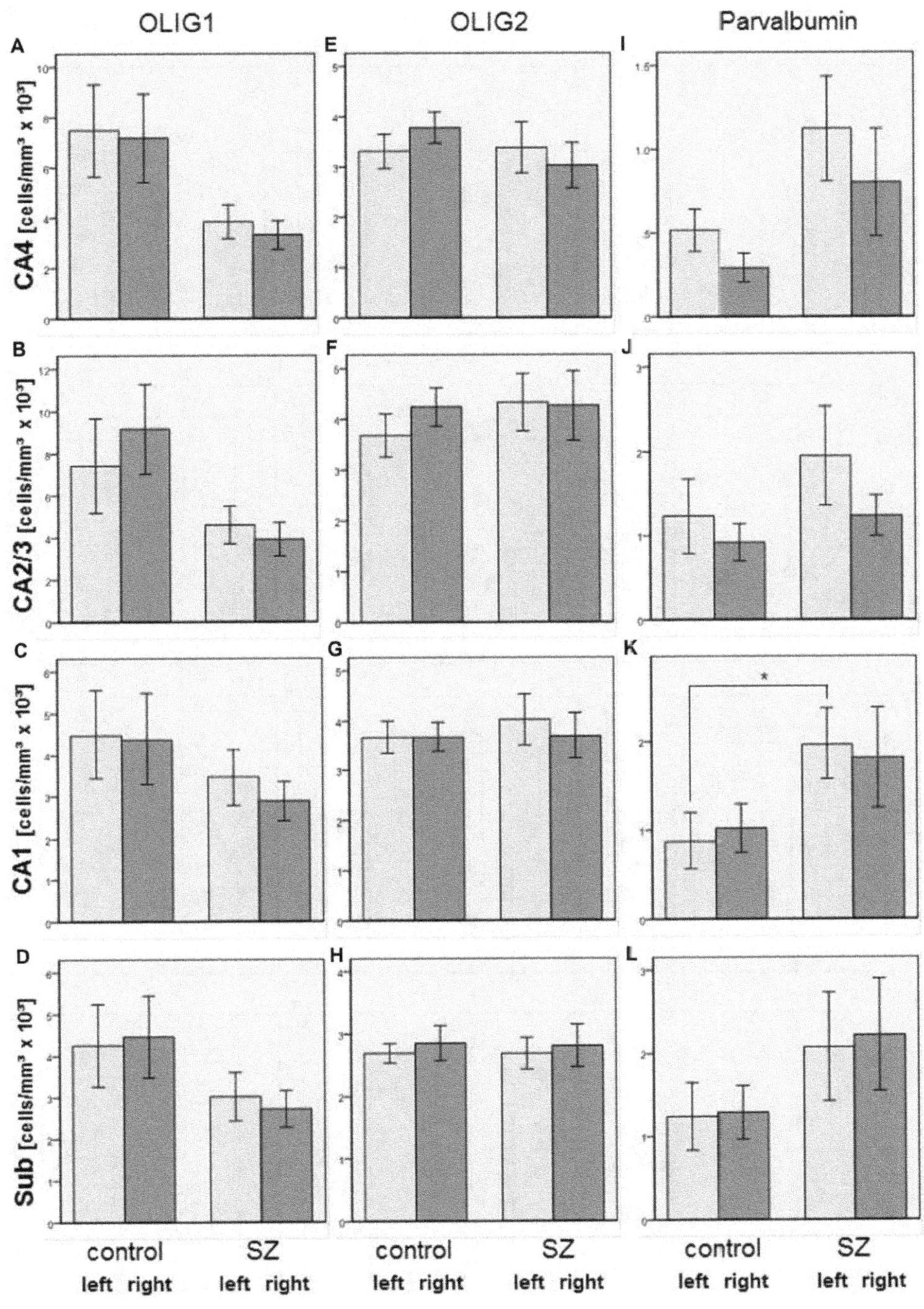


**FIGURE 4 | Left column (A–D): Cell density (cells/mm$^3$ × 10$^3$) in CA4 (A), CA2/3 (B), CA1 (C), and subiculum (Sub, [D]) of Olig1-positive oligodendrocytes in SZ patients and controls.** Columns represent mean cell density, and bars represent standard error of the mean. Light gray columns: left hemisphere; dark gray columns: right hemisphere. Middle column **(E–H)**: Cell density (cells/mm$^3$ × 10$^3$) in CA4 **(E)** CA2/3 **(F)**, CA1 **(G)**, and Sub **(H)** of Olig2-positive oligodendrocytes in SZ and controls. Columns represent mean cell density, and bars represent standard error of the mean. Light gray columns: left hemisphere; dark gray columns: right hemisphere. Right column **(I–L)**: Cell density (cells/mm$^3$ × 10$^3$) in CA4 **(I)**, CA2/3 **(J)**, CA1 **(K)**, and Sub **(L)** of parvalbumin-positive interneurons in SZ and controls. Columns represent mean cell density, and bars represent standard error of the mean. Light gray columns: left hemisphere; dark gray columns: right hemisphere. Increased density of parvalbumin-stained cells in SZ compared to controls was observed in left CA1. *$p < 0.05$.

the anterior from the posterior part of the hippocampus. Moreover, two-dimensional counting of cell density in only a few sections without considering the volume of the region has methodological limitations because of the influence of volume differences and tissue shrinkage resulting from fixation and staining procedures. Bias may be caused also by cutting of

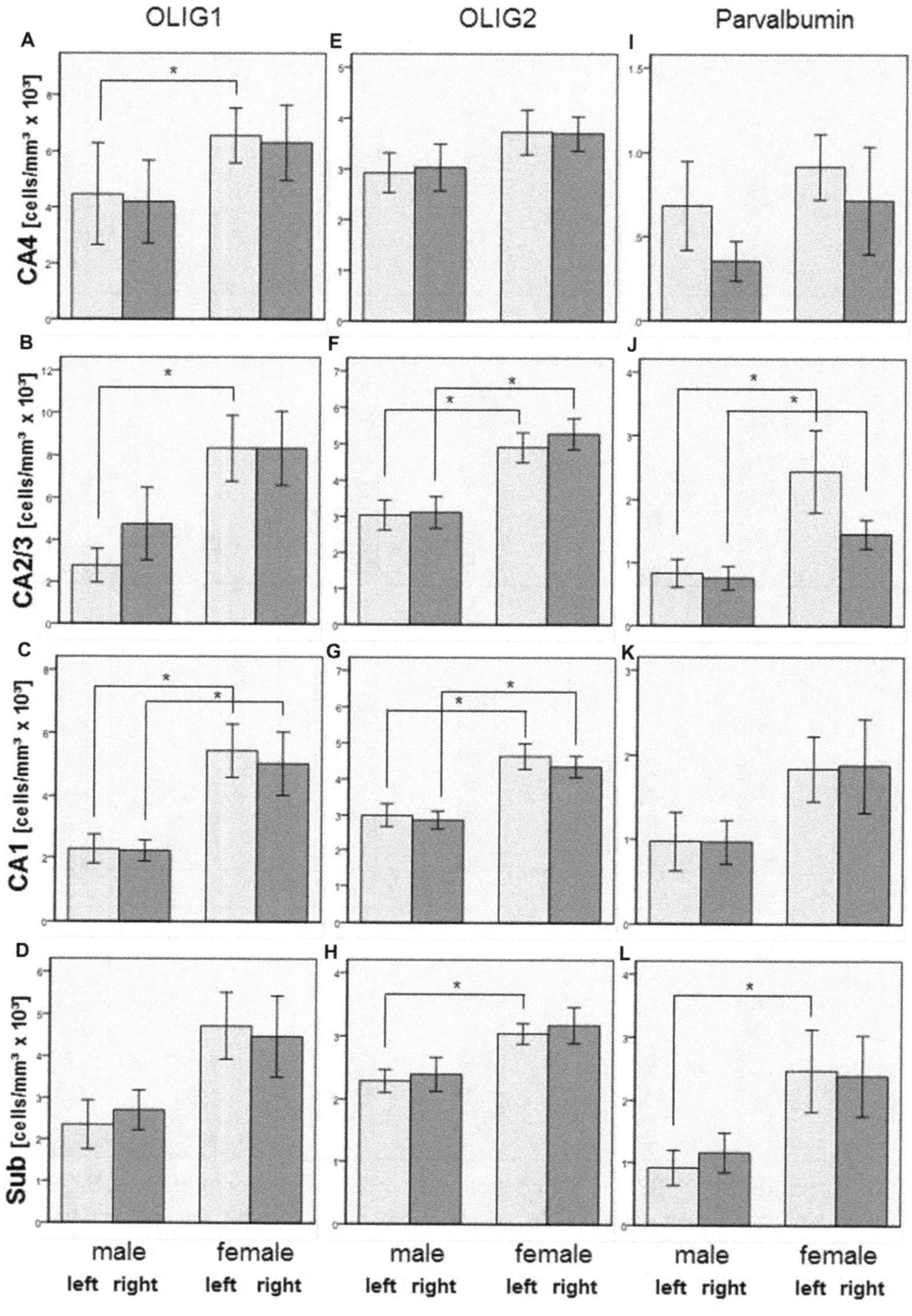


**FIGURE 5 | Left column (A–D): Cell density (cells/mm$^3$ × 10$^3$) in CA4 (A), CA2/3 (B), CA1 (C), and subiculum (Sub, [D]) of Olig1-positive oligodendrocytes in male and female subjects in the posterior hippocampus.** Columns represent mean cell density, and bars represent standard error of the mean. Light gray columns: left hemisphere; dark gray columns: right hemisphere. Increased Olig1-positive oligodendrocytes in females compared to males were observed in left and right CA1, in left CA2/3 and in left CA4. *$p < 0.05$. Middle column **(E–H)**: Cell density (cells/mm$^3$ × 10$^3$) in CA4 **(E)**, CA2/3 **(F)**, CA1 **(G)**, and subiculum **(H)** of Olig2-positive oligodendrocytes in males and females in the posterior hippocampus. Columns represent mean cell density, and bars represent standard error of the mean. Light gray columns: left hemisphere; dark gray columns: right hemisphere. Increased density of Olig2-positive oligodendrocytes in females compared to males were observed in left and right CA1, left and right CA2/3 and in left subiculum (Sub) *$p < 0.05$. Right column **(I–L)**: Cell density (cells/mm$^3$ × 10$^3$) in CA4 **(I)**, CA2/3 **(J)**, CA1 **(K)**, and subiculum **(L)** of parvalbumin-positive interneurons in males and females in the posterior hippocampus. Columns represent mean cell density, and bars represent standard error of the mean. Light gray columns: left hemisphere; dark gray columns: right hemisphere. Increased density of parvalbumin-stained cells in females compared to males has been detected in left and right CA2/3 and in left subiculum (Sub) *$p < 0.05$.

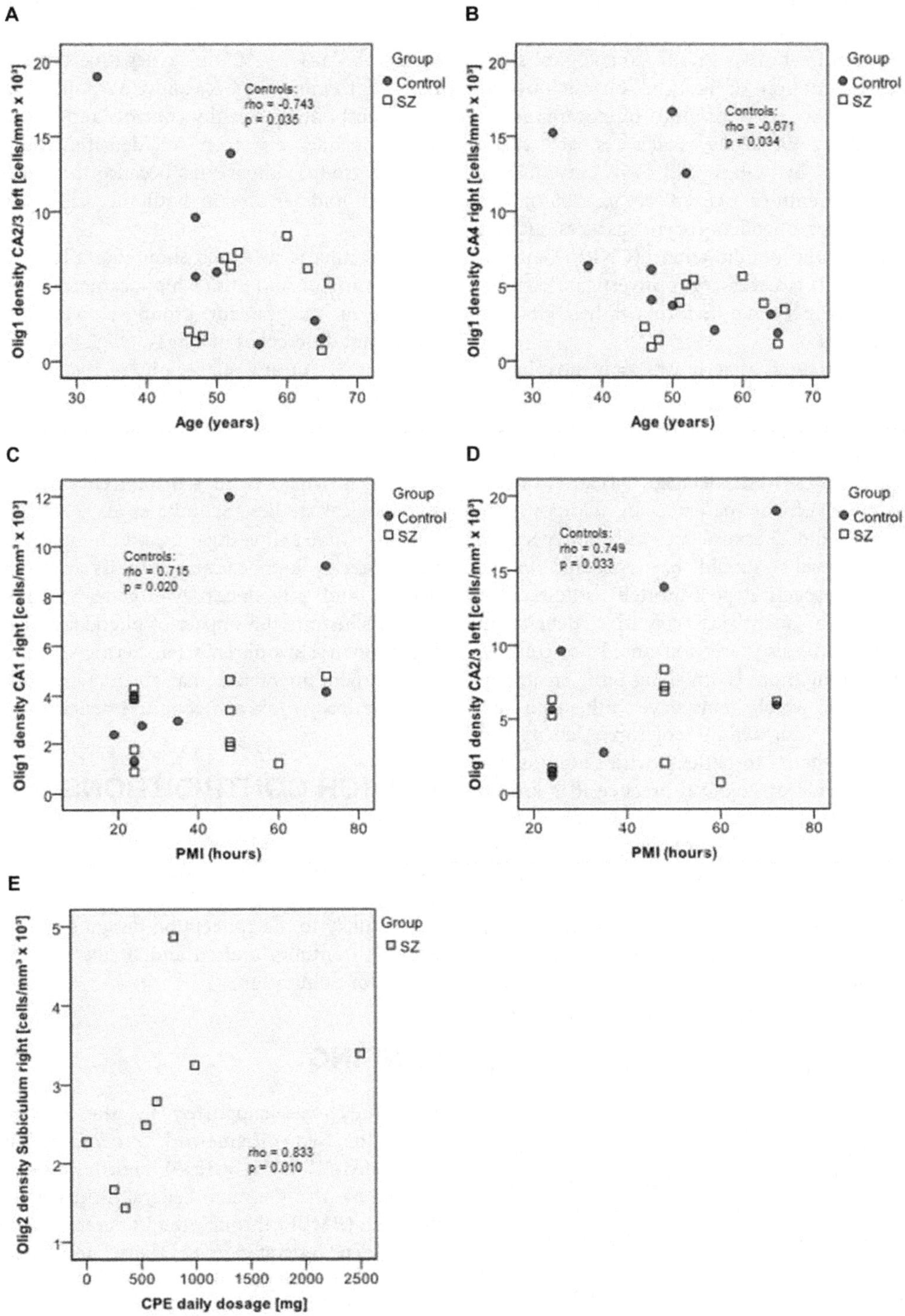


**FIGURE 6 | Upper section (A–B): scatterplots showing the relation between age and Olig1 densities in CA2/3 left (A) and in CA4 right (B).** Middle section **(C–D)**: scatterplots showing the relation between post mortem interval (PMI) and Olig1 densities in CA1 right **(C)** and CA2/3 left **(D)**. Bottom **(E)**: scatterplot showing the relation between chlorpromazine equivalents (CPE) and Olig2 density in the right subiculum. Control subjects appear as dark circles, SZ appear as light squares.

cells during sectioning, non-random orientation, and irregular cell shape and size (Williams and Rakic, 1988). Therefore, design-based stereological studies of the posterior part of the hippocampus are necessary to elucidate the impact of decreased inhibition by a marked deficit of subclasses of interneurons.

Although the reduction of Olig1-positive oligodendrocytes in CA4 did not reach significance, the trend towards significant reduction is in the same direction as in our stereological study and partly supports the notion of reduced oligodendrocyte numbers in the posterior part of the hippocampus in schizophrenia (Schmitt et al., 2009; Falkai et al., 2016). Oligodendrocytes stained by Olig1 represent myelinating and oligodendrocyte progenitors (Arnett et al., 2004), and immunolabeling with other oligodendrocyte markers such as 2',3'-cyclic nucleotide 3'-phosphodiesterase (CNP), GalC or myelin basic protein (MBP) is necessary to investigate possible myelin damage or whether more mature forms of these glia cells are altered in schizophrenia.

A limitation of our study is that it was only possible to identify cognitive deficits by evaluating medical records, and no structured neuropsychological *in vivo* test results were available. However, the rater (J. Steiner) is an experienced psychiatrist, and case notes were detailed, because of the long-term hospitalization of the patients. In addition, the sample size was small and, because we did not perform Bonferroni correction, results should be replicated in an independent sample. Prospective post-mortem studies that use standardized tests to investigate cognitive deficits in brain donors before death also are warranted to confirm our results. A further limitation is the long-term treatment with typical neuroleptics, which may have influenced our results. The patient group with definite cognitive deficits had received higher doses compared to patients with only possible cognitive deficits. However, from clinical practice it is known that patients with persisting symptoms receive higher doses of antipsychotics than patients in remission. Additionally, neuroleptic treatment may have influenced cell densities in our study. Haloperidol is known to increase expression of Olig2 in the hippocampus and cerebral cortex, whereas quetiapine and olanzapine increase expression of both Olig1 and Olig2 (Wang et al., 2010; Fang et al., 2013). Additionally, haloperidol and clozapine have been shown to be protective for energy-deprived immature oligodendrocytes (Steiner et al., 2011). Moreover, after cuprizione-induced demyelination, quetiapine enhanced oligodendrocyte regeneration and myelin repair (Zhang et al., 2012). Thus, the unchanged density of Olig1- and Olig2-positive cells in the SZ in our study may be a consequence of increased expression of oligodendrocytes due to long-term antipsychotic treatment, which counteracted the decreased expression of oligodendrocytes previously reported in these patients (Schmitt et al., 2009; Falkai et al., 2016). Moreover, the high variance in the data for the SZ may be due to treatment with different neuroleptics. However, because some variances in density were significantly higher in controls than in SZ, e.g., Olig1 densities in CA2/3 and CA4 (compare **Figure 4**) it would be speculative to explain this high variance by the type of antipsychotic medication and dosage. In addition, the density of parvalbumin-positive interneurons may also have been affected by treatment, because risperidone has been found to normalize loss of this cell population after prenatal immune activation in rats (Piontkewitz et al., 2012). However, in healthy animals haloperidol and clozapine did not change the density of parvalbumin-stained interneurons (Cahir et al., 2005). Finally, age may have influenced our results, because we found a negative correlation between age and Olig1 density in CA4 and CA2/3; however, this correlation was found only in healthy controls and not in SZ. We detected a clear gender effect on cell densities, but this is irrelevant for our group comparisons because there were equal numbers of males and females in both the schizophrenia and control groups.

In summary, we could show that a loss of oligodendrocytes in the anterior and entire hippocampus is related to cognitive deficits in this patient group. However, we did not find significant differences in Olig1-, Olig2-, or parvalbumin-positive cell densities in any subregions of the posterior hippocampus in SZ compared to healthy controls. Here, we did find a trend towards a reduction of Olig1-stained cells in CA4, which points in the same direction as the decrease of oligodendrocyte number in this area in schizophrenia found in our previous stereological studies (Schmitt et al., 2009; Falkai et al., 2016). Further studies investigating white matter tract integrity of the posterior hippocampus and its relationship to cognitive deficits and oligodendrocyte gene variants are needed to further illustrate the impact of oligodendrocyte dysfunction on cognition in schizophrenia. Furthermore, animal models of gene-environment interaction may elucidate the relationship between oligodendrocyte loss and cognitive deficits.

## AUTHOR CONTRIBUTIONS

JSt, JSh, AK, TS-A, TK, H-GB, AH, BB, PF, BM and AS were involved in data acquisition, statistical evaluation, and manuscript preparation. PF, BM, JSt, AS, and BB contributed substantially to the conception design and interpretation of the work. All authors drafted and finally approved the work and agreed for publication.

## FUNDING

The study was supported by the European Commission under the Sixth Framework Programme (BrainNet Europe II, LSHM-CT-2004-503039). Furthermore, this work was funded by the German Federal Ministry of Education and Research (BMBF) through the Integrated Network IntegraMent (Integrated Understanding of Causes and Mechanisms in Mental Disorders) under the auspices of the e:Med Programme (grant number 01ZX1314I to PF and TK). Additionally, work was funded by the EU project IN-SENS FP7-PEOPLE-2013-ITN (607616). The article reflects only the views of the authors and the Community is not liable for any use that may be made of it.

## ACKNOWLEDGMENTS

The authors wish to thank Jacquie Klesing, Board-certified Editor in the Life Sciences (ELS), for her valuable assistance with language revision.

## REFERENCES

Abdul-Rahman, M. F., Qiu, A., and Sim, K. (2011). Regionally specific white matter disruptions of fornix and cingulum in schizophrenia. *PLoS One* 6:e18652. doi: 10.1371/journal.pone.0018652

an der Heiden, W., and Häfner, H. (2011). "Course and Outcome," in *Schizophrenia*, 3rd Edn., eds D. Weinberger and P. J. Harrison. (Oxford, UK: Blackwell Publishing), 104–141.

Arnett, H. A., Fancy, S. P., Alberta, J. A., Zhao, C., Plant, S. R., Kaing, S., et al. (2004). bHLH transcription factor Oligl is required to repair demyelinated lesions in the CNS. *Science* 306, 2111–2115. doi: 10.1126/science. 1103709

Benes, F. M., Kwok, E. W., Vincent, S. L., and Todtenkopf, M. S. (1998). A reduction of nonpyramidal cells in sector CA2 of schizophrenics and manic depressives. *Biol. Psychiatry.* 44, 88–97. doi: 10.1016/s0006-3223(98) 00138-3

Bernstein, H. G., Krause, S., Krell, D., Dobrowolny, H., Wolter, M., Stauch, R., et al. (2007). Strongly reduced number of parvalbumin-immunoreactive projection neurons in the mammillary bodies in schizophrenia: further evidence for limbic neuropathology. *Ann. N. Y. Acad. Sci.* 1096, 120–127. doi: 10.1196/annals.13 97.077

Bogerts, B., Falkai, P., Haupts, M., Greve, B., Ernst, S., Tapernon-Franz, U., et al. (1990). Post-mortem volume measurements of limbic system and basal ganglia structures in chronic schizophrenics. Initial results from a new brain collection. *Schizophr. Res.* 3, 295–301. doi: 10.1016/0920-9964(90) 90013-w

Cahir, M., Costello, I., King, D. J., and Reynolds, G. P. (2005). Chronic haloperidol or clozapine treatment does not alter parvalbumin immunoreactivity in the rat frontal cortex or hippocampus. *Neurosci. Lett.* 373, 57–60. doi: 10.1016/j.neulet. 2004.09.057

Cassoli, J. C., Guest, P. C., Malchow, B., Schmitt, A., Falkai, P., and Martins-de-Souza, D. (2015). Disturbed macro-connectivity in schizophrenia linked to oligodendrocyte dysfunction: from structural findings to molecules. *npj. Schizophrenia* 1:15034. doi: 10.1038/npjschz. 2015.34

Desamericq, G., Schurhoff, F., Meary, A., Szoke, A., Macquin-Mavier, I., Bachoud-Levi, A. C., et al. (2014). Long-term neurocognitive effects of antipsychotics in schizophrenia: a network meta-analysis. *Eur. J. Clin. Pharmacol.* 70, 127–134. doi: 10.1007/s00228-013-1600-y

Falkai, P., Malchow, B., Wetzestein, K., Nowastowski, V., Bernstein, H. G., Steiner, J., et al. (2016). Decreased oligodendrocyte and neuron number in anterior hippocampal areas and the entire hippocampus in schizophrenia: A stereological post-mortem study. *Schizophr. Bull.* (in press).

Falkai, P., Schmitt, A., and Cannon, T. D. (2011). "Pathophysiology of Schizophrenia," in *Schizophrenia: Current Science and Clinical Practice*, ed. W. Gaebel (New Jersey: Wiley-Blackwell), 31–65.

Fang, F., Zhang, H., Zhang, Y., Xu, H., Huang, Q., Adilijiang, A., et al. (2013). Antipsychotics promote the differentiation of oligodendrocyte progenitor cells by regulating oligodendrocyte lineage transcription factors 1 and 2. *Life Sci.* 93, 429–434. doi: 10.1016/j.lfs.2013.08.004

Fitzsimmons, J., Hamoda, H. M., Swisher, T., Terry, D., Rosenberger, G., Seidman, L. J., et al. (2014). Diffusion tensor imaging study of the fornix in first episode schizophrenia and in healthy controls. *Schizophr. Res.* 156, 157–160. doi: 10. 1016/j.schres.2014.04.022

Freund, T. F., and Buzsaki, G. (1996). Interneurons of the hippocampus. *Hippocampus* 6, 347–470.

Fusar-Poli, P., Papanastasiou, E., Stahl, D., Rocchetti, M., Carpenter, W., Shergill, S., et al. (2015). Treatments of negative symptoms in schizophrenia: meta-analysis of 168 randomized placebo-controlled trials. *Schizophr. Bull.* 41, 892–899. doi: 10.1093/schbul/sbu170

Geisler, D., Walton, E., Naylor, M., Roessner, V., Lim, K. O., Charles Schulz, S., et al. (2015). Brain structure and function correlates of cognitive subtypes in schizophrenia. *Psychiatry Res.* 234, 74–83. doi: 10.1016/j.pscychresns.2015. 08.008

Hasan, A., Falkai, P., Wobrock, T., Lieberman, J., Glenthoj, B., Gattaz, W. F., et al. (2012). World Federation of Societies of Biological Psychiatry (WFSBP) Guidelines for Biological Treatment of Schizophrenia, part 1: update 2012 on the acute treatment of schizophrenia and the management of treatment resistance. *World J. Biol. Psychiatry* 13, 318–378. doi: 10.3109/15622975.2012. 696143

Hasan, A., Wobrock, T., Falkai, P., Schneider-Axmann, T., Guse, B., Backens, M., et al. (2014). Hippocampal integrity and neurocognition in first-episode schizophrenia: a multidimensional study. *World J. Biol. Psychiatry* 15, 188–199. doi: 10.3109/15622975.2011.620002

Haukvik, U. K., Westlye, L. T., Morch-Johnsen, L., Jorgensen, K. N., Lange, E. H., Dale, A. M., et al. (2015). In vivo hippocampal subfield volumes in schizophrenia and bipolar disorder. *Biol. Psychiatry* 77, 581–588. doi: 10.1016/j. biopsych.2014.06.020

Heckers, S., and Konradi, C. (2015). GABAergic mechanisms of hippocampal hyperactivity in schizophrenia. *Schizophr. Res.* 167, 4–11. doi: 10.1016/j.schres. 2014.09.041

Hutcheson, N. L., Sreenivasan, K. R., Deshpande, G., Reid, M. A., Hadley, J., White, D. M., et al. (2015). Effective connectivity during episodic memory retrieval in schizophrenia participants before and after antipsychotic medication. *Hum. Brain Mapp.* 36, 1442–1457. doi: 10.1002/hbm.22714

Knable, M. B., Barci, B. M., Webster, M. J., Meador-Woodruff, J., and Torrey, E. F. (2004). Molecular abnormalities of the hippocampus in severe psychiatric illness: postmortem findings from the Stanley Neuropathology Consortium. *Mol. Psychiatry* 9, 609–620. doi: 10.1038/sj.mp.4001471

Konradi, C., Yang, C. K., Zimmerman, E. I., Lohmann, K. M., Gresch, P., Pantazopoulos, H., et al. (2011). Hippocampal interneurons are abnormal in schizophrenia. *Schizophr. Res.* 131, 165–173. doi: 10.1016/j.schres.2011. 06.007

Kunimatsu, N., Aoki, S., Kunimatsu, A., Abe, O., Yamada, H., Masutani, Y., et al. (2012). Tract-specific analysis of white matter integrity disruption in schizophrenia. *Psychiatry Res* 201, 136–143. doi: 10.1016/j.pscychresns.2011. 07.010

Kuroki, N., Kubicki, M., Nestor, P. G., Salisbury, D. F., Park, H. J., Levitt, J. J., et al. (2006). Fornix integrity and hippocampal volume in male schizophrenic patients. *Biol. Psychiatry* 60, 22–31. doi: 10.1016/j.biopsych.2005.09.021

Lim, K. O., Ardekani, B. A., Nierenberg, J., Butler, P. D., Javitt, D. C., and Hoptman, M. J. (2006). Voxelwise correlational analyses of white matter integrity in multiple cognitive domains in schizophrenia. *Am. J. Psychiatry* 163, 2008–2010. doi: 10.1176/appi.ajp.163.11.2008

Mitterauer, B. J. (2011). Possible role of glia in cognitive impairment in schizophrenia. *CNS Neurosci. Ther.* 17, 333–344. doi: 10.1111/j.1755-5949. 2009.00113.x

Mosebach, J., Keilhoff, G., Gos T., Schiltz, K., Schoeneck, L., Dobrowolny, H., et al. (2013). Increased nuclear Olig1-expression in the pregenual anterior cingulate white matter of patients with major depression: a regenerative attempt to compensate oligodendrocyte loss?. *J. Psychiatr. Res.* 47, 1069–1079. doi: 10. 1016/j.jpsychires.2013.03.018

Nestor, P. G., Kubicki, M., Kuroki, N., Gurrera, R. J., Niznikiewicz, M., Shenton, M. E., et al. (2007). Episodic memory and neuroimaging of hippocampus and fornix in chronic schizophrenia. *Psychiatry Res.* 155, 21–28. doi: 10.1016/j. pscychresns.2006.12.020

Nuechterlein, K. H., Barch, D. M., Gold, J. M., Goldberg, T. E., Green, M. F., and Heaton, R. K. (2004). Identification of separable cognitive factors in schizophrenia. *Schizophr. Res.* 72, 29–39. doi: 10.1016/j.schres.2004. 09.007

Ortakov, V., Mancevski, B., Keilp, J., Oppenheim, S., and Dwork, A. J. (1999). Application of cognitive scales to medical records of schizophrenia inpatients. *Schizophr. Res.* 35, 131–140. doi: 10.1016/s0920-9964(98)00086-3

Piontkewitz, Y., Bernstein, H. G., Dobrowolny, H., Bogerts, B., Weiner, I., and Keilhoff, G. (2012). Effects of risperidone treatment in adolescence on hippocampal neurogenesis, parvalbumin expression and vascularization following prenatal immune activation in rats. *Brain Behav. Immun.* 26, 353–363. doi: 10.1016/j.bbi.2011.11.004

Rametti, G., Junque, C., Falcon, C., Bargallo, N., Catalan, R., Penades, R., et al. (2009). A voxel-based diffusion tensor imaging study of temporal white matter in patients with schizophrenia. *Psychiatry Res.* 171, 166–176. doi: 10.1016/j. pscychresns.2008.05.003

Rey, M. J., Schulz, P., Costa, C., Dick, P., and Tissot, R. (1989). Guidelines for the dosage of neuroleptics. I: chlorpromazine equivalents of orally administered neuroleptics. *Int. Clin. Psychopharmacol.* 4, 95–104. doi: 10.1097/00004850-198904000-00001

Saia-Cereda, V. M., Cassoli, J. S., Schmitt, A., Falkai, P., Nascimento, J. M., and Martins-de-Souza, D. (2015). Proteomics of the corpus callosum unravel pivotal players in the dysfunction of cell signaling, structure and myelination in schizophrenia brains. *Eur. Arch. Psychiatry Clin. Neurosci.* 265, 601–612. doi: 10.1007/s00406-015-0621-1

Schmitt, A., Steyskal, C., Bernstein, H. G., Schneider-Axmann, T., Parlapani, E., Schaeffer, E. L., et al. (2009). Stereologic investigation of the posterior part of the hippocampus in schizophrenia. *Acta Neuropathol.* 117, 395–407. doi: 10.1007/s00401-008-0430-y

Steiner, J., Sarnyai, Z., Westphal, S., Gos, T., Bernstein, H. G., Bogerts, B., et al. (2011). Protective effects of haloperidol and clozapine on energy-deprived OLN-93 oligodendrocytes. *Eur. Arch. Psychiatry Clin. Neurosci.* 261, 477–482. doi: 10.1007/s00406-011-0197-3

Voineskos, A. N., Felsky, D., Kovacevic, N., Tiwari, A. K., Zai, C., Chakravarty, M. M., et al. (2013). Oligodendrocyte genes, white matter tract integrity and cognition in schizophrenia. *Cereb. Cortex* 23, 2044–2057. doi: 10.1093/cercor/bhs188

Wang, H., Xu, H., Niu, J., Mei, F., Li, X., Kong, J., et al. (2010). Haloperidol activates quiescent oligodendroglia precursor cells in the adult mouse brain. *Schizophr. Res.* 119, 164–174. doi: 10.1016/j.schres.2010.02.1068

Williams, R. W., and Rakic, P. (1988). Three-dimensional counting: an accurate and direct method to estimate numbers of cells in sectioned material. *J. Comp. Neurol.* 278, 344–352. doi: 10.1002/cne.902780305

Zhang, Y., Zhang, H., Wang, L., Jiang, W., Xu, H., Xiao, L., et al. (2012). Quetiapine enhances oligodendrocyte regeneration and myelin repair after cuprizone-induced demyelination. *Schizophr. Res.* 138, 8–17. doi: 10.1016/j.schres.2012.04.006

Zhang, Z. J., and Reynolds, G. P. (2002). A selective decrease in the relative density of parvalbumin-immunoreactive neurons in the hippocampus in schizophrenia. *Schizophr. Res.* 55, 1–10. doi: 10.1016/s0920-9964(01)00188-8

5

# Quetiapine Inhibits Microglial Activation by Neutralizing Abnormal STIM1-Mediated Intercellular Calcium Homeostasis and Promotes Myelin Repair in a Cuprizone-Induced Mouse Model of Demyelination

*Hanzhi Wang[1], Shubao Liu[1], Yanping Tian[1], Xiyan Wu[1], Yangtao He[1], Chengren Li[1], Michael Namaka[2,3,4], Jiming Kong[2,3], Hongli Li[1]* and Lan Xiao[1]**

[1] Chongqing Key Laboratory of Neurobiology, Department of Histology and Embryology, Third Military Medical University, Chongqing, China, [2] College of Pharmacy and Medicine, Joint Laboratory of Biological Psychiatry Between Shantou University Medical College and College of Medicine, University of Manitoba, Winnipeg, MB, Canada, [3] Department of Human Anatomy and Cell Science, College of Medicine, University of Manitoba, Winnipeg, MB, Canada, [4] Department of Rehabilitation Medicine, Health Sciences Centre (HSC), Winnipeg, MB, Canada

***Correspondence:**
Hongli Li
lihongli@tmmu.edu.cn;
Lan Xiao
xiaolan35@hotmail.com

Microglial activation has been considered as a crucial process in the pathogenesis of neuroinflammation and psychiatric disorders. Several antipsychotic drugs (APDs) have been shown to display inhibitory effects on microglial activation *in vitro*, possibly through the suppression of elevated intracellular calcium ($Ca^{2+}$) concentration. However, the exact underlying mechanisms still remain elusive. In this study, we aimed to investigate the inhibitory effects of quetiapine (Que), an atypical APD, on microglial activation. We utilized a chronic cuprizone (CPZ)-induced demyelination mouse model to determine the direct effect of Que on microglial activation. Our results showed that treatment with Que significantly reduced recruitment and activation of microglia/macrophage in the lesion of corpus callosum and promoted remyelination after CPZ withdrawal. Our *in vitro* studies also confirmed the direct effect of Que on lipopolysaccharide (LPS)-induced activation of microglial N9 cells, whereby Que significantly inhibited the release of nitric oxide (NO) and tumor necrosis factor α (TNF-α). Moreover, we demonstrated that pretreatment with Que, neutralized the up-regulation of STIM1 induced by LPS and declined both LPS and thapsigargin (Tg)-induced store-operated $Ca^{2+}$ entry (SOCE). Finally, we found that pretreatment with Que significantly reduced the translocation of nuclear factor kappa B (NF-κB) p65 subunit from cytoplasm to nuclei in LPS-activated primary microglial cells. Overall, our data suggested that Que may inhibit microglial activation by neutralization of the LPS-induced abnormal STIM1-mediated intercellular calcium homeostasis.

**Keywords: quetiapine, microglia, calcium homeostasis, stored-operated calcium entry, stromal interaction molecule 1**

## INTRODUCTION

Microglia represents an abundant portion of cells that comprise the central nervous system (CNS). They are exclusively distributed in brain and spinal cord and represent about 5–20% of the total glial cell population (Lawson et al., 1990). CNS microglia cells are resident immune cells of the brain that constantly monitor the cerebral microenvironment to resist pathogens and heal injuries (Perry et al., 1993). Recent research demonstrates that microglial activation has a critical role in pathogenesis of neuroinflammatory diseases such as multiple sclerosis (MS) (Jack et al., 2005), neurodegenerative diseases, such as Alzheimer's disease (AD) (Wang et al., 2015) or Parkinson's disease (PD) (Qian et al., 2010), by producing various proinflammatory cytokines and free radicals (Kettenmann et al., 2011; Smith and Dragunow, 2014; Streit et al., 2014; Probert, 2015). In addition, other studies have also linked the importance of microglial activation to the pathogenesis associated with schizophrenia (SZ) (Monji et al., 2009; Busse et al., 2012; Monji et al., 2013; Al-Hakeim et al., 2015; An et al., 2015). Specifically, it has been shown that an elevated microglial density or microglial activation has been observed in the brains of patients with SZ (Steiner et al., 2008; Doorduin et al., 2009; Kato et al., 2013; Watkins and Andrews, 2015). Atypical antipsychotic drugs (APDs), such as risperidone, olanzapine, and aripiprazole have been reported to reduce the secretion of TNF-α and nitric oxide (NO) from activated microglia (Hou et al., 2006; Bian et al., 2008; Kato et al., 2008). These studies suggested that the pharmacological action of the antipsychotics on microglia may underlie the reported benefits associated with the use of these agents in patients with SZ (Kato et al., 2011).

Recently, accumulating evidence points to oligodendroglia dysfunction in regard to the demyelination known to be involved in the pathogenesis of SZ. As such, drugs that target oligodendroglia function are being investigated for their potential benefit in SZ (Ren et al., 2013; Roussos and Haroutunian, 2014). Que is an atypical APD that has been demonstrated to have superior therapeutic effects on cognitive symptoms displayed by patients with SZ as well as other neurological disorders (Kasper and Muller-Spahn, 2000; Riedel et al., 2007). It has been found that Que can protect mice from CPZ-induced microglial activation and myelin breakdown (Zhang et al., 2008; Shao et al., 2015). Que has also been shown to modulate immune responses in an experimental autoimmune encephalomyelitis (EAE) model of MS (Mei et al., 2012). It has also been shown to inhibit release of proinflammatory factors from activated microglia in culture (Bian et al., 2008). However, the underlying mechanism by which Que regulates microglial activation remains elusive. Meanwhile, it is also unclear as to the specific actions of Que on microglial activation during remyelination.

Interestingly, research has suggested that the elevation of intracellular calcium ($Ca^{2+}$) is critical in cell proliferation, migration, or ramification (Mizoguchi et al., 2014). Previous studies reported that pretreatment with APDs (Kato et al., 2008; Mizoguchi et al., 2014) significantly inhibited the release of proinflammatory cytokines and/or NO from activated microglia by suppression of elevation of intracellular calcium concentration ($[Ca^{2+}]_i$). Henceforth, it is possible that Que may also inhibit microglial activation *via* suppression of $[Ca^{2+}]_i$ elevation; however, the molecular pathway for this proposed effect is yet to be defined. Among $Ca^{2+}$ regulation in non-excitable cells, the main $Ca^{2+}$ influx mechanism is called store-operated $Ca^{2+}$ entry (SOCE) (Hoffmann et al., 2003; Qian et al., 2010; Kettenmann et al., 2011; Brawek and Garaschuk, 2013; Heo et al., 2015). Studies also reported that $Ca^{2+}$ release from SOCE stimulates an intercellular proinflammatory signal (Ohana et al., 2009; Mizoguchi et al., 2011), indicating that SOCE may contribute to the release of proinflammatory substances during microglial activation (Kraft, 2015; Michaelis et al., 2015; Moccia et al., 2015). However, to the best of our knowledge, there is currently no study that has addressed this issue.

In the present study, using a CPZ-induced chronic demyelination mouse model, as well an *in vitro* systems using lipopolysaccharide (LPS)-induced activated microglial, we demonstrated that Que dramatically attenuated microglial activation and promoted myelin repair. We also found that Que can neutralize the STIM1-mediated elevation of $Ca^{2+}$ entry (SOCE) and subsequent NFκB activation in LPS-induced activated microglia.

## MATERIALS AND METHODS

### Animals and Experimental Manipulations

C57BL/6 mice (male, 6 weeks old, 22–25 g) were obtained from the Animal Facility Centre of the Third Military Medical University, PR China. The animals were housed at this facility with a 12-h dark/12-h light cycle, at a constant temperature of 22 ± 1°C and a relative humidity of 60%. All procedures were performed in accordance with the guidelines set and approved by the Laboratory Animal Welfare and Ethics Committee of the Third Military Medical University.

C57BL/6 mice were randomly assigned to one of the following four groups: control (*CTL*), in which mice fed regular chow and drank distilled water for 12 weeks; *CPZ*, in which mice fed 0.2% CPZ for 12 weeks to induce a chronic demyelination (Matsushima and Morell, 2001); *Veh*, in which mice fed 0.2% CPZ for 12 weeks, then fed regular chow, and drank vehicle water for 2 weeks; *Que*, in which mice fed 0.2% CPZ for 12 weeks, and then fed regular chow, and drank Que-containing water for 2 weeks.

### Drug Treatments

Cuprizone (bis-cyclohexanone oxaldihydrazone) was purchased from Sigma-Aldrich (St. Louis, MO, USA). As previously described in other studies, 0.2% CPZ was mixed into the ground standard rodent chow. Que was provided by Astra Zeneca (Wilmington, DE, USA) and dissolved in distilled water. The mice ingested 10 mg/kg/day of Que according to our previously established in house methods with this model (Xiao et al., 2008; Zhang et al., 2008).

Lipopolysaccharide (*Escherichia coli*, E5:055) was purchased from Sigma (St. Louis, MO, USA). Fetal bovine serum (FBS) was purchased from Hyclone (Logan, UT, USA). Thiazolylblue (MTT) was from Beyotime Institute of Biotechnology, China (Shanghai, China). Iscove's Modified Dulbecco's medium (IMDM) was from Hyclone (Logan, UT, USA) and Dulbecco's

Modified Eagle Medium (DMEM) was from Gibco (Life technologies).

Que was dissolved into 20 mM of dimethyl sulfoxide (DMSO) and then diluted into 2 mM of PBS for experiments. The concentrations of Que were 0.1, 1, 10, and 50 μM.

## Histology and Immunohistochemistry

Histology and immunohistochemistry were performed as previously described (Wang et al., 2010). Briefly, 20 μm serial frozen sections between bregma −0.94 and bregma −1.8 [according to mouse atlas by Paxinos and Franklin (2004)] were analyzed. Sections were stained for myelin with Luxol fast blue (LFB)/ periodic acid-Schiff (PAS) base. For immunohistochemistry, sections were quenched with $H_2O_2$ blocked for 30 min in PBS containing 3% bovine serum albumin, 0.1% Triton X-100, and then incubated overnight with primary antibody. The primary antibody myelin basic protein (MBP) (Goat IgG; Santa Cruz) was used as a myelin protein. After washing, sections were further incubated with biotinylated secondary antibody (Daco) for 1 h, followed by peroxidase-coupled avidin–biotin complex (ABC kit, Vector Laboratories).

## N9 Cell Culture

The murine microglial cell line N9 (Provided by Prof. Yun Bai, Department of Medical Genetics, TMMU, China) were grown in DMEM supplemented with 10% heat-inactivated FBS, 100 U/ml penicillin, 100 μg/ml streptomycin, and 2 mM glutamine in humidified atmosphere of 95% air and 5% $CO_2$ at 37°C. The medium was changed every 2 days. Cells were plated at a density of $4 \times 10^4$ cells/well onto 96-well microtiter plates for MTT and nitrite assay. Que with or without LPS (100 ng/ml) was added to the culture medium of N9 cells for 24 h.

## Primary Microglial Cell Culture

Primary microglia cultures from C57BL/6 mice, cells were prepared from postnatal days 1–3. The brain tissue was dissociated in ice-cold HBSS. After removal of the cerebellum and subcortical tissue, meninges and blood vessels were dissociated under a dissecting microscope. The cortex was placed in an additional petri dish with precooled DMEM/F12 medium. The petri dish was placed on ice. The cerebral cortex was cut into about 1 $mm^3$ blocks, digested in 0.125% trypsin at 37°C for 5 min, and agitated into a cell suspension. Cell aggregates were collected by centrifugation (1000 × *g*, 5 min), resuspended in DMEM/F12, containing 10% FBS and antibiotics (40 U/ml penicillin and 40 μg/ml streptomycin) and cultured in 95% air and 5% $CO_2$ at 37°C. Floating microglia were harvested every week (between 2 and 7 weeks) and reseeded into 75 $cm^2$ culture flask to give pure microglia cultures. The medium was replaced once every 3 days.

## MTT Assay

Cell viability was evaluated by the MTT reduction assay as described previously (Niu et al., 2010). The cells were seeded in a 96-well plate for 24 h before being exposed to Que alone (10 μm) or Que with LPS (100 ng/ml) for 24 h. MTT solution (0.5 mg/ml, Beyotime, Nantong, China) was then added to each well and the cells were incubated for 1 h at 37°C and in 5% $CO_2$. Subsequently, the supernatant was removed and the formation of farmazan was solubilized with DMSO and measured at 540 nm with SpectraMax M2e spectrophotometer (Molecular Devices, Sunnyvale, CA, USA).

## Nitrite Production Assessment

Accumulation of nitrite ($NO_2^-$) in the culture media, an indicator of NO synthase activity, was measured by Griess Reaction. Cells at density of $3 \times 10^4$ cells/well were plated onto 96-well microtiter plates. Que with or without LPS (100 ng/ml) were added to the culture medium of N9 microglial cells for 48 h. Fifty microliters of culture supernatants were mixed with 50 μl Griess reagents (Part I: 1% sulfanilamide; Part II: 0.1% naphthylethylene diamide dihydrochlride and 2% phosphoric acid) at room temperature at 540 nm using the microplate reader. Nitrite concentration was calculated with reference to a standard curve of sodium nitrite.

## Immunofluorescent Staining

Cells on glass cover slips were fixed with 4% paraformaldehyde (PFA), rinsed with 0.01M PBS, incubated with 0.3% TritonX-100 for 5 min and blocked in 3% BSA for 60 min. Then glass cover slips were incubated in following primary antibodies overnight at 4°C: for NFκB p65 (rabbit IgG; Santa Cruz), for microglia CD11b (mouse IgG; Chemico), washed with PBS, and incubated with fluorescence-conjugated second antibodies at 4°C overnight. The method used for brain sections has been described previously (Wang et al., 2010). The immunoreactivity was determined using a 20× objective lens on a fluorescence microscope (Olympus BX-60) and a TCS SP5 confocal laser scanning microscope (Leica) with an excitation wavelength appropriate for 488 or 528 nm. Cell nuclei were stained with DAPI (Sigma, 0.1 μg/ml in PBS) at room temperature for 15 min. Cell counting was conducted on nine randomly chosen fields for each cover slip by using the densitometer Image Pro Plus image analysis system. There were two cover slips in each group.

## Intracellular $Ca^{2+}$ Imaging

Microglial N9 cells were plated at $1 \times 10^6$ cells on poly-D-lysine-coated, glass-bottomed culture dishes. Cells were incubated in medium containing 2 μM Fura-3 for 15 min at 37°C. Before $Ca^{2+}$ measurements were conducted, the culture dishes were washed with $Ca^{2+}$-free standard extracellular solution (SES) buffer. Cells were incubated with medium alone and 50 nM Que for 20 min before addition of LPS or thapsigargin (Tg). Tg is non-competitive inhibitor of the sarco/endoplasmic reticulum (ER) $Ca^{2+}$ ATPase (SERCA). During fluorescent measurements, the cells were continually perfused with a regular solution (37°C) containing 150 mM NaCl, 5 mM KCl, 1 mM $MaCl_2$, 10 mM glucose, and 10 mM HEPES at pH 7.4 with NaOH and either 1–2 mM $CaCl_2$ or 0.5 mM EGTA ($Ca^{2+}$-free). Fluorescent measurements were performed by imaging the Fluo-3 AM-loaded microglia using a laser scanning confocal microscope (Olympus IV 1000). Images were acquired using an olympus fluoview Ver.2.1c Viewer software. Relative average intracellular $Ca^{2+}$ concentration values were obtained from at least 20–30 microglial cells and the results obtained from at least three or four individual experiments.

## Quantitative RT-PCR

RNA was isolated from cultures using TRIzol Reagent (Invitrogen) and total RNA (5 mg) was reverse transcribed using PrimeScript™ RT-PCR Kit (Takara) according to the manufacturer's instructions. The cDNA was analyzed by real-time PCR with the Rotor Gene6000 (Corbertt Research, Australia) according to the protocol provided by the manufacturer and $2^{-\Delta\Delta Ct}$ method. Briefly, PCRs were performed using SYBR premix Ex Taq (Takara) in a final volume of 20 μl. The specific primers of target genes were as follows: TNF-α (5′-GACGTGGAACTGG CAGAAGAG-3′, 5′-TGCCACAAGCAGGAATGAGA-3′), Stim1 (5′-TCTFCATGACCTTCAGGAAA-3′, 5′-GGTGGACCTTCTC TACTTCCAC-3′), Stim2 (5′-AGTTGCCCTGCTCTGTATCG-3′, 5′-TGAAGCTGTTGTCTGGCACTT-3′), Orai1 (5′-TACTTAAG CCGCGCCAAG-3′, 5′-ACTTCCACCATCGCTACCA-3′), and GAPDH (5′-CAGCAAGGACACTGAGCAAGA-3′, 5′-GCCCCT CCTGTTATTATGGGG-3′).

## Statistical Analysis

One-way or two-way analysis of variance (ANOVA) was used to test statistical significance of three or more experimental groups, which was followed by Dunnett's *post hoc* or Tukey's *post hoc* test. Comparison between two experimental groups was made by the Student's *t*-test. A probability of $P < 0.05$ was considered statistically significant.

# RESULTS

## Que Inhibits the Activation of Microglia/ Macrophage in Corpus Callosum Lesions

To investigate the effect of Que on microglial activation involved in myelin defects, we used long-term CPZ-treated mice to mimic the neuroinflammation and white matter deterioration known to occur in the chronic disease phase (**Figure 1A**). Fast blue-staining results showed that almost no myelin fibers could be detected in corpus callosum (CC) in CPZ group vs. the control group (CTL) (**Figure 1B**). After CPZ withdrawal, remyelination was observed. However, the extent of myelin repair of CC was much higher in the Que group compared to that in the Veh group (**Figure 1C**). Similar demyelination and remyelination trends were observed in MBP-positive immunostaining (**Figures 1B,C**). Statistical analysis revealed a significant difference between CTL and CPZ group in terms of the optical density of MBP immunostaining, while Que group significantly increased in optical density of MBP staining compared to Veh group (**Figure 1D**). Interestingly, the accumulation of activated microglia/macrophages was observed by CD11b staining in the CC of CPZ group while only sporadically seen in CTL group (**Figure 1B**). After CPZ withdrawal, the density of $CD11^{+}$ cells (active microglia) decreased slightly but still remained at an elevated level that was not seen in the Que group (**Figures 1C,E**). These data suggest that Que can alleviate the recruitment and activation of microglia and promote myelin repair in CPZ-induced chronic mouse model of demyelination.

## Que Decreases the Release of NO and TNF-α from Activated N9 Microglial Cells Induced by LPS

To exclude non-specific effects of Que on microglial cells, MTT assay was performed to observe cell viabilities of N9 microglial cells treated with or without Que. Results showed that Que had no significant effect on cell viabilities at various concentrations under 100 μM, in which significant toxicity could be observed (**Figure 2A**). In addition, cell viability of N9 cells were tested after exposure to LPS at various concentrations (0, 0.1, 1, 10, 100, and 1000 ng/ml). The results displayed that LPS had no significant effect on cell viabilities (**Figure 2B**, $P > 0.05$). However, NO release in medium was increased by LPS in concentration-dependent manner, which was dramatically inhibited by pretreatment of Que (10 μM) (**Figure 2C**). Similar inhibitory effects of Que on TNF-α synthesis were also observed (**Figure 2D**). As such, our results demonstrated that Que did not affect N9 microglia cells viability, but decreased the release of NO and TNF-α from N9 microglial cells induced by LPS.

## Que Inhibits $Ca^{2+}$ Elevation in N9 Cells Induced by LPS and Thapsigargin (Tg)

To determine if Que might affect the $Ca^{2+}$ signaling pathway, which is very important for microglial activation, we utilized $Ca^{2+}$ imaging to measure alterations of $[Ca^{2+}]_i$ in N9 cells after stimulation. It was found that LPS induced sustained $[Ca^{2+}]_i$ elevation due to release of internal ER $Ca^{2+}$ (left peak, arrow) in $Ca^{2+}$-free imaging buffer. After washing, 2 mM $Ca^{2+}$ buffer induced $[Ca^{2+}]_i$ elevation (right peak, arrow) due to $Ca^{2+}$ influx through the PM, namely SOCE (**Figure 3A**). Pretreatment of Que for 15 min showed a significant decrease in the $[Ca^{2+}]_i$ level in response to LPS stimulation (**Figure 3B**). These results suggested that Que may reduce LPS-stimulated $[Ca^{2+}]_i$ by inhibiting activation-induced $Ca^{2+}$ channel in PM and $Ca^{2+}$ influx. In addition, in order to verify whether Que affect SOCE in N9 cells, or to examine the specificity of Que effects on $Ca^{2+}$ influx, we investigated the effect of Que on TG-induced activation of $[Ca^{2+}]_i$. Stimulation of Tg on N9 cells induced both $Ca^{2+}$ release in ER (left peak in **Figure 3C**) and $Ca^{2+}$ influx in PM (right peak in **Figure 3C**); pre-treated with Que, however, decreased TG-induced $Ca^{2+}$ turn over (**Figures 3C,D**). Our results suggest that Que inhibits $Ca^{2+}$ elevation likely by modulation SOCE in N9 microglial cells induced by LPS or Tg.

## Que Inhibits Upregulation of STIM1 in N9 Cells Exposed to LPS

In order to identify the SOCE channels which can be regulated by Que treatment in microglial cells, qRT-PCR was performed to analyze the mRNA levels for SOCE channel proteins STIM and Orai. These SOCE channel proteins were chosen because the interaction of STIM on ER and Orai1 on PM was essential for SOCE activation (Luik et al., 2006). It was found that LPS-exposed cells displayed a significant increase in STIM1 (**Figure 4A**), STIM2 (**Figure 4C**), and Orai1 (**Figure 4B**) expression as compared to controls (CTLs). Que pretreatment significantly reduced the

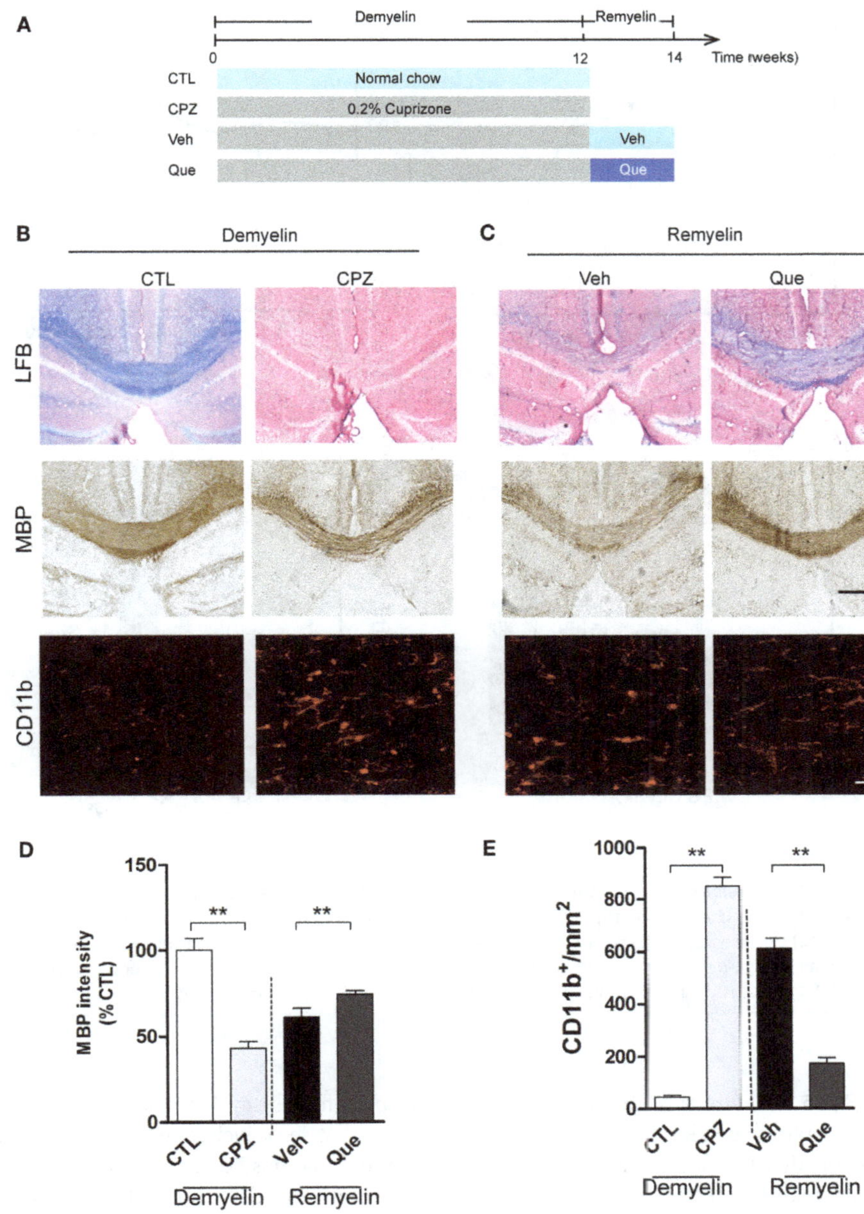


**FIGURE 1 | Effect of Que on microglial activation and remyelination in CPZ-induced chronic demyelinating mouse model.** **(A)** Schematic diagram displaying the time course and Que (10 mg/kg/day) treatment on CPZ-induced demyelination and remyelination. C57BL/6 mice were given CPZ for 12 weeks for chronic demyelination and start remyelination after CPZ withdrawal. **(B)** Representative Luxol fast blue staining, MBP and CD11b IF staining for corpus callosum (CC) mediolateral area of mice fed with or without CPZ. **(C)** Representative Luxol fast blue staining, MBP and CD11b IF staining for CC mediolateral areas of mice fed with or without Que after CPZ withdraw. **(D)** Quantification for optical density of MBP expression in CC of indicated groups. **(E)** Quantification of CD11b+ cells (activated microglia) in CC. The scale bars are 200 μm and 20 μm, respectively. Data represent means ± SEM ($n = 6$ in each group), $^{**}p < 0.01$ between indicated group.

upregulation of STIM1 (**Figure 4A**), but produced no effect on Orai1 and/or STIM2 expression (**Figures 4B,C**).

## Que Inhibits the Translocation of NF-kB p65 in LPS-Activated Microglial Cells

To further investigate the downstream mechanism of Que inhibition effect on N9 cell activation, we examined alteration of nuclear factor NF-κB activation, which has been implicated in LPS-induced microglial activation (Fan et al., 2015). Immunofluorescence staining revealed that the NF-κB p65 subunits were mainly expressed in cytoplasm and were barely detectable in the nucleus of control (CTL) and Que-treated groups (Que). However, NF-κB p65 subunits were intensively expressed in nucleus after LPS treatment (**Figure 5A**). However, Que pretreatment significantly reduced the translocation of p65 to nuclei when exposed to LPS (**Figures 5A,D**). Furthermore, we also examined the effect of Que

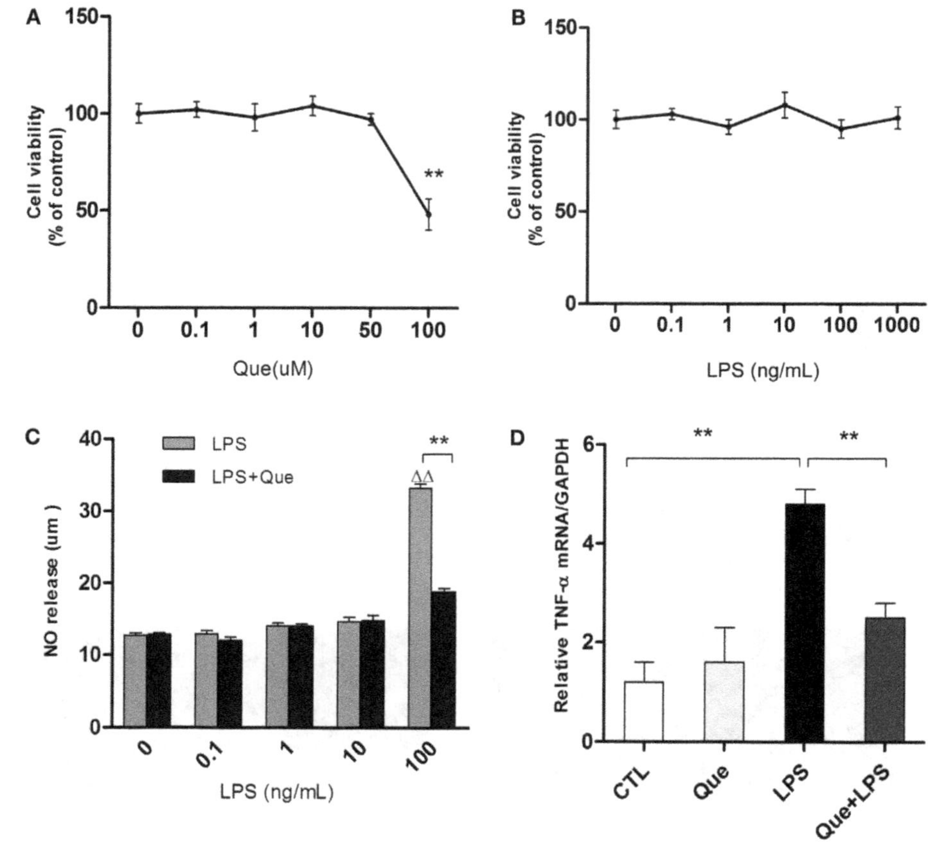


**FIGURE 2 | Effect of Que on NO and TNF-α release from N9 cells induced by LPS. (A)** MTT assay, cell viability of N9 microglial cells treated with various concentrations (0, 0.1, 1, 10, 50, and 100 μM) of Que for 24 h. **(B)** MTT assay, cell viability of N9 microglial cells treated with various concentrations (0, 0.1, 1, 10, 100, and 1000 ng/ml) of LPS for 24 h. **(C)** Griess assay of NO release from N9 cells exposed to various concentrations of LPS for 24 h with or without Que (10 μM) pretreatment. **(D)** qRT-PCR measurement of TNF-α mRNA expression in N9 cells exposed to LPS (100 ng/ml) for 24 h with or without Que (10 μM) pretreatment. Data are represented as means ± SEM. $^{**}p < 0.01$ vs. indicated group $^{\Delta\Delta}p < 0.01$ vs. control group (LPS=0ng/mL).

on phosphorylation of NF-κB p65, a feature of NF-κB activation. The results showed that the phosphorylated level of p65 was significantly increased from 60 min after LPS stimulation; however, Que pretreatment could attenuate this pattern (**Figures 5B,C,E**). Together, these data indicate that Que can inhibit NF-κB activation in N9 cells induced by LPS.

## DISCUSSION

In the last decade, structural and functional changes in glial cells have been becoming a major focus of interest in the research of SZ (Zheng et al., 2008). In our present study, we demonstrated that microglial activation was associated with the impairment of myelin repair in chronic CPZ-induced demyelination mouse model. In addition, we demonstrated that the atypical APD Que can inhibit the process of microglial activation and promote myelin repair. We further found that Que can suppress the abnormal STIM1-mediated elevation of $[Ca^{2+}]_i$ and inhibit the activation of NF-κB pathway in LPS-induced microglial cultures. As a result, the inhibitory effects of Que on microglial activation may have important implications for its therapeutic application in SZ.

Cuprizone or biscyclohexnaone oxalyldihydrazone is a copper chelator that selectively damages oligodendrocytes. As such, it is a model that has been widely used to induce demyelination. Interestingly, the CPZ-induced demyelination mouse model is also accepted as a SZ model, in which many cognitive functions or behavioral alterations associated with SZ patients are mapped (Makinodan et al., 2009; Xu et al., 2009; Xu et al., 2010; Xu et al., 2011; Praet et al., 2014). Que is currently used in the clinical treatment of SZ. Previous studies indicated that it prevents CPZ-induced white matter pathology and behavioral abnormalities in a short-term feeding (Zhang et al., 2008; Xu et al., 2010; Chandran et al., 2012). To understand the mechanism that may underlie the progression of white matter abnormality to a chronic state, we used the chronic CPZ treatment mouse model, in which the long-term (12 weeks) feeding of CPZ induced a series of demyelination/remyelination episodes, leading to the formation of chronic lesion in white matter (Matsushima and Morell, 2001). We found that long-term CPZ treatment induced serious demyelination and persistent microglial activation even after CPZ was withdrawn. These findings indicate that microglial activation may cause impairment of remyelination, since some

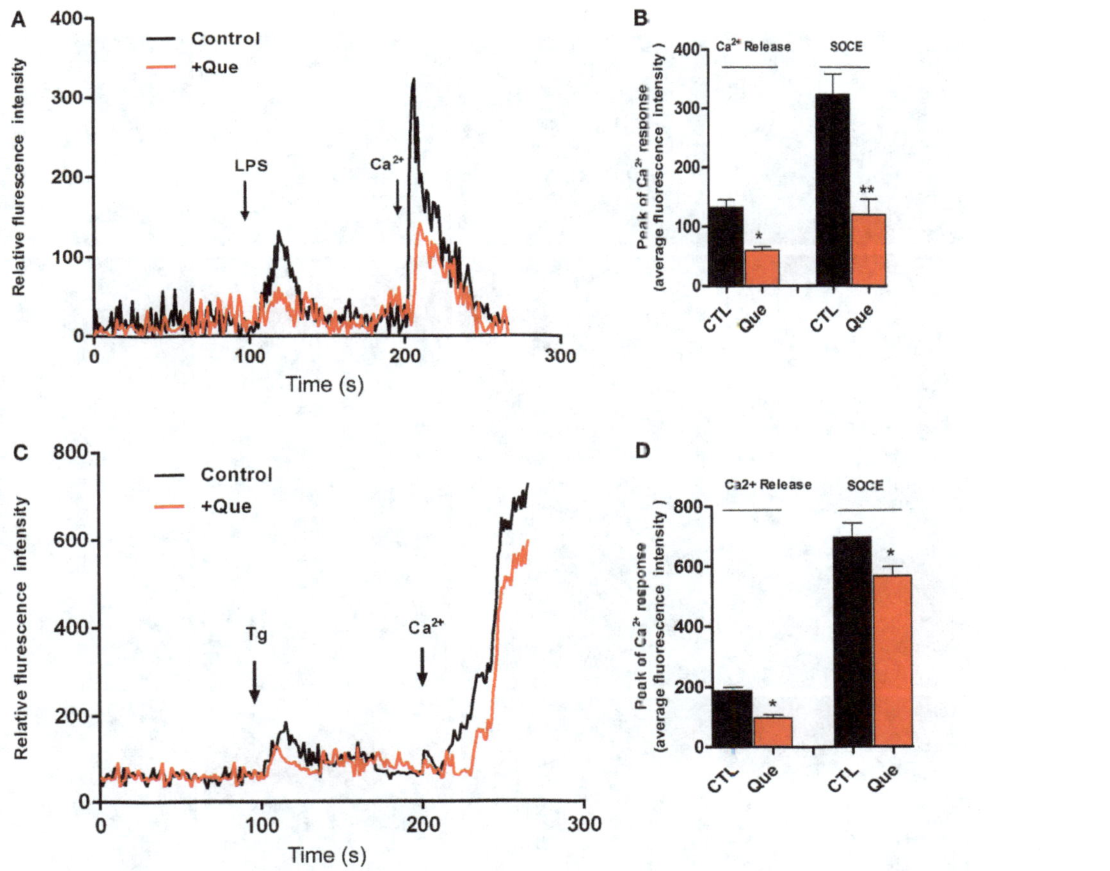


**FIGURE 3 | Effect of Que on $Ca^{2+}$ release and $Ca^{2+}$ entry in N9 cells induced by LPS or Tg. (A)** $Ca^{2+}$ image of N9 cells with LPS stimulation in $Ca^{2+}$-free medium following by $Ca^{2+}$ (2 mM) buffer incubation after wash with or without Que (10 μM) pretreatment. The first peak shows $[Ca^{2+}]_i$ elevation due to release of internal ER $Ca^{2+}$ induced by LPS; the second peak is due to $Ca^{2+}$ influx through the PM, namely ER $Ca^{2+}$ store-operated $Ca^{2+}$ entry (SOCE). Pretreatment of Que reduces the $[Ca^{2+}]_i$ elevation induced by LPS (red) (20–25 cells were analyzed in each group). **(B)** Quantification of $Ca^{2+}$ release (left peak) and store-operated $Ca^{2+}$ entry (SOCE) (right peak) in N9 cells activated by LPS with or without Que pretreatment. **(C)** $Ca^{2+}$ image of N9 cells with Tg stimulation in $Ca^{2+}$-free medium following by $Ca^{2+}$ (2 mM) buffer incubation after wash with or without Que pretreatment (20–25 cells were analyzed in each group). **(D)** Quantification of $Ca^{2+}$ release (left peak) and store-operated $Ca^{2+}$ entry (SOCE) (right peak) in N9 cells activated by Tg with or without Que pretreatment. Values are means ± SEM. $^*p < 0.05$ and $^{**}p < 0.01$ vs. CTL.

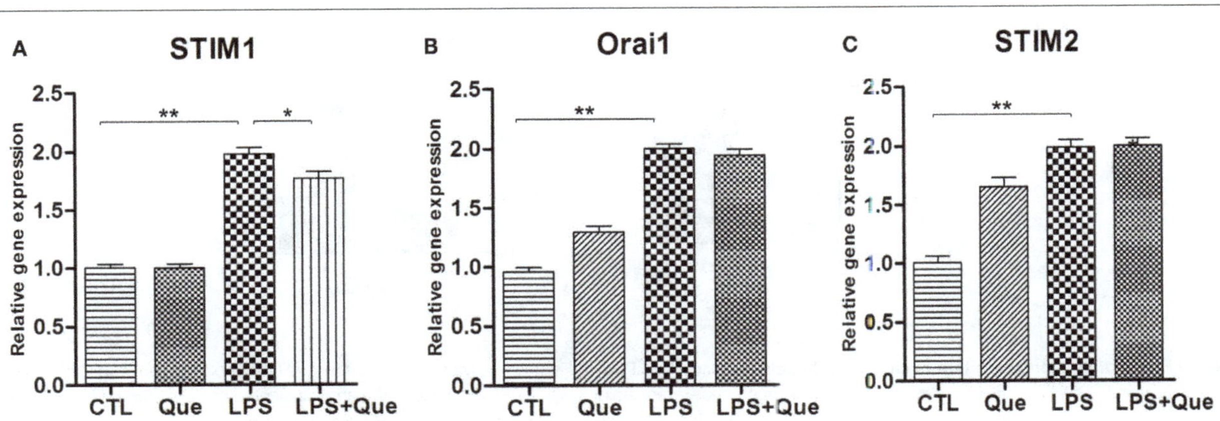


**FIGURE 4 | Effect of Que on expression of SOCE channel proteins in N9 cells exposed to LPS.** Quantification of qRT-PCR showed **(A)** STIM1 mRNA, **(B)** Orai1 mRNA, and **(C)** STIM2 mRNA in N9 cells exposed to LPS with or without 24 h of Que (10 μM) pretreatment. Values are normalized to GAPDH, a loading control. All data are means ± SEM. $^*p < 0.05$, and $^{**}p < 0.01$ vs. indicated group.

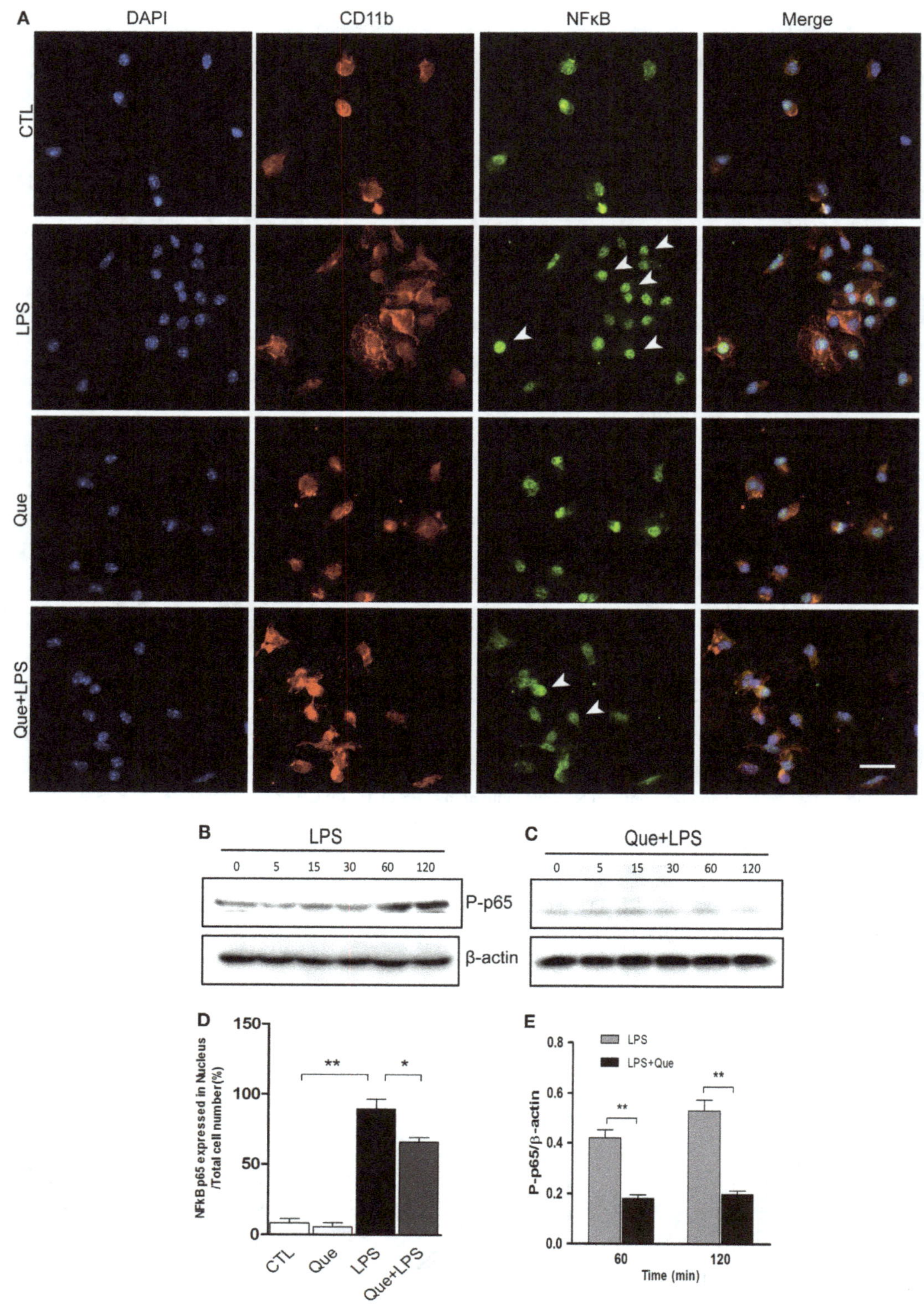


**FIGURE 5 | Effect of Que on activation of NF-κB in N9 cells induced by LPS.** **(A)** Representative double IF staining of NF-κB p65 (green) and CD11b (red) in N9 cells exposed in LPS with or without Que (10 μM) pretreatment, nuclei were stained with DAPI (blue). Note: the arrow indicated positive staining in the nucleus. Scale bars: 50 μm. **(D)** Quantification of the relative ratio of nucleus NF-κB p65 in the indicated groups. Note: LPS significantly increased the ratio of nucleus NF-κB p65, which could be reduced by Que pretreatment. **(B,C)** Western blot analysis of phosphorylated NF-κB p65 in N9 cells exposed in LPS with or without Que pretreatment at indicated time points. β-actin was used as a loading control. Note: the phosphorylated NF-κB p65 level was increased since 60 min after LPS treatment, and this pattern was attenuated by Que. **(D,E)** Quantification of the Western blot showing phosphorylated levels of NF-κB p65 in N9 cells exposed to LPS with or without Que pretreatment. Values are mean ± SEM. $^{*}p < 0.05$ and $^{**}p < 0.01$ vs. indicated group.

cytokines such as INF-γ or Interleukin-1 (IL-I) was found to inhibit oligodendroglia differentiation (Vela et al., 2002; Mana et al., 2006). The proper modulation of activated microglia, however, has been shown to be an integral step in the promotion of CNS remyelination by facilitating the increased production of neurotrophins or decreasing chemokine expression (Butovsky et al., 2006; Emmetsberger and Tsirka, 2012; Zhou et al., 2015). In our study, we demonstrate that Que treatment during the recovery period can attenuate microglial activation and enhance myelin repair. Our research findings are also supported by other researchers that have also shown the beneficial effects of Que in regard to remyelination (Zhang et al., 2012). The findings presented by these researchers suggest that the ability of Que to inhibit microglial activation may represent an important mechanism underlying its effectiveness at promoting remyelination. Normally, cytokines are virtually undetectable in the CNS. As such, when cytokines and chemokines are found in the CNS, it is usually indicative of clinical conditions involving demyelination (Schmitz et al., 2007; Puntambekar et al., 2015), brain trauma (Tasker, 2006), and/or mental disorders such as SZ (Potvin et al., 2008). Therefore, our current research further suggests that manipulating the microglial activation may be a key step in facilitating myelin repair that can be pursued as a novel treatment approach for SZ and/or other white matter disorders.

In regard to the specific mechanisms by which Que affects microglia, we demonstrate that Que can modulate STIM1-mediated intercellular calcium elevation induced by LPS. As an important second message molecule, elevation of cytosolic $Ca^{2+}$ has an essential role in microglial activation, including proliferation, migration, ramification, and release of proinflammatory cytokines and neurotrophins such as brain-derived neurotrophic factor (BDNF) (Mizoguchi et al., 2014). Although $Ca^{2+}$ entry across the plasma membrane (PM) is mediated by various channels, SOCE channels have been identified as the prevalent $Ca^{2+}$ entry mechanism in non-excitable cells, such as microglia (Laskaris et al., 2015). SOCE is controlled by stromal interaction molecule (STIM1 or STIM2) on the membrane of ER and Orail on PM. STIM1 acts as ER $Ca^{2+}$ sensor (Liou et al., 2005; Roos et al., 2005) and as such can activate $Ca^{2+}$ release-activated $Ca^{2+}$ (CARC) channels *via* interaction with Orai (Moccia et al., 2015). It has been shown that STIM1 is required for SOCE in immune cells and loss of function or null mutations in human STIM1 gene stops $Ca^{2+}$ influx in T cells resulting in immunodeficiencies in affected patients (Feske, 2009; Fuchs et al., 2012). Previous study also showed that Orail–STIM1 interaction on PM can mediate $Ca^{2+}$ influx, thereby regulating cytokine release in microglia (Sun et al., 2014; Laskaris et al., 2015). Pharmacological inhibitors and knockdown experiments using siRNA for Orail and STIM1 revealed that the inhibition of $Ca^{2+}$ influx through SOCE diminished the secretion of cytokines, TNF-α and IL-6 (Heo et al., 2015). In the present study, we demonstrate that Que did not modulate basal level of cytosolic $Ca^{2+}$; however, it can ameliorate LPS- and Tg-induced elevation of $Ca^{2+}$ influx *via* neutralizing the upregulation of STIM1. Based on our understanding in this area, it is the first time that the regulatory effect of Que on the SOCE channel that is involved in microglial activation is shown. However, the exact molecular mechanism how Que modulates SOCE still requires further investigation. Our research findings suggest that manipulating SOCE may represent a novel approach to attenuate the chronic disease progression associated with SZ. In addition, our research also suggests that STIM1 is a novel regulatory target for neutralizing microglial activation that may be advantageous in the prevention of progression of various neurodegenerative diseases or mental illness.

Following elevation of cytosolic $Ca^{2+}$, several downstream signaling pathways, such as NF-κB activation, are primarily responsible for microglial activation (Chauhan et al., 2014). NF-κB is a transcription factor that can be involved in multiple cell behaviors such as cell differentiation, survival, apoptosis, as well as immune and inflammatory response (Li and Verma, 2002; Vallabhapurapu and Karin, 2009). It has been reported that in AD or ischemia models, Que can inhibit activation of NF-κB in neurons (Bi et al., 2009; Zhao et al., 2014). Moreover, in an AD mouse model, Que was shown to attenuate glial activation and reduce the release of proinflammatory cytokines *via* inhibition NF-κB pathway (Zhu et al., 2015). In the present study, we also demonstrate that Que inhibited the translocation of NF-κB p65 and decreased the phosphorylated levels of NF-κB p65 subunits induced by LPS, indicating that the inhibition effect of Que on microglial activation may due to its effect to suppress NF-κB activation. Overall, it is likely that Que can maintain the intercellular calcium homeostasis by modulating STIM1 expression and subsequently inhibit NF-κB-dependent microglial activation.

In summary, within CPZ-induced chronic demyelination mouse model in conjunction with an *in vitro* system involving LPS-induced microglial activation cultures, we demonstrate that the atypical APD Que can inhibit microglial activation by neutralizing abnormal STIM1-mediated intercellular calcium homeostasis. In addition, our results also suggest that the ability of Que to inhibit microglial activation may also promote myelin repair. Our research findings identify a novel approach of manipulating specific calcium channels to regulate microglial activation that contributes to the underlying pathogenesis of SZ.

## AUTHOR CONTRIBUTIONS

HW, HL, and LX designed the study. HW, SL, YT, XW, YH, and HL acquired and analyzed the data. CL, JK analyzed the data. HW, HL, MN, and LX wrote the article, which all other authors reviewed. All authors approved the final version for publication.

## ACKNOWLEDGMENTS

This work is supported by the National Natural Science Foundation of China (NSCF 81471297, 31000482).

## REFERENCES


Al-Hakeim, H. K., Al-Rammahi, D. A., and Al-Dujaili, A. H. (2015). IL-6, IL-18, sIL-2R, and TNFalpha proinflammatory markers in depression and schizophrenia patients who are free of overt inflammation. *J. Affect. Disord.* 182, 106–114. doi:10.1016/j.jad.2015.04.044

An, H. M., Tan, Y. L., Shi, J., Wang, Z. R., Soars, J. C., Wu, J. Q., et al. (2015). Altered IL-2, IL-6 and IL-8 serum levels in schizophrenia patients with tardive dyskinesia. *Schizophr. Res.* 162, 261–268. doi:10.1016/j.schres.2014.12.037

Bi, X., Yan, B., Fang, S., Yang, Y., He, J., Li, X. M., et al. (2009). Quetiapine regulates neurogenesis in ischemic mice by inhibiting NF-kappaB p65/p50 expression. *Neurol. Res.* 31, 159–166. doi:10.1179/174313209X393573

Bian, Q., Kato, T., Monji, A., Hashioka, S., Mizoguchi, Y., Horikawa, H., et al. (2008). The effect of atypical antipsychotics, perospirone, ziprasidone and quetiapine on microglial activation induced by interferon-gamma. *Prog. Neuropsychopharmacol. Biol. Psychiatry* 32, 42–48. doi:10.1016/j.pnpbp.2007.06.031

Brawek, B., and Garaschuk, O. (2013). Microglial calcium signaling in the adult, aged and diseased brain. *Cell Calcium* 53, 159–169. doi:10.1016/j.ceca.2012.12.003

Busse, S., Busse, M., Schiltz, K., Bielau, H., Gos, T., Brisch, R., et al. (2012). Different distribution patterns of lymphocytes and microglia in the hippocampus of patients with residual versus paranoid schizophrenia: further evidence for disease course-related immune alterations? *Brain Behav. Immun.* 26, 1273–1279. doi:10.1016/j.bbi.2012.08.005

Butovsky, O., Landa, G., Kunis, G., Ziv, Y., Avidan, H., Greenberg, N., et al. (2006). Induction and blockage of oligodendrogenesis by differently activated microglia in an animal model of multiple sclerosis. *J. Clin. Invest.* 116, 905–915. doi:10.1172/JCI26836

Chandran, P., Upadhyay, J., Markosyan, S., Lisowski, A., Buck, W., Chin, C. L., et al. (2012). Magnetic resonance imaging and histological evidence for the blockade of cuprizone-induced demyelination in C57BL/6 mice. *Neuroscience* 202, 446–453. doi:10.1016/j.neuroscience.2011.10.051

Chauhan, A., Sun, Y., Pani, B., Quenumzangbe, F., Sharma, J., Singh, B. B., et al. (2014). Helminth induced suppression of macrophage activation is correlated with inhibition of calcium channel activity. *PLoS ONE* 9:e101023. doi:10.1371/journal.pone.0101023

Doorduin, J., De Vries, E. F., Willemsen, A. T., De Groot, J. C., Dierckx, R. A., and Klein, H. C. (2009). Neuroinflammation in schizophrenia-related psychosis: a PET study. *J. Nucl. Med.* 50, 1801–1807. doi:10.2967/jnumed.109.066647

Emmetsberger, J., and Tsirka, S. E. (2012). Microglial inhibitory factor (MIF/TKP) mitigates secondary damage following spinal cord injury. *Neurobiol. Dis.* 47, 295–309. doi:10.1016/j.nbd.2012.05.001

Fan, B., Dun, S. H., Gu, J. Q., Guo, Y., and Ikuyama, S. (2015). Pycnogenol attenuates the release of proinflammatory cytokines and expression of Perilipin 2 in lipopolysaccharide-stimulated microglia in part via inhibition of NF-kappaB and AP-1 activation. *PLoS ONE* 10:e0137837. doi:10.1371/journal.pone.0137837

Feske, S. (2009). ORAI1 and STIM1 deficiency in human and mice: roles of store-operated Ca2+ entry in the immune system and beyond. *Immunol. Rev.* 231, 189–209. doi:10.1111/j.1600-065X.2009.00818.x

Fuchs, S., Rensing-Ehl, A., Speckmann, C., Bengsch, B., Schmitt-Graeff, A., Bondzio, I., et al. (2012). Antiviral and regulatory T cell immunity in a patient with stromal interaction molecule 1 deficiency. *J. Immunol.* 188, 1523–1533. doi:10.4049/jimmunol.1102507

Heo, D. K., Lim, H. M., Nam, J. H., Lee, M. G., and Kim, J. Y. (2015). Regulation of phagocytosis and cytokine secretion by store-operated calcium entry in primary isolated murine microglia. *Cell. Signal.* 27, 177–186. doi:10.1016/j.cellsig.2014.11.003

Hoffmann, A., Kann, O., Ohlemeyer, C., Hanisch, U. K., and Kettenmann, H. (2003). Elevation of basal intracellular calcium as a central element in the activation of brain macrophages (microglia): suppression of receptor-evoked calcium signaling and control of release function. *J. Neurosci.* 23, 4410–4419.

Hou, Y., Wu, C. F., Yang, J. Y., He, X., Bi, X. L., Yu, L., et al. (2006). Effects of clozapine, olanzapine and haloperidol on nitric oxide production by lipopolysaccharide-activated N9 cells. *Prog. Neuropsychopharmacol. Biol. Psychiatry* 30, 1523–1528. doi:10.1016/j.pnpbp.2006.05.006

Jack, C., Ruffini, F., Bar-Or, A., and Antel, J. P. (2005). Microglia and multiple sclerosis. *J. Neurosci. Res.* 81, 363–373. doi:10.1002/jnr.20482

Kasper, S., and Muller-Spahn, F. (2000). Review of quetiapine and its clinical applications in schizophrenia. *Expert Opin. Pharmacother.* 1, 783–801. doi:10.1517/14656566.1.4.783

Kato, T., Mizoguchi, Y., Monji, A., Horikawa, H., Suzuki, S. O., Seki, Y., et al. (2008). Inhibitory effects of aripiprazole on interferon-gamma-induced microglial activation via intracellular Ca2+ regulation in vitro. *J. Neurochem.* 106, 815–825. doi:10.1111/j.1471-4159.2008.05435.x

Kato, T. A., Monji, A., Yasukawa, K., Mizoguchi, Y., Horikawa, H., Seki, Y., et al. (2011). Aripiprazole inhibits superoxide generation from phorbol-myristate-acetate (PMA)-stimulated microglia in vitro: implication for antioxidative psychotropic actions via microglia. *Schizophr. Res.* 129, 172–182. doi:10.1016/j.schres.2011.03.019

Kato, T. A., Yamauchi, Y., Horikawa, H., Monji, A., Mizoguchi, Y., Seki, Y., et al. (2013). Neurotransmitters, psychotropic drugs and microglia: clinical implications for psychiatry. *Curr. Med. Chem.* 20, 331–344. doi:10.2174/092986713804870800

Kettenmann, H., Hanisch, U. K., Noda, M., and Verkhratsky, A. (2011). Physiology of microglia. *Physiol. Rev.* 91, 461–553. doi:10.1152/physrev.00011.2010

Kraft, R. (2015). STIM and ORAI proteins in the nervous system. *Channels* 245–252. doi:10.1080/19336950.2015.1071747

Laskaris, L. E., Di Biase, M. A., Everall, I., Chana, G., Christopoulos, A., Skafidas, E., et al. (2015). Microglial activation and progressive brain changes in schizophrenia. *Br. J. Pharmacol.* doi:10.1111/bph.13364

Lawson, L. J., Perry, V. H., Dri, P., and Gordon, S. (1990). Heterogeneity in the distribution and morphology of microglia in the normal adult mouse brain. *Neuroscience* 39, 151–170. doi:10.1016/0306-4522(90)90229-W

Li, Q., and Verma, I. M. (2002). NF-kappaB regulation in the immune system. *Nat. Rev. Immunol.* 2, 725–734. doi:10.1038/nri968

Liou, J., Kim, M. L., Heo, W. D., Jones, J. T., Myers, J. W., Ferrell, J. E. Jr., et al. (2005). STIM is a Ca2+ sensor essential for Ca2+-store-depletion-triggered Ca2+ influx. *Curr. Biol.* 15, 1235–1241. doi:10.1016/j.cub.2005.05.055

Luik, R. M., Wu, M. M., Buchanan, J., and Lewis, R. S. (2006). The elementary unit of store-operated Ca2+ entry: local activation of CRAC channels by STIM1 at ER-plasma membrane junctions. *J. Cell Biol.* 174, 815–825. doi:10.1083/jcb.200604015

Makinodan, M., Yamauchi, T., Tatsumi, K., Okuda, H., Takeda, T., Kiuchi, K., et al. (2009). Demyelination in the juvenile period, but not in adulthood, leads to long-lasting cognitive impairment and deficient social interaction in mice. *Prog. Neuropsychopharmacol. Biol. Psychiatry* 33, 978–985. doi:10.1016/j.pnpbp.2009.05.006

Mana, P., Linares, D., Fordham, S., Staykova, M., and Willenborg, D. (2006). Deleterious role of IFNgamma in a toxic model of central nervous system demyelination. *Am. J. Pathol.* 168, 1464–1473. doi:10.2353/ajpath.2006.050799

Matsushima, G. K., and Morell, P. (2001). The neurotoxicant, cuprizone, as a model to study demyelination and remyelination in the central nervous system. *Brain Pathol.* 11, 107–116. doi:10.1111/j.1750-3639.2001.tb00385.x

Mei, F., Guo, S., He, Y., Wang, L., Wang, H., Niu, J., et al. (2012). Quetiapine, an atypical antipsychotic, is protective against autoimmune-mediated demyelination by inhibiting effector T cell proliferation. *PLoS ONE* 7:e42746. doi:10.1371/journal.pone.0042746

Michaelis, M., Nieswandt, B., Stegner, D., Eilers, J., and Kraft, R. (2015). STIM1, STIM2, and Orai1 regulate store-operated calcium entry and purinergic activation of microglia. *Glia* 63, 652–663. doi:10.1002/glia.22775

Mizoguchi, Y., Kato, T. A., Horikawa, H., and Monji, A. (2014). Microglial intracellular Ca(2+) signaling as a target of antipsychotic actions for the treatment of schizophrenia. *Front. Cell. Neurosci.* 8:370. doi:10.3389/fncel.2014.00370

Mizoguchi, Y., Monji, A., Kato, T. A., Horikawa, H., Seki, Y., Kasai, M., et al. (2011). Possible role of BDNF-induced microglial intracellular Ca(2+) elevation in the pathophysiology of neuropsychiatric disorders. *Mini Rev. Med. Chem.* 11, 575–581. doi:10.2174/138955711795906932

Moccia, F., Zuccolo, E., Soda, T., Tanzi, F., Guerra, G., Mapelli, L., et al. (2015). Stim and Orai proteins in neuronal Ca(2+) signaling and excitability. *Front. Cell. Neurosci.* 9:153. doi:10.3389/fncel.2015.00153

Monji, A., Kato, T., and Kanba, S. (2009). Cytokines and schizophrenia: microglia hypothesis of schizophrenia. *Psychiatry Clin. Neurosci.* 63, 257–265. doi:10.1111/j.1440-1819.2009.01945.x

Monji, A., Kato, T. A., Mizoguchi, Y., Horikawa, H., Seki, Y., Kasai, M., et al. (2013). Neuroinflammation in schizophrenia especially focused on the role of microglia. *Prog. Neuropsychopharmacol. Biol. Psychiatry* 42, 115–121. doi:10.1016/j.pnpbp.2011.12.002

Niu, J., Mei, F., Li, N., Wang, H., Li, X., Kong, J., et al. (2010). Haloperidol promotes proliferation but inhibits differentiation in rat oligodendrocyte progenitor cell cultures. *Biochem. Cell Biol.* 88, 611–620. doi:10.1139/O09-178

Ohana, L., Newell, E. W., Stanley, E. F., and Schlichter, L. C. (2009). The Ca2+ release-activated Ca2+ current (I(CRAC)) mediates store-operated Ca2+ entry in rat microglia. *Channels* 3, 129–139. doi:10.4161/chan.3.2.8609

Paxinos, G., and Franklin, K. B. J. (2004). *The Mouse Brain in Stereotaxic Coordinates*. Amsterdam: Elsevier Academic Press.

Perry, V. H., Andersson, P. B., and Gordon, S. (1993). Macrophages and inflammation in the central nervous system. *Trends Neurosci.* 16, 268–273. doi:10.1016/0166-2236(93)90180-T

Potvin, S., Stip, E., Sepehry, A. A., Gendron, A., Bah, R., and Kouassi, E. (2008). Inflammatory cytokine alterations in schizophrenia: a systematic quantitative review. *Biol. Psychiatry* 63, 801–808. doi:10.1016/j.biopsych.2007.09.024

Praet, J., Guglielmetti, C., Berneman, Z., Van Der Linden, A., and Ponsaerts, P. (2014). Cellular and molecular neuropathology of the cuprizone mouse model: clinical relevance for multiple sclerosis. *Neurosci. Biobehav. Rev.* 47, 485–505. doi:10.1016/j.neubiorev.2014.10.004

Probert, L. (2015). TNF and its receptors in the CNS: the essential, the desirable and the deleterious effects. *Neuroscience* 302, 2–22. doi:10.1016/j.neuroscience.2015.06.038

Puntambekar, S. S., Hinton, D. R., Yin, X., Savarin, C., Bergmann, C. C., Trapp, B. D., et al. (2015). Interleukin-10 is a critical regulator of white matter lesion containment following viral induced demyelination. *Glia.* 63, 2106–2120. doi:10.1002/glia.22880

Qian, L., Flood, P. M., and Hong, J. S. (2010). Neuroinflammation is a key player in Parkinson's disease and a prime target for therapy. *J. Neural Transm.* 117, 971–979. doi:10.1007/s00702-010-0428-1

Ren, Y., Wang, H., and Xiao, L. (2013). Improving myelin/oligodendrocyte-related dysfunction: a new mechanism of antipsychotics in the treatment of schizophrenia? *Int. J. Neuropsychopharmacol.* 16, 691–700. doi:10.1017/S1461145712001095

Riedel, M., Muller, N., Strassnig, M., Spellmann, I., Severus, E., and Moller, H. J. (2007). Quetiapine in the treatment of schizophrenia and related disorders. *Neuropsychiatr. Dis. Treat.* 3, 219–235. doi:10.2147/nedt.2007.3.2.219

Roos, J., Digregorio, P. J., Yeromin, A. V., Ohlsen, K., Lioudyno, M., Zhang, S., et al. (2005). STIM1, an essential and conserved component of store-operated Ca2+ channel function. *J. Cell Biol.* 169, 435–445. doi:10.1083/jcb.200502019

Roussos, P., and Haroutunian, V. (2014). Schizophrenia: susceptibility genes and oligodendroglial and myelin related abnormalities. *Front. Cell. Neurosci.* 8:5. doi:10.3389/fncel.2014.00005

Schmitz, T., Heep, A., Groenendaal, F., Huseman, D., Kie, S., Bartmann, P., et al. (2007). Interleukin-1beta, interleukin-18, and interferon-gamma expression in the cerebrospinal fluid of premature infants with posthemorrhagic hydrocephalus – markers of white matter damage? *Pediatr. Res.* 61, 722–726. doi:10.1203/pdr.0b013e31805341f1

Shao, Y., Peng, H., Huang, Q., Kong, J., and Xu, H. (2015). Quetiapine mitigates the neuroinflammation and oligodendrocyte loss in the brain of C57BL/6 mouse following cuprizone exposure for one week. *Eur. J. Pharmacol.* 765, 249–257. doi:10.1016/j.ejphar.2015.08.046

Smith, A. M., and Dragunow, M. (2014). The human side of microglia. *Trends Neurosci.* 37, 125–135. doi:10.1016/j.tins.2013.12.001

Steiner, J., Bielau, H., Brisch, R., Danos, P., Ullrich, O., Mawrin, C., et al. (2008). Immunological aspects in the neurobiology of suicide: elevated microglial density in schizophrenia and depression is associated with suicide. *J. Psychiatr. Res.* 42, 151–157. doi:10.1016/j.jpsychires.2006.10.013

Streit, W. J., Xue, Q. S., Tischer, J., and Bechmann, I. (2014). Microglial pathology. *Acta Neuropathol. Commun.* 2, 142. doi:10.1186/s40478-014-0142-6

Sun, Y., Chauhan, A., Sukumaran, P., Sharma, J., Singh, B. B., and Mishra, B. B. (2014). Inhibition of store-operated calcium entry in microglia by helminth factors: implications for immune suppression in neurocysticercosis. *J. Neuroinflammation* 11, 210. doi:10.1186/s12974-014-0210-7

Tasker, R. C. (2006). Changes in white matter late after severe traumatic brain injury in childhood. *Dev. Neurosci.* 28, 302–308. doi:10.1159/000094156

Vallabhapurapu, S., and Karin, M. (2009). Regulation and function of NF-kappaB transcription factors in the immune system. *Annu. Rev. Immunol.* 27, 693–733. doi:10.1146/annurev.immunol.021908.132641

Vela, J. M., Molina-Holgado, E., Arevalo-Martin, A., Almazan, G., and Guaza, C. (2002). Interleukin-1 regulates proliferation and differentiation of oligodendrocyte progenitor cells *Mol. Cell. Neurosci.* 20, 489–502. doi:10.1006/mcne.2002.1127

Wang, H., Xu, H., Niu, J., Mei, F., Li, X., Kong, J., et al. (2010). Haloperidol activates quiescent oligodendroglia precursor cells in the adult mouse brain. *Schizophr. Res.* 119, 164–174. doi:10.1016/j.schres.2010.02.1068

Wang, W. Y., Tan, M. S., Yu, J. T., and Tan, L. (2015). Role of pro-inflammatory cytokines released from microglia in Alzheimer's disease. *Ann. Transl. Med.* 3, 136. doi:10.3978/j.issn.2305-5839.2015.03.49

Watkins, C. C., and Andrews, S. R. (2015). Clinical studies of neuroinflammatory mechanisms in schizophrenia. *Schizophr. Res.* doi:10.1016/j.schres.2015.07.018

Xiao, L., Xu, H., Zhang, Y., Wei, Z., He, J., Jiang, W., et al. (2008). Quetiapine facilitates oligodendrocyte development and prevents mice from myelin breakdown and behavioral changes. *Mol. Psychiatry* 13, 697–708. doi:10.1038/sj.mp.4002064

Xu, H., Yang, H. J., Mcconomy, B., Browning, R., and Li, X. M. (2010). Behavioral and neurobiological changes in C57BL/6 mouse exposed to cuprizone: effects of antipsychotics. *Front. Behav. Neurosci.* 4:8. doi:10.3389/fnbeh.2010.00008

Xu, H., Yang, H. J., Rose, G. M., and Li, X. M. (2011). Recovery of behavioral changes and compromised white matter in C57BL/6 mice exposed to cuprizone: effects of antipsychotic drugs. *Front. Behav. Neurosci.* 5:31. doi:10.3389/fnbeh.2011.00031

Xu, H., Yang, H. J., Zhang, Y., Clough, R., Browning, R., and Li, X. M. (2009). Behavioral and neurobiological changes in C57BL/6 mice exposed to cuprizone. *Behav. Neurosci.* 123, 418–429. doi:10.1037/a0014477

Zhang, Y., Xu, H., Jiang, W., Xiao, L., Yan, B., He, J., et al. (2008). Quetiapine alleviates the cuprizone-induced white matter pathology in the brain of C57BL/6 mouse. *Schizophr. Res.* 106, 182–191. doi:10.1016/j.schres.2008.09.013

Zhang, Y., Zhang, H., Wang, L., Jiang, W., Xu, H., Xiao, L., et al. (2012). Quetiapine enhances oligodendrocyte regeneration and myelin repair after cuprizone-induced demyelination. *Schizophr. Res.* 138, 8–17. doi:10.1016/j.schres.2012.04.006

Zhao, Z., Luo, G., Liu, M., Guo, H., Xue, M., Wang, X., et al. (2014). Quetiapine reduces microglial number in the hippocampus of a transgenic mouse model of Alzheimer's disease. *Neuroreport.* 25, 870–874. doi:10.1097/WNR.0000000000000209

Zheng, L. T., Hwang, J., Ock, J., Lee, M. G., Lee, W. H., and Suk, K. (2008). The antipsychotic spiperone attenuates inflammatory response in cultured microglia via the reduction of proinflammatory cytokine expression and nitric oxide production. *J. Neurochem.* 107, 1225–1235. doi:10.1111/j.1471-4159.2008.05675.x

Zhou, J., Cai, W., Jin, M., Xu, J., Wang, Y., Xiao, Y., et al. (2015). 18beta-glycyrrhetinic acid suppresses experimental autoimmune encephalomyelitis through inhibition of microglia activation and promotion of remyelination. *Sci. Rep.* 5, 13713. doi:10.1038/srep13713

Zhu, S., Shi, R., Li, V., Wang, J., Zhang, R., Tempier, A., et al. (2015). Quetiapine attenuates glial activation and proinflammatory cytokines in APP/PS1 transgenic mice via inhibition of nuclear factor-kappaB pathway. *Int. J. Neuropsychopharmacol.* 18. doi:10.1093/ijnp/pyu022

6

# Reduced Density of Glutamine Synthetase Immunoreactive Astrocytes in Different Cortical Areas in Major Depression but not in Bipolar I Disorder

**Hans-Gert Bernstein[1]*, Gabriela Meyer-Lotz[1], Henrik Dobrowolny[1], Jana Bannier[1], Johann Steiner[1], Martin Walter[1,2] and Bernhard Bogerts[1]**

[1] Department of Psychiatry, University of Magdeburg, Magdeburg, Germany, [2] Clinical Affective Neuroimaging Laboratory, University of Magdeburg, Magdeburg, Germany

***Correspondence:**
Hans-Gert Bernstein,
Department of Psychiatry, University of Magdeburg, Leipziger Strasse 44, 39120 Magdeburg, Germany
hans-gert.bernstein@med.ovgu.de

There is increasing evidence for disturbances within the glutamate system in patients with affective disorders, which involve disruptions of the glutamate–glutamine-cycle. The mainly astroglia-located enzyme glutamine synthetase (GS) catalyzes the ATP-dependent condensation of ammonia and glutamate to form glutamine, thus playing a central role in glutamate and glutamine homoeostasis. However, GS is also expressed in numerous oligodendrocytes (OLs), another class of glial cells implicated in mood disorder pathology. To learn more about the role of glia-associated GS in mental illnesses, we decided to find out if numerical densities of glial cells immunostained for the enzyme protein differ between subjects with major depressive disorder, bipolar disorder (BD), and psychically healthy control cases. Counting of GS expressing astrocytes (ACs) and OLs in eight cortical and two subcortical brain regions of subjects with mood disorder ($N = 14$), BD ($N = 15$), and controls ($N = 16$) revealed that in major depression the densities of ACs were significantly reduced in some cortical but not subcortical gray matter areas, whereas no changes were found for OLs. In BD no alterations of GS-immunoreactive glia were found. From our findings we conclude that (1) GS expressing ACs are prominently involved in glutamate-related disturbances in major depression, but not in BD and (2) GS expressing OLs, though being present in significant numbers in prefrontal cortical areas, play a minor (if any) role in mood disorder pathology. The latter assumption is supported by findings of others showing that – at least in the mouse brain cortex – GS immunoreactive oligodendroglial cells are unable to contribute to the glutamate–glutamine-cycle due to the complete lack of amino acid transporters (Takasaki et al., 2010).

**Keywords: major depression, bipolar disorder, cortex, glutamine synthetase, astroglia, oligodendroglia, immunocytochemistry**

---

**Abbreviations:** AC(s), astrocyte(s); Aic, anterior insular cortex; ANOVA, A single-factor analysis of variance; ATP, adenosine triphosphate; BD, bipolar disorder; CNS, Central Nervous System; DLPFC, dorso-lateral prefrontal cortex; GABA, γ-Aminobutyric acid; DSM-IV; Diagnostic and Statistical Manual of Mental Disorders IVth edition; GFAP; glial fibrillary acidic protein; Glx, glutamate-glutamine-GABA complex; GS, glutamine synthetase; MANOVA, Multivariate analysis of covariance; MDD, major depression disorder; MSR, Magnetic Resonance Spectroscopy; OL(s), oligodendrocyte(s); n.a., not available; NAc, Nuc. Accumbens; pACC, pregenual anterior cingulate; PBS, Phosphate buffered saline; sACC, subgenual anterior cingulate cortex.

## Introduction

Initially, search for the possible cellular substrate of mood disorder pathology had focused on neurons (Rajkowska, 2000, 2002; Cotter et al., 2001a,b, 2002; Manji et al., 2001). However, during the last years a wave of information appeared to suggest that glial cells prominently, and in many ways, contribute to brain structural and functional changes in mood disorders. In numerous histological postmortem investigations both significantly reduced (Öngür et al., 1998; Rajkowska, 2000; Cotter et al., 2001a,b; Hamidi et al., 2004; Uranova et al., 2004; Rajkowska and Miguel-Hidalgo, 2007; Altshuler et al., 2010; Gos et al., 2013) and increased (Davis et al., 2002; Mosebach et al., 2013; Malchow et al., 2014) glial cell numbers and numerical densities have been observed in prefrontal cortex areas and limbic regions. In addition, characteristic changes in gene expression patterns and metabolic pathways of glial cells have been found in affective disorders (reviewed in Barley et al., 2009; Steiner et al., 2012; Mosebach et al., 2013; Duncan et al., 2014; Schroeter et al., 2014; Bernstein et al., 2015). Of note, each of the three glial cell classes (i.e., ACs, OLs, and microglia) appears to confer its unique contribution to the pathophysiology of affective disorders. Moreover, their impact may be different in MDD (Verkhratsky et al., 2014) and in BD, (Savitz et al., 2014; Dong and Zhen, 2015). In this context, much attention has been paid to the possible role of ACs in MDD and BD pathology. Being the most prevalent cell type in the human brain, ACs serve a wide range of different functions in the CNS. They play important roles in synaptic transmission, control of neuronal metabolism, sensing of brain microenvironment, maintenance of blood-brain barrier integrity, brain defense and inflammatory processes (Sofroniew and Vinters, 2010; Teschemacher et al., 2015). Since synaptic, metabolic and inflammatory dysregulation are reported in MDD and BD (Harrison, 2002; Si et al., 2004; Kato et al., 2013; Duman, 2014; Maletic and Raison, 2014; and others), AC abnormalities may be implicated in these disorders. ACs exert influence on cerebral information processing mainly in two ways: (1) they release, by exocytosis, gliotransmitters (glutamate, D-serine, GABA and ATP, Sahlender et al., 2014), which facilitate the communication between neurons and neuron-glia crosstalk, and (2) they remove glutamate from extracellular space and provide glutamatergic and GABAergic neurons with glutamine, which they synthesize from glutamate, ammonia and ATP (Anlauf and Derouiche, 2013). Theoretically, impaired release of gliotransmitters (Van Horn et al., 2013) and/or compromised glutamate uptake and recycling by ACs might significantly contribute to anomalies of glutamatergic (and, most probably, GABAergic) neurotransmission reported in MDD and BD (for reviews, see Walter et al., 2009; Brennan et al., 2010; Gigante et al., 2012; Salvadore et al., 2012; Bernstein et al., 2013; Dou et al., 2013; Duman, 2014; Arnone et al., 2015; Pehrson and Sanchez, 2015). However, while knowledge about the possible impact of gliotransmitters on mood disorder pathology is still fragmentary (Etiévant et al., 2013), there is some good evidence in favor of impaired AC-related glutamate-glutamine cycling as an important contributing factor in affective disorders (reviewed in detail by Bernstein et al., 2013 and Rajkowska and Stockmeier, 2013). Due to its central position in the glutamate–glutamine–GABA cycle, the glutamine-synthesizing enzyme GS (aka glutamate-ammonia ligase, EC 6.3.1.2) came early into focus of research, and a number of papers have meanwhile been published about alterations in GS in MDD and BD. In subjects with MDD a majority of studies show a decrease of cerebral GS. The expression of GS mRNA was reported to be down-regulated in the prefrontal cortex, the premotor cortex, and the amygdala of depressed suicide victims but not in suicide completers without depression (Choudary et al., 2005; Sequeira et al., 2009), whereas GS protein was found to be reduced in the anterior cingulate cortex and the orbitofrontal cortex (Choudary et al., 2005; Beasley et al., 2006; Miguel-Hidalgo et al., 2010; Rajkowska and Stockmeier, 2013). However, no alterations in cortical GS of MDD subjects were found by others (Toro et al., 2006). The implication of GS for BD is less well explored, and the sparse data are inconsistent. GS expression was reported unchanged (Toro et al., 2006) or decreased (Choudary et al., 2005) in the prefrontal cortex of bipolar subjects. Remarkably, all but one (Toro et al., 2006) studies on GS expression in mood disorders used biochemical techniques. Thus, little attention has yet been paid to the type of GS-expressing cells, although there is evidence that GS can also be detected in extra-astroglial localizations [i.e., in numerous OLs and even in some neurons (Takasaki et al., 2010; Iwata et al., 2013; Bernstein et al., 2014 and others)]. Thus, theoretically, disease-related alterations of GS expression might involve non-astroglial cells, too. We, therefore, counted GS expressing glial cells in ten different cortical and subcortical brain areas of subjects with MDD, BD, and psychically healthy controls and show herein that (1) significantly reduced densities of GS-immunoreactive glial cells occur in cortical areas of MDD, but not BD subjects and (2) these changes are restricted to GS expressing ACs, whereas GS expressing OLs are normal in mood disorders.

## Materials and Methods

### Subjects

All brains were obtained from the New Magdeburg brain collection. Case recruitment, acquisition of personal data, performance of autopsy, and handling of autoptic material were conducted in strict accordance with the Declaration of Helsinki, and have been approved by the responsible Ethical Committee of Magdeburg. Written consent was obtained from the next-of-kin. Information for clinical diagnoses was obtained from clinical records and/or structural interviews of physicians involved in treatment or relatives (Bielau et al., 2005).

Brains of 29 human subjects with mood disorders according to DSM-IV were studied. Of these individuals 14 (8 female, 6 male; mean age: 46.9 ± 11.4 years) had suffered from a MDD and 15 (5 female, 10 male; mean age: 53.5 ± 10.4 years) had a BD. Sixteen control individuals (9 female, 7 male; mean age: 50.4 ± 11.0 years) without a history of neuropsychiatric disorder were also investigated. None of the patients or controls had a history of substance abuse or alcoholism. Neuropathological changes due to neurodegenerative or traumatic processes were ruled out by an experienced neuropathologist as previously described (Bielau et al., 2005). These cases were matched with respect to age, gender, and autolysis time. The matching processes were done prior to all analyses. For demographical, clinical, and psychopharmacological details see **Tables 1** and **2**. The mean daily doses of psychotropic medication taken by patients during the last 90 lifetime days were established according to the clinical files. Since our brain bank has been established about 25 years ago, patients received tricyclic antidepressants instead of selective serotonin or noradrenalin reuptake inhibitors (for detailed considerations, see Mosebach et al., 2013).

## Tissue Processing

Brains were removed within 4–96 h after death and fixed in toto in 8% phosphate-buffered formaldehyde for at least 2 months ($pH = 7.0$, $T = 15–20°C$).

Frontal and occipital poles were separated by coronal cuts 0.9 cm anterior to the genu and posterior to the splenium of the corpus callosum. After embedding of all parts of the brains in paraffin, serial coronal sections of the prefrontal and the middle blocks were cut (20 $\mu$m) and mounted. The shrinkage factor caused by fixation and embedding of the brains was calculated by a method described previously (Bernstein et al., 1998a). The mean volume shrinkage factor for patients with affective disorders and controls was 2.21. No significant differences in the shrinkage factors among the three groups MDD, BP, and controls were found. Every 50th section was Nissl and myelin stained as described previously (Bernstein et al., 1998b).

## Glutamine Synthetase Immunohistochemistry

For immunohistochemical stainings, whole brain sections were collected at intervals of about 0.2 cm between 1.8 and 1 cm rostral to the genu of the corpus callosum. The pACC, (Brodmann Area 32) and dorsolateral prefrontal (DLPFC, Brodmann Area 9) cortices were easily identifiable using the "Atlas of the Human Brain" by Mai et al. (2003). Sections containing the left and right sACC, Aic, (Brodmann area 14), and the NAc were selected at intervals of 0.2 cm. To immunolocalize GS, we employed a well-characterized, monospecific polyclonal antiserum generated in rabbits against human GS (Prestige Antibody HPA 007316; Lot C 81287; from Sigma-Aldrich, Munich, Germany). Since different lots of the same antibody may considerably differ with regard to their staining properties (Couchman, 2009), we tested three different lots of the GS antiserum HPA 007316 (namely A42599, C81287, R04375). In our hands all three lots were of the same superior quality, and we decided to continue working with Lot C 81287. After dewaxing antigen demasking was carried out by boiling the sections for 4 min in 10 mM citrate buffer (pH 6.0). Thereafter, the sections were pre-incubated with methanol/$H_2O_2$ to suppress endogenous peroxidases and repeatedly washed with PBS. Subsequently, the primary GS antibody was applied at a dilution of 1:500 for 72 h at 4°C. Sections were then incubated with a biotinylated anti rabbit IgG (Amersham Bioscience, Buckinghamshire, GB), followed by the streptavidin horse radish complex for the application of the streptavidin–biotin technique (Amersham). The chromogen 3,3′-diaminobenzidine was used to visualize the reaction product. Subsequently, ammonium nickel sulfate hexahydrate was added to enhance the immunoreaction (Bernstein et al., 2013). For control purposes, the primary antiserum was replaced by either buffer or normal serum. Further control experiments involved the application of the GS antiserum after preabsorption with GS protein (recombinant human GS, charge number CE02; from Novoprotein, Shanghai, China) as described earlier in detail (Bernstein et al., 2014). When these controls were done the investigated regions did not show any specific immunostaining.

## Glial Fibrillary Acidic Protein (GFAP) Immunohistochemistry

For reasons of comparison and better delineation of cortical gray matter areas sections adjacent to GS immunostained ones were immunolabeled for GFAP. A monoclonal antibody (diluted 1:100 in PBS, from DAKO) was used. The secondary antibody was an anti-mouse peroxidase (from Biozol, Eching, Germany; dilution 1:50). The working dilution was 1:2000. Visualization was as described for GS. Controls involved replacement of the primary antiserum by either buffer or normal serum.

## Cell Countings

The actual section thickness after the histological procedures was 18.9 $\pm$ 1.0 $\mu$m (mean $\pm$ SD). The optical disector cell-counting method was employed. Cell countings were performed in two coronal sections per brain area under blind conditions. A counting grid was used to define a three-dimensional box within the thickness of the section as described previously (Bernstein et al., 1998b) allowing at least 4 $\mu$M guard zones at the top and bottom of the section, and to apply a direct, three-dimensional counting method. Fifteen consecutive boxes per left and right cortical area were positioned, spanning the layers I and II, layer III, and another 15 spanning the layers IV, V, and VI, thus subdividing cortical gray matter regions into superficial and deep layers as proposed by Katsel et al. (2011). To count immunostained cells in the NAc we used 15 boxes per section and hemisphere. The packing densities of glial cells are noted as the number of cells $\times 10^3/mm^3$. The product of the volume and glial cell density provided the total cell number estimates. The inter-rater reliability was about 0.87. In a few cases we observed some local tissue damage in the brain region of interest. Cell counts of these particular regions were rigorously excluded from further calculations, which resulted in smaller cohorts than nominally indicated (for example, number of right NAc in MDD subjects: 12 instead of 14 cases).

## Statistical Analysis

A single-factor analysis of variance was performed using diagnostic groups as a three-level independent variable (MDD patients versus BD versus non-psychiatric controls) and measured and calculated parameters were treated as dependent variables. MANOVA was performed with diagnosis and side, ie., left and right hemisphere, as independent variables (repeated measures). Effect sizes were determined for 3-group comparisons

**TABLE 1 | Demographical data of patients and controls.**

| Diagnosis case | Gender | Age (years) | Postmortem autolysis time (h) | Duration of illness/years | Cause of death |
|---|---|---|---|---|---|
| **MDD ($n = 14$)** | | | | | |
| 1 | Male | 42 | 5 | n.a. | Suicide (hanging) |
| 2 | Female | 39 | 48 | 7 | Suicide (benzodiazepines overdose) |
| 3 | Female | 46 | 48 | 11 | Suicide (hanging) |
| 4 | Female | 53 | 48 | n.a. | Suicide (hanging) |
| 5 | Female | 63 | 17 | 2 | Pulmonary embolism |
| 6 | Female | 61 | 70 | 11 | Heart failure |
| 8 | Male | 35 | 24 | 2 | Suicide (slitting of the wrists) |
| 9 | Male | 36 | 48 | 1 | Suicide (hanging) |
| 10 | Male | 42 | 24 | n.a. | Acute pancreatitis |
| 11 | Male | 30 | 24 | n.a. | Suicide (hanging) |
| 12 | Female | 60 | 24 | 1 | Suicide (hanging) |
| 13 | Female | 59 | 48 | 4 | Suicide (hanging) |
| 14 | Female | 35 | 24 | n.a. | Suicide (strangulation) |
| 15 | Male | 55 | 24 | n.a. | Suicide (strangulation) |
| | **8 Female/6 Male** | **46.9 ± 11.4** | **34.0 ± 17.6** | **4.9 ± 4.3** | |
| **BD ($n = 15$)** | | | | | |
| 16 | Male | 47 | 24 | 9 | Suicide (stabbing) |
| 17 | Female | 46 | 4 | 13 | Suicide (tablet intoxication) |
| 18 | Male | 42 | 12 | 16 | Suicide (hanging) |
| 19 | Female | 62 | 72 | 11 | Pulmonary embolism |
| 21 | Male | 39 | 24 | 2 | Pulmonary embolism |
| 22 | Female | 59 | 72 | 24 | Suicide (tablet intoxication) |
| 23 | Male | 39 | 56 | 14 | Myocardial infarction |
| 24 | Male | 69 | 48 | 26 | Pulmonary embolism |
| 25 | Male | 69 | 24 | 18 | Heart failure, pulmonary embolism |
| 26 | Female | 52 | 24 | 16 | Heart failure, pulmonary embolism |
| 27 | Female | 65 | 52 | 25 | Heart failure |
| 28 | Male | 44 | 96 | 6 | Trombosis after myocardial infarction |
| 29 | Male | 57 | 48 | n.a. | Suicide (strangulation) |
| 30 | Male | 60 | 24 | 5 | Suicide (strangulation) |
| 31 | Male | 53 | 24 | 1 | Suicide (strangulation) |
| | **5 female/10 Male** | **53.5 ± 10.4** | **40.3 ± 25.8** | **13.3 ± 8.2** | |
| **Depression** | **13 female/16 Male** | **50.3 ± 11.2** | **37.2 ± 22.1** | **10.2 ± 8.1** | |
| **Controls ($n = 16$)** | | | | | |
| 31 | Male | 56 | 48 | 0 | Retroperitoneal hemorrhage |
| 34 | Female | 52 | 24 | 0 | Heart failure, renal insufficiency |
| 35 | Female | 48 | 48 | 0 | Status asthmaticus |
| 38 | Female | 33 | 72 | 0 | Aortic embolism |
| 39 | Female | 50 | 72 | 0 | Ruptured aortic aneurysm |
| 40 | Male | 40 | 96 | 0 | Myocardial infarction |
| 41 | Male | 64 | 36 | 0 | Ruptured aortic aneurysm |
| 42 | Female | 48 | 26 | 0 | Pulmonary embolism |
| 43 | Male | 56 | 24 | 0 | Myocardial infarction |
| 44 | Female | 65 | 24 | 0 | Heart failure |
| 45 | Female | 30 | 48 | 0 | Pulmonary embolism |
| 46 | Male | 63 | 48 | 0 | Heart failure (after heart surgery) |
| 47 | Female | 38 | 24 | 0 | Heart failure |
| 48 | Male | 54 | 24 | 0 | Pulmonary embolism |
| 49 | Male | 46 | 24 | 0 | Heart failure, cancer |
| 50 | Female | 63 | 24 | 0 | Myocardial infarction |
| | **9 Female/7 Male** | **50.4 ± 11.0** | **41.4 ± 22.2** | – | |

**TABLE 2 | Psychopharmacological treatment.**

| Case | Mean antidepressiva dose of the last days [mg] | Mean neuroleptics dose of the last days [mg] | Mean benzodiazepine dose of the last days [mg] | Mean carbamazepine dose of the last days [mg] | Mean lithium dose of the last days [mg] |
|---|---|---|---|---|---|
| **MDD ($n = 14$)** | | | | | |
| 1 | n.a. | n.a. | n.a. | n.a. | n.a. |
| 2 | 93 | 0 | 3 | 0 | 560 |
| 3 | 124 | 109 | 0 | 0 | 0 |
| 4 | 0 | 0 | 0 | 0 | 0 |
| 5 | 50 | 0 | 0 | 0 | 0 |
| 6 | 30 | 111 | 16 | 0 | 0 |
| 8 | 0 | 0 | 0 | 0 | 0 |
| 9 | 0 | 0 | 0 | 0 | 0 |
| 10 | 200 | 200 | n.a. | n.a. | n.a. |
| 11 | 100 | 100 | n.a. | n.a. | n.a. |
| 12 | 100 | 440 | 0 | 0 | 0 |
| 13 | n.a. | n.a. | n.a. | n.a. | n.a. |
| 14 | n.a. | n.a. | n.a. | n.a. | n.a. |
| **BD ($n = 15$)** | | | | | |
| 16 | 20 | 0 | 0 | 0 | 0 |
| 17 | 133 | 327 | 3 | 0 | 558 |
| 18 | 95 | 47 | 18 | 0 | 565 |
| 19 | 0 | 110 | 18 | 0 | 0 |
| 21 | 0 | 280 | 0 | 0 | 0 |
| 22 | 112 | 0 | 10 | 600 | 0 |
| 23 | 0 | 221 | 1 | 0 | 740 |
| 24 | 0 | 0 | 7 | 0 | 0 |
| 25 | 0 | 0 | 2 | 0 | 280 |
| 26 | 0 | n.a. | n.a. | n.a. | n.a. |
| 27 | 93 | 117 | 4 | 0 | 0 |
| 28 | n.a. | n.a. | n.a. | n.a. | n.a. |
| 29 | n.a. | n.a. | n.a. | n.a. | n.a. |
| 30 | n.a. | n.a. | n.a. | n.a. | n.a. |
| 31 | 150 | 200 | 0 | 200 | 0 |

(major depressive disorder, BD, controls). Confounding variables including whole brain volume were primarily tested on normality by use of the Kolmogorov–Smirnov test. A *post hoc* Tukey HSD test was conducted to determine which variables were significantly different from each other. Pearson correlation tests were carried out to investigate effects of postmortem delay, time of fixation, illness duration, number of illness episodes, and psychotropic medication (i.e., antidepressants, neuroleptics, benzodiazepines, and lithium) on data. In addition, emphasis was given to suicide as possible confounding factor. $P$-values less than 0.05 were deemed to be statistically significant.

## Results

### Qualitative Observations

#### Glutamine Synthetase Immunostaining

##### *Astrocytes*

Glutamine synthetase -immunoreactive ACs were abundantly present in the cerebral cortex and the NAc. Their morphology was remarkably consistent. Astrocytic somata and processes were prominently stained for GS. In addition, an intense immunostaining was observed in the neuropil. Numerous blood vessels were surrounded by GS-immunoreactive AC endfeet.

##### *Oligodendrocytes*

Gray matter GS-immunoreactive OLs were easily identifiable based on their typical morphology. The immunoreaction was confined to the cell somata. Short processes were only infrequently immunolabeled. Immunopositive OLs were fairly uniformly distributed throughout prefrontal cerebral cortex. However, in the AiC and the NAc GS-expressing OLs were relatively rarely found. Therefore, we did not count them separately in the latter two brain regions. Examples for the immunolocalization of GS in ACs and OLs are given in **Figures 1A–I. Figure 1J** shows a control reaction.

#### GFAP Immunostaining

In all cortical areas GFAP protein was expressed in a majority of ACs. Their distribution showed a laminar pattern. The highest package density of GFAP was found in layers I (where ACs abut at the pial surface of the brain, Miguel-Hidalgo et al., 2010) and

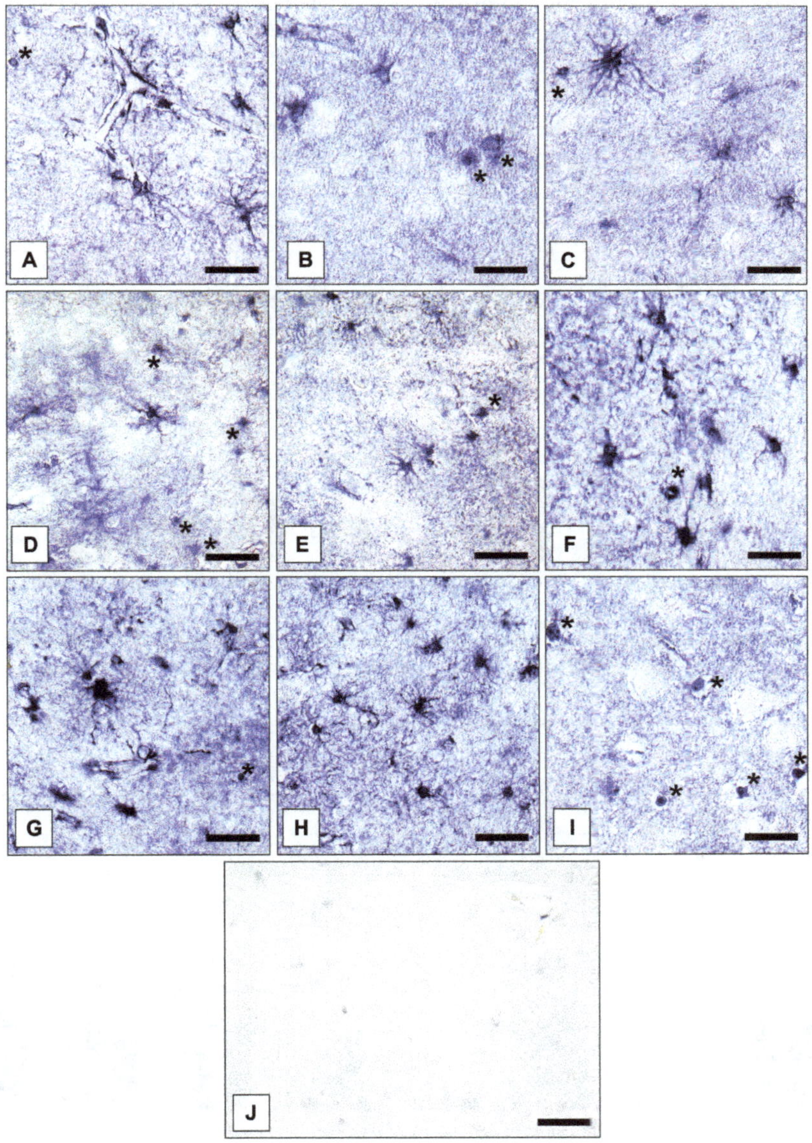

**FIGURE 1 | Immunolocalization of GS in cortical and subcortical human brain glial cells in MDD, BD, and controls. (A)** GS-immunoreactive ACs and OLs (asterisk) in the pACC (control case). Bar = 20 μm. **(B)** GS-immunoreactive ACs and OLs (asterisks) in the pACC (MDD subject). Bar = 20 μm. **(C)** GS-immunoreactive ACs and OLs (asterisk) in the pACC (BD subject). Bar = 20 μm. **(D)** GS-immunoreactive ACs and OLs (asterisks) in the sACC (control case). Bar = 20 μm.**(E)** GS-expressing ACs and OLs (asterisk) in the sACC (MDD subject). Bar = 20 μm.**(F)** GS-expressing ACs and OLs (asterisk) in the DLPFC (BD subject). Bar = 20 μm. **(G)** GS-immunopositive ACs in the AiC (control case). Bar = 20 μm. **(H)** GS-expressing ACs in the NAc (control case). Bar = 24 μm. **(I)** GS-immunoreactive OLs (asterisks) in the pACC (control case). Bar = 20 μm. **(J)** Specificity control reaction. After preabsorption of the primary antiserum with recombinant GS protein no specific immunostaining is visible. Bar = 30 μm.

II. In the NAc an even distribution of GFAP immunolabeled cell elements was observed. OLs did not express GFAP.

## Quantitative Estimates

We could replicate our own findings (Bernstein et al., 2014) as well as results previously published by others (Toro et al., 2006) that there is a higher density of GS-expressing cells in superficial cortical layers I–III than in deeper cortical layers IV–VI. It is therefore justified to count superficial and deeper layers separately.

In subjects with mood disorder significantly reduced numerical densities of GS immunoreactive ACs were found the DLPFC (left side, layers I–III, $p = 0.029$; $F = 4.487$ and right side, layers I–III; $p = 0.046$; $F = 3.647$), sACC (left side, layers I–III, $p = 0.021$; $F = 4.304$), AiC (left side, layers I–III, $p = 0.002$; $F = 7.893$; right side, layers I–III, $p = 0.001$; $F = 9.789$; ride side, layers IV–VI, $p = 0.015$; $F = 5.136$). No significant changes were detectable in the pACC and the NAc. All but one (DLPCC right side, layers I–III) significant changes survived Tukey's HSD *post hoc* tests. Notably, no significant alterations in the numerical densities of OLs were found. Results of the morphometric analyses are shown in **Figures 2–6**.

## MDD vs. controls

Compared with controls a significant reduction in the numerical densities of GS-immunopositive ACs was found in MDD in five of the 10 cortical and subcortical brain regions studied: DLPFC (left side, layers I–III, $p = 0.024$), sACC (left side, layers I–III, $p = 0.018$); AiC (left side, layers I–III; $p = 0.002$; right side, layers I–III; $p = 0.001$; $F = 9.962$; right side, layers IV–VI, $p = 0.012$).

## BD vs. controls

In BD cases the numerical densities of GS-expressing ACs and OLs did not significantly differ from those of controls.

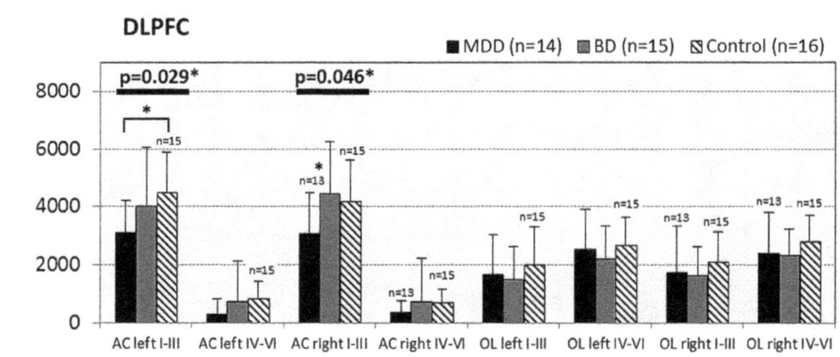


**FIGURE 2 | Numerical densities of GS-expressing glial cells (ACs and OLs) in the DLPFC of subjects with MDD, BD, and controls.** Compared with controls the density of GS-expressing ACs is significantly reduced in MDD cases (AC left I–III, $p = 0.029$; AC right I–III, $p = 0.046$).

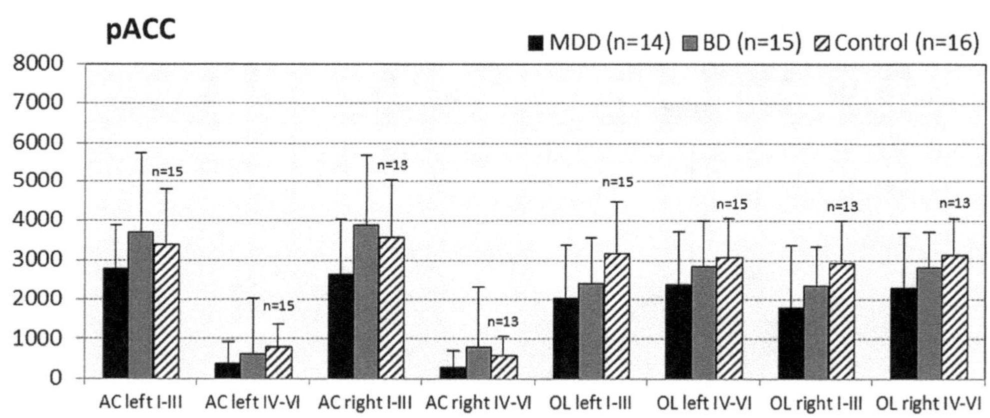


**FIGURE 3 | Numerical densities of GS-expressing glial cells (ACs and OLs) in the pACC of subjects with MDD, BD, and controls.** No significant alterations were found in this brain region.

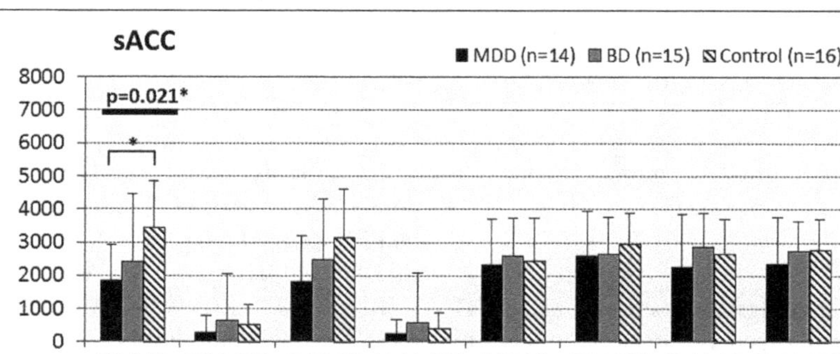


**FIGURE 4 | Numerical densities of GS-expressing glial cells (ACs and OLs) in the sACC of subjects with MDD, BD, and controls.** Compared with controls the density of GS-expressing ACs is significantly reduced in MDD cases (AC left I–III, $p = 0.021$).

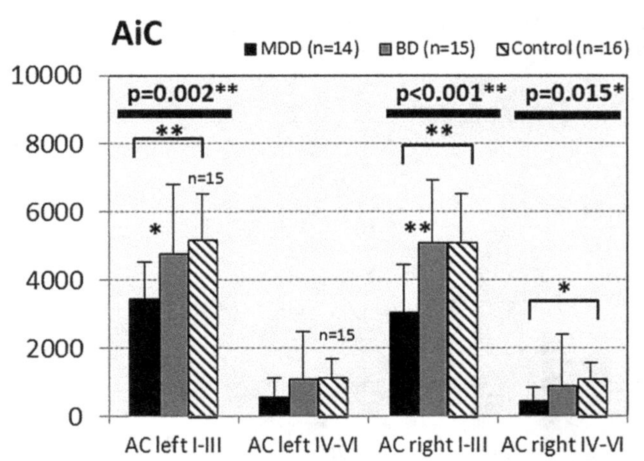


**FIGURE 5 | Numerical densities of GS-expressing glial cells (ACs and OLs) in the AiC of subjects with MDD, BD, and controls.** Compared with controls the density of GS-expressing ACs is significantly reduced in MDD cases (AiC left I–III, $p = 0.002$; AiC right I–III, $p = 0.001$; AiC right IV–VI, $p = 0.015$).

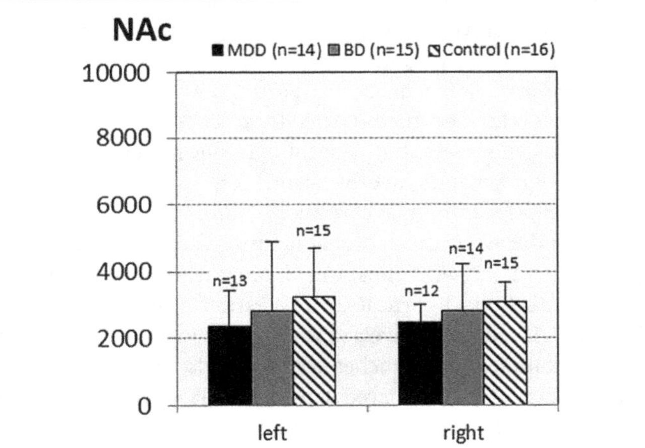


**FIGURE 6 | Numerical densities of GS-expressing glial cells (ACs and OLs) in the NAc of subjects with MDD, BD, and controls.** No significant alterations were found in this brain region.

### MDD vs. BD

Compared with BD cases subjects with MDD showed significantly decreased densities of GS-immunopositive ACs in the DLPFC (right side, layers I–III, $P = 0.047$), in the AiC (left side, layers I–III, $p = 0.024$; right side, layers IV.IV; $p = 0.001$).

### Impact of Completed Suicide on Cell Densities

Since there are reports showing that GS expression is altered in brains of suicide victims with and without mood disorder (Kim et al., 2007; Sequeira et al., 2009; Bernstein et al., 2013) we next analyzed the influence of the confounding factor "death by suicide" on the densities of GS immunoreactive ACs in the brain regions under study. For this purpose we divided MDD and BD cases into subgroups of suicide victims (MDD: $N = 11$; BD: $N = 7$) and depressed subjects who died of natural causes (MDD: $N = 3$; BD: $N = 8$). With regard to MDD cases in none of the brain regions there appeared significant differences in the densities of GS-expressing cells between depressed subjects dying by suicide and non-suicidal individuals with MDD. The same holds true for subjects with BD: Suicidal and non-suicidal BD cases did not significantly differ with regard to glial cell densities in any of the regions studied, as exemplified for the AiC in **Figure 7**. It should be emphasized, however, that the subgroup of non-suicidal subjects with MDD is too small ($N = 3$) to come to far-reaching conclusions from these data.

### The Influence of Other Confounding Factors

Analysis of the potential confounding factors on the test results revealed no significant influence of age, gender, duration of disease, or psychotropic medication. Especially the lack of correlation between the age and the density of GS-expressing ACs is interesting, because Rajkowska and Stockmeier (2013) have hypothesized the glial pathology appears to apply mostly to younger and middle age subjects with MDD (<60 years of age).

### Possible Influence of Hemispheric Asymmetry on GS Cell Distribution in Human Brain

There is evidence in the for structural, functional, and physiological asymmetries in the two hemispheres of human brain (comprehensively reviewed in Jayasundar and Raghunathan, 1997), which involve aspects of glutamate and GABA metabolism in health and mood disorder (MDD: Pfleiderer et al., 2003; Bajbouj et al., 2006; Gos et al., 2012; BD: Gos et al., 2012; Xu et al., 2013). The latter might in part result from left–right hemispheric differences in the distribution of GS immunoreactivity (Bernstein et al., 2013), Unfortunately, knowledge about the catalytic activity and distribution of human brain GS comes mainly from studies of only one (namely the left) brain hemisphere (Burbaeva et al., 2003; Rajkowska and Miguel-Hidalgo, 2007; Miguel-Hidalgo et al., 2010). To exclude a possible left–right asymmetry of GS, we counted left and right hemispheres separately. No evidence was found for a significant left–right asymmetry, neither in controls, nor in subjects with affective disorder.

## Discussion

Major depression disorder and BD are serious mental illnesses with multifactorial pathophysiologic characteristics. The past years have witnessed a remarkable extension of our understanding of the neurobiology of affective disorders, adding the glutamatergic and the GABAergic hypotheses to "classical" monoaminergic theories of mood dysregulation (Delgado, 2000; Skolnick et al., 2009; Catena-Dell'Osso et al., 2013; Dou et al., 2013; Hertz et al., 2014; Pehrson and Sanchez, 2015; Schitine et al., 2015). Besides other indicators of compromised amino acidergic neurotransmission in depression, two large meta-analyses of neuroimaging findings have demonstrated decreased levels of the Glx in adult MDD patients, whereas in the brains of BD patients increased, decreased, and unchanged

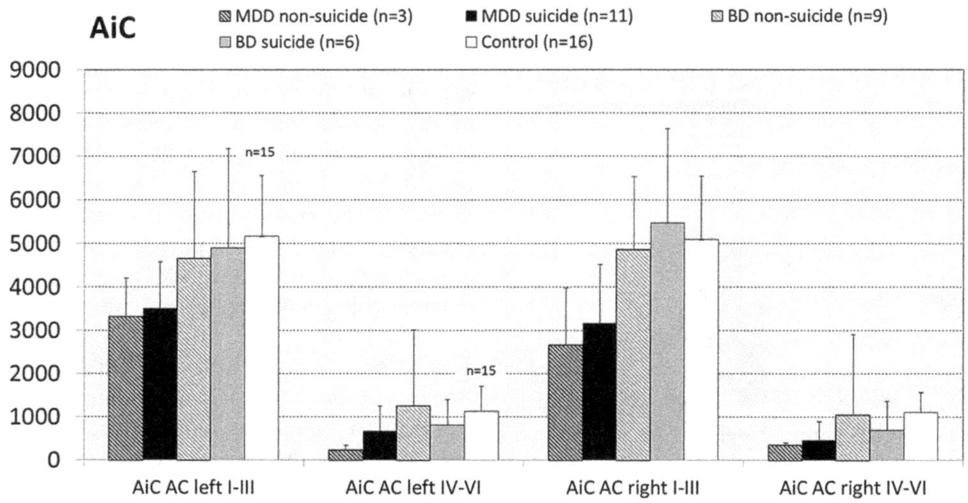


**FIGURE 7 | Numerical densities of GS-expressing glial cells in the AiC of suicide completers with MDD, non-suicide completers with MDD, suicide completers with BD, non-suicide completers with BD, and controls.** No significant alterations were found.

glutamate and reduced glutamine levels have been measured (Yüksel and Öngür, 2010; Gigante et al., 2012; Luykx et al., 2012). Moreover, the NMDA receptor antagonist ketamine has been shown in clinical trials to act as a rapid antidepressant in MDD (for recent considerations, see DeWilde et al., 2015). The acceptance of a crucial role of glutamate in the pathology of mental disorders entails the obligatory implication of glial cells (Arnone et al., 2015). Being part of the glutamatergic tripartite synapse, intact ACs are central to a proper functioning of glutamatergic neurotransmission, and imbalances in the neuron-AC communication at the synaptic level might significantly contribute to affective disorders, such as mania and depression (Mitterauer, 2015; Thompson et al., 2015). The enzyme GS, which is highly expressed in, but in its expression not restricted to, ACs, is required to synthesize the non-toxic glutamine from the re-uptake of either glutamate or GABA. Besides, in human brain an immunologically and enzymatically very closely related "sister" enzyme of (GS-like protein) of unknown cellular localization was found (Boksha et al., 2000), which shows altered expressions in schizophrenia and Alzheimer's disease (Burbaeva et al., 2003; Burbaeva et al., 2014). The possible implication of GS-like enzyme for mood disorders is unexplored, however. Keeping this in mind when designing this study, we morphometrically analyzed GS-immunoreactive glial cells located in various cortical and subcortical gray matter areas of subjects with MDD and BD, thereby counting, wherever possible, ACs and OLs separately. Significantly reduced densities of GS immunopositive ACs were found in the prefrontal areas DLPFC and sACC as well as in the AiC of subjects with MDD. Remarkably, the densities of GS-immunopositive OLs were normal in all regions studied, although a significant loss of perineuronal OLs was found in prefrontal cortex sublayers IIIa, b, and c in mood disorder by others (Vostrikov et al., 2007). When carefully analyzing cortical GS-expressing OLs in mice, Takasaki et al. (2010) found that the enzyme protein is mainly expressed in perineuronal OLs, with roughly half of them being GS-immunopositive. However, these GS-immunoreactive OLs lack plasmalemmal glutamate transporters GLAST and GLT-1, thus apparently being unable to participate in the glutamate-glutamine cycle. The reason why these cells even so express GS remains enigmatic, but is seemingly not directly related to glutamatergic synaptic neurotransmission (possibly playing a role in cellular ammonia clearance and/or certain metabolic support to the associating cortical neurons, Takasaki et al., 2010; Bernstein et al., 2014). Thus, our data clearly show a cell-type specific reduction in cortical GS expression in individuals with MDD, which cannot be revealed when analyzing total GS protein in brain samples with biochemical methods. Interestingly, we found no indication for altered densities of GS-expressing ACs in the NAc, although this brain region plays a central role in MDD (Thompson et al., 2015) and has therefore been chosen as a target structure for deep brain stimulation in cases of therapy-resistant MMD (Bewernick et al., 2012). Although ACs play a critical role in controlling the excitability of NAc neurons via activation of glutamatergic receptors (Fellin et al., 2007; Thompson et al., 2015), their possible implication for "human" depression" yet is poorly explored. However, the number of ACs in the NAc was found to be unchanged in a developmental "toxic stress" model of depression (Shende et al., 2015).

Unlike in MDD, no alterations in the density of GS-expressing glial cells were found in BD cases. This is in agreement with earlier findings by Toro et al. (2006), but in contrast to reduced GS expression in prefrontal area of BD subjects as reported by Choudary et al. (2005). Two possible conclusions may be drawn from our data: either (1) glia associated-GS is normal, because GS does not play a prominent role in the pathophysiology of BD, and/or (2) GS expression was "normalized" (most probably up-regulated) by long-term treatment of the disease. Given the latter possibility, two putative factors might have increased GS expression in brains of BD subjects: administration of lithium

(Kalkman, 2011) and treatment with antidepressants (Hashioka et al., 2013; Liu et al., 2015). Our calculations, however, did not reveal significant positive correlations of numerical densities of GS expressing glial cells and either of the aforementioned two factors. Hence we tend to believe that GS is not a major contributing factor to BD neuropathology. It should be stated, however, that disease-related alterations in the cerebral expression of GS do not always exert a direct influence on the glutamate–glutamine–GABA ratio. So, for example, a strong upregulation of GS protein was reported for the anterior cingulate cortex of female but not male individuals with schizophrenia (Martins-de-Souza et al., 2010), whereas no such gender-specific change in the Glx ratio was found in schizophrenia patients by MRS (Rowland et al., 2013). Thus, further studies are clearly needed to learn more about the impact of GS on glutamate metabolites in the brain.

### Limitations of the Study

Since a major limitation of post-mortem studies is underpowered sample size, we have tried to increase the three cohorts (controls, $N = 16$; BD, $N = 15$, MDD, $N = 14$). A consequence from doing so is to accept the lack of data on the cumulative antidepressant exposure of some patients with MDD and BD. A further limitation of the this study is that, as in all immunocytochemistry-based morphometric studies, it cannot be said with ultimate certainty, whether the observed disease-related changes are due to glial cell loss, or to reduced intracellular expression of the protein (below the detection threshold of the method) in still existing cells, or both. Lastly, a limitation may arise from the fact that the decreased expression of GS protein does not necessarily mean reduced activity of the enzyme. Unfortunately, it is impossible to reveal the catalytic activity of the AC-located GS enzyme because of the lack of a specific enzyme histochemical method for GS.

## Conclusion

In MDD but not in BD there is a glia cell-type specific (astroglial) reduction of cortical GS protein expression, which might constitute a cellular correlate of lower cortical Glx levels reported for subjects with MDD in MSR studies.

## Author Contributions

H-GB analyzed the data, researched, wrote, and edited the manuscript. GM-L analyzed the data. HD carried out statistical calculations and contributed to photography. JB analyzed the data. JS wrote, and edited the manuscript. MW wrote and edited the manuscript. BB wrote and edited the manuscript.

## Acknowledgments

We are grateful to Bianca Jerzykiewicz for excellent technical assistance. This research project was financially supported by SFB 779, project number A06 of the Deutsche Forschungsgemeinschaft (Germany).

## References

Altshuler, L. L., Abulseoud, O. A., Foland-Ross, L., Bartzokis, G., Chang, S., Mintz, J., et al. (2010). Amygdala astrocyte reduction in subjects with major depression but not bipolar disorder. *Bipolar Disord.* 1, 451–549. doi: 10.1111/j.1399-5618.2010.00838.x

Anlauf, E., and Derouiche, A. (2013). Glutamine synthetase as an astrocytic marker: its cell type and vesicle localization. *Front. Endocrinol.* 4:144. doi: 10.3389/fendo.2013.00144

Arnone, D., Mumuni, A. N., Jauhar, S., Condon, B., and Cavanagh, J. (2015). Indirect evidence of selective glial involvement in glutamate-based mechanisms of mood regulation in depression: meta-analysis of absolute prefrontal neuro-metabolic concentrations. *Eur. Neuropsychopharmacol.* doi: 10.1016/j.euroneuro.2015.04.016 [Epub ahead of print].

Bajbouj, M., Lisanby, S. H., Lang, U. E., Danker-Hopfe, H., Heuser, I., and Neu, P. (2006). Evidence for impaired cortical inhibition in patients with unipolar major depression. *Biol. Psychiatry* 59, 395–400. doi: 10.1016/j.biopsych.2005.07.036

Barley, K., Dracheva, S., and Byne, W. (2009). Subcortical oligodendrocyte- and astrocyte-associated gene expression in subjects with schizophrenia, major depression and bipolar disorder. *Schizophr. Res.* 112, 54–64. doi: 10.1016/j.schres.2009.04.01

Beasley, C. L., Pennington, K., Behan, A., Wait, R., Dunn, M. J., and Cotter, D. (2006). Proteomic analysis of the anterior cingulate cortex in the major psychiatric disorders: evidence for disease-associated changes. *Proteomics* 6, 3414–3425. doi: 10.1002/pmic.200500069

Bernstein, H. G., Bannier, J., Meyer-Lotz, G., Steiner, J., Keilhoff, G., Dobrowolny, H., et al. (2014). Distribution of immunoreactive glutamine synthetase in the adult human and mouse brain. Qualitative and quantitative observations with special emphasis on extra-astroglial protein localization. *J. Chem. Neuroanat.* 61–62, 33–50. doi: 10.1016/j.jchemneu.2014.07.003

Bernstein, H. G., Krell, D., Baumann, B., Danos, P., Falkai, P., Diekmann, S., et al. (1998a). Morphometric studies of the entorhinal cortex in neuropsychiatric patients and controls: clusters of heterotopically displaced lamina II neurons are not indicative of schizophrenia. *Schizophr. Res.* 33, 125–132. doi: 10.1016/S0920-9964(98)00071-1

Bernstein, H. G., Stanarius, A., Baumann, B., Henning, H., Krell, D., Danos, P., et al. (1998b). Nitric oxide synthase-containing neurons in the human hypothalamus: reduced number of immunoreactive cells in the paraventricular nucleus of depressive patients and schizophrenics. *Neuroscience* 83, 867–875. doi: 10.1016/S0306-4522(97)00461-2

Bernstein, H. G., Steiner, J., Guest, P. C., Dobrowolny, H., and Bogerts, B. (2015). Glial cells as key players in schizophrenia pathology: recent insights and concepts of therapy. *Schizophr. Res.* 161, 4–18. doi: 10.1016/j.schres.2014.03.035

Bernstein, H. G., Tausch, A., Wagner, R., Steiner, J., Seeleke, P., Walter, M., et al. (2013). Disruption of glutamate-glutamine-GABA cycle significantly impacts on suicidal behaviour: survey of the literature and own findings on glutamine synthetase. *CNS Neurol. Disord. Drug Targets* 12, 900–913. doi: 10.2174/18715273113129990091

Bewernick, B. H., Kayser, S., Sturm, V., and Schlaepfer, T. E. (2012). Long-term effects of nucleus accumbens deep brain stimulation in treatment-resistant depression: evidence for sustained efficacy. *Neuropsychopharmacology* 37, 1975–1985. doi: 10.1038/npp.2012.44

Bielau, H., Trübner, K., Krell, D., Agelink, M. W., Bernstein, H. G., Stauch, R., et al. (2005). Volume deficits of subcortical nuclei in mood disorders A postmortem study. *Eur. Arch. Psychiatry Clin. Neurosci.* 255, 401–412. doi: 10.1007/s00406-005-0581-y

Boksha, I. S., Tereshkina, E. B., and Burbaeva, G. S. (2000). Glutamine synthetase and glutamine synthetase-like protein from human brain: purification and comparative characterization. *J. Neurochem.* 75, 2574–2582. doi: 10.1046/j.1471-4159.2000.0752574.x

Brennan, B. P., Hudson, J. I., Jensen, J. E., McCarthy, J., Roberts, J. L., Prescot, A. P., et al. (2010). Rapid enhancement of glutamatergic neurotransmission in bipolar depression following treatment with riluzole. *Neuropsychopharmacology* 35, 834–846. doi: 10.1038/npp.2009.191

Burbaeva, G. Sh., Boksha, I. S., Tereshkina, E. B., Savushkina, O. K., Prokhorova, T. A., and Vorobyeva, E. A. (2014). Glutamate and GABA-metabolizing enzymes in post-mortem cerebellum in Alzheimer's disease: phosphate-activated glutaminase and glutamic acid decarboxylase. *Cerebellum* 13, 607–615. doi: 10.1007/s12311-014-0573-4

Burbaeva, G. Sh., Boksha, I. S., Turishcheva, M. S., Vorobyeva, E. A., Savushkina, O. K., and Tereshkina, E. B. (2003). Glutamine synthetase and glutamate dehydrogenase in the prefrontal cortex of patients with schizophrenia. *Prog. Neuropsychopharmacol. Biol. Psychiatry.* 27, 675–680. doi: 10.1016/S0278-5846(03)00078-2

Catena-Dell'Osso, M., Fagiolini, A., Rotella, F., Baroni, S., and Marazziti, D. (2013). Glutamate system as target for development of novel antidepressants. *CNS Spectr.* 18, 188–198. doi: 10.1017/S1092852912000971

Choudary, P. V., Molnar, M., Evans, S. J., Tomita, H., Li, J. Z., and Vawter, M. P. (2005). Altered cortical glutamatergic and GABAergic signal transmission with glial involvement in depression. *Proc. Natl. Acad. Sci. U.S.A.* 102, 15653–15658. doi: 10.1073/pnas.0507901102

Cotter, D., Mackay, D., Chana, G., Beasley, C., Landau, S., and Everall, I. P. (2002). Reduced neuronal size and glial cell density in area 9 of the dorsolateral prefrontal cortex in subjects with major depressive disorder. *Cereb. Cortex* 12, 386–394. doi: 10.1093/cercor/12.4.386

Cotter, D., Mackay, D., Landau, S., Kerwin, R., and Everall, I. (2001a). Reduced glial cell density and neuronal size in the anterior cingulate cortex in major depressive disorder. *Arch. Gen. Psychiatry* 58, 545–553. doi: 10.1001/archpsyc.58.6.545

Cotter, D. R., Pariante, C. M., and Everall, I. P. (2001b). Glial cell abnormalities in major psychiatric disorders: the evidence and implications. *Brain Res. Bull.* 55, 585–595. doi: 10.1016/S0361-9230(01)00527-5

Couchman, J. R. (2009). Commercial antibodies: the good, bad, and really ugly. *J. Histochem. Cytochem.* 57, 7–8. doi: 10.1369/jhc.2008.952820

Davis, S., Thomas, A., Perry, R., Oakley, A., Kalaria, R. N., and O'Brien, J. T. (2002). Glial fibrillary acidic protein in late life major depressive disorder: an immunocytochemical study. *J. Neurol. Neurosurg. Psychiatry* 73, 556–560. doi: 10.1136/jnnp.73.5.556

Delgado, P. L. (2000). Depression: the case for a monoamine deficiency. *J. Clin. Psychiatry* 61(Suppl. 6), 7–11.

DeWilde, K. E., Levitch, C. F., Murrough, J. W., Mathew, S. J., and Iosifescu, D. V. (2015). The promise of ketamine for treatment-resistant depression: current evidence and future directions. *Ann. N. Y. Acad. Sci.* 1345, 47–58. doi: 10.1111/nyas.12646

Dong, X. H., and Zhen, X. C. (2015). Glial pathology in bipolar disorder: potential therapeutic implications. *CNS Neurosci. Ther.* 21, 393–397. doi: 10.1111/cns.12390

Dou, W., Palomero-Gallagher, N., van Tol, M. J., Kaufmann, J., Zhong, K., Bernstein, H. G., et al. (2013). Systematic regional variations of GABA, glutamine, and glutamate concentrations follow receptor fingerprints of human cingulate cortex. *J. Neurosci.* 33, 12698–12704. doi: 10.1523/JNEUROSCI.1758-13.20

Duman, R. S. (2014). Neurobiology of stress, depression, and rapid acting antidepressants: remodeling synaptic connections. *Depress. Anxiety* 31, 291–296. doi: 10.1002/da.22227

Duncan, L. E., Holmans, P. A., Lee, P. H., O'Dushlaine, C. T., Kirby, A. W., Smoller, J. W., et al. (2014). Pathway analyses implicate glial cells in schizophrenia. *PLoS ONE* 9:e89441. doi: 10.1371/journal.pone.0089441

Etiévant, A., Lambás-Señas, L., Scarna, H., Lucas, G., and Haddjeri, N. (2013). Astrocytes and gliotransmitters: new players in the treatment of major depression? *Curr. Drug Targets* 14, 1295–1307. doi: 10.2174/13894501113149990197

Fellin, T., D'Ascenzo, M., and Haydon, P. G. (2007). Astrocytes control neuronal excitability in the nucleus accumbens. *ScientificWorldJournal* 7, 89–97. doi: 10.1100/tsw.2007.195

Gigante, A. D., Bond, D. J., Lafer, B., Lam, R. W., Young, L. T., and Yatham, L. N. (2012). Brain glutamate levels measured by magnetic resonance spectroscopy in patients with bipolar disorder: a meta-analysis. *Bipolar Disord.* 14, 478–487. doi: 10.1111/j.1399-5618.2012.01033.x

Gos, T., Schroeter, M. L., Lessel, W., Bernstein, H. G., Dobrowolny, H., Schiltz, K., et al. (2013). S100B-immunopositive astrocytes and oligodendrocytes in the hippocampus are differentially afflicted in unipolar and bipolar depression: a postmortem study. *J. Psychiatr. Res.* 47, 1694–1699. doi: 10.1016/j.jpsychires.2013.07.005

Gos, T., Steiner, J., Bielau, H., Dobrowoln, H., Günther, K., Mawrin, C., et al. (2012). Differences between unipolar and bipolar I depression in the quantitative analysis of glutamic acid decarboxylase-immunoreactive neuropil. *Eur. Arch. Psychiatry Clin. Neurosci.* 262, 647–655. doi: 10.1007/s00406-012-0315-x

Hamidi, M., Drevets, W. C., and Price, J. L. (2004). Glial reduction in amygdala in major depressive disorder is due to oligodendrocytes. *Biol. Psychiatry* 55, 563–569. doi: 10.1016/j.biopsych.2003.11.006

Harrison, P. J. (2002). The neuropathology of primary mood disorder. *Brain* 125, 1428–1449. doi: 10.1093/brain/awf149

Hashioka, S., Miyaoka, T., Wake, R., Furuya, M., and Horiguchi, J. (2013). Glia: an important target for anti-inflammatory and antidepressant activity. *Curr. Drug Targets* 14, 1322–1328. doi: 10.2174/13894501113146660214

Hertz, L., Song, D., Li, B., Du, T., Xu, J., Gu, L., et al. (2014). Signal transduction in astrocytes during chronic or acute treatment with drugs (SSRIs, antibipolar Drugs, GABA-ergic drugs, and benzodiazepines) ameliorating mood disorders. *J. Signal Transduct.* 2014:593934. doi: 10.1155/2014/593934

Iwata, K., Café-Mendes, C. C., Schmitt, A., Steiner, J., Manabe, T., Matsuzaki, H., et al. (2013). The human oligodendrocyte proteome. *Proteomics* 13, 3548–3553. doi: 10.1002/pmic.201300201

Jayasundar, R., and Raghunathan, P. (1997). Evidence for left-right asymmetries in the proton MRS of brain in normal volunteers. *Magn. Reson. Imaging* 15, 223–234. doi: 10.1016/S0730-725X(96)00342-6

Kalkman, H. O. (2011). Circumstantial evidence for a role of glutamine-synthetase in suicide. *Med. Hypotheses* 76, 905–907. doi: 10.1016/j.mehy.2011.03.005

Kato, T. A., Watabe, M., and Kanba, S. (2013). Neuron-glia interaction as a possible glue to translate the mind-brain gap: a novel multi-dimensional approach toward psychology and psychiatry. *Front. Psychiatry* 4:139. doi: 10.3389/fpsyt.2013.00139

Katsel, P., Byne, W., Roussos, P., Tan, W., Siever, L., and Haroutunian, V. (2011). Astrocyte and glutamate markers in the superficial, deep and white matter layers of the anterior cingulate gyrus in schizophrenia. *Neuropsychopharmacology* 36, 1171–1177. doi: 10.1038/npp.2010.252

Kim, S., Choi, K. H., Baykiz, A. F., and Gershenfeld, H. K. (2007). Suicide candidate genes associated with bipolar disorder and schizophrenia: an exploratory gene expression profiling analysis of post-mortem prefrontal cortex. *BMC Genomics* 8:413. doi: 10.1186/1471-2164-8-413

Liu, Z., Song, D., Yan, E., Verkhratsky, A., and Peng, L. (2015). Chronic treatment with anti-bipolar drugs suppresses glutamate release from astroglial cultures. *Amino Acids* 47, 1045–1051. doi: 10.1007/s00726-015-1936-y

Luykx, J. J., Laban, K. G., van den Heuvel, M. P., Boks, M. P., Mandl, R. C., Kahn, R. S., et al. (2012). Region and state specific glutamate downregulation in major depressive disorder: a meta-analysis of (1)H-MRS findings. *Neurosci. Biobehav. Rev.* 36, 198–205. doi: 10.1016/j.neubiorev.2011.05.014

Mai, J. K., Paxinos, G., and Assheuer, J. K. (2003). *Atlas of the Human Brain.* Amsterdam: Elsevier Academic Press.

Malchow, B., Strocka, S., Frank, F., Bernstein, H. G., Steiner, J., Schneider-Axmann, T., et al. (2014). Stereological investigation of the posterior hippocampus in affective disorders. *J. Neural Transm.* doi: 10.1007/s00702-014-1316-x [Epub ahead of print].

Maletic, V., and Raison, C. (2014). Integrated neurobiology of bipolar disorder. *Front. Psychiatry* 5:98. doi: 10.3389/fpsyt.2014.00098

Manji, H. K., Drevets, W. C., and Charney, D. S. (2001). The cellular neurobiology of depression. *Nat. Med.* 7, 541–547. doi: 10.1038/87865

Martins-de-Souza, D., Schmitt, A., Röder, R., Lebar, M., Schneider-Axmann, T., Falkai, P., et al. (2010). Sex-specific proteome differences in the anterior cingulate cortex of schizophrenia. *J. Psychiatr. Res.* 44, 989–991. doi: 10.1016/j.jpsychires.2010.03.003

Miguel-Hidalgo, J. J., Waltzer, R., Whittom, A. A., Austin, M. C., Rajkowska, G., and Stockmeier, C. A. (2010). Glial and glutamatergic markers in depression, alcoholism, and their comorbidity. *J. Affect. Disord.* 127, 230–240. doi: 10.1016/j.jad.2010.06.003

Mitterauer, B. J. (2015). Balancing and imbalancing effects of astrocytic receptors in tripartite synapses. Common pathophysiological model of mental disorders and epilepsy. *Med. Hypotheses* 84, 315–320. doi: 10.1016/j.mehy.2015.01.025

Mosebach, J., Keilhoff, G., Gos, T., Schiltz, K., Schoeneck, L., Dobrowolny, H., et al. (2013). Increased nuclear Olig1-expression in the pregenual anterior cingulate white matter of patients with major depression: a regenerative attempt to compensate oligodendrocyte loss? *J. Psychiatr. Res.* 47, 1069–1079. doi: 10.1016/j.jpsychires.2013.03.018

Öngür, D., Drevets, W. C., and Price, J. L. (1998). Glial reduction in the subgenual prefrontal cortex in mood disorders. *Proc. Natl. Acad. Sci. U.S.A.* 95, 13290–13295. doi: 10.1073/pnas.95.22.13290

Pehrson, A. L., and Sanchez, C. (2015). Altered γ-aminobutyric acid neurotransmission in major depressive disorder: a critical review of the supporting evidence and the influence of serotonergic antidepressants. *Drug Des. Devel. Ther.* 9, 603–624. doi: 10.2147/DDDT.S62912

Pfleiderer, B., Michael, N., Erfurth, A., Ohrmann, P., Hohmann, U., Wolgast, M., et al. (2003). Effective electroconvulsive therapy reverses glutamate/glutamine deficit in the left anterior cingulum of unipolar depressed patients. *Psychiatry Res.* 122, 185–192. doi: 10.1016/S0925-4927(03)00003-9

Rajkowska, G. (2000). Dysfunction in neural circuits involved in the pathophysiology of mood disorders: postmortem studies in mood disorders indicate altered numbers of neurons and glial cells. *Biol. Psychiatry* 48, 766–777. doi: 10.1016/S0006-3223(00)00950-1

Rajkowska, G. (2002). Cell pathology in mood disorders. *Semin. Clin. Neuropsychiatry* 7, 281–292. doi: 10.1053/scnp.2002.35228

Rajkowska, G., and Miguel-Hidalgo, J. J. (2007). Gliogenesis and glial pathology in depression. *CNS Neurol. Disord. Drug Targets* 6, 219–233. doi: 10.2174/187152707780619326

Rajkowska, G., and Stockmeier, C. A. (2013). Astrocyte pathology in major depressive disorder: insights from human postmortem brain tissue. *Curr. Drug Targets* 14, 1225–1236. doi: 10.2174/13894501113149990156

Rowland, L. M., Kontson, K., West, J., Edden, R. A., Zhu, H., Wijtenburg, S. A., et al. (2013). In vivo measurements of glutamate, GABA, and NAAG in schizophrenia. *Schizophr. Bull.* 39, 1096–1104. doi: 10.1093/schbul/sbs092

Sahlender, D. A., Savtchouk, I., and Volterra, A. (2014). What do we know about gliotransmitter release from astrocytes? *Philos. Trans. R. Soc. Lond. B Biol. Sci.* 369:20130592. doi: 10.1098/rstb.2013.0592

Salvadore, G., van der Veen, J. W., Zhang, Y., Marenco, S., Machado-Vieira, R., Baumann, J., et al. (2012). An investigation of amino-acid neurotransmitters as potential predictors of clinical improvement to ketamine in depression. *Int. J. Neuropsychopharmacol.* 15, 1063–1072. doi: 10.1017/S1461145711001593

Savitz, J. B., Price, J. L., and Drevets, W. C. (2014). Neuropathological and neuromorphometric abnormalities in bipolar disorder: view from the medial prefrontal cortical network. *Neurosci. Biobehav. Rev.* 42, 132–147. doi: 10.1016/j.neubiorev.2014.02.008

Schitine, C., Nogaroli, L., Costa, M. R., and Hedin-Pereira, C. (2015). Astrocyte heterogeneity in the brain: from development to disease. *Front. Cell. Neurosci.* 9:76. doi: 10.3389/fncel.2015.00076

Schroeter, M. L., Steiner, J., Schönknecht, P., and Mueller, K. (2014). Further evidence for a role of S100B in mood disorders: a human gene expression mega-analysis. *J. Psychiatr. Res.* 53, 84–86. doi: 10.1016/j.jpsychires.2014.02.021

Sequeira, A., Mamdani, F., Ernst, C., Vawter, M. P., Bunney, W. E., Lebel, V., et al. (2009). Global brain gene expression analysis links glutamatergic and GABAergic alterations to suicide and major depression. *PLoS ONE* 4:e6585. doi: 10.1371/journal.pone.0006585

Shende, V. H., McArthur, S., Gillies, G. E., and Opacka-Juffry, J. (2015). Astroglial plasticity is implicated in hippocampal remodelling in adult rats exposed to antenatal dexamethasone. *Neural Plast.* (in press). doi: 10.1155/2015/694347

Si, X., Miguel-Hidalgo, J. J., O'Dwyer, G., Stockmeier, C. A., and Rajkowska, G. (2004). Age-dependent reductions in the level of glial fibrillary acidic protein in the prefrontal cortex in major depression. *Neuropsychopharmacology* 29, 2088–2096. doi: 10.1038/sj.npp.1300525

Skolnick, P., Popik, P., and Trullas, R. (2009). Glutamate-based antidepressants: 20 years on. *Trends Pharmacol. Sci.* 30, 563–569. doi: 10.1016/j.tips.2009.09.002

Sofroniew, M. V., and Vinters, H. V. (2010). Astrocytes: biology and pathology. *Acta Neuropathol.* 119, 7–35. doi: 10.1007/s00401-009-0619-8

Steiner, J., Bogerts, B., Sarnyai, Z., Walter, M., Gos, T., Bernstein, H. G., et al. (2012). Bridging the gap between the immune and glutamate hypotheses of schizophrenia and major depression: potential role of glial NMDA receptor modulators and impaired blood-brain barrier integrity. *World J. Biol. Psychiatry* 13, 482–492. doi: 10.3109/15622975.2011.583941

Takasaki, C., Yamasaki, M., Uchigashima, M., Konno, K., Yanagawa, Y., and Watanabe, M. (2010). Cytochemical and cytological properties of perineuronal oligodendrocytes in the mouse cortex. *Eur. J. Neurosci.* 32, 1326–1336. doi: 10.1111/j.1460-9568.2010.07377.x

Teschemacher, A. G., Gourine, A. V., and Kasparov, S. (2015). A role for astrocytes in sensing the brain microenvironment and neuro-metabolic integration. *Neurochem. Res.* doi: 10.1007/s11064-015-1562-9 [Epub ahead of print]

Thompson, S. M., Kallarackal, A. J., Kvarta, M. D., Van Dyke, A. M., LeGates, T. A., and Cai, X. (2015). An excitatory synapse hypothesis of depression. *Trends Neurosci.* 38, 279–294. doi: 10.1016/j.tins.2015.03.003

Toro, C. T., Hallak, J. E., Dunham, J. S., and Deakin, J. F. (2006). Glial fibrillary acidic protein and glutamine synthetase in subregions of prefrontal cortex in schizophrenia and mood disorder. *Neurosci. Lett.* 404, 276–281. doi: 10.1016/j.neulet.2006.05.067

Uranova, N. A., Vostrikov, V. M., Orlovskaya, D. D., and Rachmanova, V. I. (2004). Oligodendroglial density in the prefrontal cortex in schizophrenia and mood disorders: a study from the Stanley Neuropathology Consortium. *Schizophr. Res.* 67, 269–275. doi: 10.1016/S0920-9964(03)00181-6

Van Horn, M. R., Sild, M., and Ruthazer, E. S. (2013). D-serine as a gliotransmitter and its roles in brain development and disease. *Front. Cell. Neurosci.* 7:39. doi: 10.3389/fncel.2013.00039

Verkhratsky, A., Rodríguez, J. J., and Steardo, L. (2014). Astrogliopathology: a central element of neuropsychiatric diseases? *Neuroscientist* 20, 576–588. doi: 10.1177/1073858413510208

Vostrikov, V. M., Uranova, N. A., and Orlovskaya, D. D. (2007). Deficit of perineuronal oligodendrocytes in the prefrontal cortex in schizophrenia and mood disorders. *Schizophr. Res.* 94, 273–280. doi: 10.1016/j.schres.2007.04.014

Walter, M., Henning, A., Grimm, S., Schulte, R. F., Beck, J., Dydak, U., et al. (2009). The relationship between aberrant neuronal activation in the pregenual anterior cingulate, altered glutamatergic metabolism, and anhedonia in major depression. *Arch. Gen. Psychiatry* 66, 478–486. doi: 10.1001/archgenpsychiatry.2009.39

Xu, J., Dydak, U., Harezlak, J., Nixon, J., Dzemidzic, M., Gunn, A. D., et al. (2013). Neurochemical abnormalities in unmedicated bipolar depression and mania: a 2D 1H MRS investigation. *Psychiatry Res.* 30, 235–241. doi: 10.1016/j.pscychresns.2013.02.008

Yüksel, C., and Öngür, D. (2010). Magnetic resonance spectroscopy studies of glutamate-related abnormalities in mood disorders. *Biol. Psychiatry* 68, 785–794. doi: 10.1016/j.biopsych.2010.06.016

7

# Serum S100B is Related to Illness Duration and Clinical Symptoms in Schizophrenia—A Meta-Regression Analysis

*Katharina Schümberg[1]*, Maryna Polyakova[1], Johann Steiner[2] and Matthias L. Schroeter[1,3,4,5]*

[1] Department of Cognitive Neurology, Max Planck Institute for Human Cognitive and Brain Sciences, Leipzig, Germany, [2] Department of Psychiatry, University of Magdeburg, Magdeburg, Germany, [3] Clinic for Cognitive Neurology, University of Leipzig, Leipzig, Germany, [4] LIFE—Leipzig Research Center for Civilization Diseases, University of Leipzig, Leipzig, Germany, [5] German Consortium for Frontotemporal Lobar Degeneration, Ulm, Germany

***Correspondence:**
Katharina Schümberg
schuemberg@cbs.mpg.de

S100B has been linked to glial pathology in several psychiatric disorders. Previous studies found higher S100B serum levels in patients with schizophrenia compared to healthy controls, and a number of covariates influencing the size of this effect have been proposed in the literature. Here, we conducted a meta-analysis and meta-regression analysis on alterations of serum S100B in schizophrenia in comparison with healthy control subjects. The meta-analysis followed the Preferred Reporting Items for Systematic Reviews and Meta-Analyses (PRISMA) statement to guarantee a high quality and reproducibility. With strict inclusion criteria 19 original studies could be included in the quantitative meta-analysis, comprising a total of 766 patients and 607 healthy control subjects. The meta-analysis confirmed higher values of the glial serum marker S100B in schizophrenia if compared with control subjects. Meta-regression analyses revealed significant effects of illness duration and clinical symptomatology, in particular the total score of the Positive and Negative Syndrome Scale (PANSS), on serum S100B levels in schizophrenia. In sum, results confirm glial pathology in schizophrenia that is modulated by illness duration and related to clinical symptomatology. Further studies are needed to investigate mechanisms and mediating factors related to these findings.

**Keywords: glia, meta-analysis, S100B, schizophrenia, serum marker**

## INTRODUCTION

S100B is a calcium-binding protein which can be secreted by astroglia and oligodendroglia (e.g., Donato, 2001; Steiner et al., 2007, 2008; Donato et al., 2009). In the brain, it is generally assumed to be neurotrophic in nanomolar concentrations due to its activation of neural growth factor pathways and up-regulation of anti-apoptotic factors. In micromolar concentrations however, it becomes neurotoxic, interacting with pro-inflammatory cytokines like interleukin (IL)-1, IL-6, tumor necrosis factor (TNF) alpha, up-regulating the expression of pro-apoptotic factors as well as inducing nitric oxide synthase and cyclooxygenase 2 expression (Donato, 2001; Van Eldik and Wainwright, 2003; Donato et al., 2009; Bianchi et al., 2010).

Thus, S100B has been linked to the presence of inflammatory processes in the brain, either after injury or due to primary inflammation (Sen and Belli, 2007). Furthermore, certain neuropsychiatric disorders, among them schizophrenia, have been found to be associated with elevated serum and cerebrospinal fluid (CSF) levels of S100B (e.g., Rothermundt et al., 2004a), thus implying immunoreactive glial processes as important in either their genesis or progression. Although serum S100B might be associated with other conditions such as blood-brain barrier disruption, weight changes or neurological diseases, S100B changes in schizophrenia are lower than would be expected in neurological diseases with brain injury (Schroeter et al., 2009; Steiner et al., 2010b).

Here, we conducted a systematic and quantitative meta-analysis of changes in serum S100B in schizophrenia, which extends former meta-analyses on this issue (Schroeter et al., 2003, 2009; Schroeter and Steiner, 2009; Aleksovska et al., 2014) by including further studies and accordingly, increasing statistical power and evidence. Based on previous studies, we hypothesized higher S100B in schizophrenia when compared to healthy controls. Additionally, we investigated effects of medication and applied meta-regression analyses to investigate effects of clinical parameters on serum S100B. We hypothesized here an association of S100B with the duration of illness as recent studies have shown progression of astrocytes' dystrophy/swelling and of oligodendrocyte-related disturbances of cerebral connectivity with duration of illness (Kolomeets and Uranova, 2010; Bernstein et al., 2015; Yao et al., 2015). Moreover, we hypothesized an association of S100B with negative symptoms as shown in previous studies (Rothermundt et al., 2001, 2004b; Schroeter et al., 2003; Schmitt et al., 2005).

## MATERIALS AND METHODS

### General Study Selection Criteria

The meta-analysis was conducted according to the Preferred Reporting Items for Systematic Reviews and Meta-Analyses (PRISMA) statement to guarantee a high quality and reproducibility of the meta-analysis (Moher et al., 2009). The search terms [S100 or S-100] as well as [S100B or S-100B] and [schizophrenia] were used to identify original studies published between 1970 and October 2015 in PubMed, Web of Science, Ovid and Scopus databases. Studies had to meet the following inclusion criteria: peer-reviewed, patients diagnosed with schizophrenia according to International Classification of Diseases (ICD-10) and/or Diagnostic and Statistical Manual of Mental Disorders (DSM-IV) standards, original studies, comparison with age-matched control subjects. Studies were checked for eligibility and selected by two persons (KS and MP). We pooled plasma and serum studies under the assumption that calculation of effect sizes normalizes absolute differences between patients and control subjects and thus, eliminates differences in methodological approaches.

### Data Synthesis

S100B levels were extracted from the articles along with information on additional covariates as examined and reported by the investigators. In case exact values were not given in the article or if data were only illustrated in plots, authors were contacted to obtain detailed information. To adjust for systematic measurement effects in the several original studies, we calculated effect sizes. Standard deviations (SD) were calculated from standard error of the mean (SEM) using the formula $SD = SEM^* \sqrt{n}$ if necessary. Following a conservative approach, the Comprehensive Meta-Analysis software package (versions 2 and 3, Biostat, Inc., Englewood, NJ, USA[1]) was then used to compute Hedges' g corrected for small sample size effects under a random effects model, with effect sizes of 0.2 signifying a small, 0.5 a medium, and 0.8 and larger a strong effect (Cohen, 1988; Lakens, 2013). This software has already been used in several other meta-analytic studies (e.g., Gami et al., 2007; Hofmann and Smits, 2008; Howren et al., 2009; Leucht et al., 2009).

Besides investigating differences between patients with schizophrenia and healthy control subjects *per se*, we conducted subgroup analyses comparing drug-free with medicated patients. Additionally, we checked for possible effects of clinical covariates on effect size via meta-regression, applying the Method of Moments (DerSimonian and Laird, 1986). Potential covariates included illness duration, age at onset of the disorder, male-to-female ratio, severity of clinical symptoms as measured with the clinical symptom scales Brief Psychiatric Rating Scale (BPRS, total score), and Positive And Negative Syndrome Scale (PANSS, total score as well as positive, negative and general psychopathology subscores), as well as an index of risk of bias for cross-sectional studies published in Polyakova et al. (2015). Note that mean age was not included in this analysis, because in each of the included studies schizophrenia patients were compared with age-matched control subjects (see inclusion criteria). Body mass index (BMI), although of interest due to its potential effects on serum S100B (e.g., see Steiner et al., 2010a,b, 2014), could not yet be analyzed as a covariate due to lack of a sufficient number of studies reporting this measure.

## RESULTS

### Identified Studies

Details of the study selection process are illustrated in the PRISMA flow diagram in **Figure 1**. The search in PubMed yielded a total of 121 results, while Web of Science offered 149 hits, Ovid 42 and Scopus 109 results. Following exclusion of reviews, conference abstracts, oncology related papers, book chapters, errata as well as texts written in languages other than English via database settings, 312 studies remained. Further elimination by title of post-mortem, *in vitro*, animal and genetic studies, studies investigating S100B in CSF only or studies with patients other than schizophrenia resulted in 38 articles in PubMed, 39 in Web of Science, 21 in Ovid, and 43 in Scopus databases. The abstracts of these

[1] https://www.meta-analysis.com/

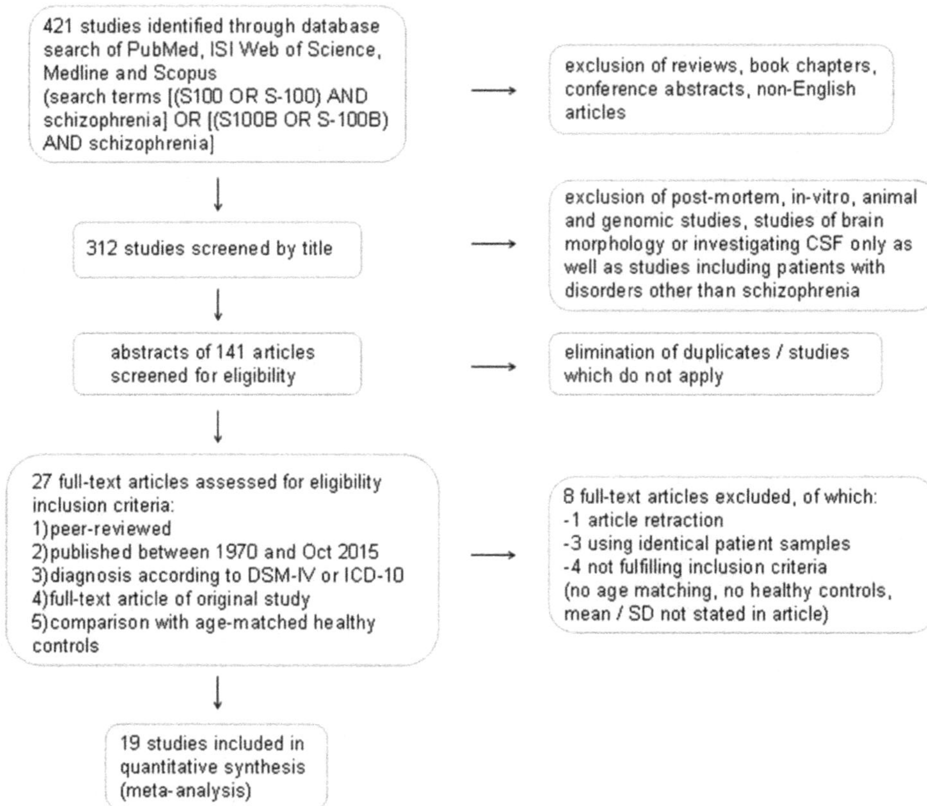


**FIGURE 1 | Flow diagram illustrating the database search process according to Preferred Reporting Items for Systematic Reviews and Meta-Analyses (PRISMA).** CSF, cerebrospinal fluid; DSM-IV, Diagnostic and Statistical Manual of Mental Disorders IV; ICD-10, International Statistical Classification of Diseases and Related Health Problems 10; SD, standard deviation.

141 articles were screened for eligibility, leading to a total of 80 articles which were then checked for duplicates, resulting in 27 full-text articles to be examined for meeting the inclusion criteria. Corresponding authors were contacted in cases where S100B levels or patient characteristics for schizophrenia-only patients were not explicitly stated in the original article. As authors did not reply, another two studies were excluded (van der Leeuw et al., 2013; Xiong et al., 2014). This resulted in an overall number of 19 original studies to be included in the quantitative meta-analysis, comprising a total of 766 patients and 607 healthy control subjects. Included studies and clinical characteristics of the study population are reported in **Table 1**.

## Main Effects

Across all included studies comparing patients suffering from schizophrenia with control subjects, Hedges' g amounted to 0.925, indicating a higher level of S100B in schizophrenia patients compared to healthy controls (**Figure 2**).

In order to analyze the influence of medication on serum S100B levels in schizophrenia there are generally two options. Firstly, one might compare medicated and unmedicated patients in a cross-sectional approach. Secondly, meta-analyzing longitudinal studies enables investigating treatment effects in the same cohort. Comparing studies including only medicated ($n$ = 249) to those including only unmedicated patients ($n$ = 244) in a subgroup meta-analysis, there was no significant difference in effect sizes between those two groups ($p$ = 0.927, **Figure 3**). Note that studies including both medicated and unmedicated patients without analyzing them separately had to be excluded from this analysis. There were, however, high levels of heterogeneity even within the two subgroups (see **Table 1**) as well as a relatively small number of studies in the subgroups (seven studies for medicated, nine for unmedicated subjects, see **Figure 3**).

Investigating effects of treatment with the longitudinal approach, thus meta-analyzing treatment studies within the same subjects (**Figure 4**), we found no significant difference in treatment effects between patient groups undergoing medication for 6 vs. for 12 weeks ($p$ = 0.281). Neither did the overall treatment effect size ($g$ = −0.135, S100B levels lower after treatment than before) reach significance ($p$ = 0.176) in a mixed effects analysis.

## Meta-Regression

The meta-regression of S100B serum levels with clinical parameters in schizophrenia revealed significant effects for the covariates illness duration ($\beta_{\text{illness duration}}$ = 0.0537,

**TABLE 1 | Study characteristics for the 19 studies included in the final meta-analysis.**

| Reference | Sample size | | Patient age (years; mean ± SD) | Illness duration (years; mean ± SD) | Serum S100B (ng/l; mean ± SD) | | Male-to-female ratio for patients | PANSS score | | | | BPRS score | Bias rating |
|---|---|---|---|---|---|---|---|---|---|---|---|---|---|
| | P | Co | | | P | Co | | Total | Positive | Negative | General | | |
| Gattaz et al. (2000) | 23 | 23 | 36.0 ± 9.0 | 17.0 ± 7.0 | 440.0 ± 270.0 | 550.0 ± 140.0 | 2.3 | | | | | 15.8 ± 15.4 | 13 |
| Ryoun Kim et al. (2007) | 60 | 30 | 37.0 ± 3.5 | 15.0 ± 6.7 | 140.0 ± 91.7 | 78.0 ± 47.0 | 0.8 | | | | | | 13 |
| Lara et al. (2001) | 20 | 20 | 31.0 ± 8.0 | 9.0 ± 7.0 | 120.0 ± 140.0 | 66.0 ± 67.0 | 1.9 | 107.0 ± 29.0 | 24.0 ± 9.0 | 29.0 ± 7.0 | 54.0 | | 14 |
| Ling et al. (2007) | 57 | 60 | 33.5 ± 11.4 | 8.0 ± 9.0 | 119.0 ± 59.0 | 67.0 ± 22.0 | 0.9 | 77.8 ± 13.8 | | 20.0 ± 6.8 | | | 14 |
| O'Connell et al. (2013) | 97 | 27 | 42.5 ± 12.2 | Only clozapine duration stated | 79.5 ± 39.8 | 67.8 ± 20.8 | 2.3 | | | | | 31.0 ± 9.0 | 14 |
| Qi et al. (2009) | 63 | 50 | 50.8 ± 6.8 | 25.4 ± 7.2 | 359.0 ± 116.0 | 123.0 ± 50.0 | 2.2 | 59.8 ± 13.1 | 13.2 ± 6.1 | 20 ± 6.2 | 26.5 ± 5.5 | | 18 |
| Rothermundt et al. (2001) | 26 | 26 | 37.0 ± 12.9 | 10.0 ± 10.4 | 98.0 ± 76.0 | 34.0 ± 17.5 | 0.6 | 86.7 ± 17.9 | 25 ± 6.3 | 19.5 ± 8.3 | 42.1 ± 9.6 | | 16 |
| Rothermundt et al. (2004a) | 21 | 21 | 32.5 ± 13.0 | | 65.0 ± 31.0 | 38.0 ± 8.0 | 4.3 | 97.7 ± 25.6 | | | | | 13 |
| Rothermundt et al. (2004b) | 98 | 98 | 42.1 ± 11.1 | | 73.0 ± 32.0 | 44.0 ± 15.0 | 1.3 | 82.5 ± 17.1 | 14.8 ± 5.2 | 27.3 ± 5.3 | 40.3 ± 10.6 | | 16 |
| Rothermundt et al. (2007) | 12 | 12 | 25.3 ± 4.8 | 1.9 ± 1.4 | 85.0 ± 70.0 | 38.0 ± 8.0 | 11 | 81.2 ± 20.1 | 19.3 ± 7.4 | 19.6 ± 7.8 | 42.4 ± 11.1 | | 18 |
| Sarandol et al. (2007) | 40 | 35 | 34.0 ± 9.9 | 6.7 ± 6.4 | 46.1 ± 43.6 | 23.6 ± 14.9 | 0.8 | | | | | 21.0 ± 6.1 | 15 |
| Schmitt et al. (2005) | 41 | 23 | 63.3 ± 7.0 | 35.3 ± 11.4 | 132.2 ± 43.0 | 61.0 ± 26.0 | 1.4 | | | | | 46.2 ± 14.9 | 16 |
| Schroeter et al. (2003) | 30 | 15 | 34.8 ± 12.4 | 8.9 ± 8.8 | 180.3 ± 129.5 | 112.8 ± 53.4 | 0.9 | | | | | 45.3 ± 12.6 | 12 |
| Schroeter et al. (2009) | 20 | 10 | 34.6 ± 12.7 | 8.4 ± 9.6 | 73.4 ± 72.1 | 42.1 ± 69.7 | 0.8 | | | | | 47.6 ± 11.9 | 15 |
| Steiner et al. (2006) | 12 | 17 | 24.0 ± 7.0 | 0.4 ± 0.2 | 90.0 ± 30.0 | 80.0 ± 20.0 | 0.7 | 87.0 ± 15.0 | 24.0 ± 6.0 | 21.0 ± 6.0 | 42.0 ± 8.0 | | 14 |
| Steiner et al. (2009) | 26 | 32 | 34.7 ± 11.3 | 8.0 ± 9.0 | 72.0 ± 38.0 | 52.0 ± 18.0 | 1.9 | 84.8 ± 11.2 | 20.1 ± 4.9 | 22.1 ± 6.5 | 42.7 ± 5.6 | | 16 |
| Uzbay et al. (2013) | 18 | 19 | 37.4 ± 12.6 | 9.8 ± 10.11 | 7.8 ± 10.6 | 6.3 ± 7.8 | 1.6 | 87.2 ± 13.3 | | | | | 16 |
| Wiesmann et al. (1999) | 20 | 20 | 35.7 ± 10.7 | 8.0 ± 5.0 | 165.0 ± 138.0 | 54.0 ± 31.0 | 0.7 | | | | | | 16 |
| Zhang et al. (2010) | 82 | 60 | 50.9 ± 7.2 | 26.6 ± 8.7 | 445.3 ± 196.0 | 122.0 ± 76.0 | 2.3 | 58.4 ± 13.2 | 12.2 ± 5.9 | 19.9 ± 6.5 | 26.2 ± 5.4 | | 18 |
| Total study population | 766 | 607 | 37.8 ± 9.2 | 12.4 ± 9.4 | 146.9 ± 126.9 | 88.4 ± 119.7 | 2.0 ± 2.4 | 82.3 ± 14.2 | 19.1 ± 5.1 | 22.0 ± 3.6 | 39.3 ± 6.3 | 34.5 ± 13.9 | 15.1 ± 1.8 |

*Note: BPRS, Brief Psychiatric Rating Scale; Co, control subjects; P, patients; PANSS, Positive And Negative Syndrome Scale; SD, standard deviation.*

| Study | Hedges's g | Standard error | Variance | Lower limit | Upper limit | Z-Value | p-Value |
|---|---|---|---|---|---|---|---|
| Gattaz et al. 2000 | -0,503 | 0,295 | 0,087 | -1,080 | 0,075 | -1,707 | 0,088 |
| Kim et al. 2007 | 0,770 | 0,229 | 0,052 | 0,321 | 1,219 | 3,363 | 0,001 |
| Lara et al. 2001 | 0,482 | 0,315 | 0,099 | -0,134 | 1,099 | 1,533 | 0,125 |
| Ling et al. 2007 | 1,172 | 0,199 | 0,040 | 0,782 | 1,562 | 5,886 | 0,000 |
| O'Connell et al. 2013 | 0,318 | 0,217 | 0,047 | -0,108 | 0,744 | 1,463 | 0,143 |
| Qi et al. 2009 | 2,525 | 0,252 | 0,064 | 2,030 | 3,019 | 10,012 | 0,000 |
| Rothermundt et al. 2001 | 1,143 | 0,295 | 0,087 | 0,564 | 1,722 | 3,871 | 0,000 |
| Rothermundt et al. 2004a | 1,170 | 0,329 | 0,108 | 0,526 | 1,814 | 3,561 | 0,000 |
| Rothermundt et al. 2004b | 1,156 | 0,154 | 0,024 | 0,854 | 1,457 | 7,515 | 0,000 |
| Rothermundt et al. 2007 | 0,911 | 0,416 | 0,173 | 0,096 | 1,725 | 2,192 | 0,028 |
| Sarandöl et al. 2007 | 0,664 | 0,235 | 0,055 | 0,203 | 1,126 | 2,822 | 0,005 |
| Schmitt et al. 2005 | 1,858 | 0,305 | 0,093 | 1,260 | 2,457 | 6,086 | 0,000 |
| Schroeter et al. 2003 | 0,600 | 0,317 | 0,101 | -0,022 | 1,221 | 1,892 | 0,058 |
| Schroeter et al. 2009 | 0,432 | 0,318 | 0,101 | -0,190 | 1,055 | 1,361 | 0,174 |
| Steiner et al. 2006 | 0,396 | 0,370 | 0,137 | -0,330 | 1,121 | 1,069 | 0,285 |
| Steiner et al. 2009 | 0,687 | 0,268 | 0,072 | 0,162 | 1,213 | 2,563 | 0,010 |
| Uzbay et al. 2013 | 0,163 | 0,322 | 0,104 | -0,469 | 0,795 | 0,506 | 0,613 |
| Wiesmann et al. 1999 | 1,088 | 0,333 | 0,111 | 0,435 | 1,740 | 3,267 | 0,001 |
| Zhang et al. 2010 | 2,325 | 0,218 | 0,048 | 1,898 | 2,753 | 10,659 | 0,000 |
| | 0,925 | 0,170 | 0,029 | 0,591 | 1,259 | 5,429 | 0,000 |

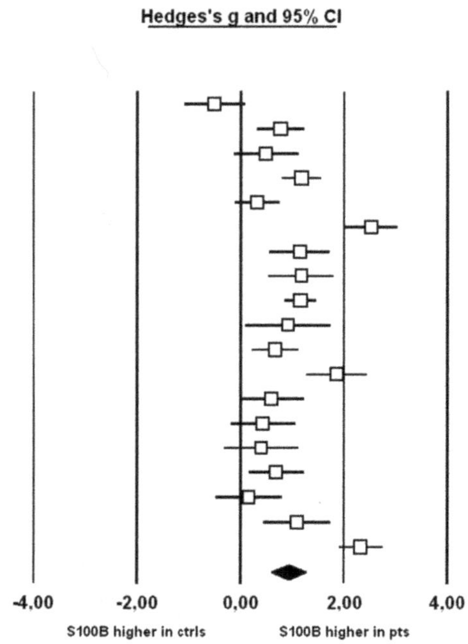


Meta Analysis of serum / plasma S100B levels in schizophrenic patients compared to healthy controls

**FIGURE 2 | Forest plot for the meta-analysis of serum S100B levels in schizophrenic patients compared to healthy control subjects.** Hedges' g was used as an estimate of effect size under a random effects model. CI, confidence interval.

| Group by medication | Study name | Hedges's g | Standard error | Variance | Lower limit | Upper limit | Z-Value | p-Value |
|---|---|---|---|---|---|---|---|---|
| medicated | Gattaz et al. 2000 | -0,503 | 0,295 | 0,087 | -1,080 | 0,075 | -1,707 | 0,088 |
| medicated | Kim et al. 2007_groupb | 1,204 | 0,278 | 0,077 | 0,660 | 1,748 | 4,340 | 0,000 |
| medicated | O'Connell et al. 2013 | 0,318 | 0,217 | 0,047 | -0,108 | 0,744 | 1,463 | 0,143 |
| medicated | Qi et al. 2009 | 0,428 | 0,318 | 0,101 | -0,195 | 1,050 | 1,346 | 0,178 |
| medicated | Schroeter et al. 2003_groupb | 1,138 | 0,358 | 0,128 | 0,436 | 1,841 | 3,177 | 0,001 |
| medicated | Wiesmann et al. 1999 | 1,088 | 0,333 | 0,111 | 0,435 | 1,740 | 3,267 | 0,001 |
| medicated | Zhang et al. 2010 | 2,325 | 0,218 | 0,048 | 1,898 | 2,753 | 10,659 | 0,000 |
| medicated | | 0,861 | 0,376 | 0,141 | 0,125 | 1,598 | 2,293 | 0,022 |
| unmedicated | Kim et al. 2007 | 1,807 | 0,304 | 0,092 | 1,212 | 2,402 | 5,952 | 0,000 |
| unmedicated | Lara et al. 2001 | 0,482 | 0,315 | 0,099 | -0,134 | 1,099 | 1,533 | 0,125 |
| unmedicated | Ling et al. 2007 | 1,172 | 0,199 | 0,040 | 0,782 | 1,562 | 5,886 | 0,000 |
| unmedicated | Rothermundt et al. 2001 | 1,285 | 0,301 | 0,090 | 0,695 | 1,875 | 4,271 | 0,000 |
| unmedicated | Rothermundt et al. 2004a | 1,170 | 0,329 | 0,108 | 0,526 | 1,814 | 3,561 | 0,000 |
| unmedicated | Rothermundt et al. 2004b | 1,156 | 0,154 | 0,024 | 0,854 | 1,457 | 7,515 | 0,000 |
| unmedicated | Sarandöl et al. 2007 | 0,664 | 0,235 | 0,055 | 0,203 | 1,126 | 2,822 | 0,005 |
| unmedicated | Schroeter et al. 2003 | -0,030 | 0,344 | 0,118 | -0,703 | 0,644 | -0,087 | 0,931 |
| unmedicated | Uzbay et al. 2013 | 0,163 | 0,322 | 0,104 | -0,469 | 0,795 | 0,506 | 0,613 |
| unmedicated | | 0,899 | 0,170 | 0,029 | 0,565 | 1,233 | 5,282 | 0,000 |
| Overall | | 0,893 | 0,155 | 0,024 | 0,589 | 1,196 | 5,757 | 0,000 |

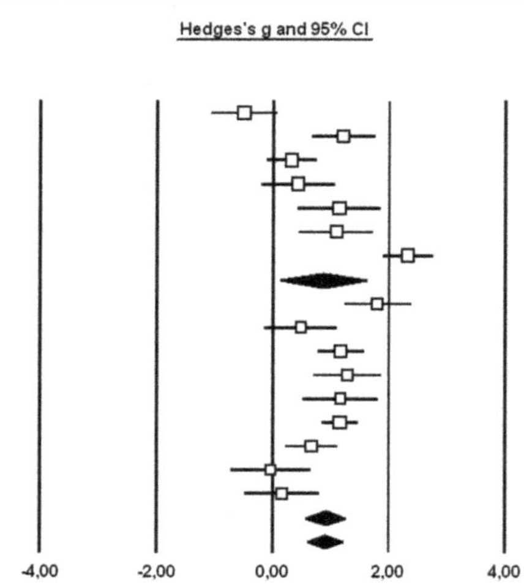


Meta Analysis of S100B levels grouped by medication status of patients

**FIGURE 3 | Forest plot for the meta-analysis of serum S100B levels in medicated vs. unmedicated patients in a cross-sectional design.** Hedges' g was used as an estimate of effect size under a random effects model. CI, confidence interval.

$p = 0.01$), bias index ($\beta_{\text{bias index}} = 0.3023$, $p = 0.001$) as well as PANSS total ($\beta_{\text{PANSS total}} = -0.0435$, $p = 0.001$), positive ($\beta_{\text{PANSS positive}} = -0.1273$, $p = 0.02$) and general psychopathology ($\beta_{\text{PANSS general}} = -0.0965$, $p < 0.001$) scores, but not for any of the other regressions calculated (see **Table 2**, **Figure 5**).

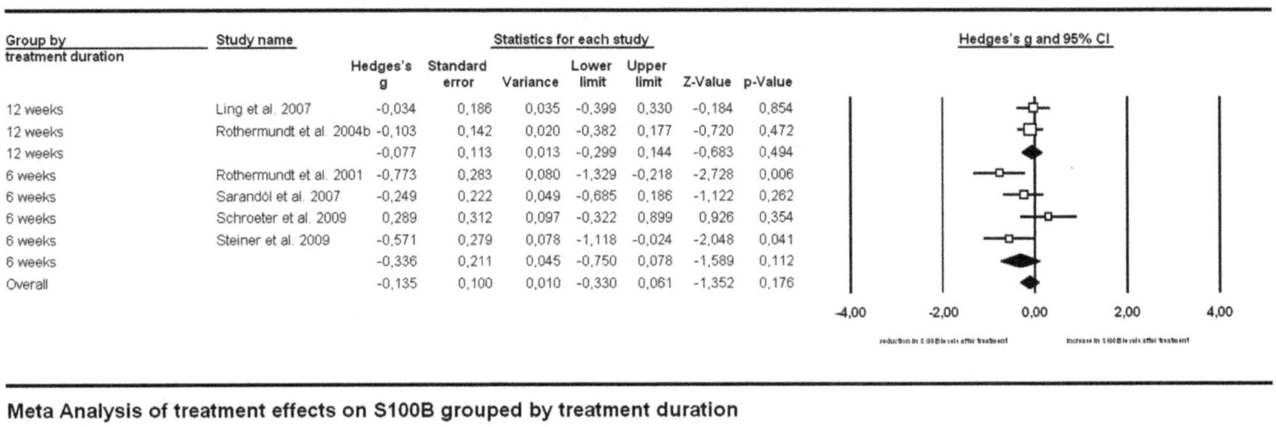


**FIGURE 4 | Forest plot for the meta-analysis of serum S100B levels before vs. after neuroleptic/antipsychotic treatment in longitudinal studies.** Hedges' g was used as an estimate of effect size under a random effects model. Effect sizes are shown for each treatment duration separately as well as the overall effect of treatment regardless of duration. CI, confidence interval.

**TABLE 2 | Results of simple meta-regression of covariates with serum S100B effect size.**

| Covariate | Number of studies | Coefficient (β) | $r^2$ | p |
|---|---|---|---|---|
| Mean age | 19 | 0.0573 | 0.52 | 0.0026 |
| Illness duration | 16 | 0.0537 | 0.46 | 0.0086 |
| Mean age at onset | 16 | 0.1022 | 0 | 0.2329 |
| Male-to-female ratio | 19 | 0.0161 | 0 | 0.8444 |
| PANSS total score | 11 | −0.0435 | 0.82 | 0.0014 |
| PANSS positive | 8 | −0.1273 | 0.55 | 0.0228 |
| PANSS negative | 9 | −0.0856 | 0 | 0.2766 |
| PANSS general | 7 | −0.0965 | 1 | 0.0008 |
| BPRS score | 6 | 0.0339 | 0.25 | 0.1859 |
| Bias index | 19 | 0.3023 | 0.61 | 0.0010 |

*Note: BPRS, Brief Psychiatric Rating Scale; PANSS, Positive And Negative Syndrome Scale.*

Subsequent multiple meta-regression of the PANSS subscores was then performed to obtain an impression of the influence of the individual factors while partialling out the impact of the other subscales. Results are illustrated in **Table 3**.

A multiple meta-regression analysis including the factors illness duration and age at onset revealed a significant influence of the former ($\beta_{\text{illness duration}} = 0.0538$, $p < 0.01$), while the latter failed to meet significance criteria ($\beta_{\text{age at onset}} = 0.0997$, $p = 0.12$, n.s., see **Table 3**). A model including the positive and the negative subscale showed a significant effect of the PANSS positive score on predicting effect sizes in the individual studies, whereas testing the influence of the negative subscale as a predictor while holding PANSS positive constant did not lead to this factor becoming significant ($\beta_{\text{PANSS positive}} = -0.1203$, $p = 0.01$, $\beta_{\text{PANSS negative}} = -0.0797$, $p = 0.13$, n.s.). A model including the positive and the general subscale revealed the factor general psychopathology to remain significant ($\beta_{\text{PANSS general}} = -0.0911$, $p < 0.01$) while the positive subscale lost its predictive value ($\beta_{\text{PANSS positive}} = -0.0127$, $p = 0.69$, n.s.). No individual factor remained significant in an analysis including all three subscales ($\beta_{\text{PANSS positive}} = -0.0038$, $p = 0.96$, n.s., $\beta_{\text{PANSS negative}} = 0.0095$, $p = 0.91$, n.s., $\beta_{\text{PANSS general}} = -0.0977$, $p = 0.16$, n.s.).

# DISCUSSION

Our comprehensive meta-analysis, including 19 original studies with 766 patients and 607 healthy control subjects revealed elevated levels of the glial marker protein S100B in serum in schizophrenia, which is related to illness duration and to clinical symptomatology. In the following we want to discuss these findings in detail.

## Serum S100B is Increased in Schizophrenia without Influences of Medication

Regarding the comparison of patient vs. control group, the outcome of a Hedges' g of 0.925 constitutes a rather strong effect (**Figure 2**), thus confirming the result of previous meta-analyses indicating higher levels of S100B in serum of patients compared to healthy control subjects (Schroeter et al., 2003; Schroeter and Steiner, 2009; Aleksovska et al., 2014). Testing the influence of risk of bias on effect size by meta-regression of a measure of bias published in Polyakova et al. (2015), we found that higher S100B effects were related to a lower likelihood of bias, as indicated by a high score in this bias index (**Figure 5**). Thus, studies with higher methodological quality tend to show higher S100B serum levels in patients compared to healthy controls, suggesting that this effect is not overestimated. Differences in included studies in comparison to the meta-analysis by Aleksovska et al. (2014) are related to more conservative inclusion criteria in our study, in particular the stricter age-matching of control cohorts.

Medication effects were investigated with two complementary approaches in our meta-analysis. Both the cross-sectional and the longitudinal approach revealed no significant effect of neuroleptic treatment on serum S100B levels in

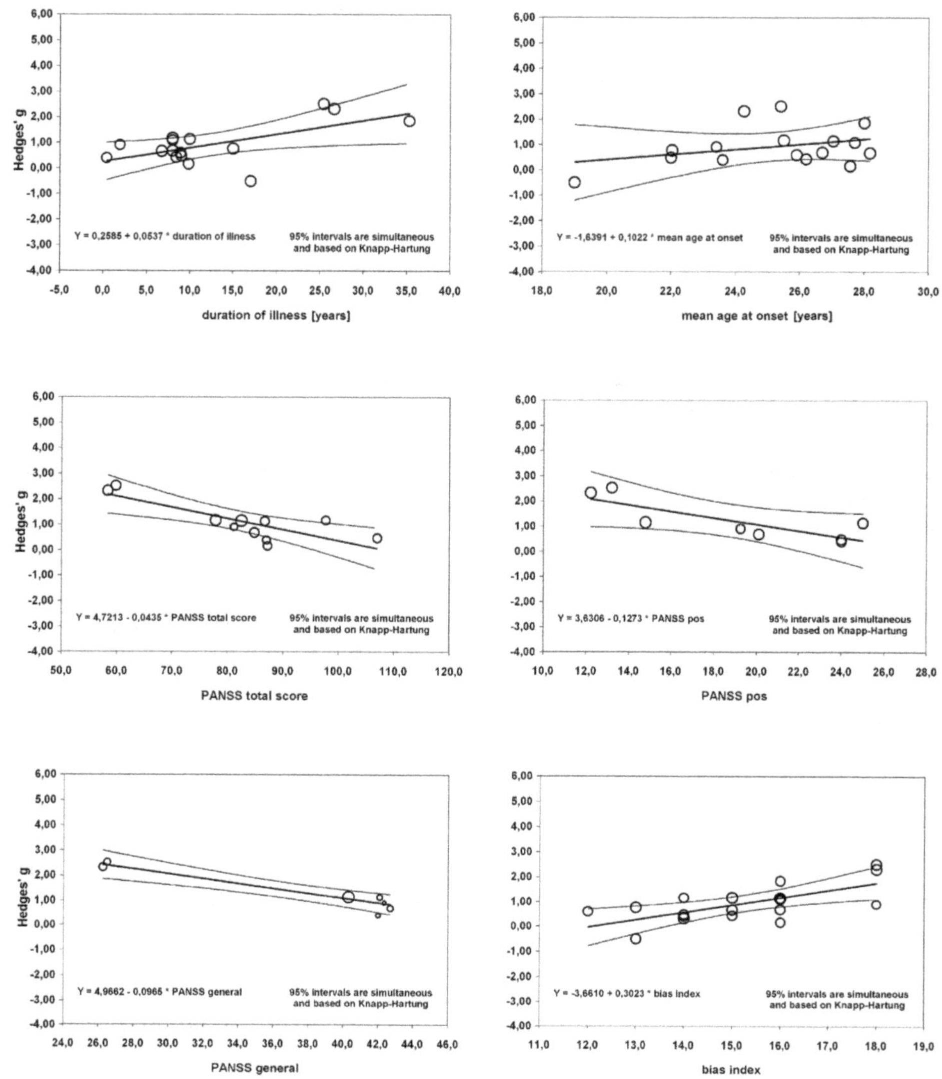


**FIGURE 5 | Results of a meta-regression analysis investigating the influence of duration of illness, age at onset, PANSS total and positive score, PANSS general subscale score and bias index on effect size of serum S100B levels in schizophrenia**. PANSS, Positive And Negative Syndrome Scale.

schizophrenia. Regarding the cross-sectional analysis one has to take into account that the lack of a between-group effect when comparing studies with only medicated to those including only unmedicated subjects could be due to a high heterogeneity both within and between studies in both groups. Unmedicated subjects encompassed never-medicated as well as patients off neuroleptics/antipsychotics for a minimum of 1 week, whereas medicated subjects widely differed in the type of neuroleptic/antipsychotic drug they were administered. Additionally, information on further psychoactive co-medication or either licit (tobacco or alcohol) or illicit drug use was not consistently supplied across studies. Similarly, the longitudinal approach also included a mixture of drug-naïve patients and such with prior neuroleptic medication but drug-free at the time of investigation. Subsequent treatment likewise consisted of different types of neuroleptics. Moreover, only six longitudinal studies were available for meta-analysis, hence lack of statistical power might be an important factor to be considered here. Accordingly, future better-controlled studies are required to disentangle the impact of medication and disease.

In sum, our meta-analyses indicate higher S100B serum levels in schizophrenia when compared to control subjects without any evidence for treatment effects to date. Our results confirm elevated S100B serum levels as an indicator of glial pathology in schizophrenia (Rothermundt et al., 2004a; Schroeter et al., 2009; Aleksovska et al., 2014), although this finding does not seem to be disease-specific, i.e., serum S100B seems to be elevated also in other psychiatric disorders such as mood disorders (Schroeter and Steiner, 2009), as

**TABLE 3 | Results of multiple meta-regression analysis with serum S100B effect size.**

| Covariate | Number of studies | Coefficient (β) | $r^2$ of combined model | $p$ |
|---|---|---|---|---|
| Illness duration | 16 | 0.0538 | 0.54 | 0.0062 |
| Mean age at onset | | 0.0997 | | 0.1171 |
| PANSS positive | 7 | −0.0038 | 0.98 | 0.9635 |
| PANSS negative | | 0.0095 | | 0.9128 |
| PANSS general | | −0.0977 | | 0.1561 |
| PANSS positive | 8 | −0.1203 | 0.80 | 0.0136 |
| PANSS negative | | −0.0797 | | 0.1316 |
| PANSS positive | 7 | −0.0127 | 1.00 | 0.6925 |
| PANSS general | | −0.0911 | | 0.0077 |
| Illness duration | 9 | 0.0446 | 0.96 | 0.0685 |
| PANSS total | | −0.0284 | | 0.0606 |

*Note: BPRS, Brief Psychiatric Rating Scale; PANSS, Positive And Negative Syndrome Scale.*

shown in recent meta-analyses (Schroeter et al., 2008, 2010, 2011, 2013). In contrast to antidepressant drugs, where S100B serum levels have been discussed as indicators/biomarkers for successful treatment (Schroeter et al., 2008), as of yet there is no meta-analytic evidence for serum S100B being related to treatment success of neuroleptics/antipsychotics in schizophrenia.

## Illness Duration and Clinical Symptoms are Correlated with Serum S100B Levels in Schizophrenia

There was a strong positive correlation between effect size of S100B with duration of illness, whereas the correlation analysis with age at onset did not show significant effects. This analysis included 16 original studies, and accordingly, has to be regarded as a highly consistent and relevant finding. A multiple meta-regression analysis including illness duration and age at onset confirmed the impact of the first factor on serum S100B in schizophrenia (**Table 3**). Although effect sizes of serum S100B levels also correlated with mean age of schizophrenia subjects (**Table 2**), this effect seems to be related to illness duration ($r_{\text{mean age/illness duration}} = 0.96$, $p < 0.001$; correlation according to Pearson, two-tailed $p$) since S100B effects sizes were calculated by comparing schizophrenia subjects to age-matched control subjects, hence excluding any impact of age *per se*. Therefore, mean age was excluded from the aforementioned multiple meta-regression analysis.

Contrary to earlier studies we observed a significant correlation of serum S100B effect size with PANSS total, positive and general psychopathology, yet not with PANSS negative scores (Rothermundt et al., 2001, 2004b; Schroeter et al., 2003; Schmitt et al., 2005). A high intercorrelation of the positive subscale with the total score also suggests that the effect of the PANSS total score might be driven by high scores in the positive subscale ($r_{\text{PANSS total/PANSS positive}} = 0.83$, $p = 0.01$). An additional multiple meta-regression analysis (**Table 3**) including positive and negative symptoms as measured with the PANSS confirmed the impact of PANSS positive scores on serum S100B levels, whereas the same analysis with the PANSS general score included additionally revealed no significant result.

While the correlation of S100B levels with the general psychopathology subscale was even stronger than with the positive subscale, it has to be noted that only seven studies contributed to the former, whereas there was one more for the latter. Furthermore, as illustrated in **Figure 5**, two studies seem to predominantly drive this effect, with the other five being distributed rather evenly. Thus, at the moment it is not possible to estimate whether there truly is any relation of the general psychopathology scale to S100B levels.

Seeing that the recommended minimum number of original studies for meta-regression to gain validity has been estimated at around ten (Borenstein et al., 2009), these subscale analyses for positive, negative, and general symptoms so far remain highly speculative as they all include less than ten studies (**Table 2**). The analysis for the PANSS total score on the other hand seems to be more statistically reliable with eleven studies included, and not prone to the strong effects of multicollinearity observed between the individual subscores.

In conclusion, duration of illness seems to influence serum S100B levels in schizophrenia patients, with larger differences between patients and control subjects the longer the disorder has been present on average. With regards to psychopathology, the PANSS total score and with a lower evidence, the PANSS positive symptom subscale as well as the PANSS general psychopathology score are inversely correlated with effect size, i.e., the more (total, positive or general) symptoms, the smaller the difference in S100B between patients and control subjects.

One might ask whether these effects, in particular influences of illness duration and clinical scores on serum S100B effect sizes, might be interrelated. Indeed, illness duration was negatively correlated with clinical symptoms as measured with the relevant PANSS scores across studies ($r_{\text{illness duration/PANSS total}} = -0.73$, $p = 0.03$, $r_{\text{illness duration/PANSS positive}} = -0.82$, $p = 0.03$, $r_{\text{illness duration/PANSS general}} = -0.91$, $p = 0.03$, in contrast $r_{\text{illness duration/PANSS negative}} = -0.15$, $p = 0.72$). Accordingly, studies examining patients with longer duration of illness find lower psychopathology scores, which might be related to medication/treatment effects in the long-term or disease course itself. Multiple meta-regression including both duration of illness and the most reliable measure for clinical symptoms, the PANSS total score, led to both factors just narrowly missing significance, indicating some shared variance (**Table 3**).

The relative increase of serum S100B levels in the course of schizophrenia could be explained with dynamic glial alterations in the course of the disease. Both astrocytes and oligodendrocytes contain S100B, which may be released under conditions of reduced energy supply or cell damage (Steiner et al., 2007, 2008). Accordingly, in the context of schizophrenia, both dystrophy and swelling of astrocytes were found to progress with the duration of illness in an electron microscopic study (Kolomeets and Uranova, 2010; Bernstein et al., 2015). Moreover, oligodendrocyte-related disturbances of cerebral connectivity (Yao et al., 2015) and white matter pathology also progress over time, including a disturbed connectome organization which has been related to longitudinal changes in general functioning in schizophrenia (Whitford et al., 2007; Collin et al., 2015). Decreases in white matter volume are more pronounced than gray matter changes in the course of schizophrenia (Andreasen et al., 2011). Furthermore, in this study, white matter changes were also associated with the psychotic but not the negative symptom dimension. Interestingly, serum S100B correlates with white and not gray matter parameters in healthy subjects (Streitbürger et al., 2012).

Alternatively, these findings might be related to treatment, as patients taking neuroleptic/antipsychotic medication for longer time tend to be less symptomatic compared to recent-onset schizophrenia, thus showing lower PANSS scores but possibly also elevated S100B levels with longer duration of illness. However, so far no significant medication effect could be detected in our meta-analyses of either the cross-sectional or the few longitudinal studies, and tendencies so far seem to show a reduction of serum S100B through medication (Rothermundt et al., 2001, 2004b; Ling et al., 2007; Sarandol et al., 2007; Schroeter et al., 2009; Steiner et al., 2009, 2010c; de Souza et al., 2009; Nardin et al., 2011).

A possible explanation integrating all these findings could be a mediating effect of BMI, as long-term use of neuroleptics/antipsychotics tends to lead to weight gain, and adipocytes are among the cell types secreting S100B. This explanation is well in line with results found by Steiner et al. (2010a,b, 2014), also linking this effect to changes in insulin metabolism (Steiner et al., 2010d). Alternatively, the progression of the schizophrenic disorder itself could cause metabolic changes leading to both weight gain and altered S100B secretion (see Steiner et al., 2014). In fact, Steiner et al. (2010d), found that in their group of patients, schizophrenia was generally associated with impaired glucose tolerance, irrespective of medication status or BMI.

Unfortunately, the influence of BMI as a covariate could not yet be investigated in this meta-analysis, as there are currently only three studies (Qi et al., 2009; Steiner et al., 2009; O'Connell et al., 2013) offering that kind of information. Other correlates of adipocyte or insulin metabolism so far have only been published for the patient group of Steiner et al. (2009). Consequently, although metabolic changes associated with schizophrenia seem to offer a plausible explanation for the meta-regression findings in this analysis, further research in that direction will be needed to elucidate the exact determinants of serum S100B levels as well as the precise function of this protein in schizophrenia.

## CONCLUSION

In summary, our comprehensive meta-analysis including 19 original studies with a total of 766 patients and 607 healthy control subjects confirms higher values of the glial serum marker protein S100B in schizophrenia compared to control subjects. Meta-regression analyses revealed significant effects of illness duration, with higher S100B serum levels in the disorder's course, and an impact of clinical symptomatology, in particular a negative correlation of the total score of the PANSS with serum S100B levels in schizophrenia. Accordingly, results are in line with glial pathology in schizophrenia that is modulated by illness duration and related to clinical symptomatology. Further studies are needed to investigate mechanisms and mediating factors for these findings, and replicate findings for subscales measuring clinical psychopathology by including more studies.

## AUTHOR CONTRIBUTIONS

KS and MLS have designed the study, analyzed and interpreted the data, drafted and revised the manuscript content; KS and MP have conducted the search for relevant studies and selected studies included in the meta-analysis according to inclusion and exclusion criteria. All authors have critically reviewed the manuscript and approved its final version. All authors agree to be accountable for all aspects of the work in ensuring that questions related to the accuracy or integrity of any part of the work are appropriately investigated and resolved.

## ACKNOWLEDGMENTS

We thank Dr. Christoph Engel from the Institute for Medical Informatics, Statistics, and Epidemiology (IMISE) at the University of Leipzig for statistical advice. MP has been supported by the German Max Planck Society (International Max Planck Research School on Neuroscience of Communication—IMPRS NeuroCom). MLS has been supported by LIFE—Leipzig Research Center for Civilization Diseases at the University of Leipzig—funded by the European Union, European Regional Development Fund and by the Free State of Saxony within the framework of the excellence initiative, by the German Consortium for Frontotemporal Lobar Degeneration, funded by the German Federal Ministry of Education and Research, by the Parkinson's Disease Foundation (Grant No. PDF-IRG-1307), and by the Michael J Fox Foundation (Grant No. 11362).

## REFERENCES

Aleksovska, K., Leoncini, E., Bonassi, S., Cesario, A., Boccia, S., and Frustaci, A. (2014). Systematic review and meta-analysis of circulating S100B blood levels in schizophrenia. *PLoS One* 9:e106342. doi: 10.1371/journal.pone.0106342

Andreasen, N. C., Nopoulos, P., Magnotta, V., Pierson, R., Ziebell, S., and Ho, B.-C. (2011). Progressive brain change in schizophrenia: a prospective longitudinal study of first-episode schizophrenia. *Biol. Psychiatry* 70, 672–679. doi: 10.1016/j.biopsych.2011.05.017

Bernstein, H.-G., Steiner, J., Guest, P. C., Dobrowolny, H., and Bogerts, B. (2015). Glial cells as key players in schizophrenia pathology: recent insights and concepts of therapy. *Schizophr. Res.* 161, 4–18. doi: 10.1016/j.schres.2014.03.035

Bianchi, R., Giambanco, I., and Donato, R. (2010). S100B/RAGE-dependent activation of microglia via NF-kappaB and AP-1 Co-regulation of COX-2 expression by S100B, IL-1beta and TNF-alpha. *Neurobiol. Aging* 31, 665–677. doi: 10.1016/j.neurobiolaging.2008.05.017

Borenstein, M., Hedges, L. V., Higgins, J. P. T., and Rothstein, H. R. (2009). *Introduction to Meta-Analysis*, 1st Edn. (Hoboken, NJ: John Wiley & Sons, Ltd.), 452.

Cohen, J. (1988). *Statistical Power Analysis for the Behavioral Sciences*. New York, NY: Routledge Academic.

Collin, G., de Nijs, J., Hulshoff Pol, H. E., Cahn, W., and van den Heuvel, M. P. (2015). Connectome organization is related to longitudinal changes in general functioning, symptoms and IQ in chronic schizophrenia. *Schizophr. Res.* doi: 10.1016/j.schres.2015.03.012 [Epub ahead of print].

DerSimonian, R., and Laird, N. (1986). Meta-analysis in clinical trials. *Control. Clin. Trials* 7, 177–188. doi: 10.1016/0197-2456(86)90046-2

de Souza, D. F., Leite, M. C., Quincozes-Santos, A., Nardin, P., Tortorelli, L. S., Rigo, M. M., et al. (2009). S100B secretion is stimulated by IL-1beta in glial cultures and hippocampal slices of rats: likely involvement of MAPK pathway. *J. Neuroimmunol.* 206, 52–57. doi: 10.1016/j.jneuroim.2008.10.012

Donato, R. (2001). S100: a multigenic family of calcium-modulated proteins of the EF-hand type with intracellular and extracellular functional roles. *Int. J. Biochem. Cell Biol.* 33, 637–668. doi: 10.1016/s1357-2725(01)00046-2

Donato, R., Sorci, G., Riuzzi, F., Arcuri, C., Bianchi, R., Brozzi, F., et al. (2009). S100B's double life: intracellular regulator and extracellular signal. *Biochim. Biophys. Acta* 1793, 1008–1022. doi: 10.1016/j.bbamcr.2008.11.009

Gami, A. S., Witt, B. J., Howard, D. E., Erwin, P. J., Gami, L. A., Somers, V. K., et al. (2007). Metabolic syndrome and risk of incident cardiovascular events and death: a systematic review and meta-analysis of longitudinal studies. *J. Am. Coll. Cardiol.* 49, 403–414. doi: 10.1016/j.jacc.2006.09.032

Gattaz, W. F., Lara, D. R., Elkis, H., Portela, L. V., Gonçalves, C. A., Tort, A. B., et al. (2000). Decreased S100-beta protein in schizophrenia: preliminary evidence. *Schizophr. Res.* 43, 91–95. doi: 10.1016/s0920-9964(99)00146-2

Hofmann, S. G., and Smits, J. A. J. (2008). Cognitive-behavioral therapy for adult anxiety disorders: a meta-analysis of randomized placebo-controlled trials. *J. Clin. Psychiatry* 69, 621–632. doi: 10.4088/jcp.v69n0415

Howren, M. B., Lamkin, D. M., and Suls, J. (2009). Associations of depression with C-reactive protein, IL-1 and IL-6: a meta-analysis. *Psychosom. Med.* 71, 171–186. doi: 10.1097/psy.0b013e3181907c1b

Kolomeets, N. S., and Uranova, N. (2010). Ultrastructural abnormalities of astrocytes in the hippocampus in schizophrenia and duration of illness: a postortem morphometric study. *World J. Biol. Psychiatry* 11, 282–292. doi: 10.3109/15622970902806124

Lakens, D. (2013). Calculating and reporting effect sizes to facilitate cumulative science: a practical primer for *t*-tests and ANOVAs. *Front. Psychol.* 4:863. doi: 10.3389/fpsyg.2013.00863

Lara, D. R., Gama, C. S., Belmonte-de-Abreu, P., Portela, L. V. C., Gonçalves, C. A., Fonseca, M., et al. (2001). Increased serum S100B protein in schizophrenia: a study in medication-free patients. *J. Psychiatr. Res.* 35, 11–14. doi: 10.1016/s0022-3956(01)00003-6

Leucht, S., Corves, C., Arbter, D., Engel, R. R., Li, C., and Davis, J. M. (2009). Second-generation versus first-generation antipsychotic drugs for schizophrenia: a meta-analysis. *Lancet* 373, 31–41. doi: 10.1016/S0140-6736(08)61764-X

Ling, S., Tang, Y., Jiang, F., Wiste, A., Guo, S., Weng, Y., et al. (2007). Plasma S-100B protein in Chinese patients with schizophrenia: comparison with healthy controls and effect of antipsychotics treatment. *J. Psychiatr. Res.* 41, 36–42. doi: 10.1016/j.jpsychires.2005.11.006

Moher, D., Liberati, A., Tetzlaff, J., Altman, D. G., and PRISMA Group, T. (2009). Preferred reporting items for systematic reviews and meta-analyses: the PRISMA statement. *Ann. Intern. Med.* 151, 264–269. doi: 10.7326/0003-4819-151-4-200908180-00135

Nardin, P., Tramontina, A. C., Quincozes-Santos, A., Tortorelli, L. S., Lunardi, P., Klein, P. R., et al. (2011). *In vitro* S100B secretion is reduced by apomorphine: effects of antipsychotics and antioxidants. *Prog. Neuropsychopharmacol. Biol. Psychiatry* 35, 1291–1296. doi: 10.1016/j.pnpbp.2011.04.004

O'Connell, K., Thakore, J., and Dev, K. K. (2013). Levels of S100B are raised in female patients with schizophrenia. *BMC Psychiatry* 13:146. doi: 10.1186/1471-244x-13-146

Polyakova, M., Stuke, K., Schuemberg, K., Mueller, K., Schoenknecht, P., and Schroeter, M. L. (2015). BDNF as a biomarker for successful treatment of mood disorders: a systematic and quantitative meta-analysis. *J. Affect. Disord.* 174, 432–440. doi: 10.1016/j.jad.2014.11.044

Qi, L. Y., Xiu, M. H., Chen, D. C., Wang, F., Kosten, T. A., Kosten, T. R., et al. (2009). Increased serum S100B levels in chronic schizophrenic patients on long-term clozapine or typical antipsychotics. *Neurosci. Lett.* 462, 113–117. doi: 10.1016/j.neulet.2009.06.019

Rothermundt, M., Falkai, P., Ponath, G., Abel, S., Bürkle, H., Diedrich, M., et al. (2004a). Glial cell dysfunction in schizophrenia indicated by increased S100B in the CSF. *Mol. Psychiatry* 9, 897–899. doi: 10.1038/sj.mp.4001548

Rothermundt, M., Ponath, G., Glaser, T., Hetzel, G., and Arolt, V. (2004b). S100B serum levels and long-term improvement of negative symptoms in patients with schizophrenia. *Neuropsychopharmacology* 29, 1004–1011. doi: 10.1038/sj.npp.1300403

Rothermundt, M., Missler, U., Arolt, V., Peters, M., Leadbeater, J., Wiesmann, M., et al. (2001). Increased S100B blood levels in unmedicated and treated schizophrenic patients are correlated with negative symptomatology. *Mol. Psychiatry* 6, 445–449. doi: 10.1038/sj.mp.4000889

Rothermundt, M., Ohrmann, P., Abel, S., Siegmund, A., Pedersen, A., Ponath, G., et al. (2007). Glial cell activation in a subgroup of patients with schizophrenia indicated by increased S100B serum concentrations and elevated myo-inositol. *Prog. Neuropsychopharmacol. Biol. Psychiatry* 31, 361–364. doi: 10.1016/j.pnpbp.2006.09.013

Ryoun Kim, H., Kyung Lee, M., and Park, D.-B. (2007). Increased serum S100B protein in chronic schizophrenic patients in Korea. *Clin. Chem. Lab. Med.* 45, 1561–1563. doi: 10.1515/cclm.2007.311

Sarandol, A., Kirli, S., Akkaya, C., Altin, A., Demirci, M., and Sarandol, E. (2007). Oxidative-antioxidative systems and their relation with serum S100 B levels in patients with schizophrenia: effects of short term antipsychotic treatment. *Prog. Neuropsychopharmacol. Biol. Psychiatry* 31, 1164–1169. doi: 10.1016/j.pnpbp.2007.03.008

Schmitt, A., Bertsch, T., Henning, U., Tost, H., Klimke, A., Henn, F. A., et al. (2005). Increased serum S100B in elderly, chronic schizophrenic patients: negative correlation with deficit symptoms. *Schizophr. Res.* 80, 305–313. doi: 10.1016/j.schres.2005.04.013

Schroeter, M., Abdul-Khaliq, H., Frühauf, S., Höhne, R., Schick, G., Diefenbacher, A., et al. (2003). Serum S100B is increased during early treatment with antipsychotics and in deficit schizophrenia. *Schizophr. Res.* 62, 231–236. doi: 10.1016/s0920-9964(02)00383-3

Schroeter, M. L., Abdul-Khaliq, H., Krebs, M., Diefenbacher, A., and Blasig, I. E. (2008). Serum markers support disease-specific glial pathology in major depression. *J. Affect. Disord.* 111, 271–280. doi: 10.1016/j.jad.2008.03.005

Schroeter, M. L., Abdul-Khaliq, H., Krebs, M., Diefenbacher, A., and Blasig, I. E. (2009). Neuron-specific enolase is unaltered whereas S100B is elevated in serum of patients with schizophrenia–original research and meta-analysis. *Psychiatry Res.* 167, 66–72. doi: 10.1016/j.psychres.2008.01.002

Schroeter, M. L., Abdul-Khaliq, H., Sacher, J., Steiner, J., Blasig, I. E., and Mueller, K. (2010). Mood disorders are glial disorders: evidence from *in vivo* studies. *Cardiovasc. Psychiatry Neurol.* 2010:780645. doi: 10.1155/2010/780645

Schroeter, M. L., Sacher, J., Steiner, J., Schoenknecht, P., and Mueller, K. (2013). Serum S100B represents a new biomarker for mood disorders. *Curr. Drug Targets* 14, 1237–1248. doi: 10.2174/13894501113149990014

Schroeter, M. L., and Steiner, J. (2009). Elevated serum levels of the glial marker protein S100B are not specific for schizophrenia or mood disorders. *Mol. Psychiatry* 14, 235–237. doi: 10.1038/mp.2008.85

Schroeter, M. L., Steiner, J., and Mueller, K. (2011). Glial pathology is modified by age in mood disorders–A systematic meta-analysis of serum S100B *in vivo* studies. *J. Affect. Disord.* 134, 32–38. doi: 10.1016/j.jad.2010.11.008

Sen, J., and Belli, A. (2007). S100B in neuropathologic states: the CRP of the brain? *J. Neurosci. Res.* 85, 1373–1380. doi: 10.1002/jnr.21211

Steiner, J., Bernstein, H.-G., Bielau, H., Berndt, A., Brisch, R., Mawrin, C., et al. (2007). Evidence for a wide extra-astrocytic distribution of S100B in human brain. *BMC Neurosci.* 8:2. doi: 10.1186/1471-2202-8-2

Steiner, J., Bernstein, H.-G., Bogerts, B., Gos, T., Richter-Landsberg, C., Wunderlich, M. T., et al. (2008). S100B is expressed in and released from, OLN-93 oligodendrocytes: influence of serum and glucose deprivation. *Neuroscience* 154, 496–503. doi: 10.1016/j.neuroscience.2008.03.060

Steiner, J., Bernstein, H.-G., Schiltz, K., Müller, U. J., Westphal, S., Drexhage, H. A., et al. (2014). Immune system and glucose metabolism interaction in schizophrenia: a chicken-egg dilemma. *Prog. Neuropsychopharmacol. Biol. Psychiatry* 48, 287–294. doi: 10.1016/j.pnpbp.2012.09.016

Steiner, J., Bielau, H., Bernstein, H.-G., Bogerts, B., and Wunderlich, M. T. (2006). Increased cerebrospinal fluid and serum levels of S100B in first-onset schizophrenia are not related to a degenerative release of glial fibrillar acidic protein, myelin basic protein and neurone-specific enolase from glia or neurones. *J. Neurol. Neurosurg. Psychiatry* 77, 1284–1287. doi: 10.1136/jnnp.2006.093427

Steiner, J., Myint, A. M., Schiltz, K., Westphal, S., Bernstein, H.-G., Walter, M., et al. (2010a). S100B serum levels in schizophrenia are presumably related to visceral obesity and insulin resistance. *Cardiovasc. Psychiatry Neurol.* 2010:480707. doi: 10.1155/2010/480707

Steiner, J., Schiltz, K., Walter, M., Wunderlich, M. T., Keilhoff, G., Brisch, R., et al. (2010b). S100B serum levels are closely correlated with body mass index: an important caveat in neuropsychiatric research. *Psychoneuroendocrinology* 35, 321–324. doi: 10.1016/j.psyneuen.2009.07.012

Steiner, J., Schroeter, M. L., Schiltz, K., Bernstein, H. G., Müller, U. J., Richter-Landsberg, C., et al. (2010c). Haloperidol and clozapine decrease S100B release from glial cells. *Neuroscience* 167, 1025–1031. doi: 10.1016/j.neuroscience.2010.03.010

Steiner, J., Walter, M., Guest, P., Myint, A. M., Schiltz, K., Panteli, B., et al. (2010d). Elevated S100B levels in schizophrenia are associated with insulin resistance. *Mol. Psychiatry* 15, 3–4. doi: 10.1038/mp.2009.87

Steiner, J., Walter, M., Wunderlich, M. T., Bernstein, H.-G., Panteli, B., Brauner, M., et al. (2009). A new pathophysiological aspect of S100B in schizophrenia: potential regulation of S100B by its scavenger soluble RAGE. *Biol. Psychiatry* 65, 1107–1110. doi: 10.1016/j.biopsych.2008.10.044

Streitbürger, D.-P., Arelin, K., Kratzsch, J., Thiery, J., Steiner, J., Villringer, A., et al. (2012). Validating serum S100B and neuron-specific enolase as biomarkers for the human brain – a combined serum, gene expression and MRI study. *PLoS One* 7:e43284. doi: 10.1371/journal.pone.0043284

Uzbay, T., Goktalay, G., Kayir, H., Eker, S. S., Sarandol, A., Oral, S., et al. (2013). Increased plasma agmatine levels in patients with schizophrenia. *J. Psychiatr. Res.* 47, 1054–1060. doi: 10.1016/j.jpsychires.2013.04.004

van der Leeuw, C., Marcelis, M., Peeters, S. C. T., Verbeek, M. M., Menheere, P. P. C. A., de Haan, L., et al. (2013). Replicated evidence of absence of association between serum S100B and (risk of) psychotic disorder. *PLoS One* 8:e82535. doi: 10.1371/journal.pone.0082535

Van Eldik, L. J., and Wainwright, M. S. (2003). The Janus face of glial-derived S100B: beneficial and detrimental functions in the brain. *Restor. Neurol. Neurosci.* 21, 97–108.

Whitford, T. J., Grieve, S. M., Farrow, T. F. D., Gomes, L., Brennan, J., Harris, A. W. F., et al. (2007). Volumetric white matter abnormalities in first-episode schizophrenia: a longitudinal, tensor-based morphometry study. *Am. J. Psychiatry* 164, 1082–1089. doi: 10.1176/appi.ajp.164.7.1082

Wiesmann, M., Wandinger, K. P., Missler, U., Eckhoff, D., Rothermundt, M., Arolt, V., et al. (1999). Elevated plasma levels of S-100b protein in schizophrenic patients. *Biol. Psychiatry* 45, 1508–1511. doi: 10.1016/s0006-3223(98)00217-0

Xiong, P., Zeng, Y., Wu, Q., Han Huang, D. X., Zainal, H., Xu, X., et al. (2014). Combining serum protein concentrations to diagnose schizophrenia: a preliminary exploration. *J. Clin. Psychiatry* 75, e794–e801. doi: 10.4088/jcp.13m08772

Yao, Y., Palaniyappan, L., Liddle, P., Zhang, J., Francis, S., and Feng, J. (2015). Variability of structurally constrained and unconstrained functional connectivity in schizophrenia. *Hum. Brain Mapp.* 36, 4529–4538. doi: 10.1002/hbm.22932

Zhang, X. Y., Xiu, M. H., Chen, D. C., Zhu, F. Y., Wu, G. Y., Haile, C. N., et al. (2010). Increased S100B serum levels in schizophrenic patients with tardive dyskinesia: association with dyskinetic movements. *J. Psychiatr. Res.* 44, 429–433. doi: 10.1016/j.jpsychires.2009.10.012

8

# Linking Activation of Microglia and Peripheral Monocytic Cells to the Pathophysiology of Psychiatric Disorders

*Yuta Takahashi* [1,2,3], *Zhiqian Yu* [1,2,4], *Mai Sakai* [1,2] *and Hiroaki Tomita* [1,2,4]*

[1] *Department of Disaster Psychiatry, International Research Institute of Disaster Science, Tohoku University, Sendai, Japan,* [2] *Department of Disaster Psychiatry, Graduate School of Medicine, Tohoku University, Sendai, Japan,* [3] *Department of Psychiatry, Graduate School of Medicine, Tohoku University, Sendai, Japan,* [4] *Group of Mental Health Promotion, Tohoku Medical Megabank Organization, Tohoku University, Sendai, Japan*

***Correspondence:***
*Hiroaki Tomita*
*htomita@med.tohoku.ac.jp*

A wide variety of studies have identified microglial activation in psychiatric disorders, such as schizophrenia, bipolar disorder, and major depressive disorder. Relatively fewer, but robust, studies have detected activation of peripheral monocytic cells in psychiatric disorders. Considering the origin of microglia, as well as neuropsychoimmune interactions in the context of the pathophysiology of psychiatric disorders, it is reasonable to speculate that microglia interact with peripheral monocytic cells in relevance with the pathogenesis of psychiatric disorders; however, these interactions have drawn little attention. In this review, we summarize findings relevant to activation of microglia and monocytic cells in psychiatric disorders, discuss the potential association between these cell types and disease pathogenesis, and propose perspectives for future research on these processes.

**Keywords: microglia, monocyte, mental disorder, psychoimmunology, peripheral biomarker, blood-brain barrier, schizophrenia, bipolar disorder**

## INTRODUCTION

A variety of postmortem brain studies and recent positron emission tomography (PET)-based studies have identified microglial activation in psychiatric disorders, such as schizophrenia (Bayer et al., 1999; Radewicz et al., 2000; van Berckel et al., 2008; Tang et al., 2012; Fillman et al., 2013), bipolar disorder (Haarman et al., 2014; Hercher et al., 2014), and major depressive disorder (Torres-Platas et al., 2014). Several studies have also indicated an association between alterations in monocytic features and psychiatric disorders (Rothermundt et al., 1998; Theodoropoulou et al., 2001; Padmos et al., 2008; Drexhage et al., 2011).

By contrast, peripheral monocytes can differentiate into macrophages and dendritic cells in peripheral tissues, both of which share similarities with microglia in their cellular morphology and functions, such as phagocytic activities, the expression of cell surface markers and cytokine production, and similar gene expression profiles (Schmitz et al., 2009; Beumer et al., 2012; Shechter and Schwartz, 2013; Prinz and Priller, 2014). Under pathological conditions in brain disorders, monocytes are recruited from peripheral blood into the brain, where they cooperate with

**Abbreviations:** CNS, central nervous system; LPS, lipopolysaccharide; NOD, non-obese diabetic.

microglia in immune responses (Beumer et al., 2012; Shechter and Schwartz, 2013; Prinz and Priller, 2014). Considering the similarity and potency of the interactions between these two cell types, it is reasonable to speculate that correlations and interactions exist between the activation identified in microglia and peripheral monocytic cells in patients with psychiatric disorders, although these possibilities have drawn little attention. In this review, we summarize the accumulated findings regarding microglial and peripheral monocytic activation in psychiatric disorders and discuss the potential mechanisms linking microglial and monocytic activation with the pathogenesis of psychiatric disorders. Finally, we propose directions for future research on these potential associations.

## ACCUMULATED FINDINGS OF MICROGLIAL ACTIVATION IN PSYCHIATRIC DISORDERS

Postmortem brain studies have suggested an association between psychiatric disorders and microglial activation (Bayer et al., 1999; Radewicz et al., 2000; Tang et al., 2012; Fillman et al., 2013; Hercher et al., 2014; Torres-Platas et al., 2014). Regarding the qualitative assessment of microglial morphology, Hercher et al. (2014) observed that activated microglial cells were increased in prefrontal white matter from patients with schizophrenia, but not that from patients with bipolar disorder. Torres-Platas et al. (2014) showed that primed (activated) microglia were significantly increased compared with ramified (resting) microglia in the anterior cingulate cortices obtained from patients who died of depressed suicides compared with healthy controls, whereas the total densities of ionized calcium-binding adapter molecule 1 (IBA1) positive microglia did not differ between the depressed suicide cases and controls. Bayer et al. (1999) and Radewicz et al. (2000) reported that the expression of Human Leukocyte Antigen-antigen D Related (HLA-DR), which reacts with activated microglia, was increased in the frontal cortices of patients with schizophrenia in immunostaining studies. Fillman et al. (2013) demonstrated that the interleukin-6 (*IL-6*), *IL8*, and *IL1β* mRNA transcripts were over-expressed in the dorsolateral prefrontal cortex, and the density of major histocompatibility complex class II (MHC-II) receptor-positive microglia (i.e., antigen-presenting cells) was increased in the white matter of patients with schizophrenia. Tang et al. (2012) found positive correlations among several activated microglial markers in subjects with schizophrenia. They also showed that changes in the expression of genes that encode markers of activated microglia were associated with inflammatory markers in the arachidonic acid signaling pathway in patients with schizophrenia.

Recent PET-based evaluations of microglial activation may also be applicable to psychiatric patients (Veenman and Gavish, 2000, 2012; Papadopoulos et al., 2006; van Berckel et al., 2008; Doorduin et al., 2009; Takano et al., 2010; Haarman et al., 2014). PET radioligands, such as C-PK11195 and DAA1106, are selective for the 18 kDa translocator protein/peripheral benzodiazepine receptor, which is highly expressed in activated microglia and is involved in multiple cellular processes, such as apoptosis, the regulation of cellular proliferation, immunomodulation and steroidogenesis (Veenman and Gavish, 2000, 2012; Papadopoulos et al., 2006). van Berckel et al.'s (2008) PET study showed a significant increase in microglial activation in patients with schizophrenia who had a disease onset within 5 calendar years compared with controls, although all patients were under treatment with atypical antipsychotics, and confounding effects of drug treatments remain unexcluded. Interestingly, Doorduin et al. (2009) in a PET study of patients who had recovered from psychosis, observed no significant microglial activation. Although Takano et al. (2010) found no significant difference between [$^{11}$C]DAA1106 binding in normal controls and patients with schizophrenia, the patients exhibited positive correlations between cortical [$^{11}$C]DAA1106 binding, positive symptom scores and duration of illness. Haarman et al. (2014) observed a significant increase in $^{11}$C-R-PK11195 binding potential in the right hippocampus of patients with bipolar disorder type I compared with healthy controls.

## MICROGLIAL FUNCTION AND POTENTIAL MECHANISMS UNDERLYING THE PATHOGENESIS OF PSYCHIATRIC DISORDERS

Microglia comprise ~12% of cells in the central nervous system (CNS; Vaughan and Peters, 1974); these cells are not uniformly distributed (Schmitz et al., 2009). More microglia are located close to neurons in the gray matter, with the highest concentrations in the hippocampus, olfactory telencephalon, basal ganglia, and substantia nigra (Lawson et al., 1990).

Accumulating evidence from fate-mapping studies suggests that the origin of most microglia is not the bone marrow after birth but hematopoietic stem cells in the yolk sac in the early developmental stage (Lassmann et al., 1993; Ginhoux et al., 2010; Schulz et al., 2012; Kierdorf et al., 2013; Prinz and Priller, 2014). Novel transgenic approaches have shown clear differences in the cellular characteristics of microglia and macrophages in the brain (Goldmann et al., 2013; Parkhurst et al., 2013; Yona et al., 2013). In contrast to macrophages, microglia are long-lived and are not replaced by circulating peripheral monocytes under physiological conditions.

Microglia can be polarized into two subtypes: M1 and M2, responding to certain stimuli. For examples, lipopolysaccharide (LPS) or interferon-γ induces polarization into M1, whereas IL-4 or IL-13 induces M2 phenotype (Orihuela et al., 2016). Microglia contain two subtypes: M1 and M2. The M1 subtype is characterized by the production of pro-inflammatory cytokines, such as IL-1β, IL-6, IL-8 and tumor necrosis factor alpha (TNF-α; Barger and Basile, 2001; Boche et al., 2013). The

M1 phenotype is activated by damage-associated molecular patterns, such as ATP, S100 molecules, histones, and heat shock proteins (Lu et al., 2014; Wiersinga et al., 2014). By contrast, the M2 phenotype is characterized by the production of anti-inflammatory cytokines, such as IL-10, insulin-like growth factor 1 (IGF-1), transforming growth factor beta (TGF-β), and neurotrophic factors (Ekdahl, 2012; Boche et al., 2013; Hu et al., 2015). The M2 phenotype is activated by cytokines, such as IL-4, IL-13 and IL-25 (Boche et al., 2013; Maiorino et al., 2013).

Activated microglia retract their cellular processes and transform from a ramified state into an ameboid morphology, in which they respond to external stimuli induced by various pathological conditions, such as trauma, infection, or other damage to brain tissue (Marshall et al., 2013). Activated microglial functions include phagocytosis and the production and release of cytokines, reactive oxygen species and nitrogen species (Barger and Basile, 2001; Takaki et al., 2012; Réus et al., 2015). They express a profile of cell surface marker expression that is similar to that of other mononuclear phagocytes (specifically macrophages), such as cluster of differentiation 14 (CD14), MHC molecules and chemokine receptors (Rock et al., 2004). Activation of microglia under pathological conditions in the brain may exert neuroprotective effects by reducing protein aggregates; however, they may exert cytotoxic effects by secreting neurotoxic factors (Streit et al., 1999; Schmitz et al., 2009).

## PERIPHERAL MONOCYTIC ACTIVATION IN PSYCHIATRIC DISORDERS

Several studies have suggested an association between monocyte activity and psychiatric disorders (Rothermundt et al., 1998; Theodoropoulou et al., 2001; Nikkilä et al., 2014). Some studies have shown that circulating peripheral blood monocytes are increased in patients with schizophrenia (Rothermundt et al., 1998; Theodoropoulou et al., 2001). In addition, in the cerebrospinal fluid of patients with schizophrenia, the numbers of monocytes and macrophages were increased during acute psychotic episodes (Nikkilä et al., 2014). In contrast to schizophrenia, the number and level of CD14-positive monocyte differentiation were not altered in patients with bipolar disorder compared with healthy controls (Padmos et al., 2008; Drexhage et al., 2011). Recently, Drexhage et al. (2010) conducted a series of gene expression profiling studies using monocytes from psychiatric patients (27 schizophrenia and 56 bipolar patients) and matched controls via a microarray analysis, followed by quantitative polymerase chain reaction (PCR) studies for validation (Padmos et al., 2008; Beumer et al., 2012). The authors identified two main subsets of strongly correlated genes: one subset was composed of pro-inflammatory cytokines; the other subset consisted mainly of adhesion/motility factors. The monocyte gene expression profiles of the majority of the patients with bipolar disorder showed dysregulation in both subsets, whereas the monocyte gene expression profiles of the majority of the schizophrenia patients showed dysregulation only in the subset of pro-inflammatory cytokines (Drexhage et al., 2010).

## SUBPOPULATIONS OF PERIPHERAL MONOCYTIC CELLS AND POTENTIAL PATHOGENIC MECHANISMS UNDERLYING THE INVOLVEMENT OF PERIPHERAL MONOCYTES IN PSYCHIATRIC DISORDERS

Monocytes are precursors of tissue macrophages, osteoclasts, and antigen-presenting cells (Lawson et al., 1990; Schmitz and Grandl, 2007). Monocytes, which comprise 5–10% of peripheral blood leukocytes, are derived from myelomonocytic stem cells in bone marrow and then released into the circulation, where they have a half-life of up to 3 days in humans (Whitelaw, 1972; Fogg et al., 2006). The brain harbors several types of monocyte-derived cells (Prinz and Priller, 2014). Macrophages and blood-derived dendritic cells are both present in the outer boundaries of the brain, such as the choroid plexus, perivascular space, and meninges; however, the number of blood-derived dendritic cells is small (Prinz and Priller, 2014).

There are five subsets of monocytes; they can be distinguished by different surface markers (Schmitz et al., 1997; Stöhr et al., 1998; Rothe et al., 1999; Gordon and Taylor, 2005; Beumer et al., 2012). More than half of monocytes belong to subset 1 and are characterized by surface marker profiles with abundant CD14 and a lack of CD16 expression (Schmitz et al., 1997; Stöhr et al., 1998). Both subsets 2 and 3 have CD16 expression and comprise active phagocytic cells. The expression of CD14 is increased in subset 2 compared with subset 3 (Schmitz et al., 1997; Stöhr et al., 1998). Subset 4 is a precursor of dendritic cells with high expression of CD40 (Schmitz et al., 1997; Stöhr et al., 1998). Subset 5, the smallest subset, shares many surface markers with subset 1; however, it differs in the additional expression of CD56, a marker of immature monocytes (Schmitz et al., 1997; Stöhr et al., 1998). Transformation between subsets among peripheral monocytes can occur concomitant with the differentiation of microglia in the brain under certain pathogenic conditions related to psychiatric diseases, although these possibilities remain to be elucidated.

## POTENTIAL MECHANISMS LINKING ACTIVATION OF MICROGLIAL AND PERIPHERAL MONOCYTIC CELLS TO PSYCHIATRIC DISORDERS

As previously described, many studies have investigated the association between microglia and psychiatric disorders or monocytes and psychiatric disorders. However, only a few studies have investigated the direct association or interaction between microglia and monocytes. Theoretically, there are several potential mechanisms underlying these interactions, as described below (**Figure 1**).

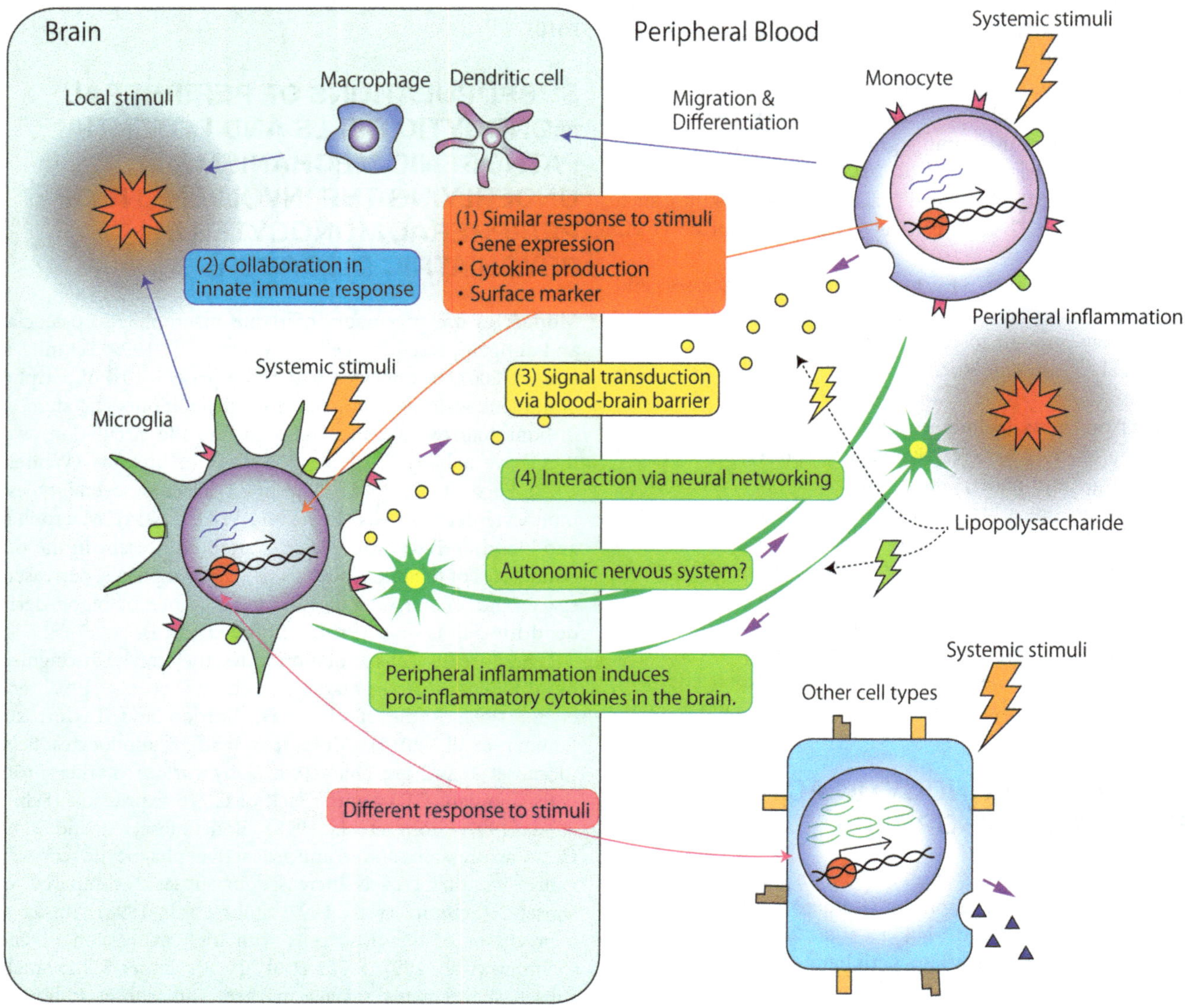


**FIGURE 1 | Potential mechanisms underlying the associations and/or interactions between microglia and monocytes. (1)** Microglia and monocytes exhibit similar responses to systemic stimuli. First, accumulated data have suggested strong associations between microglia and monocyte gene expression. Second, the two cell types show similar profiles for cytokine production, such as interleukin (IL) 1β, IL-6, IL-8 or tumor necrosis factor (TNF)-α. Third, both cell types express similar surface markers, such as cluster of differentiation 14 (CD14), major histocompatability complex (MHC) molecules, and chemokine receptors. **(2)** Local stimuli in the brain facilitate the recruitment of circulating monocyte-derived macrophage/dendritic cells into the central nervous system (CNS). Immigrant monocytic cells, which are short-lived, and localized in the outer boundaries of the brain compared with microglia (Prinz and Priller, 2014), may collaborate with microglia in the innate immune response. **(3)** Signals are transduced between microglia and circulating monocytes through the blood-brain barrier (BBB). Even relatively large molecules, such as cytokines, may comprise vehicles of signal transductions through circumventricular organs brain lymphatic pathways, BBB-relevant transporters/receptors, or abnormal permeability of BBB. **(4)** Microglia and peripheral monocytic cells may exert related biological reactions through neuronal signal transduction. Peripheral inflammation, induced by, for example, the peripheral administration of lipopolysaccharide (LPS), induces reactions in peripheral monocytic cells and also triggers the production of pro-inflammatory cytokines in the brain. Such reactions in the brain are thought to be induced by the transduction of neural excitability from peripheral nerves to the CNS because LPS rarely penetrates the BBB. Additionally, interactions between microglia and neuronal networks modulate myeloid cell proliferation through the autonomic nervous system.

## (1) Common Responses of Microglia and Peripheral Monocytic Cells to Endogenous or Exogenous Stimuli

As mentioned in the introduction, microglia and monocytes have similar functions, such as phagocytosis and the release of pro-inflammatory cytokines, as well as similar expression of surface markers, such as CD14, MHC molecules, and chemokine receptors (Schmitz et al., 2009; Beumer et al., 2012; Shechter and Schwartz, 2013; Prinz and Priller, 2014). They may also share similar epigenetic marks, in addition to having the same genomic sequence. Although limited data directly indicate epigenetic similarities between microglia and peripheral monocytic cells, several previous studies have suggested similarities in the gene expression profiles of both microglia and peripheral monocytic cells. Schmitz et al. (2009) observed over-representation of genes associated with Alzheimer's disease among the expression profiles specific to microglia and monocytes (Thomas et al., 2006; Lutter et al., 2008). The authors compared the microglial gene expression profile with the microarray data of human blood monocytes and *in vitro* macrophage colony-stimulating factor (M-CSF) differentiated macrophages to assess the expression of genes associated with Alzheimer's disease. Of 379 Alzheimer's disease-related genes, 159 were expressed in microglia, 198 in monocytes and 206 in macrophages. Of these genes, the expression of 128 Alzheimer's disease-related genes were shared by microglia, monocytes and macrophages.

In addition, we compared the gene expression profiles of mouse microglia and monocytes in our preliminary microarray study prior to evaluating the effect of lithium treatment on microglia and peripheral monocytic cells (Yu et al., 2015). These findings also suggested a strong association between microglia and monocyte gene expression patterns. Among 45,281 transcripts on the microarray, 11,597 with average signal intensities greater than 100 in microglia or monocytes were reliably detectable. Of these transcripts, 7552 genes were identified in both cell types, including 2832 that were expressed only in microglia, and 1213 that were expressed only in monocytes. The correlation coefficients among the microglia samples were 0.94–0.98, compared with 0.97–0.98 for monocytes and 0.71–0.76 between microglia and monocytes. By contrast, the alterations in the gene expression profiles following lithium treatment were quite different between the microglia and other types of monocytic cells. Yu et al. (2015) investigated the effects of lithium on two cell types: monocyte-derived dendritic cells treated with lithium and microglia separated from lithium-treated mice. They compared the gene expression profiles of these cells with those of controls. They demonstrated that the common gene significantly induced by lithium in both monocyte-derived dendritic cells and microglia was only the third component of complement. Taken together, these findings indicate that microglia and monocytes have a similar gene expression pattern under normal conditions; however, changes in the pattern of expression profiles in response to stimuli are quite different.

## (2) Collaboration of Peripheral Monocytes with Microglia in the Innate Immune Response

Damage to the CNS commonly results in the recruitment of circulating immune cells, including monocytes, which results in an innate immune response that consists of microglia and monocyte-derived macrophages/dendritic cells (Prinz and Priller, 2014). The differential roles of these myeloid cell populations in CNS disorders have only recently been acknowledged and were nicely illustrated in a recent review by Prinz and Priller (2014). In Alzheimer's disease, activated microglia have been associated with amyloid-β-induced neurotoxicity, and microglia were also damaged by amyloid species (Simard et al., 2006; Mildner et al., 2011; Prinz and Priller, 2014). Transplantation of wild-type bone marrow cells in transgenic mouse models of Alzheimer's disease causes the migration of bone marrow-derived phagocytes to the brain after CNS preconditioning. Consequently, the amyloid load in the brain is eliminated by bone marrow-derived phagocytes (Simard et al., 2006; Mildner et al., 2011; Prinz and Priller, 2014). Similarly, recovery from spinal cord injury in mice has been reported to depend more on infiltrating monocyte-derived macrophages than on resident microglia (Shechter et al., 2009).

## (3) Interactions Between Microglia and Peripheral Monocytic Cells Through the Blood-Brain Barrier

Interactions between microglia and monocytes may also be regulated by cytokines. In a mouse model of amyotrophic lateral sclerosis, Butovsky et al. (2012) demonstrated that chemokine receptor-2 (CCR2) was over-expressed in splenic Ly6C$^{hi}$ monocytes at disease onset, which was paralleled by upregulation of chemokine ligand-2 (CCL2) in CD39$^{+}$ microglia. Additionally, CCR2 was not expressed in CD39$^{+}$ microglia, and CCL2 was not expressed in Ly6C$^{hi}$ monocytes during the pathological course of the disease. Therefore, the authors suggested that the expression of CCL2 and other chemokines on microglia caused the migration of Ly6C$^{hi}$ monocytes to the CNS.

Furthermore, both microglia and monocytes are activated by and release pro-inflammatory cytokines, such as IL-1β, IL-6, IL-8 or TNF-α (Chan et al., 2007; Schmitz et al., 2009; Beumer et al., 2012). Studies have reported that these cytokines are increased in the blood of psychiatric patients (Naudin et al., 1997; Kim et al., 2000; Drexhage et al., 2008; Padmos et al., 2008; Song et al., 2009). Therefore, it is reasonable to suspect that these cytokine activation might underlie interactions between microglia and monocytes, although there has not been direct evidence to support the theory.

However, cytokines are relatively large molecules and rarely cross the blood-brain barrier (BBB). There are several known mechanisms and routes by which they can cross the barrier, such as alterations in the barrier's permeability (Esposito et al., 2001; Stamatovic et al., 2006), crossing though circumventricular organs (Anisman, 2009; Calderó et al., 2009; Banks and Erickson, 2010), or the use of specific transporters or receptors (Kastin et al., 1999; Chesnokova and Melmed, 2002; Banks and Erickson, 2010). Also, recent studies discovered functional lymphatic vessels lining the dural sinuses which can convey fluid, large molecules, and even immune cells from the brain and are connected to the deep cervical lymph nodes. Further researches into the CNS lymphatic system may facilitate understanding of interactions between microglia and peripheral monocytic cells (Iliff et al., 2015; Louveau et al., 2015).

## (4) Interactions Between Microglia and Peripheral Monocytic Cells Through Neuronal Networking

Peripheral inflammation, which is caused, for example, by peripheral administration of LPS, induces peripheral reactions among immune cells, including monocytes. LPS also induces pro-inflammatory cytokines in the brain; however, LPS rarely crosses the BBB (Hayashi et al., 2015). This phenomenon may reflect that activation of inflammatory responses in the brain is induced by transduction of neural excitability from peripheral nerves to the CNS (Banks and Robinson, 2010), as well as LPS-induced dysfunction of vascular endothelial cells at the BBB (Banks et al., 2015). These findings suggest that mild peripheral inflammation, which contributes to the pathogenesis of psychiatric disease-related events, including fatigue, may induce microglial activation through neuronal networking.

Additionally, it is possible that interactions between microglia and neuronal networks modulate myeloid cell proliferation through the autonomic nervous system, although there is little evidence (Mignini et al., 2003; Spiegel et al., 2008). Peripheral monocyte activities may reflect microglial activities through these mechanisms.

## PERSPECTIVES ON STUDIES LINKING ACTIVATION OF MICROGLIAL AND PERIPHERAL MONOCYTIC CELLS TO PSYCHIATRIC DISORDERS

Several animal models are characterized by abnormalities in both immune system function and behavior (Amrani et al., 1994; Yirmiya, 1996; Bothe et al., 2005; Frenois et al., 2007; Fu et al., 2010). These models have enabled us to observe the activation of circulating monocytes and microglia in the brain and to investigate their influence on behavior. The non-obese diabetic (NOD) mouse spontaneously develops autoimmune diabetes, which is similar to the onset of type 1 diabetes in humans. Psychiatric diseases in humans have been associated with autoimmune diseases, such as type 1 diabetes and autoimmune thyroiditis (Kupka et al., 2002; Padmos et al., 2004; Eaton et al., 2010). Interestingly, abnormal behaviors have also been observed in NOD mice (Amrani et al., 1994; Bothe et al., 2005). This model is useful for investigating associations between microglial activation and monocytes in pathological processes, as well as gene-environment interactions in this association. In addition, ion channels have recently been recognized to play important roles in the immune response of neurological disorders (Eder, 2010). Local changes in cell osmolality enable monocytes to migrate and invade the CNS parenchyma, where they further differentiate into phagocytes under pathological conditions (Fuentes et al., 1995; Bennett et al., 2003; Mahad and Ransohoff, 2003; Schwab et al., 2007). Ion channels also have important roles in the process of microglia activation (Eder, 2010). Therefore, ion channel inhibitors are good candidates for therapeutic interventions to control immune responses in psychiatric diseases (Wulff et al., 2000; Reich et al., 2005; Rangaraju et al., 2009; Eder, 2010).

## CONCLUSION

Microglia and monocytes have similar functions, surface markers, and gene expression profiles. Both cell types release pro-inflammatory cytokines when activated in response to stimuli in the brain under various pathological conditions. Accumulating data also indicate interactions between monocytes and microglia. Research into these interactions may lead to new strategies to elucidate the pathogenesis of psychiatric diseases, as well as to develop peripheral biomarkers that reflect the pathological conditions in the brain, including microglial activation related to the progression or modulation of disease.

## AUTHOR CONTRIBUTIONS

HT contributed to the design of the manuscript. YT and HT drafted the manuscript. All authors contributed to construction of the context, revision of the manuscript. All authors read and approved the final manuscript.

## ACKNOWLEDGMENTS

This work was supported by a grant-in-aid for scientific research on innovative areas (no. 24116007) from the Ministry of Education, Culture, Sports, Science, and Technology of Japan, Health and Labour Sciences Research Grants for research on psychiatric and neurological diseases and mental health (H19-kokoro-ippan-001), and an Intramural Research Grant (No. 21-9) for Neurological and Psychiatric Disorders from the National Center of Neurology and Psychiatry.

## REFERENCES

Amrani, A., Chaouloff, F., Mormede, P., Dardenne, M., and Homo-Delarche, F. (1994). Glucose, insulin and open field responses to immobilization in nonobese diabetic (NOD) mice. *Physiol. Behav.* 56, 241–246. doi: 10.1016/0031-9384(94)90190-2

Anisman, H. (2009). Cascading effects of stressors and inflammatory immune system activation: implications for major depressive disorder. *J. Psychiatry Neurosci.* 34, 4–20.

Banks, W. A., and Erickson, M. A. (2010). The blood-brain barrier and immune function and dysfunction. *Neurobiol. Dis.* 37, 26–32. doi: 10.1016/j.nbd.2009.07.031

Banks, W. A., Gray, A. M., Erickson, M. A., Salameh, T. S., Damodarasamy, M., Sheibani, N., et al. (2015). Lipopolysaccharide-induced blood-brain barrier disruption: roles of cyclooxygenase, oxidative stress, neuroinflammation and elements of the neurovascular unit. *J. Neuroinflammation* 12:223. doi: 10.1186/s12974-015-0434-1

Banks, W. A., and Robinson, S. M. (2010). Minimal penetration of lipopolysaccharide across the murine blood-brain barrier. *Brain Behav. Immun.* 24, 102–109. doi: 10.1016/j.bbi.2009.09.001

Barger, S. W., and Basile, A. S. (2001). Activation of microglia by secreted amyloid precursor protein evokes release of glutamate by cystine exchange and attenuates synaptic function. *J. Neurochem.* 76, 846–854. doi: 10.1046/j.1471-4159.2001.00075.x

Bayer, T. A., Buslei, R., Havas, L., and Falkai, P. (1999). Evidence for activation of microglia in patients with psychiatric illnesses. *Neurosci. Lett.* 271, 126–128. doi: 10.1016/s0304-3940(99)00545-5

Bennett, J. L., Elhofy, A., Dal Canto, M. C., Tani, M., Ransohoff, R. M., and Karpus, W. J. (2003). CCL2 transgene expression in the central nervous system directs diffuse infiltration of CD45highCD11b+ monocytes and enhanced Theiler's murine encephalomyelitis virus-induced demyelinating disease. *J. Neurovirol.* 9, 623–636. doi: 10.1080/714044484

Beumer, W., Gibney, S. M., Drexhage, R. C., Pont-Lezica, L., Doorduin, J., Klein, H. C., et al. (2012). The immune theory of psychiatric diseases: a key role for activated microglia and circulating monocytes. *J. Leukoc. Biol.* 92, 959–975. doi: 10.1189/jlb.0212100

Boche, D., Perry, V. H., and Nicoll, J. A. (2013). Review: activation patterns of microglia and their identification in the human brain. *Neuropathol. Appl. Neurobiol.* 39, 3–18. doi: 10.1111/nan.12011

Bothe, G. W. M., Bolivar, V. J., Vedder, M. J., and Geistfeld, J. G. (2005). Behavioral differences among fourteen inbred mouse strains commonly used as disease models. *Comp. Med.* 55, 326–334.

Butovsky, O., Siddiqui, S., Gabriely, G., Lanser, A. J., Dake, B., Murugaiyan, G., et al. (2012). Modulating inflammatory monocytes with a unique microRNA gene signature ameliorates murine ALS. *J. Clin. Invest.* 122, 3063–3087. doi: 10.1172/jci62636

Calderó, J., Brunet, N., Ciutat, D., Hereu, M., and Esquerda, J. E. (2009). Development of microglia in the chick embryo spinal cord: implications in the regulation of motoneuronal survival and death. *J. Neurosci. Res.* 87, 2447–2466. doi: 10.1002/jnr.22084

Chan, W. Y., Kohsaka, S., and Rezaie, P. (2007). The origin and cell lineage of microglia: new concepts. *Brain Res. Rev.* 53, 344–354. doi: 10.1016/j.brainresrev.2006.11.002

Chesnokova, V., and Melmed, S. (2002). Minireview: neuro-immuno-endocrine modulation of the hypothalamic-pituitary-adrenal (HPA) axis by gp130 signaling molecules. *Endocrinology* 143, 1571–1574. doi: 10.1210/en.143.5.1571

Doorduin, J., de Vries, E. F., Willemsen, A. T., de Groot, J. C., Dierckx, R. A., and Klein, H. C. (2009). Neuroinflammation in schizophrenia-related psychosis: a PET study. *J. Nucl. Med.* 50, 1801–1807. doi: 10.2967/jnumed.109.066647

Drexhage, R. C., Hoogenboezem, T. H., Versnel, M. A., Berghout, A., Nolen, W. A., and Drexhage, H. A. (2011). The activation of monocyte and T cell networks in patients with bipolar disorder. *Brain Behav. Immun.* 25, 1206–1213. doi: 10.1016/j.bbi.2011.03.013

Drexhage, R. C., Padmos, R. C., de Wit, H., Versnel, M. A., Hooijkaas, H., van der Lely, A.-J., et al. (2008). Patients with schizophrenia show raised serum levels of the pro-inflammatory chemokine CCL2: association with the metabolic syndrome in patients? *Schizophr. Res.* 102, 352–355. doi: 10.1016/j.schres.2008.03.018

Drexhage, R. C., van der Heul-Nieuwenhuijsen, L., Padmos, R. C., van Beveren, N., Cohen, D., Versnel, M. A., et al. (2010). Inflammatory gene expression in monocytes of patients with schizophrenia: overlap and difference with bipolar disorder. A study in naturalistically treated patients. *Int. J. Neuropsychopharmacol.* 13, 1369–1381. doi: 10.1017/s1461145710000799

Eaton, W. W., Pedersen, M. G., Nielsen, P. R., and Mortensen, P. B. (2010). Autoimmune diseases, bipolar disorder and non-affective psychosis. *Bipolar Disord.* 12, 638–646. doi: 10.1111/j.1399-5618.2010.00853.x

Eder, C. (2010). Ion channels in monocytes and microglia/brain macrophages: promising therapeutic targets for neurological diseases. *J. Neuroimmunol.* 224, 51–55. doi: 10.1016/j.jneuroim.2010.05.008

Ekdahl, C. T. (2012). Microglial activation-tuning and pruning adult neurogenesis. *Front. Pharmacol.* 3:41. doi: 10.3389/fphar.2012.00041

Esposito, P., Gheorghe, D., Kandere, K., Pang, X., Connolly, R., Jacobson, S., et al. (2001). Acute stress increases permeability of the blood-brain-barrier through activation of brain mast cells. *Brain Res.* 888, 117–127. doi: 10.1016/s0006-8993(00)03026-2

Fillman, S. G., Cloonan, N., Catts, V. S., Miller, L. C., Wong, J., McCrossin, T., et al. (2013). Increased inflammatory markers identified in the dorsolateral prefrontal cortex of individuals with schizophrenia. *Mol. Psychiatry* 18, 206–214. doi: 10.1038/mp.2012.110

Fogg, D. K., Sibon, C., Miled, C., Jung, S., Aucouturier, P., Littman, D. R., et al. (2006). A clonogenic bone marrow progenitor specific for macrophages and dendritic cells. *Science* 311, 83–87. doi: 10.1126/science.1117729

Frenois, F., Moreau, M., O'Connor, J., Lawson, M., Micon, C., Lestage, J., et al. (2007). Lipopolysaccharide induces delayed FosB/DeltaFosB immunostaining within the mouse extended amygdala, hippocampus and hypothalamus, that parallel the expression of depressive-like behavior. *Psychoneuroendocrinology* 32, 516–531. doi: 10.1016/j.psyneuen.2007.03.005

Fu, X., Zunich, S. M., O'Connor, J. C., Kavelaars, A., Dantzer, R., and Kelley, K. W. (2010). Central administration of lipopolysaccharide induces depressive-like behavior *in vivo* and activates brain indoleamine 2,3 dioxygenase in murine organotypic hippocampal slice cultures. *J. Neuroinflammation* 7:43. doi: 10.1186/1742-2094-7-43

Fuentes, M. E., Durham, S. K., Swerdel, M. R., Lewin, A. C., Barton, D. S., Megill, J. R., et al. (1995). Controlled recruitment of monocytes and macrophages to specific organs through transgenic expression of monocyte chemoattractant protein-1. *J. Immunol.* 155, 5769–5776.

Ginhoux, F., Greter, M., Leboeuf, M., Nandi, S., See, P., Gokhan, S., et al. (2010). Fate mapping analysis reveals that adult microglia derive from primitive macrophages. *Science* 330, 841–845. doi: 10.1126/science.1194637

Goldmann, T., Wieghofer, P., Müller, P. F., Wolf, Y., Varol, D., Yona, S., et al. (2013). A new type of microglia gene targeting shows TAK1 to be pivotal in CNS autoimmune inflammation. *Nat. Neurosci.* 16, 1618–1626. doi: 10.1038/nn.3531

Gordon, S., and Taylor, P. R. (2005). Monocyte and macrophage heterogeneity. *Nat. Rev. Immunol.* 5, 953–964. doi: 10.1038/nri1733

Haarman, B. C., Riemersma-Van der Lek, R. F., de Groot, J. C., Ruhé, H. G., Klein, H. C., Zandstra, T. E., et al. (2014). Neuroinflammation in bipolar disorder - A [(11)C]-(R)-PK11195 positron emission tomography study. *Brain Behav. Immun.* 40, 219–225. doi: 10.1016/j.bbi.2014.03.016

Hayashi, M., Takai, J., Yu, L., Motohashi, H., Moriguchi, T., and Yamamoto, M. (2015). Whole-body *in vivo* monitoring of inflammatory diseases exploiting human interleukin 6-luciferase transgenic mice. *Mol. Cell Biol.* 35, 3590–3601. doi: 10.1128/MCB.00506-15

Hercher, C., Chopra, V., and Beasley, C. L. (2014). Evidence for morphological alterations in prefrontal white matter glia in schizophrenia and bipolar disorder. *J. Psychiatry Neurosci.* 39, 376–385. doi: 10.1503/jpn.130277

Hu, X., Leak, R. K., Shi, Y., Suenaga, J., Gao, Y., Zheng, P., et al. (2015). Microglial and macrophage polarization new prospects for brain repair. *Nat. Rev. Neurol.* 11, 56–64. doi: 10.1038/nrneurol.2014.207

Iliff, J. J., Goldman, S. A., and Nedergaard, M. (2015). Implications of the discovery of brain lymphatic pathways. *Lancet Neurol.* 14, 977–979. doi: 10.1016/s1474-4422(15)00221-5

Kastin, A. J., Pan, W., Maness, L. M., and Banks, W. A. (1999). Peptides crossing the blood-brain barrier: some unusual observations. *Brain Res.* 848, 96–100. doi: 10.1016/s0006-8993(99)01961-7

Kierdorf, K., Erny, D., Goldmann, T., Sander, V., Schulz, C., Perdiguero, E. G., et al. (2013). Microglia emerge from erythromyeloid precursors via Pu.1- and Irf8-dependent pathways. *Nat. Neurosci.* 16, 273–280. doi: 10.1038/nn.3318

Kim, Y. K., Kim, L., and Lee, M. S. (2000). Relationships between interleukins, neurotransmitters and psychopathology in drug-free male schizophrenics. *Schizophr. Res.* 44, 165–175. doi: 10.1016/s0920-9964(99)00171-1

Kupka, R. W., Nolen, W. A. Post, R. M., McElroy, S. L., Altshuler, L. L., Denicoff, K. D., et al. (2002). High rate of autoimmune thyroiditis in bipolar disorder: lack of association with lithium exposure. *Biol. Psychiatry* 51, 305–311. doi: 10.1016/s0006-3223(01)01217-3

Lassmann, H., Schmied, M., Vass, K., and Hickey, W. F. (1993). Bone marrow derived elements and resident microglia in brain inflammation. *Glia* 7, 19–24. doi: 10.1002/glia.440070106

Lawson, L. J., Perry, V. H., Dri, P., and Gordon, S. (1990). Heterogeneity in the distribution and morphology of microglia in the normal adult mouse brain. *Neuroscience* 39, 151–170. doi: 10.1016/0306-4522(90)90229-w

Louveau, A., Smirnov, I., Keyes, T. J., Eccles, J. D., Rouhani, S. J., Peske, J. D., et al. (2015). Structural and functional features of central nervous system lymphatic vessels. *Nature* 523, 337–341. doi: 10.1038/nature14432

Lu, B., Wang, C., Wang, M., Li, W., Chen, F., Tracey, K. J., et al. (2014). Molecular mechanism and therapeutic modulation of high mobility group box 1 release and action: an updated review. *Expert Rev. Clin. Immunol.* 10, 713–727. doi: 10.1586/1744666X.2014.909730

Lutter, D., Ugocsai, P., Grandl, M., Orso, E., Theis, F., Lang, E. W., et al. (2008). Analyzing M-CSF dependent monocyte/macrophage differentiation: expression modes and meta-modes derived from an independent component analysis. *BMC Bioinformatics* 9:100. doi: 10.1186/1471-2105-9-100

Mahad, D. J., and Ransohoff, R. M. (2003). The role of MCP-1 (CCL2) and CCR2 in multiple sclerosis and experimental autoimmune encephalomyelitis (EAE). *Semin. Immunol.* 15, 23–32. doi: 10.1016/s1044-5323(02)00125-2

Maiorino, C., Khorooshi, R., Ruffini, F., Løbner, M., Bergami, A., Garzetti, L., et al. (2013). Lentiviral-mediated administration of IL-25 in the CNS induces alternative activation of microglia. *Gene Ther.* 20, 487–496. doi: 10.1038/gt. 2012.58

Marshall, S. A., McClain, J. A., Kelso, M. L., Hopkins, D. M., Pauly, J. R., and Nixon, K. (2013). Microglial activation is not equivalent to neuroinflammation in alcohol-induced neurodegeneration: the importance of microglia phenotype. *Neurobiol. Dis.* 54, 239–251. doi: 10.1016/j.nbd.2012.12.016

Mignini, F., Streccioni, V., and Amenta, F. (2003). Autonomic innervation of immune organs and neuroimmune modulation. *Auton. Autacoid Pharmacol.* 23, 1–25. doi: 10.1046/j.1474-8673.2003.00280.x

Mildner, A., Schlevogt, B., Kierdorf, K., Böttcher, C., Erny, D., Kummer, M. P., et al. (2011). Distinct and non-redundant roles of microglia and myeloid subsets in mouse models of Alzheimer's disease. *J. Neurosci.* 31, 11159–11171. doi: 10.1523/JNEUROSCI.6209-10.2011

Naudin, J., Capo, C., Giusano, B., Mège, J., and Azorin, J. (1997). A differential role for interleukin-6 and tumor necrosis factor-α in schizophrenia? *Schizophr. Res.* 26, 227–233. doi: 10.1016/s0920-9964(97)00059-5

Nikkilä, H. V., Müller, K., Ahokas, A., Miettinen, K., Rimón, R., and Andersson, L. C. (2014). Accumulation of macrophages in the CSF of schizophrenic patients during acute psychotic episodes. *Am. J. Psychiatry* 156, 1725–1729.

Orihuela, R., McPherson, C. A., and Harry, G. J. (2016). Microglial M1/M2 polarization and metabolic states. *Br. J. Pharmacol.* 173, 649–665. doi: 10. 1111/bph.13139

Padmos, R. C., Bekris, L., Knijff, E. M., Tiemeier, H., Kupka, R. W., Cohen, D., et al. (2004). A high prevalence of organ-specific autoimmunity in patients with bipolar disorder. *Biol. Psychiatry* 56, 476–482. doi: 10.1016/j.biopsych.2004. 07.003

Padmos, R. C., Hillegers, M. H., Knijff, E. M., Vonk, R., Bouvy, A., Staal, F. J., et al. (2008). A discriminating messenger RNA signature for bipolar disorder formed by an aberrant expression of inflammatory genes in monocytes. *Arch. Gen. Psychiatry* 65, 395–407. doi: 10.1001/archpsyc.65.4.395

Papadopoulos, V., Baraldi, M., Guilarte, T. R., Knudsen, T. B., Lacapère, J. J., Lindemann, P., et al. (2006). Translocator protein (18kDa): new nomenclature for the peripheral-type benzodiazepine receptor based on its structure and molecular function. *Trends Pharmacol. Sci.* 27, 402–409. doi: 10.1016/j.tips. 2006.06.005

Parkhurst, C. N., Yang, G., Ninan, I., Savas, J. N., Yates, J. R. III, Lafaille, J. J., et al. (2013). Microglia promote learning-dependent synapse formation through brain-derived neurotrophic factor. *Cell* 155, 1596–1609. doi: 10.1016/j.cell. 2013.11.030

Prinz, M., and Priller, J. (2014). Microglia and brain macrophages in the molecular age: from origin to neuropsychiatric disease. *Nat. Rev. Neurosci.* 15, 300–312. doi: 10.1038/nrn3722

Radewicz, K., Garey, L. J., Gentleman, S. M., and Reynolds, R. (2000). Increase in HLA-DR immunoreactive microglia in frontal and temporal cortex of chronic schizophrenics. *J. Neuropathol. Exp. Neurol.* 59, 137–150. doi: 10.1093/jnen/59. 2.137

Rangaraju, S., Chi, V., Pennington, M. W., and Chandy, K. G. (2009). Kv1. 3 potassium channels as a therapeutic target in multiple sclerosis. *Expert Opin. Ther. Targets* 13, 909–924. doi: 10.1517/14728220903018957

Reich, E. P., Cui, L., Yang, L., Pugliese-Sivo, C., Golovko, A., Petro, M., et al. (2005). Blocking ion channel KCNN4 alleviates the symptoms of experimental autoimmune encephalomyelitis in mice. *Eur. J. Immunol.* 35, 1027–1036. doi: 10.1002/eji.200425954

Réus, G. Z., Fries, G. R., Stertz, L., Badawy, M., Passos, I. C., Barichello, T., et al. (2015). The role of inflammation and microglial activation in the pathophysiology of psychiatric disorders. *Neuroscience* 300, 141–154. doi: 10. 1016/j.neuroscience.2015.05.018

Rock, R. B., Gekker, G., Hu, S., Sheng, W. S., Cheeran, M., Lokensgard, J. R., et al. (2004). Role of microglia in central nervous system infections. *Clin. Microbiol. Rev.* 17, 942–964. doi: 10.1128/cmr.17.4.942-964.2004

Rothe, G., Herr, A. S., Stöhr, J., Abletshauser, C., Weidinger, G., and Schmitz, G. (1999). A more mature phenotype of blood mononuclear phagocytes is induced by fluvastatin treatment in hypercholesterolemic patients with coronary heart disease. *Atherosclerosis* 144, 251–261. doi: 10.1016/s0021-9150(99) 00061-1

Rothermundt, M., Arolt, V., Weitzsch, C., Eckhoff, D., and Kirchner, H. (1998). Immunological dysfunction in schizophrenia: a systematic approach. *Neuropsychobiology* 37, 186–193. doi: 10.1159/000026501

Schmitz, G., and Grandl, M. (2007). Role of redox regulation and lipid rafts in macrophages during Ox-LDL-mediated foam cell formation. *Antioxid. Redox Signal.* 9, 1499–1518. doi: 10.1089/ars.2007.1663

Schmitz, G., Leuthäuser-Jaschinski, K., and Orsó, E. (2009). Are circulating monocytes as microglia orthologues appropriate biomarker targets for neuronal diseases? *Cent. Nerv. Syst. Agents Med. Chem.* 9, 307–330. doi: 10. 2174/187152409789630424

Schmitz, G., Orsó, E., Rothe, G., and Klucken, J. (1997). Scavenging, signalling and adhesion coupling in macrophages: implications for atherogenesis. *Curr. Opin. Lipidol.* 8, 287–300. doi: 10.1097/00041433-199710000-00008

Schulz, C., Gomez Perdiguero, E., Chorro, L., Szabo-Rogers, H., Cagnard, N., Kierdorf, K., et al. (2012). A lineage of myeloid cells independent of Myb and hematopoietic stem cells. *Science* 336, 86–90. doi: 10.1126/science.1219179

Schwab, A., Nechyporuk-Zloy, V., Fabian, A., and Stock, C. (2007). Cells move when ions and water flow. *Pflugers Arch.* 453, 421–432. doi: 10.1007/s00424-006-0138-6

Shechter, R., London, A., Varol, C., Raposo, C., Cusimano, M., Yovel, G., et al. (2009). Infiltrating blood-derived macrophages are vital cells playing an anti-inflammatory role in recovery from spinal cord injury in mice. *PLoS Med.* 6:e1000113. doi: 10.1371/journal.pmed.1000113

Shechter, R., and Schwartz, M. (2013). Harnessing monocyte-derived macrophages to control central nervous system pathologies: no longer 'if' but 'how'. *J. Pathol.* 229, 332–346. doi: 10.1002/path.4106

Simard, A. R., Soulet, D., Gowing, G., Julien, J. P., and Rivest, S. (2006). Bone marrow-derived microglia play a critical role in restricting senile plaque formation in Alzheimer's disease. *Neuron* 49, 489–502. doi: 10.1016/j.neuron. 2006.01.022

Song, X. Q., Lv, L. X., Li, W. Q., Hao, Y. H., and Zhao, J. P. (2009). The interaction of nuclear factor-kappa B and cytokines is associated with schizophrenia. *Biol. Psychiatry* 65, 481–488. doi: 10.1016/j.biopsych.2008.10.018

Spiegel, A., Kalinkovich, A., Shivtiel, S., Kollet, O., and Lapidot, T. (2008). Stem cell regulation via dynamic interactions of the nervous and immune systems with the microenvironment. *Cell Stem Cell* 3, 484–492. doi: 10.1016/j.stem.2008. 10.006

Stamatovic, S., Dimitrijevic, O., Keep, R., and Andjelkovic, A. (2006). "Inflammation and brain edema: new insights into the role of chemokines and their receptors," in *Brain Edema XIII*, eds J. T. Hoff, R. F. Keep, G. Xi and Y. Hua (Vienna: Springer), 444–450.

Stöhr, J., Schindler, G., Rothe, G., and Schmitz, G. (1998). Enhanced upregulation of the fc γ receptor IIIa (CD16a) during *in vitro* differentiation of ApoE4/4 monocytes. *Arterioscler. Thromb. Vasc. Biol.* 18, 1424–1432. doi: 10.1161/01. atv.18.9.1424

Streit, W. J., Walter, S. A., and Pennell, N. A. (1999). Reactive microgliosis. *Prog. Neurobiol.* 57, 563–581. doi: 10.1016/s0301-0082(98)00069-0

Takaki, J., Fujimori, K., Miura, M., Suzuki, T., Sekino, Y., and Sato, K. (2012). L-glutamate released from activated microglia downregulates astrocytic L-glutamate transporter expression in neuroinflammation: the 'collusion'hypothesis for increased extracellular L-glutamate concentration in neuroinflammation. *J. Neuroinflammation* 9:275. doi: 10.1186/1742-2094-9-275

Takano, A., Arakawa, R., Ito, H., Tateno, A., Takahashi, H., Matsumoto, R., et al. (2010). Peripheral benzodiazepine receptors in patients with chronic schizophrenia: a PET study with [11C]DAA1106. *Int. J. Neuropsychopharmacol.* 13, 943–950. doi: 10.1017/s1461145710000313

Tang, B., Capitao, C., Dean, B., and Thomas, E. A. (2012). Differential age- and disease-related effects on the expression of genes related to the arachidonic acid signaling pathway in schizophrenia. *Psychiatry Res.* 196, 201–206. doi: 10. 1016/j.psychres.2011.09.026

Theodoropoulou, S., Spanakos, G., Baxevanis, C. N., Economou, M., Gritzapis, A. D., Papamichail, M. P., et al. (2001). Cytokine serum levels, autologous mixed lymphocyte reaction and surface marker analysis in never medicated and chronically medicated schizophrenic patients. *Schizophr. Res.* 47, 13–25. doi: 10.1016/s0920-9964(00)00007-4

Thomas, D. M., Francescutti-Verbeem, D. M., and Kuhn, D. M. (2006). Gene expression profile of activated microglia under conditions associated with dopamine neuronal damage. *FASEB J.* 20, 515–517. doi: 10.1096/fj.05-4873fje

Torres-Platas, S. G., Cruceanu, C., Chen, G. G., Turecki, G., and Mechawar, N. (2014). Evidence for increased microglial priming and macrophage recruitment in the dorsal anterior cingulate white matter of depressed suicides. *Brain Behav. Immun.* 42, 50–59. doi: 10.1016/j.bbi.2014.05.007

van Berckel, B. N., Bossong, M. G., Boellaard, R., Kloet, R., Schuitemaker, A., Caspers, E., et al. (2008). Microglia activation in recent-onset schizophrenia: a quantitative (R)-[11 C] PK11195 positron emission tomography study. *Biol. Psychiatry* 64, 820–822. doi: 10.1016/j.biopsych.2008.04.025

Vaughan, D. W., and Peters, A. (1974). Neuroglial cells in the cerebral cortex of rats from young adulthood to old age: an electron microscope study. *J. Neurocytol.* 3, 405–429. doi: 10.1007/bf01098730

Veenman, L., and Gavish, M. (2000). Peripheral-type benzodiazepine receptors: their implication in brain disease. *Drug Dev. Res.* 50, 355–370. doi: 10.1002/1098-2299(200007/08)50:3/4<355::AID-DDR18>3.0.CO;2-W

Veenman, L., and Gavish, M. (2012). The role of 18 kDa mitochondrial translocator protein (TSPO) in programmed cell death and effects of steroids on TSPO expression. *Curr. Mol. Med.* 12, 398–412. doi: 10.2174/1566524011207040398

Whitelaw, D. M. (1972). Observations on human monocyte kinetics after pulse labeling. *Cell Tissue Kinet.* 5, 311–317. doi: 10.1111/j.1365-2184.1972.tb00369.x

Wiersinga, W. J., Leopold, S. J., Cranendonk, D. R., and van der Poll, T. (2014). Host innate immune responses to sepsis. *Virulence* 5, 36–44. doi: 10.4161/viru.25436

Wulff, H., Miller, M. J., Hänsel, W., Grissmer, S., Cahalan, M. D., and Chandy, K. G. (2000). Design of a potent and selective inhibitor of the intermediate-conductance $Ca^{2+}$-activated $K^+$ channel, IKCa1: a potential immunosuppressant. *Proc. Natl. Acad. Sci. U S A* 97, 8151–8156. doi: 10.1073/pnas.97.14.8151

Yirmiya, R. (1996). Endotoxin produces a depressive-like episode in rats. *Brain Res.* 711, 163–174. doi: 10.1016/0006-8993(95)01415-2

Yona, S., Kim, K. W., Wolf, Y., Mildner, A., Varol, D., Breker, M., et al. (2013). Fate mapping reveals origins and dynamics of monocytes and tissue macrophages under homeostasis. *Immunity* 38, 79–91. doi: 10.1016/j.immuni.2012.12.001

Yu, Z., Ono, C., Aiba, S., Kikuchi, Y., Sora, I., Matsuoka, H., et al. (2015). Therapeutic concentration of lithium stimulates complement C3 production in dendritic cells and microglia via GSK-3 inhibition. *Glia* 63, 257–270. doi: 10.1002/glia.22749

# 9

# Impairment of Oligodendroglia Maturation Leads to Aberrantly Increased Cortical Glutamate and Anxiety-Like Behaviors in Juvenile Mice

*Xianjun Chen[1], Weiguo Zhang[2], Tao Li[1], Yu Guo[2], Yanping Tian[1], Fei Wang[1], Shubao Liu[1], Hai-Ying Shen[3], Yue Feng[4]* and Lan Xiao[1]**

[1] Department of Histology and Embryology, Chongqing Key Laboratory of Neurobiology, Third Military Medical University, Chongqing, China, [2] Department of Radiology, Institute of Surgery Research, Daping Hospital, Third Military Medical University, Chongqing, China, [3] Robert Stone Dow Neurobiology Laboratories, Legacy Research Institute, Portland, OR, USA, [4] Department of Pharmacology, Emory University School of Medicine, Atlanta, GA, USA

***Correspondence:**
Lan Xiao
xiaolan35@hotmail.com;
Yue Feng
yfeng@emory.edu

Adolescence is the critical time for developing proper oligodendrocyte (OL)-neuron interaction and the peak of onset for many cognitive diseases, among which anxiety disorders display the highest prevalence. However, whether impairment of *de novo* OL development causes neuronal abnormalities and contributes to the early onset of anxiety phenotype in childhood still remains unexplored. In this study, we tested the hypothesis that defects in OL maturation manifests cortical neuron function and leads to anxiety-like behaviors in juvenile mice. We report here that conditional knockout of the *Olig2 gene* (*Olig2* cKO) specifically in differentiating OLs in the mouse brain preferentially impaired OL maturation in the gray matter of cerebral cortex. Interestingly, localized proton magnetic resonance spectroscopy *revealed that Olig2* cKO mice displayed abnormally elevated cortical glutamate levels. In addition, transmission electron microscopy demonstrated increased vesicle density in excitatory glutamatergic synapses in the cortex of the *Olig2* cKO mice. Moreover, juvenile *Olig2* cKO mice exhibited anxiety-like behaviors and impairment in behavioral inhibition. Taken together, our results suggest that impaired OL development affects glutamatergic neuron function in the cortex and causes anxiety-related behaviors in juvenile mice. These discoveries raise an intriguing possibility that OL defects may be a contributing mechanism for the onset of anxiety in childhood.

**Keywords: oligodendrocyte, brain development, *Olig2* knockout, cortical neurons, glutamate, anxiety behavior**

## INTRODUCTION

Adolescence is a peak time for the onset of numerous mental disorders, represented by anxiety, impulse control disorders, and schizophrenia (Paus et al., 2008). One in five children and adolescents suffers from a mental illness that persists into adulthood. Among the numerous mental disorders, the prevalence of anxiety is the highest (Kessler et al., 2005). Consistent with the emotionality, risk-taking and impulsivity characters (Butters, 2011), anxiety phenotypes often begin in childhood and early adolescence, sometimes continue into the adulthood (Lee et al., 2014). However, molecular and cellular mechanisms that lead to anxiety in adolescence remain unknown, which is a prevailing issue in understanding the early onset of mental dysfunction.

In the adolescent brain, the structure of neuronal circuits and the functional properties of neurons are highly plastic (Tau and Peterson, 2010). Not only the number and morphology of synapses are dynamically altered (Penzes et al., 2011), the availability of neurotransmitters and corresponding receptors also undergo differential regulation in various brain regions (Lee et al., 2014). Conceivably, a transient interference of neurotransmission may markedly affect the functional balance of neuronal circuitry in the young brain, thus resulting in dysregulated emotions and actions (Casey et al., 2008). Moreover, recent clinical studies revealed that aberrantly elevated glutamate levels in the anterior cingulate cortex were positively correlated with clinical symptoms of anxiety and impulsivity in patients (Phan et al., 2005; Hoerst et al., 2010; Modi et al., 2014). These findings suggest that abnormal cortical glutamate homeostasis may contribute to the pathogenesis of anxiety disorders, while the underlying mechanisms remain undefined.

Synaptic transmission and cognitive ability are tightly regulated by neuron-glia interaction (de Hoz and Simons, 2015). Emerging evidence suggests key roles of oligodendroglia (OL) in brain function and psychiatric diseases (Fields, 2008). In particular, the clinical onset of anxiety peaks during vigorous OL and myelin development in the cerebral cortex (Kessler et al., 2005; Miller et al., 2012; Young et al., 2013). Besides the classical view of OL function in myelination that is essential for saltatory conductance, recent studies revealed that OL also provides trophic factors and metabolites that are critical for modulating neuronal function and plasticity (Du and Dreyfus, 2002; Funfschilling et al., 2012; Lee et al., 2012). In fact, essential role of OL is demonstrated in higher brain function, including learning motor skills, long distance connectivity and spiking-timing-dependent plasticity (McKenzie et al., 2014; Nave and Ehrenreich, 2014). Moreover, OL impairment is frequently observed in neuropsychiatric disorders, including schizophrenia, bipolar, and major depression (Fields, 2008; Edgar and Sibille, 2012; Cassoli et al., 2015). Nonetheless, whether defects in OL development during childhood and early adolescence may affect cortical neurons and contribute to the anxiety behaviors still remain unexplored.

In this study, we explored whether specific impairment of *de novo* OL maturation may affect cortical glutamate and result in maladaptive behaviors in juvenile mice. The *Olig2* gene encodes a transcription factor essential for OL lineage specification, differentiation and myelination (Zhou et al., 2000; Lu et al., 2002; Ligon et al., 2006; Yue et al., 2006; Mei et al., 2013). We showed that conditional deletion of the *Olig2* gene specifically in differentiated OLs resulted in preferential reduction of mature OL in the cerebral cortex. Interestingly, *Olig2* cKO mice display abnormally elevated glutamate levels in the cortex and increased density of vesicles in cortical glutamatergic synapses in young mice. Moreover, juvenile *Olig2* cKO mice showed anxiety and impulsivity-like behaviors. Taking together, our results indicate that impaired OL development in the cortex interferes with glutamate function and lead to anxiety- and impulsivity-like behaviors reminiscent of adolescent mental illnesses.

## MATERIALS AND METHODS

### Animals

The *Olig2*-flox mice were previously described (Yue et al., 2006) in which the *Olig2* coding region is flanked by two inserted loxp sites. The mice that express Cre recombinase under the control of the *CNPase* (*CNP*) promoter (*CNP-Cre* mice) were also previously described (Lappe-Siefke et al., 2003) where *Cre* recombinase was knocked into one allele of the *CNP* gene locus. To delete *Olig2* in oligodendroglia lineage cells, $Olig2^{loxp/loxp}$ mice were crossed with the $CNP\text{-}Cre^{+/-}$ mice to generate both $CNP\text{-}Cre^{+}$; $Olig2^{loxp/loxp}$ offspring (*Olig2* cKO) and $CNP\text{-}Cre^{-}$; $Olig2^{loxp/loxp}$ littermates (WT).

### Ethics Statement

All animal experiments were performed according to an approved protocol from the Laboratory Animal Welfare and Ethics Committee of the Third Military Medical University.

### Immunohistochemistry

At the age of postnatal day 21 (P21), mice ($n = 6$ for each group) were deeply anesthetized with 1% sodium pentobarbital and transcardially perfused with 4% paraformaldehyde in PBS. Brains were dehydrated in 10, 20, 30% sucrose in 4% paraformaldehyde for 12 h, respectively. The frozen brains were sectioned (20 μm) on a cryostat microtome (MS 1900, Leica). Free-floating sections were incubated with primary antibodies overnight at 4°C after blocking with PBS containing 0.3% TritonX-100 and 5% bovine serum at 37°C for 1 h. Then they were incubated with secondary antibodies for 3 h following by SABC regent (1:200; VECTASTAIN) for 1h at room temperature. The antigen-antibody complexes were visualized using DAB (Boster) as the chromogen. The primary antibodies included: mouse anti-CC1 (1:500; Millipore), rabbit anti-PDGFRα (1:200; Santa Cruz Biotechnology). Biotinylated secondary antibodies to rabbit (1:1000; VECTOR BA1000) or mouse (1:1000; VECTOR BA9200) were used as indicated in the legends.

### Western Blotting

At the age of P21, mice ($n = 7$ in WT, $n = 8$ in *Olig2* cKO) were anesthetized with 1% pentobarbital. Cerebral cortex (anterior cingulated area) and corpus callosum were rapidly removed and frozen. Frozen samples were homogenized and proteins were extracted using RIPA lyses buffer with protease inhibitors (Roche). Lysates containing 40 μg protein were denatured in gel-loading buffer, separated on 10% SDS-PAGE gels, transferred to PVDF membranes and visualized by chemiluminescence (ECL plus, GE Healthcare). Quantification of band intensity was analyzed using Image-Pro Plus software 5.0 (Media Cybernetics). The following primary antibodies were used: mouse anti-Olig2 (1:500; Millipore), mouse anti-MBP (1:1000; Santa Cruz

Biotechnology) and mouse anti-β-actin (1:2000; Santa Cruz Biotechnology).

## MRI and MRS

At the age of P21, MRI and MRS were performed, as recently described (Michaelis et al., 2009), on *Olig2* cKO ($n = 7$) and WT control ($n = 6$). Mice were initially anesthetized with 5% isoflurane, subsequently incubated and kept under anesthesia with 1.75% isoflurane in ambient air. *In vivo* localized proton MRS (PRESS, TR/TE = 3,000/20 ms) in cerebral cortex (2.5 mm × 1 mm × 2.5 mm) was performed at 7.0T (Bruker BioSpec 70/20 USR). T2-weighted MRI (Turbo-RARE, TR/TE = 1,500/35ms, 8 echoes, slice thickness 500 μm) in axial and sagittal orientation served to ensure a proper position of volumes-of-interest. Metabolite quantification involved spectral evaluation by LCModel and calibration with brain water concentration (Provencher, 1993). Metabolites with Cramer-Rao lower bounds above 20% were excluded from further analyses.

## Quantification of Glutamate in Cerebral Cortex

At the age of P21, mice (n = 6 for each group) were initially anesthetized with 5% isoflurane. Cerebral cortex (anterior cingulate area) was removed and frozen at −80°C immediately. The brain tissues were homogenized with 100 μl glutamate assay buffer and followed the manufacturer's instruction from Glutamate assay kit (Sigma). The 10KD spin filters (Biovision) were applied. The absorbance was measured at 450 nm with Model 680 microplate reader (Bio-Rad).

## Electron Microscopy

Electron microscopy (EM) analysis was performed as previously described (Mei et al., 2013). At the age of P21, mice were initially anesthetized with 5% isoflurane. The anterior cingulate cortex of *Olig2* cKO mice ($n = 3$) and WT controls ($n = 3$) were removed rapidly and fixed in fresh fixative overnight at 4°C. Tissue cubes (1 mm × 1 mm × 1 mm) were rinsed in PBS, postfixed in 1% OsO4 in PBS for 2 h, counterstained with uranyl acetate, dehydrated in a graded ethanol series, infiltrated with propylene oxide, and embedded in Epon. Ultrathin sections (~60 nm) were generated by an ultramicrotome (LKB-V, LKB Produkter AB, Bromma) and were viewed with a transmission electron microscope (TECNAI10, Philips). Three sections from each mouse were investigated at a comparable location from *Olig2* cKO and WT control mice under magnification of 60k. Digital images were acquired with an AMT XR-60 CCD Digital Camera System and analyzed using Image-Pro Plus software 5.0 (Media Cybernetics).

## Behavioral Tests

*Olig2* cKO mice and WT littermates were housed in a controlled environment (25°C) with free access to food and water and maintained on a 12 h/12 h day/night cycle. Behavioral tests were conducted on sex-balanced groups of experimentally naive mice at P21. All tests were done from 10:00 h to 18:00 h. One group of mice were tested in open-field test (between 10:00 h and 12:00 h) and elevated plus-maze test (between 15:00 h and 18:00 h) on the same day to measure anxiety. Another group of mice were only tested in cliff avoidance reaction (CAR) test (between 10:00 h and 18:00 h) to measure impulsivity. After each experiment, all the apparatuses were wiped clean with 70% ethanol to prevent a bias due to olfactory cues. For all behavioral experiments, investigators were blinded for genotype and mice were gently handled to avoid stress.

Open field test was performed using an open-field activity system (Biowill, Shanghai, China), as described (Wang et al., 2013). Briefly, mice ($n = 26$ in WT, $n = 18$ in *Olig2* cKO) were placed in the center of the open-field box (50 cm × 50 cm × 50 cm), and activity was recorded during a period of 10 min. The total and center-area travel distances were measured and the time spent in the central area was recorded.

Elevated plus-maze test was conducted as previously described (Katayama et al., 2010). Briefly, mice ($n = 24$ in WT, $n = 15$ in *Olig2* cKO) were tested on a plus-maze apparatus (Biowill, Shanghai, China) [closed arms, 25 × 5 × 15 (H) cm; open arms 25 × 5 × 0.3 (H) cm] arranged orthogonally 60 cm above the floor. Each mouse was initially placed in the center area facing an open arm, and then allowed to move freely in the maze for 5 min. The total travel distance on the maze, time spent on any arms and entries into any arms were recorded.

Cliff avoidance reaction test was conducted as previously described with slight modification (Yamashita et al., 2013). Mice ($n = 14$ in WT, $n = 15$ in *Olig2* cKO) were assessed using a round platform (diameter, 16 cm; height, 50 cm). The test was initiated by gently placing an animal on the platform with the forelimbs approached the edge. If the animal fell from the platform during the 20 min test, it was judged to have impaired CAR. The latency from an initial placement on the platform until falling was recorded. The incidence of impaired CAR was calculated as a percentage index for each group: % (CAR) = (the number of intact CAR mice (which did not fall from platform)/total number of tested mice) × 100. Duration of each entry into the edge area, which was defined as an outer ring with a width of 2 cm, was recorded before the mouse fell off.

## Statistical Analysis

We performed statistical analyses using the SPSS software version 13.0. All the data were confirmed to be normal distribution, as tested by the Kolmogorov–Smirnov test. For between-group comparisons, we used the Independent-Samples *t*-test with Welch correction, if the variance was unequal. We considered results to be significant at $p < 0.05$.

# RESULTS

## The Loss of *Olig2* Preferentially Impaired OL Maturation in the Cerebral Cortex

To explore the consequence of impaired OL development on brain function, conditional deletion of the *Olig2* gene was achieved in differentiated OL during neonatal development by introducing expression of the cre recombinase under transcriptional control of the *CNPase* promoter (*CNP-Cre*) in the *Olig2-loxp* mice (**Figure 1A**). The offspring were genotyped by PCR at postnatal day 7 (P7) to identify *Olig2*$^{loxp/loxp}$ mice that carry the *CNP-Cre* allele (*Olig2* cKO) and *Olig2*$^{loxp/loxp}$ littermates that lack the *CNP-Cre* allele (WT control) (**Figure 1B**). The knockout efficiency of *Olig2* was confirmed by the diminished expression of the *Olig2* protein in both the corpus callosum and cerebral cortex of the *Olig2* cKO mice at P21 (**Figure 1C**). To investigate the effects of *Olig2* loss on OL development, we quantified oligodendroglia progenitor cells (OPCs) marked by immunohistochemistry staining of PDGF receptor α (PDGFRα) and mature OL marked by CC1. As shown in **Figure 2**, the numbers of CC1$^+$ mature OL in *Olig2* cKO mice were significantly decreased by 85.6% in the cortex (250 ± 13 in WT vs. 36 ± 2.8 in *Olig2* cKO) and 36.1% (521 ± 40 in WT vs. 333 ± 47 in *Olig2* cKO) in the corpus callosum, respectively (**Figures 2A,B**). In contrast, the density of PDGFRα$^+$ OPCs was not affected (**Figures 2C,D**). These results suggest that OL maturation is preferentially affected in the cerebral cortex of the *Olig2* cKO. Such a conclusion is further supported by the observation that myelin basic protein (MBP) was reduced 94% in the *Olig2* cKO cortex (100 ± 12.3% in WT vs. 6.6 ± 3.0% in *Olig2* cKO), but only reduced 60% in the *Olig2* cKO corpus callosum (100 ± 15.1% in WT vs. 40.0 ± 7.3% in *Olig2* cKO) (**Figures 2E,F**).

## The Cerebral Cortex of *Olig2* cKO Mice Harbored Abnormally Higher Levels of Glutamate

To explore whether and how impaired OL maturation may interfere with neuronal function in the juvenile brain, we examined the spectrum of neurochemicals in the cortex of WT and *Olig2* cKO mice at the age of P21 using proton magnetic resonance spectroscopy (1H MRS). T2-weighted MRI images in axial and sagittal orientation were used to ensure the volume-of-interest (**Figure 3A**). Representative MRS spectrums showed resonance of various neurochemicals (**Figure 3B**). *N*-acetylaspartate (NAA) and glutamate (Glu) are the two most abundant neurochemicals in the brain. The peak areas for NAA and Glu were normalized to that of creatine (Cr) for quantitative comparison between the genotypes. Interestingly, the *Olig2* cKO cortex harbors a moderate yet statistically significant increase of Glu/Cr than WT littermates (0.83 ± 0.02 in WT vs. 0.93 ± 0.03 in *Olig2* cKO, $P = 0.01$) (**Figure 3D**). In contrast, the ratio of NAA/Cr, which is thought to reflect neuronal health or viability (Urenjak et al., 1993), was not altered in the *Olig2* cKO mutant ($P = 0.379$) (**Figure 3C**). In addition, choline (Cho) level showed a trend of decrease in the *Olig2* cKO cortex, although no statistical significance was achieved (data not shown). The increase of glutamate in *Olig2* cKO cortex was further validated by enzymatic assay, in which a significant increase of total glutamate in the cortex of *Olig2* cKO mice was observed (1.32 ± 0.06 μg/mg in WT vs. 1.53 ± 0.06 μg/mg in *Olig2* cKO, $P = 0.029$) (**Figure 3E**). These results demonstrated that impaired OL maturation specifically leads to an abnormal increase of glutamate in the cortex without altering neuronal viability.

## Glutamatergic Synapses of *Olig2* cKO Cortical Neurons Contained Higher Density of Synaptic Vehicles

Glutamate is the primary excitatory neurotransmitter, which is largely stored in synaptic vesicles in pyramidal neurons and released upon synaptic stimulation in the cortex (Fonnum, 1984). The long axonal projections of cortical glutamatergic neurons are the primary target for myelination (Tomassy et al., 2014). Moreover, most non-myelinating cortical OLs form contacts with the soma of glutamatergic neurons (Takasaki et al., 2010). Thus, we next questioned whether OL impairment caused by the loss of *Olig2* may affect glutamatergic synapses. Transmission EM images were captured in randomly selected

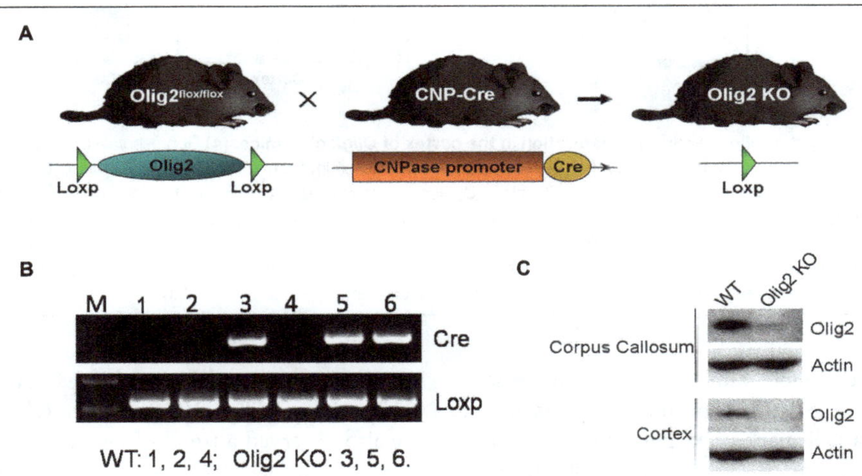


**FIGURE 1 | Generating *Olig2* conditional knockout mice. (A)** Diagram shows *Olig2*$^{flox/flox}$ mice were crossed with mice that express *Cre* recombinase under the control of the *CNPase* promoter to generate *Olig2* cKO mice. **(B)** The offspring were genotyped by PCR for cnp-cre and floxed Olig2 alleles. **(C)** Western Blot analyses showed an absence of Olig2 protein in cortex and corpus callosum of *Olig2* cKO mice.

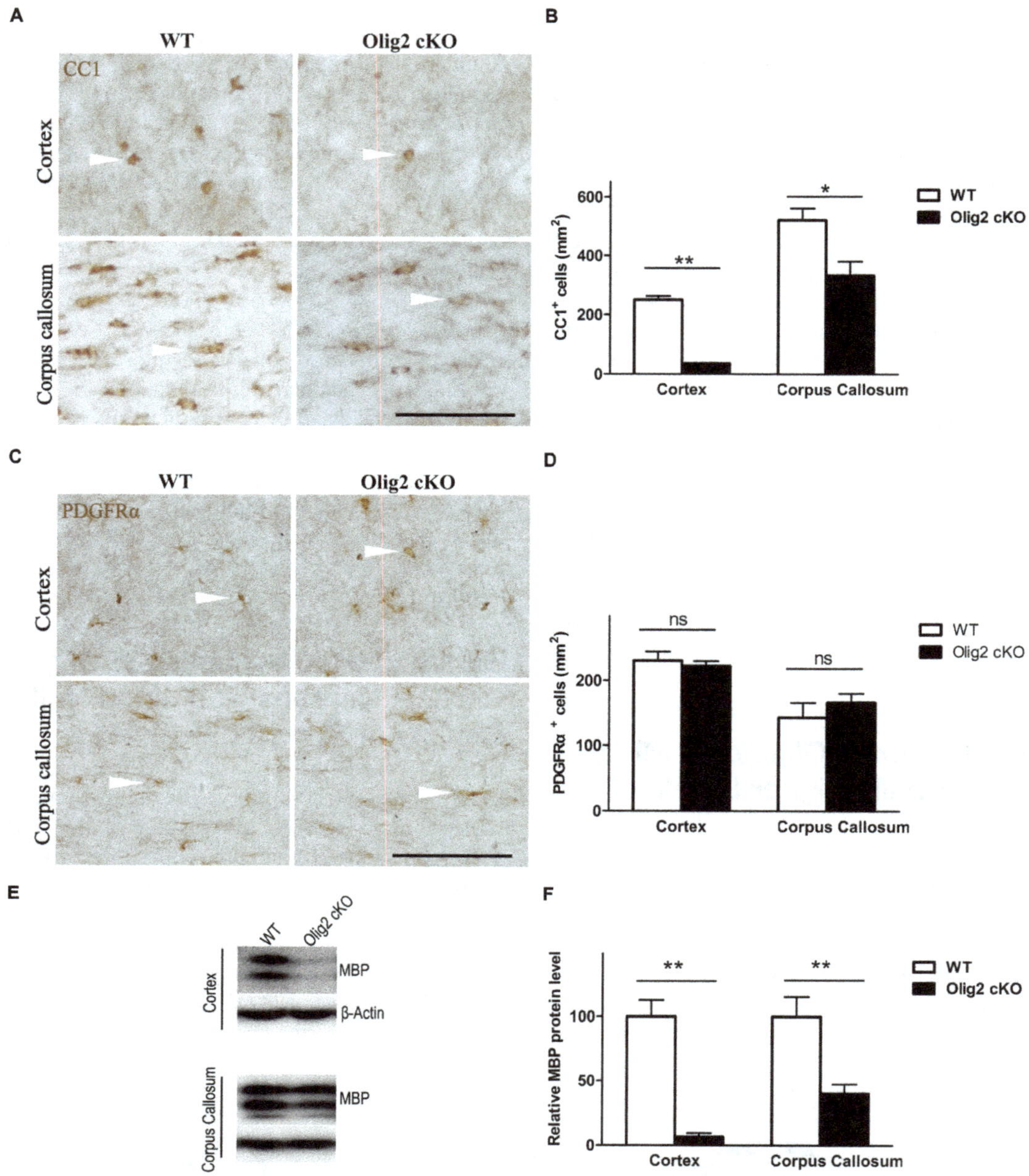


**FIGURE 2 | Preferential impairment of oligodendroglia maturation in the cortex of *Olig2* cKO mice. (A)** Representative images of immunohistochemistry of CC1 showing mature oligodendrocytes (OLs) (white arrow head) in the cortex and corpus callosum from WT and *Olig2* cKO mice. **(B)** Quantification of the density of CC1+ cells in the cortex and corpus callosum from WT and *Olig2* cKO mice. **(C)** Representative images of immunohistochemistry of PDGFRα+ showing oligodendroglia progenitor cells (OPCs) in the cortex and corpus callosum from WT and *Olig2* cKO mice. **(D)** Quantification of the density of PDGFRα+ cells in the cortex and corpus callosum from WT and *Olig2* cKO mice. **(E)** Representative Western blot of MBP expression in the cortex and corpus callosum from WT or *Olig2* cKO mice. **(F)** Quantification of MBP signal on the immunoblot of the cortex and corpus callosum from WT or *Olig2* cKO mice normalized to β-actin as a loading control. Scale bars = 100 μm. Data are presented as mean ± SEM. ns, no significant different; $*P < 0.05$; $**P < 0.01$.

sections and subjected to double blind analysis. The vesicles in each asymmetric synapse with a prominent postsynaptic density (PSD), which is a hall mark of excitatory glutamatergic synapses, were counted in all EM images. Consistent with the increase of overall glutamate levels in the cortex of *Olig2* cKO mice (**Figure 3**), the density of synaptic vesicles within the excitatory presynaptic boutons in the cotex of *Olig2* cKO mice was significantly increased as compared to WT controls (97.2 ± 4.1 in WT vs. 125.2 ± 4.5 in *Olig2* cKO) (**Figures 4A,B**). We also observed a trend of increase in the numbers of docked vesicles at the active zone of *Olig2* cKO boutons (1.53 ± 0.18 in WT vs. 1.97 ± 0.18 in *Olig2* cKO, $P = 0.096$) (**Figure 4C**). No significant difference was detected in the length of PSD between WT and *Olig2* cKO (282.5 ± 17.7 in WT vs. 260.2 ± 12.5 in

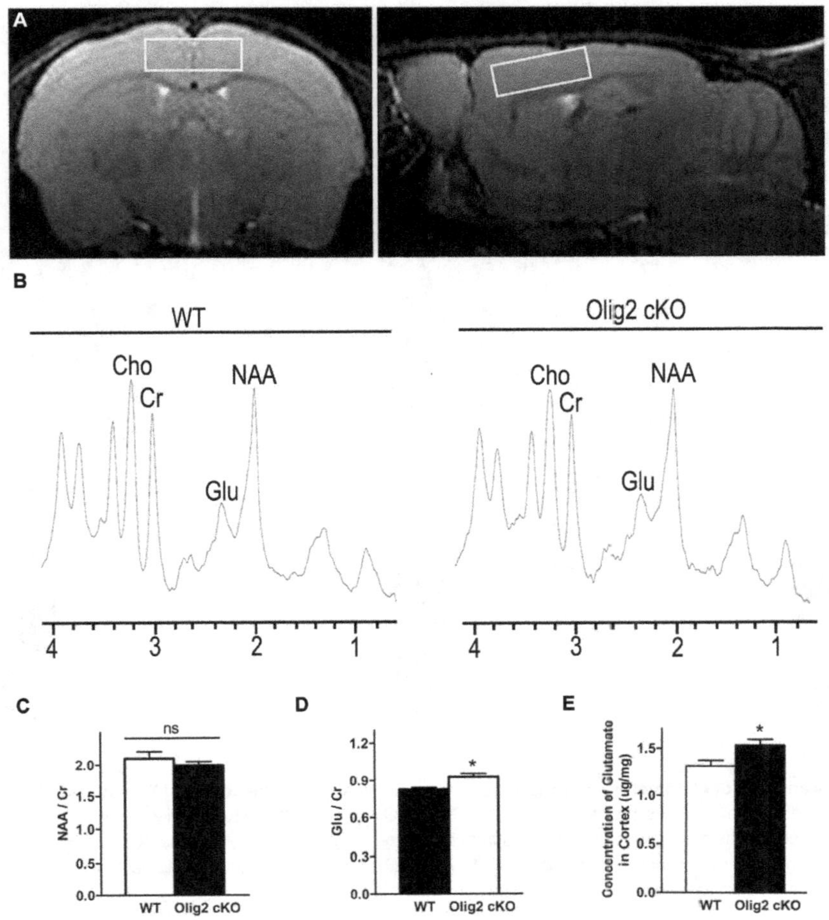


**FIGURE 3 | Aberrantly increased glutamate level in the cortex of *Olig2* cKO mice. (A)** Representative axial and sagittal T2-weighted MR images indicate the position and orientation of point-resolved spectroscopy voxel in the cortex (white rectangle). **(B)** Localized proton magnetic resonance spectra of the cortex from WT or *Olig2* cKO mice, respectively. NAA, *N*-acetylaspartate; Glu, Glutamate; Cr, total creatine; ppm, parts per million. **(C)** Quantification of the ratio of NAA/Cr in the cortex of WT or *Olig2* cKO mice. **(D)** Quantification of the ratio of Glu/Cr in the cortex of WT or *Olig2* cKO mice. **(E)** Quantification of glutamate concentration in the cortex by the enzymatic assay from WT or *Olig2* cKO mice. Data are mean ± SEM. ns, no significant difference. $^{*}P < 0.05$.

*Olig2* cKO, $P = 0.293$) (**Figure 4D**). These results suggest that OL impairment caused by the loss of *Olig2* may lead to aberrantly increased glutamate vesicles within synapses and likely increased glutamate release upon synaptic activation.

## *Olig2* cKO Mice Displayed Anxiety-like Behaviors and Deficits in Behavioral Inhibition

We next tested whether OL impairment and glutamate abnormalities may lead to maladaptive behaviors in juvenile mice. We first chose the open field test and elevated plus maze test, which are non-conditioned procedures commonly used for assessing anxiety-like behaviors in rodents (Bourin et al., 2007). In the open field test, juvenile *Olig2* cKO mice showed a significantly lower ratio of travel distance within central area to total travel distance, as compared with WT controls (13.8 ± 1.2% in WT vs. 9.0 ± 0.8% in *Olig2* cKO, $P = 0.004$) (**Figure 5A**) and spent more time in the central area (30.8 ± 3.6 sec in WT vs. 51.1 ± 4.1 sec in *Olig2* cKO, $P = 0.001$) (**Figure 5B**) during the 10-min test, indicating an anxious phenotype. In addition, in the elevated plus maze test, the numbers of entry into the open arms and time spent on the open arms were previously shown to be inversely related with the anxiety level (Xu et al., 2014), hence used to identify anxiety-like behaviors (Brunner et al., 2014). The time spent on the open arms and entries into the open arms were expressed as a percentage of the total time on any arms and entries into any arms during the test. We found that *Olig2* cKO mice showed less entries into the open arms (51.9 ± 2.0% in WT vs. 43.4 ± 3.1% in *Olig2* cKO, $P = 0.021$) (**Figure 5C**) and spent less time on open arms (34.1 ± 3.2% in WT vs. 22.2 ± 2.3% in *Olig2* cKO, $P = 0.011$) (**Figure 5D**), again indicating a more anxious behavior. We also assessed locomotor activity of the animals on the maze by the total distance traveled on both open and closed arms. We found that *Olig2* cKO mice traveled a significantly longer distance than WT controls (6663 ± 404.5 cm in WT vs. 8264 ± 444.3 cm in *Olig2* cKO, $P = 0.014$) (**Figure 5E**), suggesting a higher locomotor activity

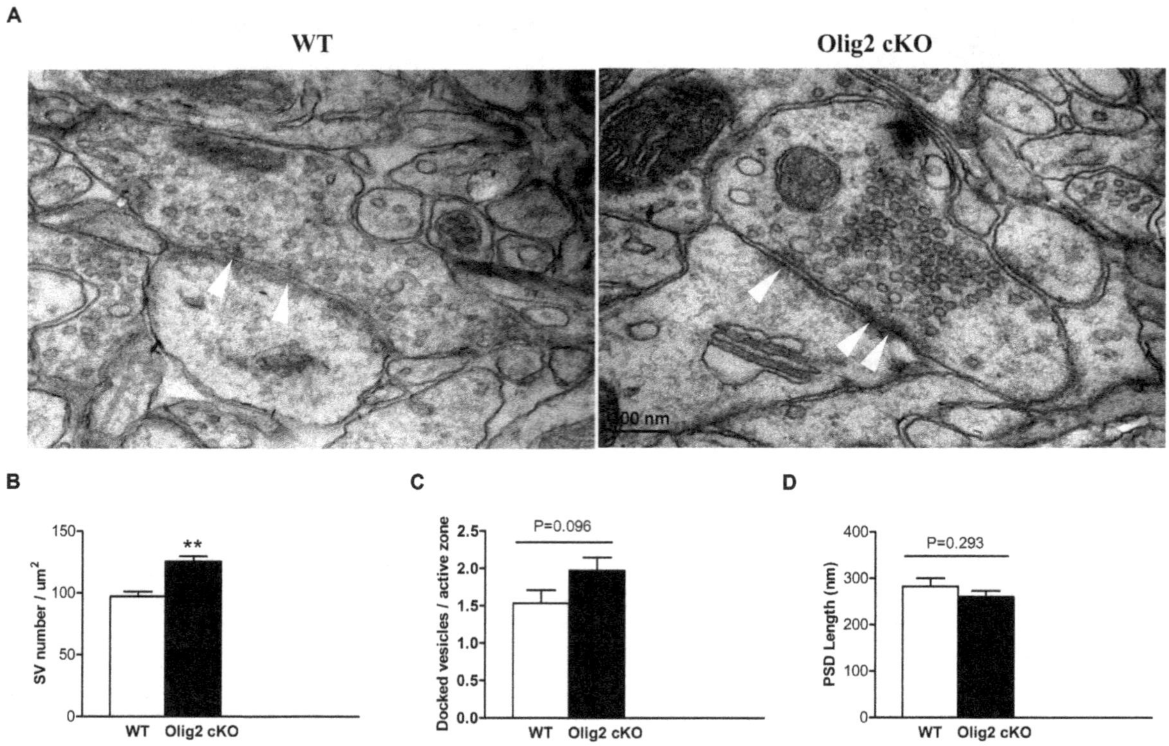


**FIGURE 4 | Electronmicrocopy analysis of glutamatergic synapses and synaptic vesicles in the cortex of WT and *Olig2* cKO mice. (A)** Representative electron microscopy micrographs show an excitatory synapse in the WT and *Olig2* cKO cortices. White arrows indicate docked vesicles. **(B)** Quantification of the density of synaptic vesicles in cortical glutamatergic presynaptic boutons from EM images of WT or *Olig2* cKO mice. **(C)** Quantification of the number of docked vesicles per active zone in WT or *Olig2* cKO excitatory synapses. **(D)** Quantification of the length of the postsynaptic density (PSD) in WT or *Olig2* cKO excitatory synapses. Scale bar = 200 nm, Data are given as mean ± SEM, $^{**}P < 0.01$.

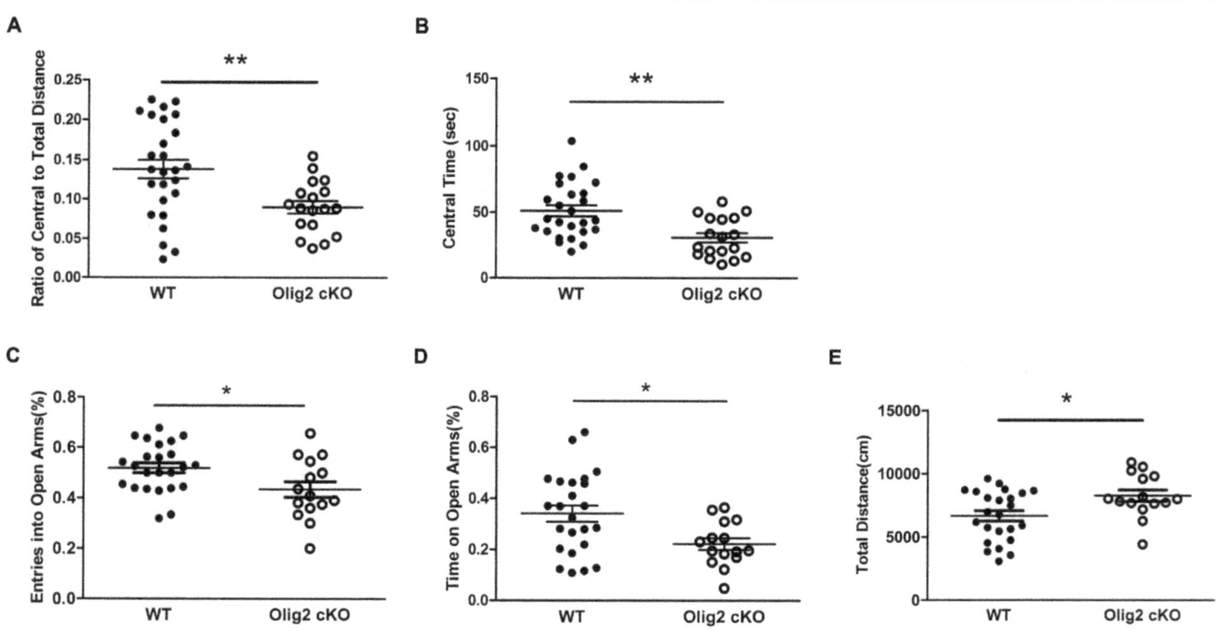


**FIGURE 5 | Anxiety-like behavior tests on WT and *Olig2* cKO mice.** Open field test **(A,B)**: Graphs showed ratio of central to total distance **(A)** and center time **(B)** in WT and *Olig2* cKO mice. Elevated plus maze test **(C–E)**: Graphs showed number of entries into open arms **(C)**, time spent on the open arms **(D)** and total distance traveled on the arms **(E)**, Data are given as mean ± SEM. $^{*}P < 0.05$, $^{**}P < 0.01$.

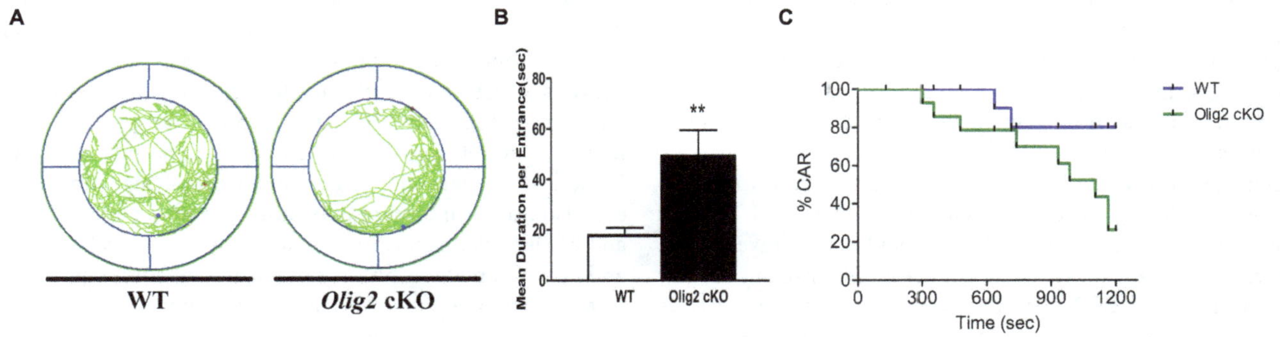


**FIGURE 6 | Impulsivity-like behavior analyses on WT and *Olig2* cKO mice.** Cliff avoidance reaction test **(A–C)**: an example of the travel pathway of WT and *Olig2* cKO on the elevated platform **(A)**. *Olig2* cKO mice failed to avoid the cliff actively by spending significantly more time around the cliff **(B)**. Graphs represent the time course of CAR measurement in WT and *Olig2* cKO mice **(C)**. Data are given as mean ± SEM. $^{**}P < 0.01$.

of *Olig2* cKO mice on the maze. Together, all the aforementioned behavior tests consistently demonstrated anxiety-like behaviors in juvenile *Olig2* cKO mice.

Impulsivity is defined as a failure in controlling and inhibiting the emotion for appropriate actions and behaviors (Dalley et al., 2008), which is also a typical tendency in adolescence. Recent studies suggest that certain types of functional impulsivity may be linked with anxiety (Taylor et al., 2008). Thus, we explored whether the loss of *Olig2* may also lead to impulsivity-like behavior in juvenile mice. CAR impairment is thought to represent impulsivity-like behaviors in rodents (Matsuoka et al., 2005). Unlike many classical mouse impulsivity tests that require lengthy training, the CAR test can be readily applied to juvenile mice. We found *Olig2* cKO mice traveled more and spent longer time than WT control in the edge area in the CAR test (17.7 ± 3.1 s in WT vs. 49.4 ± 10.2 s in *Olig2* cKO, $P = 0.007$) (**Figures 6A,B**). Moreover, 60% of *Olig2* cKO mice failed to avoid a potential fall from a height, whereas only 14.3% of WT controls fell (**Figure 6C**).These results suggest that the defects in OL maturation due to the loss of *Olig2* also lead to impulsivity-like behaviors.

## DISCUSSION

Using the *Olig2* cKO mouse model, our studies demonstrated that impaired OL maturation can affect glutamate levels in the cerebral cortex and synaptic vesicle density in glutamatergic presynaptic boutons. Furthermore, *Olig2* cKO mice display anxiety-related maladaptive behaviors. To our knowledge, it is the first evidence that demonstrates behavioral abnormalities of *Olig2* cKO mice. These results suggests that OL-neuron interaction in the cortex plays important roles in governing synaptic function and raises an intriguing possibility that impaired *de novo* OL maturation in adolescence may contribute to the early onset of anxiety.

Proton magnetic resonance spectroscopy (1H MRS) is a non-invasive technique that provides great advantages in studying biochemical concentrations of neurotransmitters *in vivo* (Soares and Law, 2009). Specifically, glutamate, which is measured by 1H MRS, has been suggested as an index of cortical excitability (Stagg et al., 2009, 2011). In multiple clinical MRS studies, increased cortical glutamate levels were positively correlated with anxiety symptoms in patients (Phan et al., 2005; Modi et al., 2014). These observations suggest that hyperfunction of cortical glutamatergic neurons may be an important contributing factor for the etiology of anxiety and related disorders. Extensive studies have demonstrated that a wide variety of molecular and cellular mechanisms in neurons and nearby glia cells tightly control glutamate homeostasis and synaptic release (Deitmer et al., 2003; DeSilva et al., 2009). However, which mechanism(s) is dysregulated that underlie the increased glutamate in the cortex of anxiety disorder patients still remains elusive.

Cortical OL maturation occurs concurrently with the most frequent onset of anxiety disorders (Kessler et al., 2005; Miller et al., 2012; Young et al., 2013). In addition, OL and myelin development overlaps with the time for peak binding of cortical glutamate to NMDA receptors in early adolescence (Kornhuber et al., 1988). Therefore, we explored whether selective impairment of OL maturation may affect glutamatergic neurons and behavior in juvenile mice. The *CNP-Cre* mouse line was used in previous studies for specific deletion of genes in mature OL (Wahl et al., 2014; Zou et al., 2014). We employed this mouse line for conditionally deleting the *Olig2* gene that encodes a transcription factor critical for OL development (Zhou et al., 2000; Lu et al., 2002; Ligon et al., 2006; Yue et al., 2006; Mei et al., 2013). Interestingly, *Olig2* cKO mice displayed preferential reduction of cortical mature OLs at P21, whereas OLs in the corpus callosum were much less severely affected. Hence, despite the undefined mechanism that underlies the preferential impairment of OL maturation in the cortex of *Olig2* cKO mouse, this genetic model provides a reasonable tool for dissecting the role of OL maturation in modulating cortical neuronal function during juvenile age. Importantly, using 1H MRS, we detected an overall increase of glutamate in the cortex of *Olig2* cKO mice, suggesting elevated cortical excitability. In addition, we detected increased vesicles in glutamatergic synapses, which further supported glutamatergic hyperfunction as a result of defects in OL maturation. Moreover, juvenile *Olig2* cKO mice displayed anxiety-related behaviors. Together, these observations suggest that normal OL development plays essential roles in governing glutamate signaling and adolescence behavior, and defects in *de novo* OL maturation in early postnatal life could cause aberrant glutamate function and maladaptive behaviors.

Oligodendroglia impairment may affect cortical neurons through multiple distinct mechanisms that still remain elusive. Because the loss of *Olig2* could affect myelination and axonal conductance (Baumann and Pham-Dinh, 2001), neurons in *Olig2* cKO cortex may increase synaptic vesicles as a compensatory adaptation. This may especially affect glutamatergic neurons, because their axons are mostly myelinated by OLs (Tomassy et al., 2014). However, several lines of evidence argue that myelination defects alone do not necessarily cause glutamatergic hyperfunction. For instance, cortical glutamate levels were maintained normal in the heterozygous shiverer mutant mouse that lacked one copy of the *MBP* gene thus displaying hypomyelination without affecting mature OL density (Takanashi et al., 2014). Thus, the preferential impairment of *de novo* OL maturation in the cortex may be a specific mechanism that underlies the aberrant increase of cortical glutamate.

Unlike white matter OLs that perform primary roles in myelin formation, cortical OLs display a radial gradient distribution and differentially myelinate the long-range projections of glutamatergic pyramidal neurons in distinct cortical layers (Tomassy et al., 2014). Besides myelination, the majority of mature OLs reside in deep layers of cerebral cortex are attached with the soma of pyramidal neurons, rather than GABAergic neurons (Takasaki et al., 2010). Although the function of these perineuronal OLs in the cortex still remains unknown, accumulating evidence suggest that OLs can provide metabolic and neurotrophic support (Du and Dreyfus, 2002). In addition, OLs are known to express several glutamate transporters (Domercq et al., 1999; Karadottir et al., 2005), and can uptake glutamate in the gray matter of the developing brain (DeSilva et al., 2009). More importantly, cortical perineuronal oligodendroglia, but not white matter oligodendroglia, express glutamine synthetase (GS) for converting glutamate to glutamine (Damelio et al., 1990). It is well established that glutamine produced by astrocyte GS from the up-taken glutamate can be recycled into neurons, which plays key roles in controlling glutamate recycling (Deitmer et al., 2003). In this regard, cortical gray matter OLs may play important roles in controlling glutamate homeostasis, in parallel with the known function of astrocytes in modulating glutamatergic function.

It is also important to note that besides aberrant glutamate, abnormalities in other neurotransmitters, including GABA, dopamine, serotonin and norepinephrine, are also thought to contribute to anxiety (Kent et al., 2002). Because our understanding of the functional interplay between OLs and neurons is still at its infancy, the types of neurons affected by OL defects still remain undefined. It is conceivable that OL defects in *Olig2* cKO mice could also affect the function of other neuronal cell types in addition to glutamatergic pyramidal neurons, which could contribute to the anxiety-like behaviors we observed in this study. In fact, dopamine transporter knockout mice are severely impaired in CAR test (Yamashita et al., 2013). In addition, disturbing neuregulin-1-ErbB4 signaling in OLs can also lead to increased dopamine receptors and transporters and anxiety-like behaviors in mice (Roy et al., 2007). Whether and how OL maturation may modulate dopaminergic function is a challenging question for future studies. Moreover, the symptoms of anxiety are shared by some other psychiatric disorders, like schizophrenia (Buckley et al., 2009), suggesting that the anxiety like behavior found in Olig2 cKO mice may also contribute to other psychiatric disorders. In fact, ErbB signaling pathway has been considered as a potential therapeutic target for schizophrenia (Deng et al., 2013), which conceivably modulates OL function. However, many well-established behavioral tests for cognitive abnormalities require lengthy training hence could not be applied to juvenile mice. This limits our ability in the current study that aims to identify juvenile abnormalities caused by defects of OL maturation. Future studies may need more specific behavior tests utilized in both young and adult mice to explore whether OL maturation affects higher cognitive function.

## CONCLUSION

Our studies demonstrate that impaired OL maturation by conditional deleting the *Olig2* gene in differentiated OL can aberrantly increase cortical glutamate, which likely leads to glutamatergic hyperfunction. Moreover, the defects in *de novo* OL maturation clearly result in anxiety-like behaviors and deficits of behavioral inhibition in juvenile mice. Our findings prompt future studies to investigate the intriguing possibility whether defects in OL and/or myelin development in childhood may contribute to the pathogenesis of anxiety in humans.

## AUTHOR CONTRIBUTIONS

XC, LX, and YF designed the study. XC, WZ and YG acquired and analyzed the data. TL, YT and SL also acquired the data. H-YS analyzed the data. XC, YF and LX wrote the article, which all other authors reviewed. All authors approved the final version for publication.

## ACKNOWLEDGMENTS

This work is supported by the National Natural Science Foundation of China (NSCF 81471297), and Chongqing Science Foundation to LX. We thank Mrs. Yu Sun for her assistance in ultrathin sections.

## REFERENCES


Baumann, N., and Pham-Dinh, D. (2001). Biology of oligodendrocyte and myelin in the mammalian central nervous system. *Physiol. Rev.* 81, 871–927.

Bourin, M., Petit-Demouliere, B., Dhonnchadha, B. N., and Hascoet, M. (2007). Animal models of anxiety in mice. *Fundam. Clin. Pharmacol.* 21, 567–574. doi: 10.1111/j.1472-8206.2007.00526.x

Brunner, S. M., Farzi, A., Locker, F., Holub, B. S., Drexel, M., Reichmann, F., et al. (2014). GAL3 receptor KO mice exhibit an anxiety-like phenotype. *Proc. Natl. Acad. Sci. U.S.A.* 111, 7138–7143. doi: 10.1073/pnas.1318066111

Buckley, P. F., Miller, B. J., Lehrer, D. S., and Castle, D. J. (2009). Psychiatric comorbidities and schizophrenia. *Schizophr. Bull.* 35, 383–402. doi: 10.1093/schbul/sbn135

Butters, R. P. (2011). The behavioral neuroscience of adolescence. *Clin. Soc. Work J.* 39, 315–317. doi: 10.1007/s10615-011-0320-y

Casey, B. J., Getz, S., and Galvan, A. (2008). The adolescent brain. *Dev. Rev.* 28, 62–77. doi: 10.1016/j.dr.2007.08.003

Cassoli, J. S., Guest, P. C., Malchow, B., Schmitt, A., Falkai, P., and Martins-de-Souza, D. (2015). Disturbed macro-connectivity in schizophrenia linked to oligodendrocyte dysfunction: from structural findings to molecules. *NPJ Schizophr.* 1:15034. doi: 10.1038/npjschz.2015.34

Dalley, J. W., Mar, A. C., Economidou, D., and Robbins, T. W. (2008). Neurobehavioral mechanisms of impulsivity: fronto-striatal systems and functional neurochemistry. *Pharmacol. Biochem. Behav.* 90, 250–260. doi: 10.1016/j.pbb.2007.12.021

Damelio, F., Eng, L. F., and Gibbs, M. A. (1990). Glutamine-synthetase immunoreactivity is present in oligodendroglia of various regions of the central-nervous-system. *Glia* 3, 335–341. doi: 10.1002/glia.440030504

de Hoz, L., and Simons, M. (2015). The emerging functions of oligodendrocytes in regulating neuronal network behaviour. *Bioessays* 37, 60–69. doi: 10.1002/bies.201400127

Deitmer, J. W., Broer, A., and Broer, S. (2003). Glutamine efflux from astrocytes is mediated by multiple pathways. *J. Neurochem.* 87, 127–135. doi: 10.1046/j.1471-4159.2003.01981.x

Deng, C., Pan, B., Engel, M., and Huang, X. F. (2013). Neuregulin-1 signalling and antipsychotic treatment: potential therapeutic targets in a schizophrenia candidate signalling pathway. *Psychopharmacology (Berl)* 226, 201–215. doi: 10.1007/s00213-013-3003-2

DeSilva, T. M., Kabakov, A. Y., Goldhoff, P. E., Volpe, J. J., and Rosenberg, P. A. (2009). Regulation of glutamate transport in developing rat oligodendrocytes. *J. Neurosci.* 29, 7898–7908. doi: 10.1523/Jneurosci.6129-08.2009

Domercq, M., Sanchez-Gomez, M. V., Areso, P., and Matute, C. (1999). Expression of glutamate transporters in rat optic nerve oligodendrocytes. *Eur. J. Neurosci.* 11, 2226–2236. doi: 10.1046/j.1460-9568.1999.00639.x

Du, Y. Z., and Dreyfus, C. F. (2002). Oligodendrocytes as providers of growth factors. *J. Neurosci. Res.* 68, 647–654. doi: 10.1002/jnr.10245

Edgar, N., and Sibille, E. (2012). A putative functional role for oligodendrocytes in mood regulation. *Transl. Psychiatry* 2:e102. doi: 10.1038/tp.2012.34

Fields, R. D. (2008). White matter in learning, cognition and psychiatric disorders. *Trends Neurosci.* 31, 361–370. doi: 10.1016/j.tins.2008.04.001

Fonnum, F. (1984). Glutamate - a neurotransmitter in mammalian Brain. *J. Neurochem.* 42, 1–11. doi: 10.1111/j.1471-4159.1984.tb09689.x

Funfschilling, U., Supplie, L. M., Mahad, D., Boretius, S., Saab, A. S., Edgar, J., et al. (2012). Glycolytic oligodendrocytes maintain myelin and long-term axonal integrity. *Nature* 485, 517–521. doi: 10.1038/nature11007

Hoerst, M., Weber-Fahr, W., Tunc-Skarka, N., Ruf, M., Bohus, M., Schmahl, C., et al. (2010). Correlation of glutamate levels in the anterior cingulate cortex with self-reported impulsivity in patients with borderline personality disorder and healthy controls. *Arch. Gen. Psychiatry* 67, 946–954. doi: 10.1001/archgenpsychiatry.2010.93

Karadottir, R., Cavelier, P., Bergersen, L. H., and Attwell, D. (2005). NMDA receptors are expressed in oligodendrocytes and activated in ischaemia. *Nature* 438, 1162–1166. doi: 10.1038/nature04302

Katayama, K., Yamada, K., Ornthanalai, V. G., Inoue, T., Ota, M., Murphy, N. P., et al. (2010). Slitrk1-deficient mice display elevated anxiety-like behavior and noradrenergic abnormalities. *Mol. Psychiatry* 15, 177–184. doi: 10.1038/mp.2008.97

Kent, J. M., Mathew, S. J., and Gorman, J. M. (2002). Molecular targets in the treatment of anxiety. *Biol. Psychiatry* 52, 1008–1030. doi: 10.1016/S0006-3223(02)01672-4

Kessler, R. C., Berglund, P., Demler, O., Jin, R., and Walters, E. E. (2005). Lifetime prevalence and age-of-onset distributions' of DSM-IV disorders in the national comorbidity survey replication. *Arch. Gen. Psychiatry* 62, 593–602. doi: 10.1001/archpsyc.62.6.593

Kornhuber, J., Retz, W., Riederer, P., Heinsen, H., and Fritze, J. (1988). Effect of antemortem and postmortem factors on [3H] glutamate binding in the human brain. *Neurosci. Lett.* 93, 312–317. doi: 10.1016/0304-3940(88)90101-2

Lappe-Siefke, C., Goebbels, S., Gravel, M., Nicksch, E., Lee, J., Braun, P. E., et al. (2003). Disruption of Cnp1 uncouples oligodendroglial functions in axonal support and myelination. *Nat. Genet.* 33, 366–374. doi: 10.1038/ng1095

Lee, F. S., Heimer, H., Giedd, J. N., Lein, E. S., Sestan, N., Weinberger, D. R., et al. (2014). Adolescent mental health-Opportunity and obligation. *Science* 346, 547–549. doi: 10.1126/science.1260497

Lee, Y. J., Morrison, B. M., Li, Y., Lengacher, S., Farah, M. H., Hoffman, P. N., et al. (2012). Oligodendroglia metabolically support axons and contribute to neurodegeneration. *Nature* 487, 443–448. doi: 10.1038/nature11314

Ligon, K. L., Kesari, S., Kitada, M., Sun, T., Arnett, H. A., Alberta, J. A., et al. (2006). Development of NG2 neural progenitor cells requires Olig gene function. *Proc. Natl. Acad. Sci. U.S.A.* 103, 7853–7858. doi: 10.1073/pnas.0511001103

Lu, Q. R., Sun, T., Zhu, Z. M., Ma, N., Garcia, M., Stiles, C. D., et al. (2002). Common developmental requirement for Olig function indicates a motor neuron/oligodendrocyte connection. *Cell* 109, 75–86. doi: 10.1016/S0092-8674(02)00678-5

Matsuoka, Y., Furuyashiki, T., Yamada, K., Nagai, T., Bito, H., Tanaka, Y., et al. (2005). Prostaglandin E receptor EP1 controls impulsive behavior under stress. *Proc. Natl. Acad. Sci. U.S.A.* 102, 16066–16071. doi: 10.1073/pnas.0504908102

McKenzie, I. A., Ohayon, D., Li, H. L., de Faria, J. P., Emery, B., Tohyama, K., et al. (2014). Motor skill learning requires active central myelination. *Science* 346, 318–322. doi: 10.1126/science.1254960

Mei, F., Wang, H. K., Liu, S. B., Niu, J. Q., Wang, L. Y., He, Y. T., et al. (2013). Stage-Specific deletion of olig2 conveys opposing functions on differentiation and maturation of oligodendrocytes. *J. Neurosci.* 33, 8454–8462. doi: 10.1523/Jneurosci.2453-12.2013

Michaelis, T., Boretius, S., and Frahm, J. (2009). Localized proton MRS of animal brain in vivo: models of human disorders. *Progr. Nuclear Magn. Reson. Spectrosc.* 55, 1–34. doi: 10.1016/j.pnmrs.2008.11.001

Miller, D. J., Duka, T., Stimpson, C. D., Schapiro, S. J., Baze, W. B., McArthur, M. J., et al. (2012). Prolonged myelination in human neocortical evolution. *Proc. Natl. Acad. Sci. U.S.A.* 109, 16480–16485. doi: 10.1073/pnas.1117943109

Modi, S., Rana, P., Kaur, P., Rani, N., and Khushu, S. (2014). Glutamate level in anterior cingulate predicts anxiety in healthy humans: a magnetic resonance spectroscopy study. *Psychiatry Res.* 224, 34–41. doi: 10.1016/j.pscychresns.2014.03.001

Nave, K. A., and Ehrenreich, H. (2014). Myelination and Oligodendrocyte functions in psychiatric diseases. *JAMA Psychiatry* 71, 582–584. doi: 10.1001/jamapsychiatry.2014.189

Paus, T., Keshavan, M., and Giedd, J. N. (2008). OPINION why do many psychiatric disorders emerge during adolescence? *Nat. Rev. Neurosci.* 9, 947–957. doi: 10.1038/nrn2513

Penzes, P., Cahill, M. E., Jones, K. A., VanLeeuwen, J. E., and Woolfrey, K. M. (2011). Dendritic spine pathology in neuropsychiatric disorders. *Nat. Neurosci.* 14, 285–293. doi: 10.1038/nn.2741

Phan, K. L., Fitzgerald, D. A., Cortese, B. M., Seraji-Bozorgzad, N., Tancer, M. E., and Moore, G. J. (2005). Anterior cingulate neurochemistry in social anxiety disorder: 1H-MRS at 4 Tesla. *Neuroreport* 16, 183–186. doi: 10.1097/00001756-200502080-00024

Provencher, S. W. (1993). Estimation of metabolite concentrations from localized in-vivo proton nmr-spectra. *Magn. Reson. Med.* 30, 672–679. doi: 10.1002/mrm.1910300604

Roy, K., Murtie, J. C., El Khodort, B. F., Edgar, N., Sardi, S. P., Hooks, B. M., et al. (2007). Loss of erbB signaling in oligodendrocytes alters myelin and dopaminergic function, a potential mechanism for neuropsychiatric disorders. *Proc. Natl. Acad. Sci. U.S.A.* 104, 8131–8136. doi: 10.1073/pnas.0702157104

Soares, D. P., and Law, M. (2009). Magnetic resonance spectroscopy of the brain: review of metabolites and clinical applications. *Clin. Radiol.* 64, 12–21. doi: 10.1016/j.crad.2008.07.002

Stagg, C. J., Bestmann, S., Constantinescu, A. O., Moreno, L. M., Allman, C., Mekle, R., et al. (2011). Relationship between physiological measures of excitability and levels of glutamate and GABA in the human motor cortex. *J. Physiol. Lond.* 589, 5845–5855. doi: 10.1113/jphysiol.2011.216978

Stagg, C. J., Wylezinska, M., Matthews, P. M., Johansen-Berg, H., Jezzard, P., Rothwell, J. C., et al. (2009). Neurochemical effects of theta burst stimulation as assessed by magnetic resonance spectroscopy. *J. Neurophysiol.* 101, 2872–2877. doi: 10.1152/jn.91060.2008

Takanashi, J., Nitta, N., Iwasaki, N., Saito, S., Tanaka, R., Barkovich, A. J., et al. (2014). Neurochemistry in shiverer mouse depicted on MR spectroscopy. *J. Magn. Reson. Imaging* 39, 1550–1557. doi: 10.1002/jmri.24306

Takasaki, C., Yamasaki, M., Uchigashima, M., Konno, K., Yanagawa, Y., and Watanabe, M. (2010). Cytochemical and cytological properties of perineuronal oligodendrocytes in the mouse cortex. *Eur. J. Neurosci.* 32, 1326–1336. doi: 10.1111/j.1460-9568.2010.07377.x

Tau, G. Z., and Peterson, B. S. (2010). Normal development of brain circuits. *Neuropsychopharmacology* 35, 147–168. doi: 10.1038/npp.2009.115

Taylor, C. T., Hirshfeld-Becker, D. R., Ostacher, M. J., Chow, C. W., LeBeau, R. T., Pollack, M. H., et al. (2008). Anxiety is associated with impulsivity in bipolar disorder. *J. Anxiety Disord.* 22, 868–876. doi: 10.1016/j.janxdis.2007.09.001

Tomassy, G. S., Berger, D. R., Chen, H. H., Kasthuri, N., Hayworth, K. J., Vercelli, A., et al. (2014). Distinct profiles of myelin distribution along single axons of pyramidal neurons in the neocortex. *Science* 344, 319–324. doi: 10.1126/science.1249766

Urenjak, J., Williams, S. R., Gadian, D. G., and Noble, M. (1993). Proton nuclear-magnetic-resonance spectroscopy unambiguously identifies different neural cell-types. *J. Neurosci.* 13, 981–989.

Wahl, S. E., McLane, L. E., Bercury, K. K., Macklin, W. B., and Wood, T. L. (2014). Mammalian target of rapamycin promotes oligodendrocyte differentiation, initiation and extent of CNS myelination. *J. Neurosci.* 34, 4453–4465. doi: 10.1523/JNEUROSCI.4311-13.2014

Wang, H. K., Li, C. R., Wang, H. Z., Mei, F., Liu, Z., Shen, H. Y., et al. (2013). Cuprizone-induced demyelination in mice: age-related vulnerability and exploratory behavior deficit. *Neurosci. Bull.* 29, 251–259. doi: 10.1007/s12264-013-1323-1321

Xu, P., Xu, H., Tang, X., Xu, L., Wang, Y., Guo, L., et al. (2014). Liver X receptor beta is essential for the differentiation of radial glial cells to oligodendrocytes in the dorsal cortex. *Mol. Psychiatry* 19, 947–957. doi: 10.1038/mp.2014.60

Yamashita, M., Sakakibara, Y., Hall, F. S., Numachi, Y., Yoshida, S., Kobayashi, H., et al. (2013). Impaired cliff avoidance reaction in dopamine transporter knockout mice. *Psychopharmacology (Berl)* 227, 741–749. doi: 10.1007/s00213-013-3009

Young, K. M., Psachoulia, K., Tripathi, R. B., Dunn, S. J., Cossell, L., Attwell, D., et al. (2013). Oligodendrocyte dynamics in the healthy adult CNS: evidence for myelin remodeling. *Neuron* 77, 873–885. doi: 10.1016/j.neuron.2013.01.006

Yue, T., Xian, K., Hurlock, E., Xin, M., Kernie, S. G., Parada, L. F., et al. (2006). A critical role for dorsal progenitors in cortical myelination. *J. Neurosci.* 26, 1275–1280. doi: 10.1523/Jneurosci.4717-05.2006

Zhou, Q., Wang, S. L., and Anderson, D. J. (2000). Identification of a novel family of oligodendrocyte lineage-specific basic helix-loop-helix transcription factors. *Neuron* 25, 331–343. doi: 10.1016/S0896-6273(00)80898-3

Zou, Y., Jiang, W., Wang, J., Li, Z., Zhang, J., Bu, J., et al. (2014). Oligodendrocyte precursor cell-intrinsic effect of Rheb1 controls differentiation and mediates mTORC1-dependent myelination in brain. *J. Neurosci.* 34, 15764–15778. doi: 10.1523/JNEUROSCI.2267-14.2014

# 10

# Long-Term NMDAR Antagonism Correlates Reduced Astrocytic Glutamate Uptake with Anxiety-Like Phenotype

***Eduardo R. Zimmer[1], Vitor R. Torrez[1], Eduardo Kalinine[1,2], Marina C. Augustin[1], Kamila C. Zenki[1], Roberto F. Almeida[1], Gisele Hansel[1], Alexandre P. Muller[1,3], Diogo O. Souza[1], Rodrigo Machado-Vieira[4,5,6] and Luis V. Portela[1]****

*[1] Department of Biochemistry, Universidade Federal do Rio Grande do Sul, Porto Alegre, Brazil, [2] Department of Physiology, Universidade Federal de Sergipe, São Cristovão, Brazil, [3] Laboratory of Exercise, Biochemistry and Physiology, Universidade do Extremo Sul Catarinense, Criciúma, Brazil, [4] Laboratory of Neuroscience, LIM-27, Institute and Department of Psychiatry, Universidade de São Paulo, São Paulo, Brazil, [5] Center for Interdisciplinary Research on Applied Neurosciences (NAPNA), Universidade de São Paulo, São Paulo, Brazil, [6] Experimental Therapeutics and Pathophysiology Branch, National Institute of Mental Health, National Institutes of Health, Bethesda, MD, USA*

***Correspondence:***
*Luis V. Portela,*
*Department of Biochemistry,*
*Universidade Federal do Rio Grande do Sul, 2600 Ramiro Barcelos Street, 90035-003, Porto Alegre, Rio Grande do Sul, Brazil*
*roskaportela@gmail.com*

The role of glutamate *N*-methyl-D-aspartate receptor (NMDAR) hypofunction has been extensively studied in schizophrenia; however, less is known about its role in anxiety disorders. Recently, it was demonstrated that astrocytic GLT-1 blockade leads to an anxiety-like phenotype. Although astrocytes are capable of modulating NMDAR activity through glutamate uptake transporters, the relationship between astrocytic glutamate uptake and the development of an anxiety phenotype remains poorly explored. Here, we aimed to investigative whether long-term antagonism of NMDAR impacts anxiety-related behaviors and astrocytic glutamate uptake. Memantine, an NMDAR antagonist, was administered daily for 24 days to healthy adult CF-1 mice by oral gavage at doses of 5, 10, or 20 mg/kg. The mice were submitted to a sequential battery of behavioral tests (open field, light–dark box and elevated plus-maze tests). We then evaluated glutamate uptake activity and the immunocontents of glutamate transporters in the frontoparietal cortex and hippocampus. Our results demonstrated that long-term administration of memantine induces anxiety-like behavior in mice in the light–dark box and elevated plus-maze paradigms. Additionally, the administration of memantine decreased glutamate uptake activity in both the frontoparietal cortex and hippocampus without altering the immunocontent of either GLT-1 or GLAST. Remarkably, the memantine-induced reduction in glutamate uptake was correlated with enhancement of an anxiety-like phenotype. In conclusion, long-term NMDAR antagonism with memantine induces anxiety-like behavior that is associated with reduced glutamate uptake activity but that is not dependent on GLT-1 or GLAST protein expression. Our study suggests that NMDAR and glutamate uptake hypofunction may contribute to the development of conditions that fall within the category of anxiety disorders.

**Keywords: anxiety, astrocytes, behavior, glutamate, memantine**

## Introduction

Anxiety disorders are among the most prevalent psychiatric conditions worldwide. These disorders have been associated with social isolation, alcoholism, and increased suicide attempts and are also considered to be risk factors for the development of additional psychiatric disorders (Gross and Hen, 2004). Hence, it is imperative to understand the neurobiological mechanisms that are associated with anxiety disorders. It has recently been proposed that a functional imbalance of the tripartite glutamatergic synapse plays a role in anxiety disorders (Clement and Chapouthier, 1998; Nutt and Malizia, 2001; Nemeroff, 2003; Machado-Vieira et al., 2009, 2012). Indeed, glutamatergic neurotransmission offers multiple potential pharmacological targets for treating anxiety-related disorders, such as postsynaptic receptor signaling, presynaptic glutamate release, and astrocytic glutamate uptake (Szabo et al., 2009; Zarate et al., 2010; Riaza Bermudo-Soriano et al., 2012; Pilc et al., 2013).

Currently, antagonism of *N*-methyl-D-aspartate receptor (NMDAR) has been proposed as a feasible strategy for reducing the major symptoms that are linked to anxiety-like behavior (Cortese and Phan, 2005). Indeed, when memantine, an NMDAR antagonist, is administered to patients presenting with depression, anxiety or obsessive-compulsive disorder, their neuropsychiatric symptoms appear to be relieved (Tariot et al., 2004; Sani et al., 2012). By contrast, a recent work demonstrated that chronic antagonism of NMDAR induces elevated anxiety in healthy mice (Hanson et al., 2014). Overall, the current data that are available regarding the association between the use of NMDAR antagonists and the presentation of anxiety-related behaviors refute a simple model of dose-effect and instead seem to be closely related to the regimen, type of drug, or route of administration (Silvestre et al., 1997; Riaza Bermudo-Soriano et al., 2012; Schwartz et al., 2012). Additionally, it is prudent to consider that glutamatergic neurotransmission involves not only neuronal receptors (ionotropic and metabotropic) but also astroglial transporters that participate in neuron-astrocyte coupling.

Two major astroglial $Na^+$-dependent glutamate transporters, glutamate transporter 1 (GLT-1, also known as EAAT2) and glutamate aspartate transporter (GLAST, also known as EAAT1), take up glutamate from synapses to maintain the homeostasis that is necessary to orchestrate the physiological activity of receptors (Danbolt, 2001). Remarkably, cerebral GLT-1 and GLAST are predominately localized in astrocytes, with very low expression in other cell types (Zhou and Danbolt, 2014). Moreover, astrocytes account for 95% of the glutamate uptake activity in the brain (Danbolt et al., 1992; Lehre and Danbolt, 1998). Importantly, a recent work demonstrated that cerebral microinjection of the GLT-1 inhibitor, dihydrokainic acid (DHK), induced anhedonia and anxiety in rats (John et al., 2015). Thus, one could claim that astrocytic dysfunction may have a considerable impact on the expression of anxiety-like phenotypes (Bechtholt-Gompf et al., 2010; Schroeter et al., 2010; Lee et al., 2013). Based on the principles of neuron-astrocyte coupling, we hypothesized that long-term antagonism of NMDAR would impact astrocytic function and that this would likely affect anxiety phenotype.

In this study, we aimed to investigate the impact of long-term NMDAR antagonism by memantine on anxiety-related paradigms and their potential association with astrocytic glutamate transport.

## Materials and Methods

### Animals

Three-month-old CF-1 mice were housed in standard cages (48 cm × 26 cm). The animals were kept in a room with controlled temperature (22°C) under a 12 h light/12 h dark cycle (lights on at 7 am) and had free access to food and water. The mice ($n = 40$) were randomized into four groups: control (CO), memantine 5 mg (MN5), memantine 10 mg (MN10), and memantine 20 mg (MN20). To avoid social isolation, we maintained two animals per cage (Leasure and Decker, 2009). All behavioral tests were performed between 1:00 pm and 5:00 pm. All experiments were conducted in accordance with official governmental guidelines in compliance with the Federation of Brazilian Societies for Experimental Biology and were approved by the Ethical Committee of the Federal University of Rio Grande do Sul, Brazil.

### Drug Administration

Memantine (Sigma, USA) was dissolved in distilled water at three different concentrations (0.5, 1.0, and 2.0 mg/mL) to standardize the volume used for oral administration and reach the desired dose. For 24 days, the animals received daily administration of either 5, 10, or 20 mg/kg of memantine, or an equivalent volume of distilled water, via oral gavage. Body weight and food intake were monitored. All groups received oral gavage at 1 h after each behavioral task.

### Open Field Test

On the 22nd day, the animals were submitted to an open field task to evaluate spontaneous locomotion and exploratory activity. The apparatus was made of a black-painted box measuring 50 cm × 50 cm and was surrounded by 50 cm high walls. The experiments were conducted in a quiet room under low-intensity light (12 lx). Each mouse ($n = 10$ per group) was placed in the center of the arena, and the distance traveled (total and central zone), time spent in the central zone, and mean speed were measured over a course of 10 min (Muller et al., 2012). The experiment was recorded with a video camera that was positioned above the arena. The analysis was performed using a computer-operated tracking system (Any-maze, Stoelting, Woods Dale, IL, USA).

### Light–Dark Task

On the 23rd day, the light–dark task was performed as previously described (Crawley and Goodwin, 1980) with some modifications to analyze anxiety profiles. The light–dark apparatus consisted of a wood rectangular box with two separated chambers. One chamber had black walls and floor (50 cm × 50 cm × 50 cm) and was not illuminated. The other side had white walls and floor (50 cm × 50 cm × 50 cm) and was illuminated by a 100 W white lamp that was placed overhead. The two compartments were separated by a wall, which had a small opening at floor level. For each experiment, an animal ($n = 10$ per group) was initially placed in the white chamber and then allowed to explore the two-chamber area for a duration of 5 min. The following parameters were recorded by a trained and blinded-to-treatment observer: number of transitions between the two chambers, time spent in the light chamber, and risk assessment behavior. After each experiment, the apparatus was cleaned with 70% alcohol and dried before being used with the next animal.

### Elevated Plus-Maze Task

On the 24th day, the animals were submitted to an elevated plus-maze task to evaluate further signs of anxiety-like behavior. The elevated plus-maze was performed as previously described (Pellow, 1986). The elevated plus-maze apparatus consisted of two open arms (30 cm × 5 cm) and two enclosed arms (30 cm × 5 cm × 10 cm), which were separated by a central platform (5 cm × 5 cm) with the two identical arms of each type being placed opposite to each other. The height of the maze was 70 cm, and the experiments were conducted under dim red light in a quiet room. Each mouse ($n = 10$ per group) was individually placed onto the central platform of the plus-maze, facing one of the open arms, and was observed/recorded for 5 min by a trained and blinded-to-treatment observer. The time spent in the open arms and the total distance traveled were used for further analysis. After each session, the maze was cleaned with 70% ethanol. Data analysis was performed using a computer-operated tracking system (Any-maze, Stoelting, Woods Dale, IL, USA).

### Glutamate Uptake Assay

On the 25th day, the animals ($n = 6$ per group) were sacrificed/dissected and left hippocampal and left frontoparietal cortical brain slices were taken for use in a glutamate uptake assay. The glutamate uptake assay was performed according to Thomazi et al. (2004). Brain hippocampal and frontoparietal cortical slices (0.4 mm) were obtained using a McIlwain tissue chopper and were pre-incubated for 15 min at 37°C in Hank's balanced salt solution (HBSS), containing 137 mM NaCl, 0.63 mM $Na_2HPO_4$, 4.17 mM $NaHCO_3$, 5.36 mM KCl, 0.44 mM $KH_2PO_4$, 1.26 mM $CaCl_2$, 0.41 mM $MgSO_4$, 0.49 mM $MgCl_2$, and 1.11 mM glucose, at pH 7.2. Afterward, 0.66 and 0.33 Ci $ml^{-1}$ L-[$^3$H]glutamate were added to a final 100 M concentration of glutamate for incubation with hippocampal and cortical samples, respectively. The incubations were stopped after 5 and 7 min for the hippocampal and cortical samples, respectively, with two ice-cold washes of 1 ml HBSS, which were immediately followed by the addition of 0.5 N NaOH. The samples were kept in this solution overnight. Nonspecific uptake was measured using the same protocol as described above, with differences in temperature (4°C) and medium composition (*N*-methyl-D-glucamine instead of sodium chloride). $Na^+$-dependent uptake was considered as the difference between the total uptake and the non-specific uptake. Note that astrocytic transport mediated by GLAST and GLT-1 is responsible for the $Na^+$-dependent glutamate uptake (Anderson and Swanson, 2000). Both uptakes were performed in triplicate. Any radioactivity that was incorporated into the slices was measured using a liquid scintillation counter.

### Western Blotting

For western blot analysis, right hippocampal and right frontoparietal cortical homogenates ($n = 6$, per group) were prepared in PIK buffer (1% NP-40, 150 mM NaCl, 20 mM Tris, pH 7.4, 10% glycerol, 1 mM $CaCl_2$, 1 mM $MgCl_2$, 400 µM sodium vanadate, 0.2 mM PMSF, 1 µg/ml leupeptin, 1 µg/ml aprotinin, and 0.1% phosphatase inhibitor cocktails I and II from Sigma–Aldrich) and centrifuged (Zimmer et al., 2012). Supernatants were collected and total protein was measured using Peterson's method (Peterson, 1977). Samples containing 20 µg of protein from the hippocampal homogenate were separated by electrophoresis on a polyacrylamide gel and electrotransferred to PVDF membranes. Protein bands within each sample lane were compared to standard molecular weight markers (Precision Plus Protein$^{TM}$ Dual Color Standards, Bio-Rad), which were used to identify the molecular weights of proteins of interest. Non-specific binding sites were blocked using Tween–Tris buffered saline (TTBS, 100 mM Tris–HCl, pH 7.5) with 5% albumin for 2 h. Samples were incubated overnight at 4°C with primary antibodies against GLT-1 (Abcam, 1:1000), GLAST (Abcam, 1:1000), and β-actin (Sigma, 1:5000). Following primary antibody incubation, the membranes were incubated with secondary antibodies (anti-rabbit, GE life sciences, 1:3000; anti-mouse, GE life sciences, 1:5000) for 2 h at room temperature. Films were scanned, and band intensity was analyzed using Image J software (Abramoff et al., 2004).

### Statistical Analysis

Differences between groups were analyzed with analysis of variance (ANOVA) followed by Tukey's *post hoc* test. Correlations between behavioral assessments and glutamate uptake were analyzed by Pearson's correlation coefficient. The results are presented as mean values ± SEM. Differences were considered significant at $p < 0.05$.

## Results

### Long-Term NMDAR Antagonism does not Alter Spontaneous Locomotion but Induces Anxiety-Like Behavior

Administration of memantine did not cause significant changes in either distance traveled [**Figure 1A**; $F_{(3,36)} = 1.642$, $p = 0.1967$] or time spent in the central zone [**Figure 1B**; $F_{(3,36)} = 0.1697$, $p = 0.9162$] in the open field. Occupancy plots are used to illustrate the similarities between groups in the open field test (**Figure 1C**).

### Long-Term NMDAR Antagonism Reduced Time Spent in the Light Compartment of the Light–Dark Box

In the light–dark box (**Figure 1G**), all of the doses of memantine that were tested significantly reduced the time spent in the light compartment by the memantine-administered mice compared to the CO group [**Figure 1D**; $F_{(3,36)} = 7.364$, MN5: $p = 0.03$, MN10: $p = 0.002$, MN20: $p = 0.01$]. However, transition numbers (light to dark) were unrelated to memantine administration [**Figure 1E**; $F_{(3,36)} = 0.8257$, $p = 0.4884$]. Additionally, there were no differences among groups in risk assessment index [**Figure 1F**; $F_{(3,36)} = 1.129$, $p = 0.3519$].

### Long-Term NMDAR Antagonism Decreased Time Spent in the Open Arms of the Elevated Plus-Maze

The administration of memantine reduced the time spent by mice in the open arms of the elevated plus-maze (**Figure 1J**) when compared to the CO group [**Figure 1H**; $F_{(3,36)} = 6.974$, MN5: $p = 0.007$, MN10: $p = 0.002$, MN20: $p = 0.004$]; however, there were no changes in total distance traveled [**Figure 1I**; $F_{(3,36)} = 2.227$, $p = 0.1018$].

### Long-Term NMDAR Antagonism Decreased Glutamate Uptake in the Frontoparietal Cortex and Hippocampus without Affecting the Immunocontents of GLAST and GLT-1

The administration of memantine significantly decreased glutamate uptake in slices of frontoparietal cortex [**Figure 2A**; $F_{(3,20)} = 11.458$, MN5: $p = 0.026$, MN10: $p < 0.001$, MN20: $p < 0.001$] and hippocampus [**Figure 2D**; $F_{(3,20)} = 15.008$, MN5: $p = 0.015$, MN10: $p < 0.001$, MN20: $p < 0.001$]. However, memantine did not alter the immunocontent of GLAST in either the frontoparietal cortex [**Figure 2B**; $F_{(3,20)} = 1.300$, $p = 0.3020$] or the hippocampus [**Figure 2E**; $F_{(3,20)} = 0.6174$, $p = 0.6118$]. Additionally, no alterations were found in the immunocontent of GLT-1 in either the frontoparietal cortex [**Figure 2C**; $F_{(3,20)} = 2.225$, $p = 0.1167$] or the hippocampus [**Figure 2F**; $F_{(3,20)} = 0.1520$, $p = 0.9272$].

### Correlation Between Anxiety-Like Behavior and Glutamate Uptake

A positive correlation was found between time spent in the light compartment of the light dark-box and glutamate uptake in the frontoparietal cortex (**Figure 3A**; $p < 0.0001$, $R = 0.7289$) and hippocampus (**Figure 3C**; $p = 0.03$, $R = 0.4337$). Time spent in the open arms of the elevated plus-maze test was also correlated with glutamate uptake in the frontoparietal cortex (**Figure 3B**; $p = 0.03$, $R = 0.4313$) and hippocampus (**Figure 3D**; $p = 0.01$, $R = 0.4815$).

## Discussion

Our results demonstrated that long-term antagonism of NMDAR by memantine induces anxiety-like behavior in healthy CF-1 mice. Additionally, memantine decreased glutamate uptake activity in the frontoparietal cortex and in the hippocampus

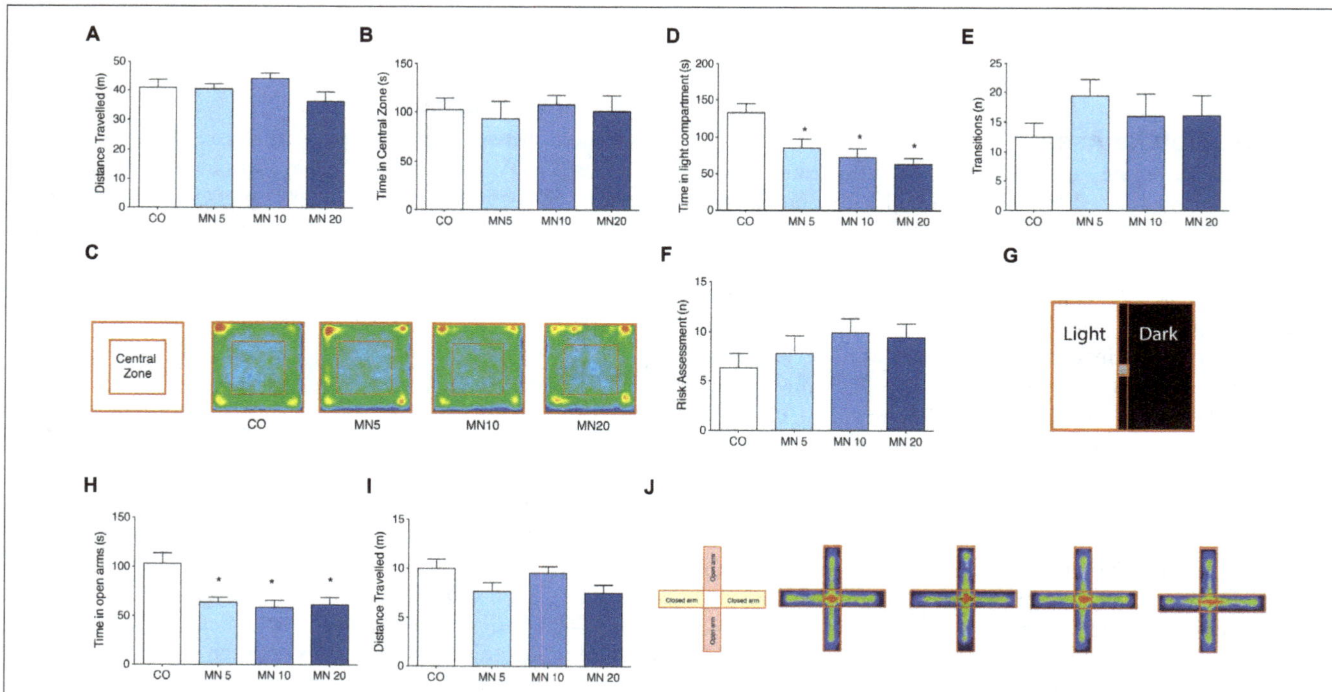


**FIGURE 1 | Long-term NMDAR antagonism does not alter spontaneous locomotor and exploratory behavior, but induces anxiety-like behavior. (A)** Total distance traveled in the open field. **(B)** Time in central zone in the open field. **(C)** Open field apparatus and occupancy plots. **(D)** Time in light compartment in the light–dark box. **(E)** Number of transitions in the light–dark box. **(F)** Risk assessment index in the light–dark box. **(G)** Light–dark box apparatus. **(H)** Time in open arms in the elevated plus-maze. **(I)** Distance traveled in the elevated plus-maze. **(J)** Elevated plus-maze apparatus and occupancy plots. Groups: control (CO), memantine 5 mg (MN 5), memantine 10 mg (MN 10), and memantine 20 mg (MN 20); $n = 10$ per group. Data are presented as mean values ± SEM.

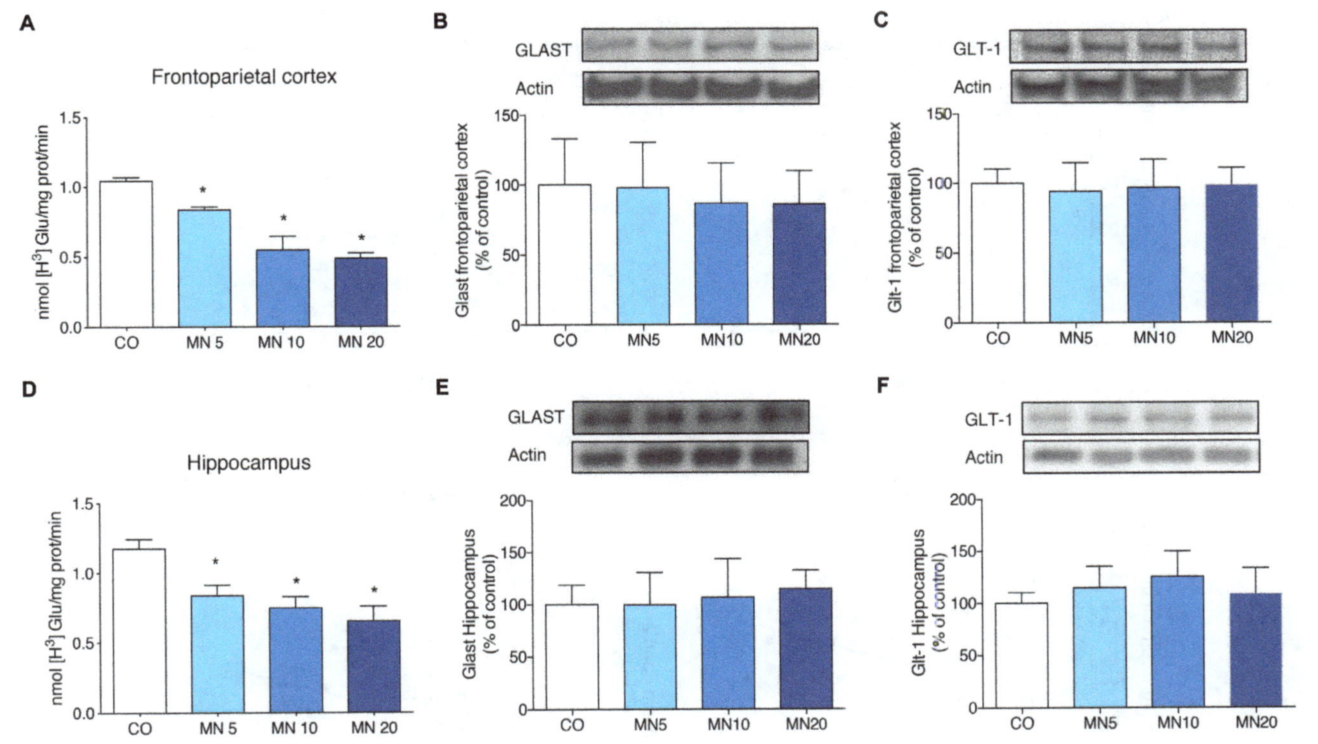


**FIGURE 2 | Long-term NMDAR antagonism decreases glutamate uptake in the frontoparietal cortex and hippocampus, but does not alter astroglial transporter immunocontent. (A)** Glutamate uptake in slices of frontoparietal cortex. **(B)** Immunocontent of GLAST in the frontoparietal cortex. **(C)** Immunocontent of GLT-1 in the frontoparietal cortex. **(D)** Glutamate uptake in slices of hippocampus. **(E)** Immunocontent of GLAST in the frontoparietal cortex. **(F)** Immunocontent of GLT-1T in the frontoparietal cortex. Groups: CO, memantine 5 mg (MN 5), memantine 10 mg (MN 10), and memantine 20 mg (MN 20); $n = 6$ per group. Data are presented as mean values ± SEM. $^*p < 0.05$ among groups.

with this phenomenon correlating with anxiety-like behavior. By contrast, the immunocontents of the astroglial glutamate transporters GLT-1 and GLAST were not affected.

Long-term administration of memantine did not induce significant changes in the spontaneous locomotion and exploratory activity of mice in the open field test. These findings imply that neither the dose nor the regimen of memantine that was used in our work led to non-specific effects such as sedation, which can potentially impair performance in anxiety-like tasks. This finding is in agreement with previous reports that have demonstrated that memantine administration does not alter locomotion or exploratory profiles (Reus et al., 2010). Conversely, we also showed that long-term memantine administration at doses of 5, 10, or 20 mg/kg leads to an anxiogenic phenotype that is manifested by decreased time spent in the light compartment (light–dark box) and reduced time spent in open arms (elevated plus-maze). Interestingly, a previous work showed that the administration of MK801, another non-competitive NMDAR antagonist, to rats induced an anxiety-like phenotype in the elevated plus-maze (Solati, 2011). In contrast to MK801, high doses of memantine (100 mg/kg) increased time spent in open arms, implying an anxiolytic effect. However, doses ranging from 10 to 30 mg/kg decreased time spent in open arms (~40%), without reaching statistical significance, which suggests a trend representative of an anxiogenic-like effect (Minkeviciene et al., 2008). Additionally, chronic antagonism of NMDAR with piperine18 exacerbated anxiogenic symptoms in C57BL/6 mice (Hanson et al., 2014). Indeed, it would appear that the antagonism of NMDAR does not follow a linear dose-response effect in terms of modulating anxiety-like behavior.

It has also been shown that memantine plays a role in controlling synaptic glutamate release. In fact, Lu et al. (2010) have shown that memantine suppresses glutamate release in cortical synaptosomes. In this study, however, we showed that long-term administration of memantine reduces glutamate uptake without affecting the glutamate transporters expression, GLT-1 and GLAST, in the frontoparietal cortex and hippocampus. Based on these findings, one could argue that memantine-induced reduction of glutamate uptake by astrocytes is a direct adaptive response to the reduced release of glutamate by neurons. This assumption reinforces a theoretical framework in which neurons and astrocytes are capable of sensing each other while regulating tripartite glutamatergic synapses (Wade et al., 2013; Karus et al., 2015). However, further studies using additional methodologies, such as immunostaining and electron microscopy, are necessary to better understand neuron-astrocyte coupling in the context of anxiety-like phenotypes.

Interestingly, a recent work demonstrated that blockade of GLT-1 in the central amygdala was also capable of inducing anxiety-like behavior, which reinforces the association between

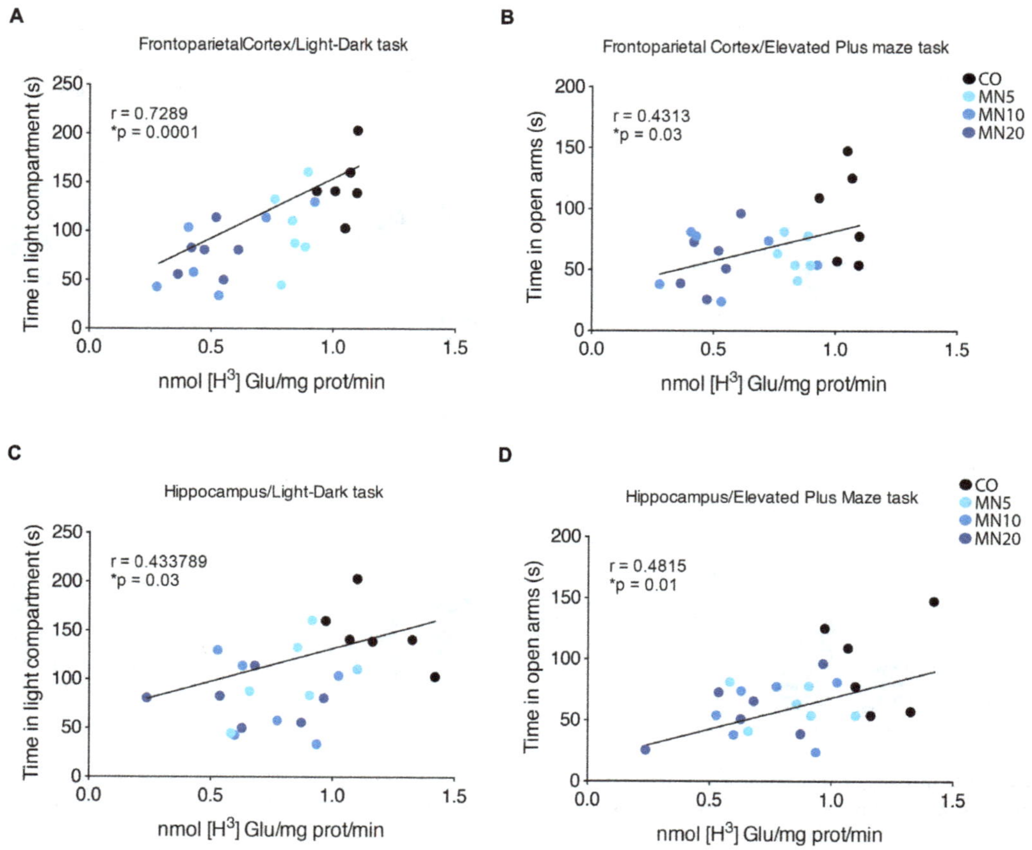


**FIGURE 3 | Anxiety-like behavior correlates with glutamate uptake.** **(A)** Linear correlation between time spent in light compartment during the light/dark task and glutamate uptake in slices of frontoparietal cortex. **(B)** Linear correlation between time spent in open arms and glutamate uptake in slices of frontoparietal cortex. **(C)** Linear correlation between time spent in light compartment during light/dark task and glutamate uptake in slices of hippocampus. **(D)** Linear correlation between time spent in open arms in elevated plus-maze test and glutamate uptake in slices of hippocampus. Groups: CO, memantine 5 mg (MN 5), memantine 10 mg (MN 10), and memantine 20 mg (MN 20); $n = 24$. Data presented by one animal per point. $^{*}p < 0.05$.

astrocytic glutamate uptake activity and the development of an anxiety phenotype (John et al., 2015). Remarkably, we were able to show through linear correlation that decreased glutamate uptake activity in the hippocampus and frontoparietal cortex was significantly correlated with an increased anxiety-like response.

## Conclusion

Long-term NMDAR antagonism by memantine induces an anxiety phenotype that is associated with reduced glutamate uptake activity in healthy CF-1 mice, which suggests that interactions between neurons and astrocytes can shape anxiety-related behavior.

## Author Contributions

EZ was responsible for the design, acquisition, analysis, interpretation, drafting, and approval of the final version of the manuscript. VT, EK, MA, KZ, RA, and GH were responsible for acquisition, analysis, interpretation, and approval of the final version of the manuscript. AM, DS, and RV were responsible for interpretation, drafting, critical revision, and approval of the final version of the manuscript. LV was responsible for the design, interpretation, drafting, critical revision, and approval of the final version of the manuscript.

## Acknowledgments

This work was supported by the following Brazilian agencies and grants: National Counsel of Technological and Scientific Development (CNPq), CAPES, FAPERGS, Brazilian Institute of Neuroscience (IBNnet), FINEP, and National Institute of Science and Technology (INCT) – Excitotoxicity and Neuroprotection.

## References


Abramoff, M. D., Magalhaes, P. J., and Ram, S. J. (2004). Processing with ImageJ. *Biophotonics Intern.* 11, 36–42.

Anderson, C. M., and Swanson, R. A. (2000). Astrocyte glutamate transport: review of properties, regulation, and physiological functions. *Glia* 32, 1–14. doi: 10.1002/1098-1136(200010)32:1<1::AID-GLIA10>3.0.CO;2-W

Bechtholt-Gompf, A. J., Walther, H. V., Adams, M. A., Carlezon, W. A. Jr., Ongur, D., and Cohen, B. M. (2010). Blockade of astrocytic glutamate uptake in rats induces signs of anhedonia and impaired spatial memory. *Neuropsychopharmacology* 35, 2049–2059. doi: 10.1038/npp.2010.74

Clement, Y., and Chapouthier, G. (1998). Biological bases of anxiety. *Neurosci. Biobehav. Rev.* 22, 623–633. doi: 10.1016/S0149-7634(97)00058-4

Cortese, B. M., and Phan, K. L. (2005). The role of glutamate in anxiety and related disorders. *CNS Spectr.* 10, 820–830.

Crawley, J., and Goodwin, F. K. (1980). Preliminary report of a simple animal behavior model for the anxiolytic effects of benzodiazepines. *Pharmacol. Biochem. Behav.* 13, 167–170. doi: 10.1016/0091-3057(80)90067-2

Danbolt, N. C. (2001). Glutamate uptake. *Prog. Neurobiol.* 65, 1–105. doi: 10.1016/S0301-0082(00)00067-8

Danbolt, N. C., Storm-Mathisen, J., and Kanner, B. I. (1992). An [$Na^+$ + $K^+$]coupled L-glutamate transporter purified from rat brain is located in glial cell processes. *Neuroscience* 51, 295–310. doi: 10.1016/0306-4522(92)90316-T

Gross, C., and Hen, R. (2004). The developmental origins of anxiety. *Nat. Rev. Neurosci.* 5, 545–552. doi: 10.1038/nrn1429

Hanson, J. E., Meilandt, W. J., Gogineni, A., Reynen, P., Herrington, J., Weimer, R. M., et al. (2014). Chronic GluN2B antagonism disrupts behavior in wild-type mice without protecting against synapse loss or memory impairment in Alzheimer's disease mouse models. *J. Neurosci.* 34, 8277–8288. doi: 10.1523/JNEUROSCI.5106-13.2014

John, C. S., Sypek, E. I., Carlezon, W. A., Cohen, B. M., Ongur, D., and Bechtholt, A. J. (2015). Blockade of the GLT-1 transporter in the central nucleus of the amygdala induces both anxiety and depressive-like symptoms. *Neuropsychopharmacology* 40, 1700–1708. doi: 10.1038/npp.2015.16

Karus, C., Mondragao, M. A., Ziemens, D., and Rose, C. R. (2015). Astrocytes restrict discharge duration and neuronal sodium loads during recurrent network activity. *Glia* 63, 936–957. doi: 10.1002/glia.22793

Leasure, J. L., and Decker, L. (2009). Social isolation prevents exercise-induced proliferation of hippocampal progenitor cells in female rats. *Hippocampus* 19, 907–912. doi: 10.1002/hipo.20563

Lee, Y., Son, H., Kim, G., Kim, S., Lee, D. H., Roh, G. S., et al. (2013). Glutamine deficiency in the prefrontal cortex increases depressive-like behaviours in male mice. *J. Psychiatry Neurosci.* 38, 183–191. doi: 10.1503/jpn.120024

Lehre, K. P., and Danbolt, N. C. (1998). The number of glutamate transporter subtype molecules at glutamatergic synapses: chemical and stereological quantification in young adult rat brain. *J. Neurosci.* 18, 8751–8757.

Lu, C. W., Lin, T. Y., and Wang, S. J. (2010). Memantine depresses glutamate release through inhibition of voltage-dependent $Ca^{2+}$ entry and protein kinase C in rat cerebral cortex nerve terminals: an NMDA receptor-independent mechanism. *Neurochem. Int.* 57, 168–176. doi: 10.1016/j.neuint.2010.05.010

Machado-Vieira, R., Ibrahim, L., Henter, I. D., and Zarate, C. A. Jr. (2012). Novel glutamatergic agents for major depressive disorder and bipolar disorder. *Pharmacol. Biochem. Behav.* 100, 678–687. doi: 10.1016/j.pbb.2011.09.010

Machado-Vieira, R., Manji, H. K., and Zarate, C. A. (2009). The role of the tripartite glutamatergic synapse in the pathophysiology and therapeutics of mood disorders. *Neuroscientist* 15, 525–539. doi: 10.1177/1073858409336093

Minkeviciene, R., Banerjee, P., and Tanila, H. (2008). Cognition-enhancing and anxiolytic effects of memantine. *Neuropharmacology* 54, 1079–1085. doi: 10.1016/j.neuropharm.2008.02.014

Muller, A. P., Zimmer, E. R., Kalinine, E., Haas, C. B., Oses, J. P., Martimbianco De Assis, A., et al. (2012). Physical exercise exacerbates memory deficits induced by intracerebroventricular STZ but improves insulin regulation of H2O2 production in mice synaptosomes. *J. Alzheimers Dis.* 30, 889–898. doi: 10.3233/JAD-2012-112066

Nemeroff, C. B. (2003). The role of GABA in the pathophysiology and treatment of anxiety disorders. *Psychopharmacol. Bull.* 37, 133–146.

Nutt, D. J., and Malizia, A. L. (2001). New insights into the role of the GABA(A)-benzodiazepine receptor in psychiatric disorder. *Br. J. Psychiatry* 179, 390–396. doi: 10.1192/bjp.179.5.390

Pellow, S. (1986). Anxiolytic and anxiogenic drug effects in a novel test of anxiety: are exploratory models of anxiety in rodents valid? *Methods Find Exp. Clin. Pharmacol.* 8, 557–565.

Peterson, G. L. (1977). A simplification of the protein assay method of Lowry et al. which is more generally applicable. *Anal. Biochem.* 83, 346–356. doi: 10.1016/0003-2697(77)90043-4

Pilc, A., Wierońska, J. M., and Skolnick, P. (2013). Glutamate-based antidepressants: preclinical psychopharmacology. *Biol. Psychiatry* 73, 1125–1132. doi: 10.1016/j.biopsych.2013.01.021

Reus, G. Z., Stringari, R. B., Kirsch, T. R., Fries, G. R., Kapczinski, F., Roesler, R., et al. (2010). Neurochemical and behavioural effects of acute and chronic memantine administration in rats: further support for NMDA as a new pharmacological target for the treatment of depression? *Brain Res. Bull.* 81, 585–589. doi: 10.1016/j.brainresbull.2009.11.013

Riaza Bermudo-Soriano, C., Perez-Rodriguez, M. M., Vaquero-Lorenzo, C., and Baca-Garcia, E. (2012). New perspectives in glutamate and anxiety. *Pharmacol. Biochem. Behav.* 100, 752–774. doi: 10.1016/j.pbb.2011.04.010

Sani, G., Serra, G., Kotzalidis, G. D., Romano, S., Tamorri, S. M., Manfredi, G., et al. (2012). The role of memantine in the treatment of psychiatric disorders other than the dementias: a review of current preclinical and clinical evidence. *CNS Drugs* 26, 663–690. doi: 10.2165/11634390-000000000-00000

Schroeter, M. L., Abdul-Khaliq, H., Sacher, J., Steiner, J., Blasig, I. E., and Mueller, K. (2010). Mood disorders are glial disorders: evidence from in vivo studies. *Cardiovasc. Psychiatry Neurol.* 2010:780645. doi: 10.1155/2010/780645

Schwartz, T. L., Siddiqui, U. A., and Raza, S. (2012). Memantine as an augmentation therapy for anxiety disorders. *Case Rep. Psychiatry* 2012:749796. doi: 10.1155/2012/749796

Silvestre, J. S., Nadal, R., Pallares, M., and Ferre, N. (1997). Acute effects of ketamine in the holeboard, the elevated-plus maze, and the social interaction test in Wistar rats. *Depress. Anxiety* 5, 29–33. doi: 10.1002/(SICI)1520-6394(1997)5:1<29::AID-DA5>3.0.CO;2-0

Solati, J. (2011). Dorsal hippocampal N-methyl-d-aspartate glutamatergic and delta-opioidergic systems modulate anxiety behaviors in rats in a noninteractive manner. *Kaohsiung J. Med. Sci.* 27, 485–493. doi: 10.1016/j.kjms.2011.06.011

Szabo, S. T., Machado-Vieira, R., Yuan, P., Wang, Y., Wei, Y., Falke, C., et al. (2009). Glutamate receptors as targets of protein kinase C in the pathophysiology and treatment of animal models of mania. *Neuropharmacology* 56, 47–55. doi: 10.1016/j.neuropharm.2008.08.015

Tariot, P. N., Farlow, M. R., Grossberg, G. T., Graham, S. M., Mcdonald, S., and Gergel, I. (2004). Memantine treatment in patients with moderate to severe Alzheimer disease already receiving donepezil: a randomized controlled trial. *JAMA* 291, 317–324. doi: 10.1001/jama.291.3.317

Thomazi, A. P., Godinho, G. F., Rodrigues, J. M., Schwalm, F. D., Frizzo, M. E., Moriguchi, E., et al. (2004). Ontogenetic profile of glutamate uptake in brain structures slices from rats: sensitivity to guanosine. *Mech. Ageing Dev.* 125, 475–481. doi: 10.1016/j.mad.2004.04.005

Wade, J., Mcdaid, L., Harkin, J., Crunelli, V., and Kelso, S. (2013). Biophysically based computational models of astrocyte ~ neuron coupling and their functional significance. *Front. Comput. Neurosci.* 7:44. doi: 10.3389/fncom.2013.00044

Zarate, C. Jr., Machado-Vieira, R., Henter, I., Ibrahim, L., Diazgranados, N., and Salvadore, G. (2010). Glutamatergic modulators: the future of treating mood disorders? *Harv. Rev. Psychiatry* 18, 293–303. doi: 10.3109/10673229.2010.511059

Zhou, Y., and Danbolt, N. C. (2014). Glutamate as a neurotransmitter in the healthy brain. *J. Neural. Transm.* 121, 799–817. doi: 10.1007/s00702-014-1180-8

# 11

# Possible Role of Glial Cells in the Relationship between Thyroid Dysfunction and Mental Disorders

*Mami Noda* *

*Laboratory of Pathophysiology, Graduate School of Pharmaceutical Sciences, Kyushu University, 3-1-1 Maidashi, Higashi-ku, Fukuoka, Japan*

***Correspondence:***
*Mami Noda,*
*Laboratory of Pathophysiology,*
*Graduate School of Pharmaceutical Sciences, Kyushu University,*
*3-1-1 Maidashi, Higashi-ku, Fukuoka 812-8582, Japan*
*noda@phar.kyushu-u.ac.jp*

It is widely accepted that there is a close relationship between the endocrine system and the central nervous system (CNS). Among hormones closely related to the nervous system, thyroid hormones (THs) are critical for the development and function of the CNS; not only for neuronal cells but also for glial development and differentiation. Any impairment of TH supply to the developing CNS causes severe and irreversible changes in the overall architecture and function of the human brain, leading to various neurological dysfunctions. In the adult brain, impairment of THs, such as hypothyroidism and hyperthyroidism, can cause psychiatric disorders such as schizophrenia, bipolar disorder, anxiety and depression. Although impact of hypothyroidism on synaptic transmission and plasticity is known, its effect on glial cells and related cellular mechanisms remain enigmatic. This mini-review article summarizes how THs are transported into the brain, metabolized in astrocytes and affect microglia and oligodendrocytes, demonstrating an example of glioendocrine system. Neuroglial effects may help to understand physiological and/or pathophysiological functions of THs in the CNS and how hypo- and hyper-thyroidism may cause mental disorders.

**Keywords: thyroid hormones, triiodothyronine, microglia, migration, phagocytosis**

## Introduction

Thyroid hormones (THs; Rothsschild et al., 2006) are critical for the development and function of the central nervous system (CNS; Zoeller and Rovet, 2004; Stenzel and Huttner, 2013). THs regulate development and differentiation of neurons and neuroglia (Gomes et al., 1999; Billon et al., 2001; Lima et al., 2001; Jones et al., 2003; Baxi et al., 2014; Dezonne et al., 2015). There are 2 major types of THs in the CNS represented by L-tri-iodothyronine (T3) and L-thyroxine (T4). The T4 is the major TH secreted by the follicular cells of thyroid gland; whereas T3, the most powerful TH, is mainly produced locally within the brain tissue by 5'-deiodination of T4. The T3 is an active form of the thyroid hormone (TH) essential for the development and function of the CNS.

Hyperthyroidism and hypothyroidism result from overactivation or suppression of thyroid grand leading to either excessive or insufficient production of THs. The prevalence of subclinical hyperthyroidism ranges from 1–15%, and of subclinical hypothyroidism from 3–16% in individuals aged 60 years and older was reported, which also suggested that there are differences in age, gender, and dietary iodine intake in the populations studied (Biondi and Cooper, 2008).

Any impairment of THs supply to the developing CNS causes severe and irreversible changes to the overall architecture and function of human brain, leading to various neurological dysfunctions (Di Liegro, 2008; Henrichs et al., 2010; Duntas and Maillis, 2013). Although in many respects the hypothyroid brain appears morphologically normal, clinical observations reported that hypothyroidism may be associated with both neurological and behavioral abnormalities as well as with functional impairments including mental retardation, ataxia and spasticity (Thompson and Potter, 2000). Psychiatric symptoms of hypothyroidism can include psychosis, mood instability, mania, hypersomnia, apathy, anergia, impaired memory mimicking dementia (Osterweil et al., 1992; Goh et al., 2014), psychomotor slowing, and attentional problems (Awad, 2000). The incidence of hypothyroidism increases with age, and adult-onset hypothyroidism is one of the most common causes of cognitive impairment (Mallett et al., 1995; Dugbartey, 1998).

On the other hand, hyperthyroidism may induce emotional lability, impatience and irritability, distractible overactivity, exaggerated sensitivity to noise, problems with sleep and the appetite (Awad, 2000) or depression and anxiety (Demet et al., 2002). Even at subclinical level, hyperthyroidism in the elderly is suggested to remarkably increase the risk of cognitive decline, dementia and Alzheimer's disease (AD; Kalmijn et al., 2000; van Osch et al., 2004; Wijsman et al., 2013).

Multiple studies have reported that both hypo- and hyperthyroidism may potentially increase the risk of cognitive impairment and neurodegeneration. It has been also reported that both hyper- and hypothyroidism can affect the immune system (Klecha et al., 2008; De Vito et al., 2012). Hyperthyroidism decreases the proinflammatory activities of monocytes and macrophages. On the other hand, during hypothyroidism enhancement of phagocytosis and increased levels of ROS may occur so that the expression of proinflammatory molecules such as macrophage inflammatory protein-1α and interleukin-1β increases (De Vito et al., 2011). In contrast, hypothyroidism is reported to produce opposite effects on the immune function, such as decrease in immune response, antibody production, cell migration, and lymphocyte proliferation markers (Klecha et al., 2000, 2006), antioxidant enzymes and their activity (De Vito et al., 2011). The role of microglia, an immune cell population in the CNS, in this relationship between thyroid dysfunctions and neuropsychological disorders remains to be elucidated. In addition, knowledge of how other glial cells are involved in neuropsychological disorders, especially in the TH-sensitive regions of the brain (Fonseca et al., 2013), needs to be considered.

## Transportation of THs to The Brain and Metabolism in Astrocytes

Circulating T4 is transported across the blood-brain barrier via specific transporters such as organic anion-transporting polypeptides (OATPs) containing OATP14/SLCO1C1 (OATP1c1) (Sugiyama et al., 2003; Tohyama et al., 2004) and OATP1a2 (Gao et al., 2000; Lee et al., 2005; Hagenbuch, 2007), L-type amino acid transporters (LAT1 and LAT2), mainly LAT1 (Taylor and Ritchie, 2007), and monocarboxylate transporters 8 (MCT8) (SLC16A2) (for both T3 and T4) (Roberts et al., 2008). T4 also enters into astroytes through OATP1c1 (Dezonne et al., 2015), where it is de-iodinated by type 2-deiodinase (D2) to produce T3 (Guadaño-Ferraz et al., 1997; Fliers et al., 2006; Di Liegro, 2008). Subsequently T3 is released by LAT (Francon et al., 1989; Blondeau et al., 1993), presumably LAT2, and taken by other cells via distinct transporters; For example neurons express MCT8 while microglia express OATP4a1, LAT2 and MCT10 (Braun et al., 2011; **Figure 1**).

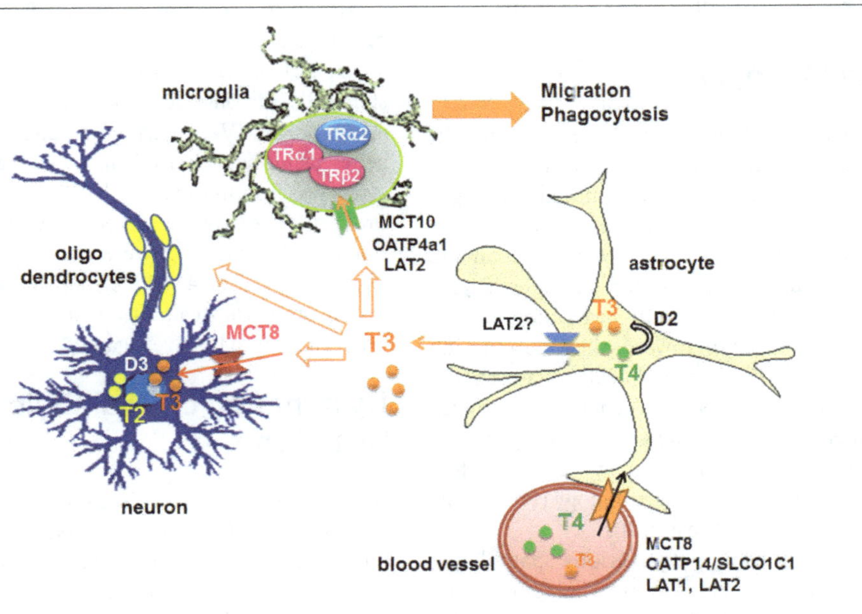


**FIGURE 1 | Transport of THs to the brains and their metabolism.** D: iodothyronine deiodinases, LAT: L-type amino acid transporter, MCT: monocarboxylate transporter, OATP: organic anion-transporting polypeptide, T2: diiodothyronines, T3: triiodothyronine, T4: thyroxine, TR: thyroid hormone receptor.

## Thyroid Hormone Receptors

The majority of TH effects are mediated through TH receptors (TRs), which belong to the members of the nuclear receptor superfamily and which function as T3-inducible transcription factors that are expressed in a tissue-specific and developmentally regulated manner (Cheng et al., 2010). In mammals, there are several TR isoforms: TRα1, TRα2, TRβ1, TRβ2a and TRβ3 (Koenig et al., 1989; Macchia et al., 2001). Among TRs, TRα1 is predominantly and widely expressed in the developing brain. The genomic actions of THs are exerted by the binding of T3 to nuclear TRs, which can either repress or activate gene expression.

Expression of TRα1 and TRβ1 have been identified in primary cultured rat microglia (Lima et al., 2001). Mutation of TRα1 in humans is associated with abnormal levels of TH but normal levels of thyrotropin as well as with growth retardation, and mildly delayed motor and cognitive development (van Mullem et al., 2012). A child with classic features of hypothyroidism with a *de novo* heterozygous nonsense mutation in a gene encoding TRα was also identified (Bochukova et al., 2012).

In addition to genomic effects of TRs, nongenomic signaling of THs through a plasma membrane–localized receptor has been recently described (Kalyanaraman et al., 2014; Mori et al., 2015). Potential mechanism for integrating regulation of development and metabolism by thyroid hormone and receptor tyrosine kinases through association of TRβ with PI3K was also suggested (Martin et al., 2014). These nongenomic effects of T3 may be important for glial function, which will be discussed later. In addition, it was suggested that the heterogeneity of TR expression throughout brain regions and between different cell types might lead to diverse effects on neuronal morphogenesis. The complexity may also result from not only the direct action of the hormone on neurons but also from indirect actions triggered by astrocytes (Dezonne et al., 2015) or other glial cell type.

## Effects of T3 on Microglia

Microglia, the resident macrophages of the CNS are generally considered the primary immune cells of the brain (Kim and de Vellis, 2005). In healthy CNS, ramified microglia are widely distributed to detect any environmental changes by their motile processes (Streit et al., 1988; Kettenmann et al., 2011). Pathological insults of multiple etiologies trigger microglial activation, represented by multi-stage and complex remodeling involving rapid migration towards the lesion site and phagocytosis of damaged cells (Becher et al., 2000; Hanisch and Kettenmann, 2007; Tanaka et al., 2009). It is generally recognized that the microglial phenotype may change depending on the microenvironment, which can be modified by various factors associated with specific types and stages of pathology (Perry et al., 1993; Scheffel et al., 2012; Solito and Sastre, 2012).

Microglial activation contribute to various pathologies (including, for example, Alzheimers disease) (El Khoury and Luster, 2008; Solito and Sastre, 2012). Recently, activated microglia have been indicated to cause also psychiatric disorders. Positron emission tomography imaging and postmortem studies have revealed microglial activation and abnormalities in schizophrenia, depression and autism (Kato et al., 2013; Mizoguchi et al., 2014; Monji et al., 2014).

T3 is important for microglial development (Lima et al., 2001), and could directly or indirectly stimulate morphological maturation of amoeboid microglial cells and limit their degeneration (Mallat et al., 2002). Recently, it has been demonstrated that T3 stimulates microglial migration and phagocytosis *in vitro and in vivo* (Mori et al., 2015). Microglial migration is mediated through T3 uptake by TH transporters and binding to the TRs. Then TH signaling in microglia involved several signaling pathways including $G_{i/o}$-protein, PI3K, and MAPK/ERK, as reported in ATP-induced microglial migration (Honda et al., 2001). T3-induced nitric oxide signaling (Kalyanaraman et al., 2014) is also present in microglia (Mori et al., 2015). In addition, $Na^+/K^+$-ATPase, $Na^+/Ca^{2+}$ exchanger operating in the reverse mode, and GABA receptors contribute to T3-induced microglial migration (**Figure 2**; Mori et al., 2015), although the precise mechanism is still unknown. Since dysfunction of T3 in the aged brain significantly affected microglial morphology (Mori, 2014), microglial dysfunction may be closely related to psychological impairment in hypo- or hyper-thyroidism in elderly patients which will be investigated in the future.

## Astrocytes and Oligodendrocytes Differentiation by T3

In developing CNS T3 exerts numerous effects regulating axonal myelination and dendritic growth (Walravens and Chase, 1969; Legrand, 1982; Porterfield and Hendrich, 1993; Bernal and Nunez, 1995; Vose et al., 2013) and astrocyte and oligodendrocyte differentiation (Martinez-Galan et al., 1997, 2004; Jones et al., 2003; Schoonover et al., 2004; Manzano et al., 2007; Dezonne et al., 2009; Baxi et al., 2014). Effects of TH on astrocytes have been recently reviewed (Dezonne et al., 2015). Also, differentiation of human cultured CD34+ stem cells into oligodendrocyte precursors under THs action was also reported (Venkatesh et al., 2014). Expression alterations of genes using hypothyroidism model rats showed that immature astrocytes immunoreactive for vimentin and glial fibrillary acidic protein (GFAP) were increased, while oligodendrocyte lineage transcription factor 2 were decreased in the corpus callosum (Shiraki et al., 2014). Effects and molecular mechanisms of T3 action on astrocytes and oligodendrocytes in matured or aged brain remain to be investigated.

## Dysfunction of Glial Cells and Psychiatric Symptoms

As mentioned above, THs are not only important for neuronal development (Rami et al., 1986; Gould and Butcher, 1989) but it also support development of microglia (Lima et al., 2001), astrocytes (Gould et al., 1990; Manzano et al., 2007) including radial glial cells (Martinez-Galan et al., 2004), and oligodendrocytes (Walravens and Chase, 1969; Jones et al., 2003). Hypothyroid animals and TR mutant mice exhibit severe deficits in glial development (Morte et al., 2004). Therefore, indirect

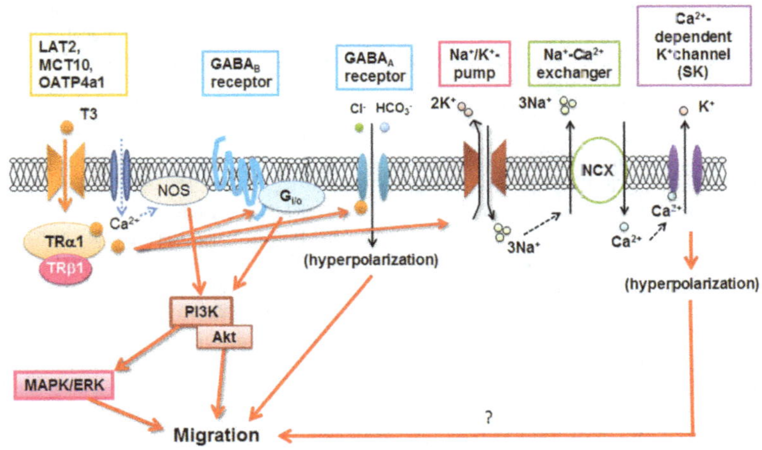


**FIGURE 2 | T3-induced signal transduction in microglia.** NOS: Nitric oxide synthase, NCX: $Na^+/Ca^{2+}$ exchanger. (Modified from Mori et al., 2015).

action of THs that occurs through astrocytes at different stages of brain development may contribute to neuronal progenitor proliferation, neuronal migration and differentiation, axonal growth and synapse function (Lima et al., 1998; Gomes et al., 1999; Martinez and Gomes, 2002; Martinez et al., 2011; Dezonne et al., 2013). Therapeutic use of THs in psychiatric disorders, mainly in depression, came to the light thus contributing to better understanding the action of THs in the brain (Weissel, 1999). Perhaps the major role of thyroxine therapy on depression might be due to hypothalamus-pituitary-thyroid axis activity and serotonin function in depressive episodes (Gomes et al., 2001). Neuroglial cells, as well as neurons contribute to psychiatric symptoms. For example, activated microglia and astrocytes in immunologically induced fatigue (Ifuku et al., 2014), microglial oxidative reactions in schizophrenia (Kato et al., 2011; Monji et al., 2013), and alteration of astrocytes or oligodendrocyte function in bipolar disorder (Dong and Zhen, 2015) have been reported. On the other hand, decreased glial density in association with glial hypotrophy in bipolar disorder or major depression (Rajkowska et al., 2001; Bowley et al., 2002) was also reported. Considering these reports, it is likely that indirect actions of THs through glial cells are important for neuronal activity and their impairment may at least in part, induce psychiatric symptoms.

These psychiatric symptoms can be seen in both hyperthyroidism and hypothyroidism. When it comes to the metabolism and balance of TH levels, it must be noted that propylthiouracyl (PTU) is a thiouracil-derived drug that inhibits thyroid peroxidase and type 1 deiodinase (D1), which is used to treat hyperthyroidism by decreasing TH level by suppression of T4 and T3 production. However, unlike D1 which is expressed mainly in the liver, kidney and testis, the major deiodinase D2 in the brain is known to be insensitive to PTU. Both mRNA concentration and activity of D2 are increased in hypothyroidism (van Doorn et al., 1982, 1983) and decreased in hyperthyroidism (Leonard et al., 1981; van Doorn et al., 1984; Croteau et al., 1996; Burmeister et al., 1997). D2 was also reported to be up-regulated in reactive astrocytes following traumatic brain injury (Zou et al., 1998). Thus, D2 is believed to serve a protective role to preserve the concentration of intracerebral T3 during states of thyroid hormone deficiency. This may explain, in part, why both hypo- and hyperthyroidism cause similar neurological symptoms.

## Conclusion

T3 is important not only for neuronal development but also for differentiation of astrocytes and oligodendrocytes, and for microglial development. In addition, T3 is an important signaling factor that affects microglial functions via complex mechanisms. Therefore, dysfunction of THs may impair glial function and thus disturb of the brain, which may cause mental disorders.

## Acknowledgments

I thank Prof. David A. Brown (UCL, UK) and Prof. Alexej Verkhratsky (University of Manchester, UK) for critical reading of the manuscript.

## References

Awad, A. G. (2000). The thyroid and the mind and emotions/thyroid dysfunction and mental disorders. *Thyrobulletin* 7, 3.e1–3.e2.

Baxi, E. G., Schott, J. T., Fairchild, A. N., Kirby, L. A., Karani, R., Uapinyoying, P., et al. (2014). A selective thyroid hormone beta receptor agonist enhances human and rodent oligodendrocyte differentiation. *Glia* 62, 1513–1529. doi: 10.1002/glia.22697

Becher, B., Prat, A., and Antel, J. P. (2000). Brain-immune connection: immuno-regulatory properties of CNS-resident cells. *Glia* 29, 293–304. doi: 10.1002/(sici)1098-1136(20000215)29:4<293::aid-glia1>3.3.co;2-1

Bernal, J., and Nunez, J. (1995). Thyroid hormones and brain development. *Eur. J. Endocrinol.* 133, 390–398. doi: 10.1530/eje.0.1330390

Billon, N., Tokumoto, Y., Forrest, D., and Raff, M. (2001). Role of thyroid hormone receptors in timing oligodendrocyte differentiation. *Dev. Biol.* 235, 110–120. doi: 10.1006/dbio.2001.0293

Biondi, B., and Cooper, D. S. (2008). The clinical significance of subclinical thyroid dysfunction. *Endocr. Rev.* 29, 76–131. doi: 10.1210/er.2006-0043

Blondeau, J. P., Beslin, A., Chantoux, F., and Francon, J. (1993). Triiodothyronine is a high-affinity inhibitor of amino acid transport system L1 in cultured astrocytes. *J. Neurochem.* 60, 1407–1413. doi: 10.1111/j.1471-4159.1993.tb03302.x

Bochukova, E., Schoenmakers, N., Agostini, M., Schoenmakers, E., Rajanayagam, O., Keogh, J. M., et al. (2012). A mutation in the thyroid hormone receptor alpha gene. *N. Engl. J. Med.* 366, 243–249. doi: 10.1056/NEJMoa1110296

Bowley, M. P., Drevets, W. C., Ongür, D., and Price, J. L. (2002). Low glial numbers in the amygdala in major depressive disorder. *Biol. Psychiatry* 52, 404–412. doi: 10.1016/s0006-3223(02)01404-x

Braun, D., Kinne, A., Bräuer, A. U., Sapin, R., Klein, M. O., Köhrle, J., et al. (2011). Developmental and cell type-specific expression of thyroid hormone transporters in the mouse brain and in primary brain cells. *Glia* 59, 463–471. doi: 10.1002/glia.21116

Burmeister, L. A., Pachucki, J., and St Germain, D. L. (1997). Thyroid hormones inhibit type 2 iodothyronine deiodinase in the rat cerebral cortex by both pre- and posttranslational mechanisms. *Endocrinology* 138, 5231–5237. doi: 10.1210/en.138.12.5231

Cheng, S. Y., Leonard, J. L., and Davis, P. J. (2010). Molecular aspects of thyroid hormone actions. *Endocr. Rev.* 31, 139–170. doi: 10.1210/er.2009-0007

Croteau, W., Davey, J. C., Galton, V. A., and St Germain, D. L. (1996). Cloning of the mammalian type II iodothyronine deiodinase. A selenoprotein differentially expressed and regulated in human and rat brain and other tissues. *J. Clin. Invest.* 98, 405–417. doi: 10.1172/jci118806

Demet, M. M., Ozmen, B., Deveci, A., Boyvada, S., Adigüzel, H., and Aydemir, O. (2002). Depression and anxiety in hyperthyroidism. *Arch. Med. Res.* 33, 552–556. doi: 10.1016/s0188-4409(02)00410-1

De Vito, P., Balducci, V., Leone, S., Percario, Z., Mangino, G., Davis, P. J., et al. (2012). Nongenomic effects of thyroid hormones on the immune system cells: new targets, old players. *Steroids* 77, 988–995. doi: 10.1016/j.steroids.2012.02.018

De Vito, P., Incerpi, S., Pedersen, J. Z., Luly, P., Davis, F. B., and Davis, P. J. (2011). Thyroid hormones as modulators of immune activities at the cellular level. *Thyroid* 21, 879–890. doi: 10.1089/thy.2010.0429

Dezonne, R. S., Lima, F. R., Trentin, A. G., and Gomes, F. C. (2015). Thyroid hormone and astroglia: endocrine control of the neural environment. *J. Neuroendocrinol.* doi: 10.1111/jne.12283 [Epub ahead of print].

Dezonne, R. S., Stipursky, J., Araujo, A. P., Nones, J., Pavão, M. S., Porcionatto, M., et al. (2013). Thyroid hormone treated astrocytes induce maturation of cerebral cortical neurons through modulation of proteoglycan levels. *Front. Cell. Neurosci.* 7:125. doi: 10.3389/fncel.2013.00125

Dezonne, R. S., Stipursky, J., and Gomes, F. C. (2009). Effect of thyroid hormone depletion on cultured murine cerebral cortex astrocytes. *Neurosci. Lett.* 467, 58–62. doi: 10.1016/j.neulet.2009.10.001

Di Liegro, I. (2008). Thyroid hormones and the central nervous system of mammals (Review). *Mol. Med. Rep.* 1, 279–295. doi: 10.3892/mmr.1.3.279

Dong, X. H., and Zhen, X. C. (2015). Glial pathology in bipolar disorder: potential therapeutic implications. *CNS Neurosci. Ther.* 21, 393–397. doi: 10.1111/cns.12390

Dugbartey, A. T. (1998). Neurocognitive aspects of hypothyroidism. *Arch. Intern. Med.* 158, 1413–1418. doi: 10.1001/archinte.158.13.1413

Duntas, L. H., and Maillis, A. (2013). Hypothyroidism and depression: salient aspects of pathogenesis and management. *Minerva Endocrinol.* 38, 365–377. doi: 10.1155/2013/312378

El Khoury, J., and Luster, A. D. (2008). Mechanisms of microglia accumulation in Alzheimer's disease: therapeutic implications. *Trends Pharmacol. Sci.* 29, 626–632. doi: 10.1016/j.tips.2008.08.004

Fliers, E., Unmehopa, U. A., and Alkemade, A. (2006). Functional neuroanatomy of thyroid hormone feedback in the human hypothalamus and pituitary gland. *Mol. Cell. Endocrinol.* 251, 1–8. doi: 10.1016/j.mce.2006.03.042

Fonseca, T. L., Correa-Medina, M., Campos, M. P. O., Wittmann, G., Werneck-de-Castro, J. P., Arrojo e Drigo, R., et al. (2013). Coordination of hypothalamic and pituitary T3 production regulates TSH expression. *J. Clin. Invest.* 123, 1492–1500. doi: 10.1172/JCI61231

Francon, J., Chantoux, F., and Blondeau, J. P. (1989). Carrier-mediated transport of thyroid hormones into rat glial cells in primary culture. *J. Neurochem.* 53, 1456–1463. doi: 10.1111/j.1471-4159.1989.tb08538.x

Gao, B., Hagenbuch, B., Kullak-Ublick, G. A., Benke, D., Aguzzi, A., and Meier, P. J. (2000). Organic anion-transporting polypeptides mediate transport of opioid peptides across blood-brain barrier. *J. Pharmacol. Exp. Ther.* 294, 73–79.

Goh, K. K., Chiu, Y. H., and Shen, W. W. (2014). Hashimoto's encephalopathy mimicking presenile dementia. *Gen. Hosp. Psychiatry* 36, 360.e9–360.e11. doi: 10.1016/j.genhosppsych.2014.01.006

Gomes, F. C., Lima, F. R., Trentin, A. G., and Moura Neto, V. (2001). Thyroid hormone role in nervous system morphogenesis. *Prog. Brain Res.* 132, 41–50. doi: 10.1016/s0079-6123(01)32064-2

Gomes, F. C., Maia, C. G., de Menezes, J. R., and Neto, V. M. (1999). Cerebellar astrocytes treated by thyroid hormone modulate neuronal proliferation. *Glia* 25, 247–255. doi: 10.1002/(sici)1098-1136(19990201)25:3<247::aid-glia5>3.3.co;2-u

Gould, E., and Butcher, L. L. (1989). Developing cholinergic basal forebrain neurons are sensitive to thyroid hormone. *J. Neurosci.* 9, 3347–3358.

Gould, E., Frankfurt, M., Westlind-Danielsson, A., and McEwen, B. S. (1990). Developing forebrain astrocytes are sensitive to thyroid hormone. *Glia* 3, 283–292. doi: 10.1002/glia.440030408

Guadaño-Ferraz, A., Obregón, M. J., StGermain, D. L., and Bernal, J. (1997). The type 2 iodothyronine deiodinase is expressed primarily in glial cells in the neonatal rat brain. *Proc. Natl. Acad. Sci. U S A* 94, 10391–10396. doi: 10.1073/pnas.94.19.10391

Hagenbuch, B. (2007). Cellular entry of thyroid hormones by organic anion transporting polypeptides. *Best Pract. Res. Clin. Endocrinol. Metab.* 21, 209–221. doi: 10.1016/j.beem.2007.03.004

Hanisch, U. K., and Kettenmann, H. (2007). Microglia: active sensor and versatile effector cells in the normal and pathologic brain. *Nat. Neurosci.* 10, 1387–1394. doi: 10.1038/nn1997

Henrichs, J., Bongers-Schokking, J. J., Schenk, J. J., Ghassabian, A., Schmidt, H. G., Visser, T. J., et al. (2010). Maternal thyroid function during early pregnancy and cognitive functioning in early childhood: the generation R study. *J. Clin. Endocrinol. Metab.* 95, 4227–4234. doi: 10.1210/jc.2010-0415

Honda, S., Sasaki, Y., Ohsawa, K., Imai, Y., Nakamura, Y., Inoue, K., et al. (2001). Extracellular ATP or ADP induce chemotaxis of cultured microglia through Gi/o-coupled P2Y receptors. *J. Neurosci.* 21, 1975–1982.

Ifuku, M., Hossain, S. M., Noda, M., and Katafuchi, T. (2014). Induction of interleukin-1beta by activated microglia is a prerequisite for immunologically induced fatigue. *Eur. J. Neurosci.* 40, 3253–3263. doi: 10.1111/ejn.12668

Jones, S. A., Jolson, D. M., Cuta, K. K., Mariash, C. N., and Anderson, G. W. (2003). Triiodothyronine is a survival factor for developing oligodendrocytes. *Mol. Cell. Endocrinol.* 199, 49–60. doi: 10.1016/s0303-7207(02)00296-4

Kalmijn, S., Mehta, K. M., Pols, H. A., Hofman, A., Drexhage, H. A., and Breteler, M. M. (2000). Subclinical hyperthyroidism and the risk of dementia. The Rotterdam study. *Clin. Endocrinol. (Oxf)* 53, 733–737. doi: 10.1046/j.1365-2265.2000.01146.x

Kalyanaraman, H., Schwappacher, R., Joshua, J., Zhuang, S., Scott, B. T., Klos, M., et al. (2014). Nongenomic thyroid hormone signaling occurs through a plasma membrane-localized receptor. *Sci. Signal.* 7:ra48. doi: 10.1126/scisignal.2004911

Kato, T. A., Monji, A., Yasukawa, K., Mizoguchi, Y., Horikawa, H., Seki, Y., et al. (2011). Aripiprazole inhibits superoxide generation from phorbol-myristate-acetate (PMA)-stimulated microglia in vitro: implication for antioxidative psychotropic actions via microglia. *Schizophr. Res.* 129, 172–182. doi: 10.1016/j.schres.2011.03.019

Kato, T. A., Yamauchi, Y., Horikawa, H., Monji, A., Mizoguchi, Y., Seki, Y., et al. (2013). Neurotransmitters, psychotropic drugs and microglia: clinical implications for psychiatry. *Curr. Med. Chem.* 20, 331–344. doi: 10.2174/0929867311320030003

Kettenmann, H., Hanisch, U. K., Noda, M., and Verkhratsky, A. (2011). Physiology of microglia. *Physiol. Rev.* 91, 461–553. doi: 10.1152/physrev.00011.2010

Kim, S. U., and de Vellis, J. (2005). Microglia in health and disease. *J. Neurosci. Res.* 81, 302–313. doi: 10.1002/jnr.20562

Klecha, A. J., Barreiro Arcos, M. L., Frick, L., Genaro, A. M., and Cremaschi, G. (2008). Immune-endocrine interactions in autoimmune thyroid diseases. *Neuroimmunomodulation* 15, 68–75. doi: 10.1159/000135626

Klecha, A. J., Genaro, A. M., Gorelik, G., Barreiro Arcos, M. L., Silberman, D. M., Schuman, M., et al. (2006). Integrative study of hypothalamus-pituitary-thyroid-immune system interaction: thyroid hormone-mediated modulation of lymphocyte activity through the protein kinase C signaling pathway. *J. Endocrinol.* 189, 45–55. doi: 10.1677/joe.1.06137

Klecha, A. J., Genaro, A. M., Lysionek, A. E., Caro, R. A., Coluccia, A. G., and Cremaschi, G. A. (2000). Experimental evidence pointing to the bidirectional interaction between the immune system and the thyroid axis. *Int. J. Immunopharmacol.* 22, 491–500. doi: 10.1016/s0192-0561(00)00012-6

Koenig, R. J., Lazar, M. A., Hodin, R. A., Brent, G. A., Larsen, P. R., Chin, W. W., et al. (1989). Inhibition of thyroid-hormone action by a non-hormone binding c-erbA protein generated by alternative mRNA Splicing. *Nature* 337, 659–661. doi: 10.1038/337659a0

Lee, W., Glaeser, H., Smith, L. H., Roberts, R. L., Moeckel, G. W., Gervasini, G., et al. (2005). Polymorphisms in human organic anion-transporting polypeptide 1A2 (OATP1A2): implications for altered drug disposition and central nervous system drug entry. *J. Biol. Chem.* 280, 9610–9617. doi: 10.1074/jbc.m411092200

Legrand, J. (1982). [Thyroid hormones and maturation of the nervous system]. *J. Physiol. (Paris)* 78, 603–652.

Leonard, J. L., Kaplan, M. M., Visser, T. J., Silva, J. E., and Larsen, P. R. (1981). Cerebral cortex responds rapidly to thyroid hormones. *Science* 214, 571–573. doi: 10.1126/science.7291997

Lima, F. R., Gervais, A., Colin, C., Izembart, M., Neto, V. M., and Mallat, M. (2001). Regulation of microglial development: a novel role for thyroid hormone. *J. Neurosci.* 21, 2028–2038.

Lima, F. R., Goncalves, N., Gomes, F. C., de Freitas, M. S., and Moura Neto, V. (1998). Thyroid hormone action on astroglial cells from distinct brain regions during development. *Int. J. Dev. Neurosci.* 16, 19–27. doi: 10.1016/s0736-5748(98)00002-1

Macchia, P. E., Takeuchi, Y., Kawai, T., Cua, K., Gauthier, K., Chassande, O., et al. (2001). Increased sensitivity to thyroid hormone in mice with complete deficiency of thyroid hormone receptor alpha. *Proc. Natl. Acad. Sci. U S A* 98, 349–354. doi: 10.1073/pnas.011306998

Mallat, M., Lima, F. R., Gervais, A., Colin, C., and Moura Neto, V. (2002). New insights into the role of thyroid hormone in the CNS: the microglial track. *Mol. Psychiatry* 7, 7–8. doi: 10.1038/sj/mp/4000988

Mallett, P., Andrew, M., Hunter, C., Smith, J., Richards, C., Othman, S., et al. (1995). Cognitive function, thyroid status and postpartum depression. *Acta Psychiatr. Scand.* 91, 243–246. doi: 10.1111/j.1600-0447.1995.tb09776.x

Manzano, J., Bernal, J., and Morte, B. (2007). Influence of thyroid hormones on maturation of rat cerebellar astrocytes. *Int. J. Dev. Neurosci.* 25, 171–179. doi: 10.1016/j.ijdevneu.2007.01.003

Martin, N. P., Marron Fernandez de Velasco, E., Mizuno, F., Scappini, E. L., Gloss, B., Erxleben, C., et al. (2014). A rapid cytoplasmic mechanism for PI3 kinase regulation by the nuclear thyroid hormone receptor, TRbeta and genetic evidence for its role in the maturation of mouse hippocampal synapses in vivo. *Endocrinology* 155, 3713–3724. doi: 10.1210/en.2013-2058

Martinez, R., Eller, C., Viana, N. B., and Gomes, F. C. (2011). Thyroid hormone induces cerebellar neuronal migration and Bergmann glia differentiation through epidermal growth factor/mitogen-activated protein kinase pathway. *Eur. J. Neurosci.* 33, 26–35. doi: 10.1111/j.1460-9568.2010.07490.x

Martinez, R., and Gomes, F. C. (2002). Neuritogenesis induced by thyroid hormone-treated astrocytes is mediated by epidermal growth factor/mitogen-activated protein kinase-phosphatidylinositol 3-kinase pathways and involves modulation of extracellular matrix proteins. *J. Biol. Chem.* 277, 49311–49318. doi: 10.1074/jbc.m209284200

Martinez-Galan, J. R., Escobar del Rey, F., Morreale de Escobar, G., Santacana, M., and Ruiz-Marcos, A. (2004). Hypothyroidism alters the development of radial glial cells in the term fetal and postnatal neocortex of the rat. *Brain Res. Dev. Brain Res.* 153, 109–114. doi: 10.1016/j.devbrainres.2004.08.002

Martinez-Galan, J. R., Pedraza, P., Santacana, M., Escobar del Ray, F., Morreale de Escobar, G., and Ruiz-Marcos, A. (1997). Early effects of iodine deficiency on radial glial cells of the hippocampus of the rat fetus. A model of neurological cretinism. *J. Clin. Invest.* 99, 2701–2709. doi: 10.1172/jci119459

Mizoguchi, Y., Kato, T. A., Horikawa, H., and Monji, A. (2014). Microglial intracellular Ca(2+) signaling as a target of antipsychotic actions for the treatment of schizophrenia. *Front. Cell. Neurosci.* 8:370. doi: 10.3389/fncel.2014.00370

Monji, A., Kato, T. A., Mizoguchi, Y., Horikawa, H., Seki, Y., Kasai, M., et al. (2013). Neuroinflammation in schizophrenia especially focused on the role of microglia. *Prog. Neuropsychopharmacol. Biol. Psychiatry* 42, 115–121. doi: 10.1016/j.pnpbp.2011.12.002

Monji, A., Mizoguchi, Y., and Kato, T. A. (2014). Microglial abnormalities in the pathophysiology of schizophrenia. *J. Neurol. Disord. Stroke* 2, 1059.e1–1059.e11.

Mori, Y. (2014). Association between thyroid hormones and brain function via regulation of microglial migration and phagocytosis. *PhD Thesis* (Kyushu University, Graduate School of Pharmaceutical Sciences), 1–60.

Mori, Y., Tomonaga, D., Kalashnikova, A., Furuya, F., Akimoto, N., Ifuku, M., et al. (2015). Effects of 3, 3', 5-triiodothyronine on microglial functions. *Glia* 63, 906–920. doi: 10.1002/glia.22792

Morte, B., Manzano, J., Scanlan, T. S., Vennstrom, B., and Bernal, J. (2004). Aberrant maturation of astrocytes in thyroid hormone receptor alpha 1 knockout mice reveals an interplay between thyroid hormone receptor isoforms. *Endocrinology* 145, 1386–1391. doi: 10.1210/en.2003-1123

Osterweil, D., Syndulko, K., Cohen, S. N., Pettler-Jennings, P. D., Hershman, J. M., Cummings, J. L., et al. (1992). Cognitive function in non-demented older adults with hypothyroidism. *J. Am. Geriatr. Soc.* 40, 325–335. doi: 10.1111/j.1532-5415.1992.tb02130.x

Perry, V. H., Matyszak, M. K., and Fearn, S. (1993). Altered antigen expression of microglia in the aged rodent CNS. *Glia* 7, 60–67. doi: 10.1002/glia.440070111

Porterfield, S. P., and Hendrich, C. E. (1993). The role of thyroid hormones in prenatal and neonatal neurological development—current perspectives. *Endocr. Rev.* 14, 94–106. doi: 10.1210/er.14.1.94

Rajkowska, G., Halaris, A., and Selemon, L. D. (2001). Reductions in neuronal and glial density characterize the dorsolateral prefrontal cortex in bipolar disorder. *Biol. Psychiatry* 49, 741–752. doi: 10.1016/s0006-3223(01)01080-0

Rami, A., Patel, A. J., and Rabié, A. (1986). Thyroid hormone and development of the rat hippocampus: morphological alterations in granule and pyramidal cells. *Neuroscience* 19, 1217–1226. doi: 10.1016/0306-4522(86)90135-1

Roberts, L. M., Woodford, K., Zhou, M., Black, D. S., Haggerty, J. E., Tate, E. H., et al. (2008). Expression of the thyroid hormone transporters monocarboxylate transporter-8 (SLC16A2) and organic ion transporter-14 (SLCO1C1) at the blood-brain barrier. *Endocrinology* 149, 6251–6261. doi: 10.1210/en.2008-0378

Rothsschild, B. L., Shim, A. H., Ammer, A. G., Kelley, L. C., Irby, K. B., Head, J. A., et al. (2006). Cortactin overexpression regulates actin-related protein 2/3 complex activity, motility and invasion in carcinomas with chromosome 11q13 amplification. *Cancer Res.* 66, 8017–8025. doi: 10.1158/0008-5472.can-05-4490

Scheffel, J., Regen, T., Van Rossum, D., Seifert, S., Ribes, S., Nau, R., et al. (2012). Toll-like receptor activation reveals developmental reorganization and unmasks responder subsets of microglia. *Glia* 60, 1930–1943. doi: 10.1002/glia.22409

Schoonover, C. M., Seibel, M. M., Jolson, D. M., Stack, M. J., Rahman, R. J., Jones, S. A., et al. (2004). Thyroid hormone regulates oligodendrocyte accumulation in developing rat brain white matter tracts. *Endocrinology* 145, 5013–5020. doi: 10.1210/en.2004-0065

Shiraki, A., Saito, F., Akane, H., Takeyoshi, M., Imatanaka, N., Itahashi, M., et al. (2014). Expression alterations of genes on both neuronal and glial development in rats after developmental exposure to 6-propyl-2-thiouracil. *Toxic. Lett.* 228, 225–234. doi: 10.1016/j.toxlet.2014.04.018

Solito, E., and Sastre, M. (2012). Microglia function in Alzheimer's disease. *Front. Pharmacol.* 3:14. doi: 10.3389/fphar.2012.00014

Stenzel, D., and Huttner, W. B. (2013). Role of maternal thyroid hormones in the developing neocortex and during human evolution. *Front. Neuroanat.* 7:19. doi: 10.3389/fnana.2013.00019

Streit, W. J., Graeber M. B., and Kreutzberg, G. W. (1988). Functional plasticity of microglia: a review. *Glia* 1, 301–307. doi: 10.1002/glia.440010502

Sugiyama, D., Kusuhara, H., Taniguchi, H., Ishikawa, S., Nozaki, Y., Aburatani, H., et al. (2003). Functional characterization of rat brain-specific organic anion transporter (Oatp14) at the blood-brain barrier: high affinity transporter for thyroxine. *J. Biol. Chem.* 278, 43489–43495. doi: 10.1074/jbc.m306933200

Tanaka, T., Ueno, M., and Yamashita, T. (2009). Engulfment of axon debris by microglia requires p38 MAPK activity. *J. Biol. Chem.* 284, 21626–21636. doi: 10.1074/jbc.m109.005603

Taylor, P. M., and Ritchie, J. W. (2007). Tissue uptake of thyroid hormone by amino acid transporters. *Best Pract. Res. Clin. Endocrinol. Metab.* 21, 237–251. doi: 10.1016/j.beem.2007.03.002

Thompson, C. C., and Potter, G. B. (2000). Thyroid hormone action in neural development. *Cereb. Cortex* 10, 939–945. doi: 10.1093/cercor/10.10.939

Tohyama, K., Kusuhara, H., and Sugiyama, Y. (2004). Involvement of multispecific organic anion transporter, Oatp14 (Slc21a14), in the transport of thyroxine across the blood-brain barrier. *Endocrinology* 145, 4384–4391. doi: 10.1210/en.2004-0058

van Doorn, J., Roelfsema, F., and van der Heide, D. (1982). Contribution fron local conversion of thyroxine to 3,5,3′-triiodothyronine to intracellular 3,5,3′-triiodothyronine in several organs in hypothyroid rats at isotope equilibrium. *Acta Endocrinol. (Copenh)* 101, 386–396. doi: 10.1530/acta.0.1010386

van Doorn, J., van der Heide, D., and Roelfsema, F. (1983). Sources and quantity of 3,5,3′-triiodothyronine in several tissues of the rat. *J. Clin. Invest.* 72, 1778–1792. doi: 10.1172/jci111138

van Doorn, J., van der Heide, D., and Roelfsema, F. (1984). The contribution of local thyroxine monodeiodination to intracellular 3,5, 3′-triiodothyronine in several tissues of hyperthyroid rats at isotopic equilibrium. *Endocrinology* 115, 174–182. doi: 10.1210/endo-115-1-174

van Mullem, A., van Heerebeek, R., Chrysis, D., Visser, E., Medici, M., Andrikoula, M., et al. (2012). Clinical phenotype and mutant TR alpha 1. *N. Engl. J. Med.* 366, 1451–1453. doi: 10.1056/NEJMc1113940

van Osch, L. A., Hogervorst, E., Combrinck, M., and Smith, A. D. (2004). Low thyroid-stimulating hormone as an independent risk factor for Alzheimer disease. *Neurology* 62, 1967–1971. doi: 10.1212/01.wnl.0000128134.84230.9f

Venkatesh, K., Srikanth, L., Vengamma, B., Chandrasekhar, C., Prasad, B. C., and Sarma, P. V. (2014). In vitro transdifferentiation of human cultured CD34+ stem cells into oligodendrocyte precursors using thyroid hormones. *Neurosci. Lett.* 588, 36–41. doi: 10.1016/j.neulet.2014.12.050

Vose, L. R., Vinukonda, G., Jo, S., Miry, O., Diamond, D., Korumilli, R., et al. (2013). Treatment with thyroxine restores myelination and clinical recovery after intraventricular hemorrhage. *J. Neurosci.* 33, 17232–17246. doi: 10.1523/jneurosci.2713-13.2013

Walravens, P., and Chase, H. P. (1969). Influence of thyroid on formation of myelin lipids. *J. Neurochem.* 16, 1477–1484. doi: 10.1111/j.1471-4159.1969.tb09900.x

Weissel, M. (1999). [Administration of thyroid hormones in therapy of psychiatric illnesses]. *Acta Med. Austriaca* 26, 129–131.

Wijsman, L. W., de Craen, A. J., Trompet, S., Gussekloo, J., Stott, D. J., Rodondi, N., et al. (2013). Subclinical thyroid dysfunction and cognitive decline in old age. *PLoS One* 8:e59199. doi: 10.1371/journal.pone.0059199

Zoeller, R. T., and Rovet, J. (2004). Timing of thyroid hormone action in the developing brain: clinical observations and experimental findings. *J. Neuroendocrinol.* 16, 809–818. doi: 10.1111/j.1365-2826.2004.01243.x

Zou, L., Burmeister, L. A., Styren, S. D., Kochanek, P. M., and DeKosky, S. T. (1998). Up-regulation of type 2 iodothyronine deiodinase mRNA in reactive astrocytes following traumatic brain injury in the rat. *J. Neurochem.* 71, 887–890. doi: 10.1046/j.1471-4159.1998.71020887.x

12

# Changes in Astroglial Markers in a Maternal Immune Activation Model of Schizophrenia in Wistar Rats are Dependent on Sex

*Daniela F. de Souza, Krista M. Wartchow, Paula S. Lunardi, Giovana Brolese, Lucas S. Tortorelli, Cristiane Batassini, Regina Biasibetti and Carlos-Alberto Gonçalves**

*Departamento de Bioquímica, Instituto de Ciências Básicas da Saúde, Universidade Federal do Rio Grande do Sul, Porto Alegre, Brazil*

***Correspondence:***
*Carlos-Alberto Gonçalves*
*casg@ufrgs.br*

Data from epidemiological studies suggest that prenatal exposure to bacterial and viral infection is an important environmental risk factor for schizophrenia. The maternal immune activation (MIA) animal model is used to study how an insult directed at the maternal host can have adverse effects on the fetus, leading to behavioral and neurochemical changes later in life. We evaluated whether the administration of LPS to rat dams during late pregnancy affects astroglial markers (S100B and GFAP) of the offspring in later life. The frontal cortex and hippocampus were compared in male and female offspring on postnatal days (PND) 30 and 60. The S100B protein exhibited an age-dependent pattern of expression, being increased in the frontal cortex and hippocampus of the MIA group at PND 60, while at PND 30, male rats presented increased S100B levels only in the frontal cortex. Considering that S100B secretion is reduced by elevation of glutamate levels, we may hypothesize that this early increment in frontal cortex tissue of males is associated with elevated extracellular levels of glutamate and glutamatergic hypofunction, an alteration commonly associated with SCZ pathology. Moreover, we also found augmented GFAP in the frontal cortex of the LPS group at PND 30, but not in the hippocampus. Taken together data indicate that astroglial changes induced by MIA are dependent on sex and brain region and that these changes could reflect astroglial dysfunction. Such alterations may contribute to our understanding of the abnormal neuronal connectivity and developmental aspects of SCZ and other psychiatric disorders.

**Keywords: animal model, astrogliosis, GFAP, lipopolysaccharide, schizophrenia, S100B**

## INTRODUCTION

Schizophrenia (SCZ) is a chronic and debilitating illness that affects about 1% of the world population, with the onset of the manifestation occurring typically in late adolescence or in early adulthood (Monji et al., 2013). The incidence of SCZ is significantly higher in men than in women (male: female ratio = 1.4) (Aleman et al., 2003; McGrath et al., 2008). Nevertheless, the etiology of SCZ remains unclear, although numerous findings indicate that neurodevelopmental factors contribute to its

---

**Abbreviations:** CNS, central nervous system; ELISA, enzyme-linked immunosorbent assay; GFAP, glial fibrillary acidic protein; GSH, glutathione; IL-6, interleukin-6; LPS, lipopolysaccharide; MIA, maternal immune activation; NeuN, neuronal nuclei; PND, postnatal day; ROS, reactive oxygen species.

pathophysiology (Murray et al., 1992; Knuesel et al., 2014). Among these factors are included prenatal exposure to infection agents such as viruses (Kneeland and Fatemi, 2012) and gram-negative bacteria (Babulas et al., 2006; Sørensen et al., 2009; Khandaker et al., 2012).

The MIA animal model is used to study how an insult directed at the maternal host can have adverse effects on the fetus, leading to behavioral and neurochemistry changes later in life, specifically within abnormal exploration and social behaviors, cytokine levels and gene regulation (Ashdown et al., 2006; Fatemi et al., 2008; Meyer et al., 2009). Interestingly, prenatal exposure to the viral mimetic polyinosinic-polycytidylic acid changed behavioral flexibility of offspring rats, in a sex-dependent manner (Zhang et al., 2012). Systemic administration of the bacterial endotoxin, LPS, is a widely used and accepted MIA model that emulates immune activation and subsequent release of immunoregulatory, cytotoxic and inflammatory cytokines secondary to gram-negative bacterial infections (Borrell et al., 2002). Furthermore, inflammatory signals have been described in the hippocampus and cerebral cortex in postmortem studies of SCZ patients and MIA models (Beumer et al., 2012).

Changes in glial cells seem to be closely related to the pathology of SCZ (Cotter et al., 2001; Bernstein et al., 2009; Beumer et al., 2012). Astrocytes, the most abundant glial cells, are involved, together with microglia, in brain immune activation, as well as antioxidant defenses and glutamatergic neurotransmission (Takuma et al., 2004; Liu et al., 2011). S100B, a protein mainly expressed and secreted by astrocytes in the CNS, has been proposed as a marker of brain damage (Marchi et al., 2004; Gonçalves et al., 2008; Koh and Lee, 2014) and several studies have suggested that S100B is altered in neurological and psychiatric disorders (Ashraf et al., 1999; Lara et al., 2001; Steiner et al., 2011). Corroborating the idea of the neuroinflammatory basis of SCZ, and the involvement of the S100B protein in its pathogenesis, we recently showed that cerebrospinal fluid (CSF) S100B is increased by intracerebroventricular or intraperitoneal LPS administration (Guerra et al., 2011). Furthermore we observed that S100B secretion stimulated by cytokines *in vitro* is prevented by antipsychotics (de Souza et al., 2013).

Brain inflammation involving astrogliosis (characterized by over expression of GFAP and/or astrocyte hypertrophy) has been observed in the offspring of models of MIA, in IL-6 or LPS-treated mothers (Samuelsson et al., 2006; Hao et al., 2010). However, the role of GFAP in SCZ is controversial; some studies have found no changes or decreased GFAP content in the cortex and cerebellum of schizophrenic patients (Falkai et al., 1999; Rajkowska et al., 2002). On the other hand, there is evidence that this protein might be significantly augmented in demented schizophrenic patients, when compared to non-demented patients (Arnold et al., 1996).

Additionally, studies suggest that the altered regulation of fundamental mechanisms of anti-oxidant defense, where astrocytes are key elements (Takuma et al., 2004), may contribute to the pathogenesis of SCZ and related disorders (Floyd, 1999; Chauhan and Chauhan, 2006; Boskovic et al., 2011). In fact, analyses of the molecular mechanisms underlying oxidative stress suggest that cognitive dysfunction may be associated with an imbalance in the generation and clearance of ROS (Bitanihirwe and Woo, 2011) and MIA models support the role of oxidative/nitrosative stress in SCZ (Venkatasubramanian and Debnath, 2013)

In this study, we evaluated whether the administration of LPS in rat dams during late pregnancy affects the main astroglial markers, S100B and GFAP, in the frontal cerebral cortex and hippocampus of the dams' offspring during later life. S100B levels were also investigated in CSF and serum. We compared the offspring at 30 and 60 days to evaluate the possible differences between juvenile and adult rats and also investigated the existence of differences between male and female offspring. We also investigated the oxidative/nitrosative stress parameters, NO and GSH contents, in this model.

## MATERIALS AND METHODS

### Animals

Female Wistar rats from our breeding colony (Department of Biochemistry, UFRGS, Porto Alegre, Brazil), weighing 216–263 g each, were used, and maintained under controlled light and environmental conditions (12 h light/12 h dark cycle at a constant temperature of 22 ± 1°C), with free access to commercial chow and water. The fertility cycle of the rats was controlled, and, when on proestrus, they were mated overnight. In the morning, vaginal secretion was collected for analysis. If spermatozoa were found in the morning, the day was designated as the first day of pregnancy. All animal experiments were carried out in accordance with the National Institute of Health Guide for the Care and Use of Laboratory Animals (NIH Publications No. 80-23) revised in 1996 and followed the regulations of the local animal housing authorities.

The study has been approved by the Comite de Etica no Uso de Animais (CEUA), UFRGS, number 18672.

### LPS Administration to Pregnant Rats

For gestational LPS treatment, timed pregnant Wistar rats were injected on days 18 and 19 of pregnancy, as follows: six pregnant rats were injected intraperitoneally with 500 μg/kg LPS (from *Escherichia coli*, serotype 055:B5, Sigma) and five were injected with a corresponding volume of sterile saline (control), once daily. Females were kept separate and with free access to their own litters. Rats from both groups (control and LPS) were born healthy and the numbers of offspring were normal. The offspring rats were weaned at 21 days old and were housed separately according to sex. The experiments were performed using male and female rats from each litter. Rats had free access to food and water. All the experiments were performed between 12:00 h and 17:00 h. In order to analyze the differences between young and adult rats, experiments were performed at PND 30 and PND 60 (Cai et al., 2000).

### Obtaining CSF, Serum and Hippocampal Samples

Animals were anesthetized with ketamine/xylazine (75 and 10 mg/kg, respectively, i.p.) and then positioned in a stereotaxic holder; CSF was obtained by cisterna magna puncture using an insulin syringe (27 gage × 1/2 inch length). The blood samples were collected by careful intracardiac puncture, using a 5-mL non-heparinized syringe to obtain 3 mL of blood. Blood samples were incubated at room temperature (25°C) for 5 min and centrifuged at 3200 rpm for 5 min to obtain serum. CSF and serum were frozen (−20°C) until further analysis, at most for 2 weeks. The animals were killed by decapitation, and the brains were removed and placed in cold saline medium with the following composition (in mM): 120 NaCl; 2 KCl; 1 CaCl2; 1 MgSO4; 25 HEPES; 1 KH2PO4 and 10 glucose, adjusted to pH 7.4. The hippocampi and frontal cortex were dissected and transverse slices of 0.3 mm were obtained using a McIlwain Tissue Chopper. Slices were then frozen at −20°C (for measurement of GFAP and S100B) or −80°C (for measurement GSH and NO), at most for 2 weeks.

## ELISA for S100B

The S100B concentration was determined in the hippocampal and cortical samples, in addition to serum and CSF from offspring at PND 30 and PND 60. S100B levels were determined by ELISA, as described previously (Leite et al., 2008). Briefly, 50 μL of sample plus 50 μL of Tris buffer were incubated for 2 h on a microtiter plate, previously coated with anti-S100B monoclonal antibody (SH-B1, from Sigma). Anti-S100 polyclonal antibody (from DAKO) was incubated for 30 min and then peroxidase-conjugated anti-rabbit antibody was added for a further 30 min. The color reaction with *o*-phenylenediamine was measured at 492 nm. The standard S100B curve ranged from 0.002 to 1 ng/mL.

## ELISA for GFAP

Enzyme-linked immunosorbent assay for GFAP was carried out by coating the microtiter plate with 100 μL samples containing 20 ng of protein for 24 h at 4°C. Incubation with a polyclonal anti-GFAP from rabbit (GE Healthcare) for 1 h was followed by incubation with a secondary antibody conjugated with peroxidase for 1 h, at room temperature. A colorimetric reaction with *o*-phenylenediamine was measured at 492 nm. The standard human GFAP (from Calbiochem) curve ranged from 0.1 to 5 ng/mL.

## Immunohistochemistry for GFAP and NeuN

Rats were anesthetized using ketamine/xylazine and were perfused through the left cardiac ventricle with 200 mL of saline solution, followed by 200 mL of 4% paraformaldehyde in 0.1 M phosphate buffer, pH 7.4. The brains were removed and left for post-fixation in the same fixative solution at 4°C for 24 h. Subsequently, the material was cryoprotected by immersing the brain in 30% sucrose in phosphate buffer at 4°C. The brains were sectioned (50 μm) on a cryostat (Leitz). The sections were then preincubated in 2% bovine serum albumin (BSA) in phosphate-buffered saline (PBS) containing 0.4% Triton X-100 for 30 min and incubated with polyclonal anti-GFAP from rabbit or -NeuN from mouse, diluted 1:500 in 0.4% BSA in PBS-Triton X-100, for 48 h at 40°C. After washing several times, tissue sections were incubated with a secondary antibody Alexa Fluor 488 (goat anti-rabbit-IgG; green fluorescence) and Alexa Fluor 568 (goat anti-mouse-IgG; red fluorescence) diluted 1:500 in PBS, at room temperature for 2 h. Afterward, the sections were mounted on slides with Fluor Save and covered with coverslips. Samples were quantified according to (Centenaro et al., 2011). Briefly, images were viewed with an Olympus microscope with a digital camera and then transferred to a computer. Then, the GFAP and NeuN immunoreactivity was evaluated by means of regional semi-quantitative optical densitometry, using Image J Software 1.42q (Wayne Rasband, National Institutes of Health, USA). Five images were analyzed in the stratum radiatum of the CA1 in the hippocampus from each animal (four fields were analyzed per section).

## Glutathione Content Assay

Glutathione levels (nmol/mg protein) were measured, as described previously (Anderson, 1985). Slices were homogenized and assayed in 10 volumes of 100 mM sodium phosphate buffer, pH 8.0, containing 5 mM EDTA and protein was precipitated with 1.7% meta-phosphoric acid. Supernatant was assayed with *o*-phthaldialdeyde (1 mg/mL methanol) at room temperature for 15 min. Fluorescence was measured using excitation and emission wavelengths of 350 and 420 nm, respectively. A calibration curve was performed with standard GSH solutions (0–500 μM).

## Nitric Oxide (NO) Production

Nitric Oxide metabolites, $NO^{3-}$ (nitrate) and $NO^{2-}$ (nitrite) were determined according to (Hu et al., 1996). Briefly, homogenates from one hippocampus were mixed with 25% trichloroacetic and centrifuged at 1,800 × *g* for 10 min. The supernatant was immediately neutralized with 2 M potassium bicarbonate. $NO^{3-}$ was reduced to $NO^{2-}$ by nitrate reductase. The total $NO^{2-}$ in the supernatant was measured by a colorimetric assay at 540 nm, based on the Griess reaction. A standard curve was performed using sodium nitrate (0–50 μM).

## Protein Determination

Protein content was measured by Lowry's method using BSA as standard (Peterson, 1977).

## Statistical Analysis

Parametric data are reported as means ± standard error and were analyzed by two-way ANOVA (followed by Bonferroni's test). Values of $p < 0.05$ were considered to be significant.

# RESULTS

## Prenatal LPS Treatment Increases S100B in the Frontal Cortex and Hippocampus of Offspring Rats

S100B content was measured in the frontal cortex and hippocampus of juvenile (PND 30) and adult (PND 60) rats born from mothers exposed to LPS during pregnancy. Prenatal LPS significantly changed only S100B levels in the frontal cortex of male juvenile rats ($p < 0.05$). However, a significant effect of sex on S100B levels in the frontal cortex [$F(1,44) = 13{,}18$; $p = 0.0007$] and in the hippocampus [$F(1,45) = 11{,}89$; $p = 0.001$] in juveniles rats was observed (**Figures 1A,B**).

In adult rats, a significant effect of prenatal LPS treatment on S100B immunocontent was observed in the frontal cortex [$F(1,25) = 9{,}77$; $p = 0.005$] and hippocampus [$F(1,24) = 4{,}58$; $p = 0.04$], but no effect of sex was observed [$F(1,25) = 3{,}23$; $p = 0.08$] and [$F(1,24) = 3{,}57$; $p = 0.07$] in these either of these regions (**Figures 1C,D**).

## Prenatal LPS Treatment Decreased S100B Levels in the CSF of Young Offspring Females

In juvenile rats, a significant interaction of (LPS treatment × sex) was observed for the CSF levels of S100B [$F(1,22) = 4{,}84$; $p = 0.003$]. *Post hoc* analysis revealed that S100B levels were significantly lower in the females of the LPS group ($p < 0.05$), when compared with the control group (**Figure 2A**). No significant alterations were observed in the serum of juvenile offspring (**Figure 2B**).

Prenatal LPS exposure did not significantly alter S100B levels in the CSF or serum of adult offspring, however, an effect of sex on the amount of S100B in the CSF was found [$F(1,23) = 5{,}96$; $p = 0.03$] (**Figures 2C,D**).

## GFAP Content is Altered in Offspring Born to LPS-Treated Dams

A significant effect of prenatal LPS treatment [$F(1,36) = 4{,}41$; $p = 0.04$] on GFAP immunocontent was observed in the frontal cortex of juvenile offspring rats, but no influence of sex was observed [$F(1,36) = 0{,}82$; $p = 0.8$] (**Figure 3A**). No effects of LPS treatment [$F(1,37) = 1{,}08$; $p = 0.30$] or sex [$F(1,37) = 0{,}68$; $p = 0.41$] were observed in the hippocampus of juvenile rats (**Figure 3B**).

No changes were found in the frontal cortex of adult rats (**Figure 3C**). However, significant effects of LPS treatment [$F(1,21) = 8{,}3$; $p = 0.008$] and sex [$F(1,21) = 5{,}94$; $p = 0.02$] were observed in the hippocampus of adult rats (**Figure 3D**).

## Immunohistochemistry for GFAP and NeuN in the CA1 Hippocampus of LPS-Offspring Rats

In order to confirm the alterations in GFAP in the hippocampus (measured by ELISA), we localized this protein in the CA1 region using immunohistochemistry and also stained for the NeuN protein in the neuronal population. Male and female rats born to LPS-exposed dams were analyzed on PND 30 and 60 (**Figure 4A**).

After quantification, significant effects of sex [$F(1,10) = 18{,}66$; $p = 0.002$] and LPS treatment [$F(1,10) = 30{,}62$; $p = 0.0002$] were observed on the GFAP immunocontent of the CA1 hippocampus in the offspring of PND 30 rats. There was also an interaction effect between treatment and sex [$F(1,10) = 10{,}51$;

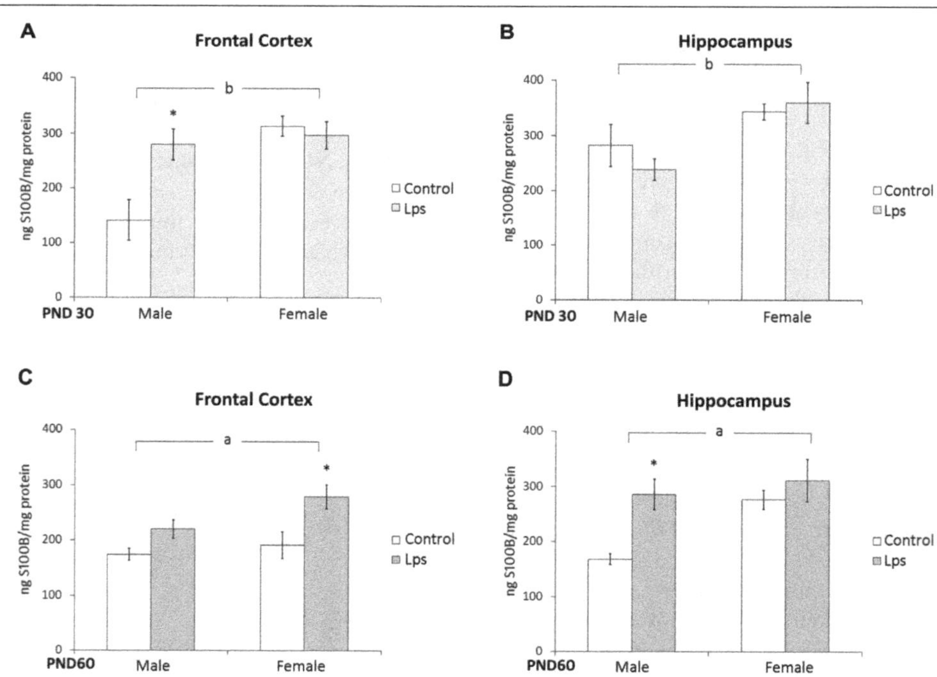


**FIGURE 1 | Prenatal LPS treatment increases S100B in the frontal cortex and hippocampus of offspring rats.** Cortical or hippocampal slices from PND 30 (**A,B**, respectively) and PND 60 Wistar rats prenatally exposed to LPS (**C,D**, respectively); S100B was measured by ELISA. Data are expressed as means ± standard error (LPS group, $N = 10$; control group, $N = 10$), the measurements were performed in triplicate. [a]Significant effect of prenatal treatment and [b]significant effect of sex (Two-way ANOVA $p < 0.05$). *Significantly different from respective control (Bonferroni's *post hoc*, $p < 0.05$).

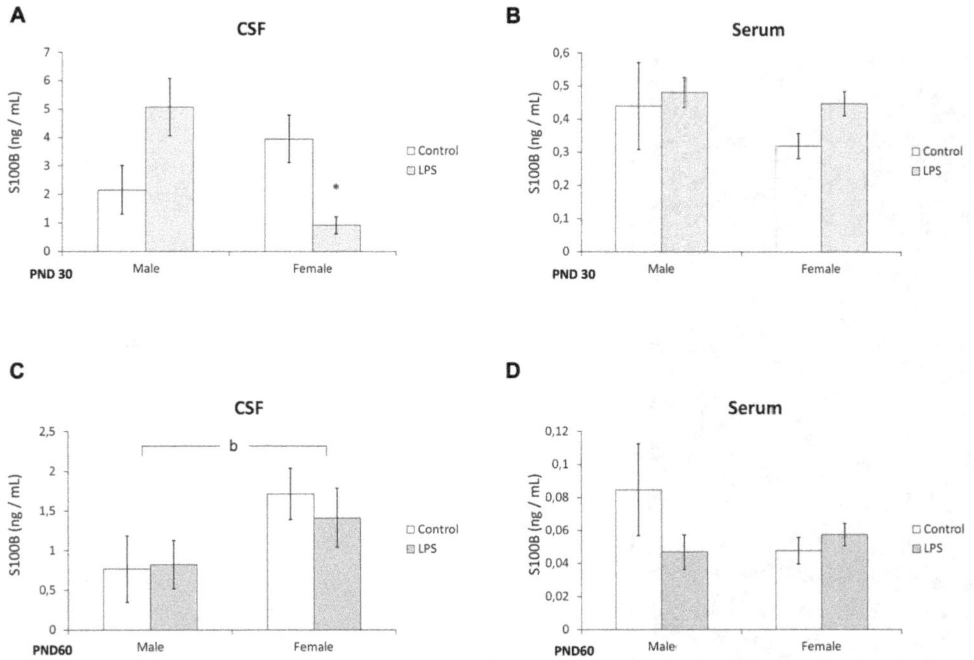


**FIGURE 2 | Prenatal LPS treatment decreases S100B levels in the CSF of juvenile offspring females.** CSF and serum from PND 30 (**A,B**, respectively) and PND 60 Wistar rats prenatally exposed to LPS (**C,D**, respectively); S100B was measured by ELISA. Data are expressed as means ± standard error (LPS group, $N = 10$; control group, $N = 10$), the measurements were performed in triplicate. [b]Significant effect of sex ($p < 0.05$) and significant interaction prenatal treatment × sex (Two-way ANOVA, $p < 0.05$). **(A)** *Significantly different from control (Two-way ANOVA followed by Bonferroni's *post hoc*, $p < 0.05$).

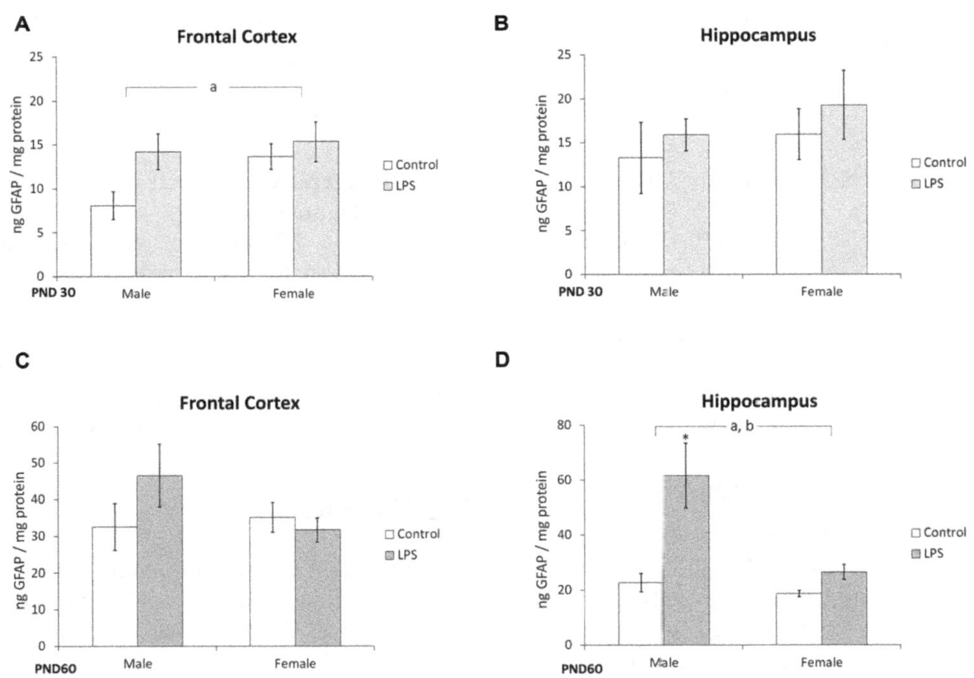


**FIGURE 3 | Glial fibrillary acidic protein content is altered in offspring born to LPS-treated dams.** Cortical or hippocampal slices from PND 30 (**A,B**, respectively) and PND 60 Wistar rats, prenatally exposed to LPS (**C,D**, respectively); GFAP was measured by ELISA. Data are expressed as means ± standard error (LPS group, $N = 10$; control group, $N = 10$); the measurements were performed in triplicate. [a]Significant effect of prenatal treatment and [b]significant effect of sex (Two-way ANOVA, $p < 0.05$). *Significantly different from control (Bonferroni's *post hoc*, $p < 0.05$).

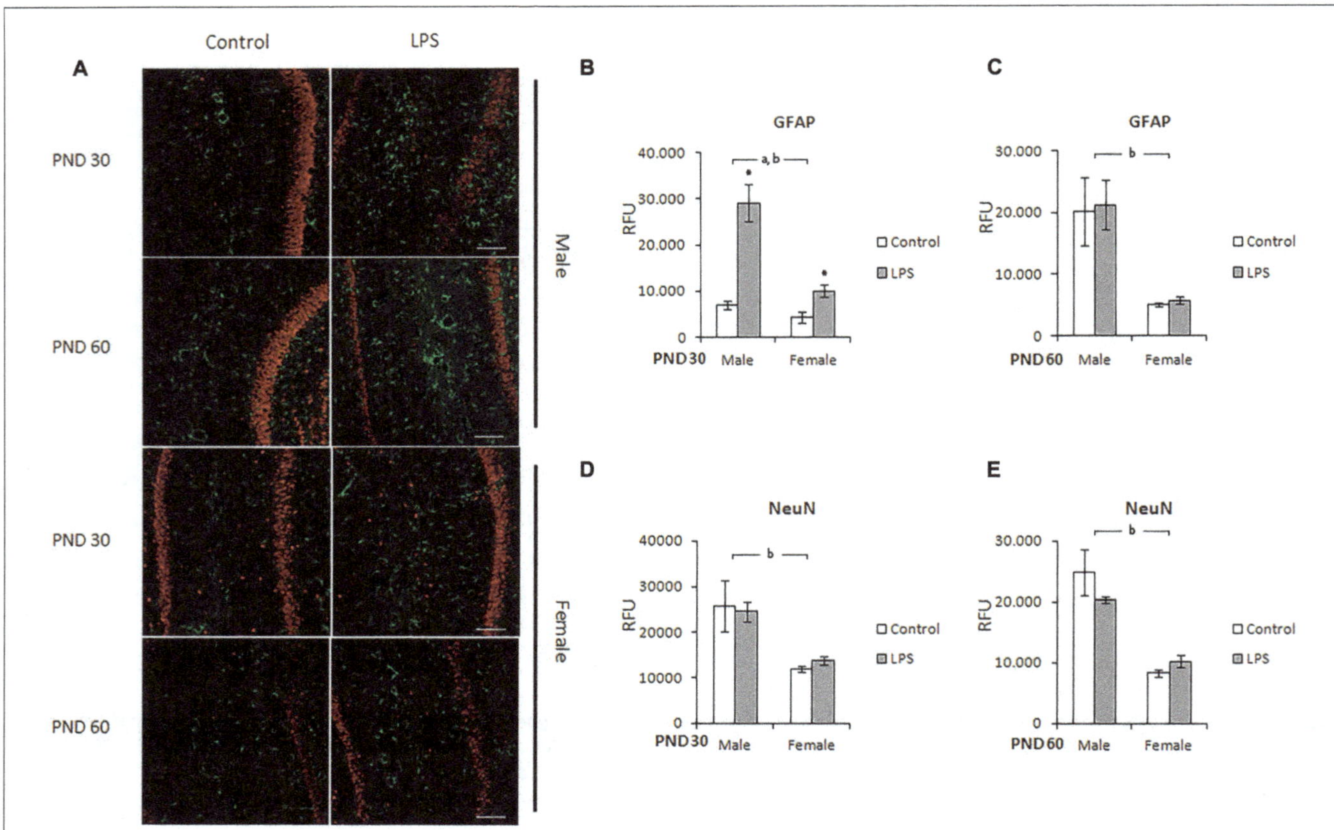


**FIGURE 4 | Immunohistochemistry for GFAP and NeuN in the CA1 hippocampus of LPS-offspring rats. (A)** Shows immunohistochemistry for GFAP (green) and NeuN (red) in hipocampal slices of 30- and 60-day old Wistar rats prenatally exposed to LPS (males and females). GFAP and NeuN were then quantified in the hippocampal slices of PND 30 (**B,D**, respectively) and PND 60 Wistar rats prenatally exposed to LPS (**C,E**, respectively). Data are expressed as means ± standard error (LPS group, $N = 5$; control group, $N = 5$); the experiments were performed in triplicate. [a]Significant effect of prenatal treatment; [b]significant effect of sex (Two-way ANOVA, $p < 0.05$). *Significantly different from control (Bonferroni's *post hoc*, $p < 0.05$). Scale bar = 10 mm.

$p = 0.008$] (**Figure 4B**). On PND 60, two-way ANOVA showed a significant effect of sex ($p = 0.0007$), but there was no effect of LPS treatment ($p = 0.23$ and 0.33, respectively) (**Figure 4C**).

Prenatal LPS did not significantly change NeuN levels in the hippocampus of juvenile or adult rats (**Figures 4D,E** respectively); however, two-way ANOVA demonstrated a significant effect of sex in both juvenile [$F(1,12) = 33{,}27$; $p < 0.0001$] and adult [$F(1,14) = 45{,}36$; $p < 0.0001$] rats.

## Offspring from LPS-Treated Dams Demonstrate Alterations in Oxidative/Nitrosative Stress

Glutathione content and NO production were used as parameters to evaluate possible oxidative stress caused by LPS prenatal exposure. Two-way ANOVA (treatment × sex) indicated no significant effect of LPS treatment or sex in the frontal cortex at PND 30 (**Figure 5A**). However, a significant effect of sex [$F(1,40) = 4{,}54$; $p = 0.03$] was seen in the hippocampus at PND 30 (**Figure 5B**).

A significant effect of LPS treatment on GSH content was observed in the frontal cortex at PND 60 [$F(1,21) = 4{,}79$; $p = 0.04$] (**Figure 5C**); no effects were found in the hippocampus at this age (**Figure 5D**).

The effect of LPS prenatal treatment on the content of NO was observed in the frontal cortex of offspring rats at PND 30 [$F(1,14) = 7{,}8$; $p < 0.014$] (**Figure 6A**). Furthermore, a significant effect of sex was observed in the hippocampus of juvenile [$F(1,12) = 33{,}27$; $p < 0.0001$] (**Figure 6B**) and adult rats [$F(1,20) = 4{,}64$; $p = 0.043$] (**Figure 6C**), where *post hoc* analysis indicated an increase in NO in adult females.

# DISCUSSION

Schizophrenia is believed to involve neurochemical, metabolic activities and connectivity impairment between several brain regions, such as the prefrontal cortex and hippocampus (Cui et al., 2009; Ledoux et al., 2014). Increasing evidence suggests that an imbalance of neurodegenerative and neuroprotective factors may play a key role in this brain disorder. Of the factors that may modulate the subtle balance between cell death and survival, a role for cytokines has been consistently reported in SCZ (Mansur et al., 2012). Previous studies indicate that astroglial dysfunction could be an important element in SCZ pathology, as indicated

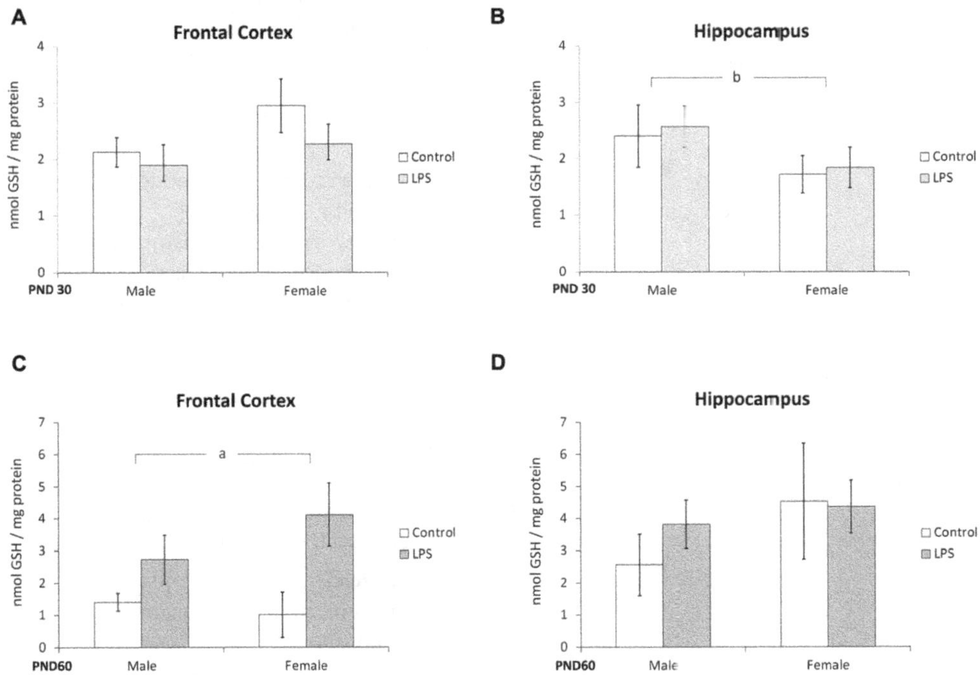


**FIGURE 5 | Glutathione content is dependent on sex and modulated by prenatal treatment with LPS.** Cortical or hippocampal slices from PND 30 (**A,B**, respectively) and PND 60 Wistar rats prenatally exposed to LPS (**C,D**, respectively). Data are expressed as means ± standard error (LPS group, $N = 10$; control group, $N = 10$), the experiments were performed in triplicate. Significant interaction prenatal treatment × sex **(A)**; [a]significant effect of prenatal treatment (Two-way ANOVA, $p < 0.05$). *Significantly different from control (Bonferroni's *post hoc*, $p < 0.05$).

by alterations in the markers GFAP and S100B (Fekkes et al., 2009).

S100B is a calcium-binding protein secreted by astrocytes into the synapse, where it is thought to participate in synaptic plasticity (Donato et al., 2009) and glutamatergic neurotransmission (Tramontina et al., 2006). The expression and secretion of this protein is modulated by cytokines, suggesting its involvement in the neuroinflammatory response (Schmitt et al., 2007; de Souza et al., 2009). In addition, we observed that cytokine-stimulated S100B secretion in astroglial cultures and hippocampal slices can be prevented by antipsychotics (de Souza et al., 2013). Herein, we showed that S100B has an age-dependent pattern of expression, and that it is increased in the frontal cortex and hippocampus of the LPS group at PND 60, when compared to control rats, while juvenile male rats present an increase in S100B levels only in the frontal cortex. It is important to mention that, at this age, behavioral alterations such as disruption of prepulse inhibition and deficient social interaction are associated with the SCZ model induced by MIA (Smith et al., 2007; de Souza, unpublished results).

As such, based on tissue S100B changes in the MIA model, we may suggest that a higher astroglial sensitivity/reactivity occurs in the frontal cortex of male offspring in response to prenatal LPS exposure. Accordingly, we found an increase in GFAP in the frontal cortex of the LPS group at PND 30, but not in the hippocampus. Considering that S100B secretion is reduced by elevation of glutamate levels in astrocyte cultures and brain slices (Goncalves et al., 2002; Büyükuysal, 2005; Nardin et al., 2009), we may speculate that this early increment in frontal cortex tissue of offspring males is associated with elevated extracellular levels of glutamate and glutamatergic hypofunction, commonly thought to be involved in SCZ pathology (Javitt, 2010). In support, an increment of glutamate levels has been reported in prefrontal cortex of male offspring in other MIA models induced by LPS (Connors et al., 2014) or polyinosinic:polycytidylic acid (Roenker et al., 2012). Furthermore, we found a decrease in CSF levels of S100B in females at PND 30 in the LPS group

These data are particularly interesting given the fact that the first signs of SCZ generally occur at the beginning of adulthood (Monji et al., 2009) and that an elevation of S100B has been observed in patients during the first onset of SCZ (Steiner et al., 2006). Elevations of serum S100B also have been described in SCZ patients (Wiesmann et al., 1999; Lara et al., 2001; Rothermundt et al., 2001), but no significant changes were observed in serum S100B levels at the ages analyzed in this MIA model. Furthermore, early CSF changes were not accompanied by serum changes. It is important to emphasize that changes in CSF S100B are not necessarily followed by changes in serum S100B (Gonçalves et al., 2008; Guerra et al., 2011), even though serum S100B, in SCZ, may be potentially modulated by peripheral S100B sources (Gonçalves et al., 2010; Steiner et al., 2010).

However, while increased S100B levels in patients with SCZ have been interpreted as a marker of structural damage or, alternatively, as a sign of astroglial dysfunction (Wiesmann et al., 1999; Rothermundt et al., 2001), the role of GFAP (a classical marker of astrogliosis) in psychiatric disease remains

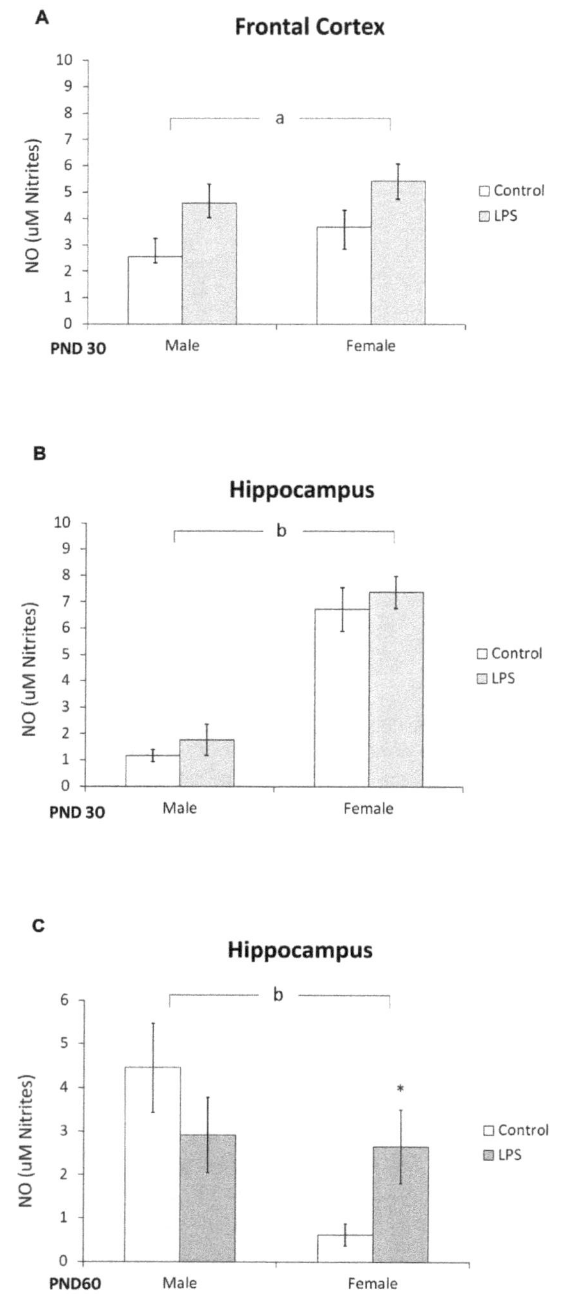


**FIGURE 6 | Nitric oxide content is dependent on sex.** Cortical **(A)** and hippocampal slices from PND 30 **(B)** and hippocampal slices from PND 60 Wistar rats prenatally exposed to LPS **(C)**. Data are expressed as means ± standard error (LPS group, $N = 10$; control group, $N = 10$); experiments were performed in triplicate. [b]Significant effect of sex (Two-way ANOVA, $p < 0.05$). *Significantly different from control (Bonferroni's *post hoc*, $p < 0.05$).

controversial (Samuelsson et al., 2006; Hao et al., 2010). We found a transitory increase of GFAP in the frontal cortex (but not in the hippocampus) at PND 30 in offspring that had been prenatally exposed to LPS, independent of sex. This hippocampal increment of GFAP was observed only at PND 60, and the effect was dependent on sex. Notably, when we looked specifically at hippocampus CA1 using immunohistochemical staining for GFAP, we found similar results at PND 60 when measuring GFAP by ELISA. Conversely, in this hippocampal region, we also observed astrogliosis at PND 30. Therefore, in spite of methodological differences, taken together these results indicate that astrogliosis in this LPS-induced MIA model is dependent on sex, time and brain region.

In parallel to immunohistochemical studies for GFAP in the CA1 hippocampus, we also stained for NeuN. We found an ontogenetic difference in this protein's levels in males and females; however, no changes were observed at PND 30 or 60 after prenatal LPS exposure. In fact, no significant changes in the number of neurons have been described in SZC patients (Heckers and Konradi, 2002) or in MIA models of SCZ (Wolff and Bilkey, 2015). It is probable that SCZ does not occur as a consequence of a reduction in neuron number, but due to alterations in the interconnectivity between them (Selemon et al., 1995). Our data reinforce the idea that alterations in astrocytes, glial cells intimately related to synaptic plasticity, could contribute to the abnormal connectivity of neurons.

In addition to glutamatergic communication, oxidative/nitrosative stress has been associated with SCZ pathology (Dadheech et al., 2008; Do et al., 2009; Venkatasubramanian and Debnath, 2013). Astrocytes are a heterogeneous group of cells involved in the production and recycling of GSH (the main antioxidant molecule in brain tissue) (Takuma et al., 2004), and also contribute to the production of NO, which can cause nitrosative stress under certain circumstances. However, nitrosative stress in the LPS-induced MIA model has not been well characterized. We observed an increase in NO in the hippocampus of female (not males) at PND 60 following prenatal exposure to LPS. Unfortunately, we were unable to measure NO metabolites in stored samples from frontal cortex at this age. Surprisingly we observed an increase in GSH in the LPS group, which was dependent on sex, in the frontal cortex, but not in the hippocampus at PND 60. The significance of these findings is unclear at moment, but the increase in GSH could indicate a compensatory mechanism to the oxidative stress that occurs in this model.

Some limitations of this study should be noted. Firstly, MIA is a risk factor, not a model, as we have mentioned throughout the text, for several developmental neuropsychiatric disorders, including SCZ, autism and bipolar disorder. Secondly, we have focused this study on astroglial cells; however, other glial cells such as oligodendrocytes and microglia should also be investigated as these also contribute to the behavioral phenotypes of MIA observed at PND 60 (DF de Souza, unpublished results). Finally, astrocytes, as mentioned, are a heterogeneous group of cells, and the differences in levels of S100B and GFAP observed in the different cerebral regions may reflect this characteristic. Furthermore, numerous other specific astroglial parameters such as glutamate transporters, glutamine synthesis and GSH synthesis should be investigated in future studies to amplify the understanding of astroglial activity in MIA and SCZ pathology for diagnosis and even therapeutic intervention.

In summary, our results show that prenatal LPS challenge leads to neurochemical abnormalities in astroglial markers during postnatal life and these findings reinforce the hypothesis that MIA may underlie SCZ pathology. The S100B protein exhibited an age-dependent pattern of expression, being increased in the frontal cortex and hippocampus of the MIA group at PND 60, while at PND 30, male rats presented an increase in S100B levels only in the frontal cortex. Considering that S100B secretion is reduced by elevation of glutamate levels, we may hypothesize that this early increment in frontal cortex tissue of males is associated with elevated extracellular levels of glutamate and glutamatergic hypofunction, an alteration commonly associated with SCZ pathology. Accordingly, we also found augmented GFAP expression in the frontal cortex of the LPS group at PND 30, but not in the hippocampus. Moreover, we found a decrease in CSF levels of S100B in females at PND 30 in the LPS group, but not later on at PND 60. Taken together, data indicate that astroglial changes induced by MIA are dependent on sex and brain region, and that such changes could reflect astroglial dysfunction. Such dysfunction could help us, in part, to understand the abnormal neuronal connectivity and developmental aspects of SCZ and other psychiatric disorders.

## AUTHOR CONTRIBUTIONS

DS and C-AG: Conception and experimental design, acquisition and analysis of data, and writing the manuscript. KW, PL, GB, LT, CB, RB: Experimental design, acquisition and analysis of data, and writing the manuscript.

## ACKNOWLEDGMENTS

This work was supported by the Conselho Nacional de Desenvolvimento Científico e Tecnológico (CNPq), Coordenação de Aperfeiçoamento de Pessoal de Nível Superior (CAPES), and INCT-National Institute of Science and Technology for Excitotoxicity and Neuroprotection.

## REFERENCES

Aleman, A., Kahn, R. S., and Selten, J.-P. (2003). Sex differences in the risk of schizophrenia: evidence from meta-analysis. *Arch. Gen. Psychiatry* 60, 565–571. doi: 10.1001/archpsyc.60.6.565

Anderson, M. (1985). Glutathione and glutathione disulfide in biological samples. *Methods Enzymol.* 113, 548–555. doi: 10.1016/S0076-6879(85)13073-9

Arnold, S. E., Franz, B. R., Trojanowski, J. Q., Moberg, P. J., and Gur, R. E. (1996). Glial fibrillary acidic protein-immunoreactive astrocytosis in elderly patients with schizophrenia and dementia. *Acta Neuropathol.* 91, 269–277. doi: 10.1007/s004010050425

Ashdown, H., Dumont, Y., Ng, M., Poole, S., Boksa, P., and Luheshi, G. N. (2006). The role of cytokines in mediating effects of prenatal infection on the fetus: implications for schizophrenia. *Mol. Psychiatry* 11, 47–55. doi: 10.1038/sj.mp.4001748

Ashraf, S., Bhattacharya, K., Tian, Y., and Watterson, K. (1999). Cytokine and S100B levels in paediatric patients undergoing corrective cardiac surgery with or without total circulatory arrest. *Eur. J. Cardiothorac. Surg.* 16, 32–37. doi: 10.1016/S1010-7940(99)00136-0

Babulas, V., Factor-Litvak, P., Goetz, R., Schaefer, C. A., and Brown, A. S. (2006). Prenatal exposure to maternal genital and reproductive infections and adult schizophrenia. *Am. J. Psychiatry* 163, 927–929. doi: 10.1176/appi.ajp.163.5.927

Bernstein, H.-G., Steiner, J., and Bogerts, B. (2009). Glial cells in schizophrenia: pathophysiological significance and possible consequences for therapy. *Expert Rev. Neurother.* 9, 1059–1071. doi: 10.1586/ern.09.59

Beumer, W., Gibney, S. M., Drexhage, R. C., Pont-Lezica, L., Doorduin, J., Klein, H. C., et al. (2012). The immune theory of psychiatric diseases: a key role for activated microglia and circulating monocytes. *J. Leukoc. Biol.* 92, 959–975. doi: 10.1189/jlb.0212100

Bitanihirwe, B. K. Y., and Woo, T. U. W. (2011). Oxidative stress in schizophrenia: an integrated approach. *Neurosci. Biobehav. Rev.* 35, 878–893. doi: 10.1016/j.neubiorev.2010.10.008

Borrell, J., Vela, J. M., Arévalo-Martin, A., Molina-Holgado, E., and Guaza, C. (2002). Prenatal immune challenge disrupts sensorimotor gating in adult rats: implications for the etiopathogenesis of schizophrenia. *Neuropsychopharmacology* 26, 204–215. doi: 10.1016/S0893-133X(01)00360-8

Boskovic, M., Vovk, T., Kores Plesnicar, B., and Grabnar, I. (2011). Oxidative stress in schizophrenia. *Curr. Neuropharmacol.* 9, 301–312. doi: 10.2174/157015911795596595

Büyükuysal, R. L. (2005). Protein S100B release from rat brain slices during and after ischemia: comparison with lactate dehydrogenase leakage. *Neurochem. Int.* 47, 580–588. doi: 10.1016/j.neuint.2005.06.009

Cai, Z., Pan, Z. L., Pang, Y., Evans, O. B., and Rhodes, P. G. (2000). Cytokine induction in fetal rat brains and brain injury in neonatal rats after maternal lipopolysaccharide administration. *Pediatr. Res.* 47, 64–72. doi: 10.1203/00006450-200001000-00013

Centenaro, L. A., Jaeger, M. D. C., Ilha, J., De Souza, M. A., Kalil-Gaspar, P. I., Cunha, N. B., et al. (2011). Olfactory and respiratory lamina propria transplantation after spinal cord transection in rats: effects on functional recovery and axonal regeneration. *Brain Res.* 1426, 54–72. doi: 10.1016/j.brainres.2011.09.054

Chauhan, V., and Chauhan, A. (2006). Oxidative stress in Alzheimer's disease. *Pathophysiology* 13, 195–208. doi: 10.1016/j.pathophys.2006.05.004

Connors, E. J., Shaik, A. N., Migliore, M. M., and Kentner, A. C. (2014). Environmental enrichment mitigates the sex-specific effects of gestational inflammation on social engagement and the hypothalamic pituitary adrenal axis-feedback system. *Brain Behav. Immun.* 42, 178–190. doi: 10.1016/j.bbi.2014.06.020

Cotter, D. R., Pariante, C. M., and Everall, I. P. (2001). Glial cell abnormalities in major psychiatric disorders: the evidence and implications. *Brain Res. Bull.* 55, 585–595. doi: 10.1016/S0361-9230(01)00527-5

Cui, K., Ashdown, H., Luheshi, G. N., and Boksa, P. (2009). Effects of prenatal immune activation on hippocampal neurogenesis in the rat. *Schizophr. Res.* 113, 288–297. doi: 10.1016/j.schres.2009.05.003

Dadheech, G., Mishra, S., Gautam, S., and Sharma, P. (2008). Evaluation of antioxidant deficit in schizophrenia. *Indian J. Psychiatry* 50, 16–20. doi: 10.4103/0019-5545.39753

de Souza, D. F., Leite, M. C., Quincozes-Santos, A., Nardin, P., Tortorelli, L. S., Rigo, M. M., et al. (2009). S100B secretion is stimulated by IL-1β in glial cultures and hippocampal slices of rats: likely involvement of MAPK pathway. *J. Neuroimmunol.* 206, 52–57. doi: 10.1016/j.jneuroim.2008.10.012

de Souza, D. F., Wartchow, K., Hansen, F., Lunardi, P., Guerra, M. C., Nardin, P., et al. (2013). Interleukin-6-induced S100B secretion is inhibited by haloperidol and risperidone. *Prog. Neuropsychopharmacol. Biol. Psychiatry* 43, 14–22. doi: 10.1016/j.pnpbp.2012.12.001

Do, K. Q., Cabungcal, J. H., Frank, A., Steullet, P., and Cuenod, M. (2009). Redox dysregulation, neurodevelopment, and schizophrenia. *Curr. Opin. Neurobiol.* 19, 220–230. doi: 10.1016/j.conb.2009.05.001

Donato, R., Sorci, G., Riuzzi, F., Arcuri, C., Bianchi, R., Brozzi, F., et al. (2009). S100B's double life: intracellular regulator and extracellular signal. *Biochim. Biophys. Acta* 1793, 1008–1022. doi: 10.1016/j.bbamcr.2008.11.009

Falkai, P., Honer, W. G., David, S., Bogerts, B., Majtenyi, C., and Bayer, T. A. (1999). No evidence for astrogliosis in brains of schizophrenic patients. A post-mortem study. *Neuropathol. Appl. Neurobiol.* 25, 48–53.

Fatemi, S. H., Reutiman, T. J., Folsom, T. D., Huang, H., Oishi, K., Mori, S., et al. (2008). Maternal infection leads to abnormal gene regulation and brain atrophy in mouse offspring: implications for genesis of neurodevelopmental disorders. *Schizophr. Res.* 99, 56–70. doi: 10.1016/j.schres.2007.11.018

Fekkes, D., Van Beveren, N. J. M., and Roder, C. H. R. (2009). Glial Fibrillary Acidic Protein (GFAP) and S100B protein serum levels in recent onset schizophrenia. *Eur. Neuropsychopharmacol.* 19, S505–S506. doi: 10.1016/S0924-977X(09)70799-0

Floyd, R. A. (1999). Antioxidants, oxidative stress, and degenerative neurological disorders. *Proc. Soc. Exp. Biol. Med.* 222, 236–245. doi: 10.1046/j.1525-1373.1999.d01-140.x

Gonçalves, C. A., Concli Leite, M., and Nardin, P. (2008). Biological and methodological features of the measurement of S100B, a putative marker of brain injury. *Clin. Biochem.* 41, 755–763. doi: 10.1016/j.clinbiochem.2008.04.003

Gonçalves, C. A., Leite, M. C., and Guerra, M. C. (2010). Adipocytes as an important source of serum S100B and possible roles of this protein in adipose tissue. *Cardiovasc. Psychiatry Neurol.* 2010, 790431. doi: 10.1155/2010/790431

Goncalves, D., Karl, J., Leite, M., Rotta, L., Salbego, C., Rocha, E., et al. (2002). High glutamate decreases S100B secretion stimulated by serum deprivation in astrocytes. *Neuroreport* 13, 1533–1535. doi: 10.1097/00001756-200208270-00009

Guerra, M., Tortorelli, L. S., Galland, F., Da Ré, C., Negri, E., Engelke, D. S., et al. (2011). Lipopolysaccharide modulates astrocytic S100B secretion: a study in cerebrospinal fluid and astrocyte cultures from rats. *J. Neuroinflammation* 8, 128. doi: 10.1186/1742-2094-8-128

Hao, L. Y., Hao, X. Q., Li, S. H., and Li, X. H. (2010). Prenatal exposure to lipopolysaccharide results in cognitive deficits in age-increasing offspring rats. *Neuroscience* 166, 763–770. doi: 10.1016/j.neuroscience.2010.01.006

Heckers, S., and Konradi, C. (2002). Hippocampal neurons in schizophrenia. *J. Neural Transm.* 109, 891–905. doi: 10.1007/s007020200073

Hu, J., Castets, F., Guevara, J. L., and Van Eldik, L. J. (1996). S100 beta stimulates inducible nitric oxide synthase activity and mRNA levels in rat cortical astrocytes. *J. Biol. Chem.* 271, 2543–2547. doi: 10.1074/jbc.271.5.2543

Javitt, D. C. (2010). Glutamatergic theories of schizophrenia. *Isr. J. Psychiatry Relat. Sci.* 47, 4–16.

Khandaker, G. M., Zimbron, J., Lewis, G., and Jones, P. B. (2012). Prenatal maternal infection, neurodevelopment and adult schizophrenia: a systematic review of population-based studies. *Psychol. Med.* 43, 1–19. doi: 10.1017/S0033291712000736

Kneeland, R. E., and Fatemi, S. H. (2012). Viral infection, inflammation and schizophrenia. *Prog. Neuropsychopharmacol. Biol. Psychiatry* 42, 35–48. doi: 10.1016/j.pnpbp.2012.02.001

Knuesel, I., Chicha, L., Britschgi, M., Schobel, S. A., Bodmer, M., Hellings, J. A., et al. (2014). Maternal immune activation and abnormal brain development across CNS disorders. *Nat. Rev. Neurol.* 10, 643–660. doi: 10.1038/nrneurol.2014.187

Koh, S. X. T., and Lee, J. K. W. (2014). S100B as a marker for brain damage and blood-brain barrier disruption following exercise. *Sports Med.* 44, 369–385. doi: 10.1007/s40279-013-0119-9

Lara, D. R., Gama, C. S., Belmonte-De-Abreu, P., Portela, L. V. C., Gonçalves, C. A., Fonseca, M., et al. (2001). Increased serum S100B protein in schizophrenia: a study in medication-free patients. *J. Psychiatr. Res.* 35, 11–14. doi: 10.1016/S0022-3956(01)00003-6

Ledoux, A.-A., Boyer, P., Phillips, J. L., Labelle, A., Smith, A., and Bohbot, V. D. (2014). Structural hippocampal anomalies in a schizophrenia population correlate with navigation performance on a wayfinding task. *Front. Behav. Neurosci.* 8:88. doi: 10.3389/fnbeh.2014.00088

Leite, M. C., Galland, F., Brolese, G., Guerra, M. C., Bortolotto, J. W., Freitas, R., et al. (2008). A simple, sensitive and widely applicable ELISA for S100B: methodological features of the measurement of this glial protein. *J. Neurosci. Methods* 169, 93–99. doi: 10.1016/j.jneumeth.2007.11.021

Liu, T., Sun, L., Xiong, Y., Shang, S., Guo, N., Teng, S., et al. (2011). Calcium triggers exocytosis from two types of organelles in a single astrocyte. *J. Neurosci.* 31, 10593–10601. doi: 10.1523/JNEUROSCI.6401-10.2011

Mansur, R. B., Zugman, A., Asevedo, E. D. M., Da Cunha, G. R., Bressan, R. A., and Brietzke, E. (2012). Cytokines in schizophrenia: possible role of anti-inflammatory medications in clinical and preclinical stages. *Psychiatry Clin. Neurosci.* 66, 247–260. doi: 10.1111/j.1440-1819.2012.02354.x

Marchi, N., Cavaglia, M., Fazio, V., Bhudia, S., Hallene, K., and Janigro, D. (2004). Peripheral markers of blood-brain barrier damage. *Clin. Chim. Acta* 342, 1–12. doi: 10.1016/j.cccn.2003.12.008

McGrath, J., Saha, S., Chant, D., and Welham, J. (2008). Schizophrenia: a concise overview of incidence, prevalence, and mortality. *Epidemiol. Rev.* 30, 67–76. doi: 10.1093/epirev/mxn001

Meyer, U., Feldon, J., and Yee, B. K. (2009). A review of the fetal brain cytokine imbalance hypothesis of schizophrenia. *Schizophr. Bull.* 35, 959–972. doi: 10.1093/schbul/sbn022

Monji, A., Kato, T., and Kanba, S. (2009). Activated microglia. *Psychiatr. Interpers Biol. Process.* 63, 257–265. doi: 10.1111/j.1440-1819.2009.01945.x

Monji, A., Kato, T. A., Mizoguchi, Y., Horikawa, H., Seki, Y., Kasai, M., et al. (2013). Neuroinflammation in schizophrenia especially focused on the role of microglia. *Prog. Neuropsychopharmacol. Biol. Psychiatry* 42, 115–121. doi: 10.1016/j.pnpbp.2011.12.002

Murray, R. M., O'Callaghan, E., Castle, D. J., and Lewis, S. W. (1992). A neurodevelopmental approach to the classification of schizophrenia. *Schizophr. Bull.* 18, 319–332. doi: 10.1093/schbul/18.2.319

Nardin, P., Tortorelli, L., Quincozes-Santos, A., De Almeida, L. M. V., Leite, M. C., Thomazi, A. P., et al. (2009). S100B secretion in acute brain slices: modulation by extracellular levels of Ca2+ and K+. *Neurochem. Res.* 34, 1603–1611. doi: 10.1007/s11064-009-9949-0

Peterson, G. L. (1977). A simplification of the protein assay method of Lowry et al. which is more generally applicable. *Anal. Biochem.* 83, 346–356. doi: 10.1016/0003-2697(77)90043-4

Rajkowska, G., Miguel-Hidalgo, J. J., Makkos, Z., Meltzer, H., Overholser, J., and Stockmeier, C. (2002). Layer-specific reductions in GFAP-reactive astroglia in the dorsolateral prefrontal cortex in schizophrenia. *Schizophr. Res.* 57, 127–138. doi: 10.1016/S0920-9964(02)00339-0

Roenker, N. L., Gudelsky, G. A., Ahlbrand, R., Horn, P. S., and Richtand, N. M. (2012). Evidence for involvement of nitric oxide and GABAB receptors in MK-801- Stimulated release of glutamate in rat prefrontal cortex. *Neuropharmacology* 63, 575–581. doi: 10.1016/j.neuropharm.2012.04.032

Rothermundt, M., Missler, U., Arolt, V., Peters, M., Leadbeater, J., Wiesmann, M., et al. (2001). Increased S100B blood levels in unmedicated and treated schizophrenic patients are correlated with negative symptomatology. *Mol. Psychiatry* 6, 445–449. doi: 10.1038/sj.mp.4000889

Samuelsson, A.-M., Jennische, E., Hansson, H.-A., and Holmäng, A. (2006). Prenatal exposure to interleukin-6 results in inflammatory neurodegeneration in hippocampus with NMDA/GABA(A) dysregulation and impaired spatial learning. *Am. J. Physiol. Regul. Integr. Comp. Physiol.* 290, R1345–R1356. doi: 10.1152/ajpregu.00268.2005

Schmitt, K. R. L., Kern, C., Lange, P. E., Berger, F., Abdul-Khaliq, H., and Hendrix, S. (2007). S100B modulates IL-6 release and cytotoxicity from hypothermic brain cells and inhibits hypothermia-induced axonal outgrowth. *Neurosci. Res.* 59, 68–73. doi: 10.1016/j.neures.2007.05.011

Selemon, L. D., Rajkowska, G., and Goldman-Rakic, P. S. (1995). Abnormally high neuronal density in the schizophrenic cortex: a morphometric analysis of prefrontal area 9 and occipital area 17. *Arch. Gen. Psychiatry* 52, 805–818. doi: 10.1001/archpsyc.1995.03950220015005

Smith, S. E. P., Li, J., Garbett, K., Mirnics, K., and Patterson, P. H. (2007). Maternal immune activation alters fetal brain development through interleukin-6. *J. Neurosci.* 27, 10695–10702. doi: 10.1523/JNEUROSCI.2178-07.2007

Sørensen, H. J., Mortensen, E. L., Reinisch, J. M., and Mednick, S. A. (2009). Association between prenatal exposure to bacterial infection and risk of Schizophrenia. *Schizophr. Bull.* 35, 631–637. doi: 10.1093/schbul/sbn121

Steiner, J., Bielau, H., Bernstein, H.-G., Bogerts, B., and Wunderlich, M. T. (2006). Increased cerebrospinal fluid and serum levels of S100B in first-onset schizophrenia are not related to a degenerative release of glial fibrillar acidic protein, myelin basic protein and neurone-specific enolase from glia or neurones. *J. Neurol. Neurosurg. Psychiatry* 77, 1284–1287. doi: 10.1136/jnnp.2006.093427

Steiner, J., Bogerts, B., Schroeter, M. L., and Bernstein, H.-G. (2011). S100B protein in neurodegenerative disorders. *Clin. Chem. Lab. Med.* 49, 409–424. doi: 10.1515/CCLM.2011.083

Steiner, J., Schiltz, K., Walter, M., Wunderlich, M. T., Keilhoff, G., Brisch, R., et al. (2010). S100B serum levels are closely correlated with body mass index: an important caveat in neuropsychiatric research. *Psychoneuroendocrinology* 35, 321–324. doi: 10.1016/j.psyneuen.2009.07.012

Takuma, K., Baba, A., and Matsuda, T. (2004). Astrocyte apoptosis: implications for neuroprotection. *Prog. Neurobiol.* 72, 111–127. doi: 10.1016/j.pneurobio.2004.02.001

Tramontina, F., Tramontina, A. C., Souza, D. F., Leite, M. C., Gottfried, C., Souza, D. O., et al. (2006). Glutamate uptake is stimulated by extracellular S100B in hippocampal astrocytes. *Cell. Mol. Neurobiol.* 26, 81–86.

Venkatasubramanian, G., and Debnath, M. (2013). The TRIPS (Toll-like receptors in immuno-inflammatory pathogenesis) Hypothesis: a novel postulate to understand schizophrenia. *Prog. Neuropsychopharmacol. Biol. Psychiatry* 44, 301–311. doi: 10.1016/j.pnpbp.2013.04.001

Wiesmann, M., Wandinger, K. P., Missler, U., Eckhoff, D., Rothermundt, M., Arolt, V., et al. (1999). Elevated plasma levels of S-100b protein in schizophrenic patients. *Biol. Psychiatry* 45, 1508–1511. doi: 10.1016/S0006-3223(98)00217-0

Wolff, A. R., and Bilkey, D. K. (2015). Prenatal immune activation alters hippocampal place cell firing characteristics in adult animals. *Brain Behav. Immun.* 48, 232–243. doi: 10.1016/j.bbi.2015.03.012

Zhang, Y., Cazakoff, B. N., Thai, C. A., and Howland, J. G. (2012). Prenatal exposure to a viral mimetic alters behavioural flexibility in male, but not female, rats. *Neuropharmacology* 62, 1299–1307. doi: 10.1016/j.neuropharm.2011.02.022

# 13

# A New Outlook on Mental Illnesses: Glial Involvement Beyond the Glue

*Maha Elsayed*[1] *and Pierre J. Magistretti*[1,2,3]*

[1] Laboratory of Neuroenergetics and Cellular Dynamics, Brain Mind Institute, Ecole Polytechnique Fédérale de Lausanne, Lausanne, Switzerland, [2] Division of Biological and Environmental Sciences and Engineering, King Abdullah University of Science and Technology, Thuwal, Saudi Arabia, [3] Department of Psychiatry, Center for Psychiatric Neurosciences, University of Lausanne, Lausanne, Switzerland

***Correspondence:**
Pierre J. Magistretti
pierre.magistretti@kaust.edu.sa

Mental illnesses have long been perceived as the exclusive consequence of abnormalities in neuronal functioning. Until recently, the role of glial cells in the pathophysiology of mental diseases has largely been overlooked. However recently, multiple lines of evidence suggest more diverse and significant functions of glia with behavior-altering effects. The newly ascribed roles of astrocytes, oligodendrocytes and microglia have led to their examination in brain pathology and mental illnesses. Indeed, abnormalities in glial function, structure and density have been observed in postmortem brain studies of subjects diagnosed with mental illnesses. In this review, we discuss the newly identified functions of glia and highlight the findings of glial abnormalities in psychiatric disorders. We discuss these preclinical and clinical findings implicating the involvement of glial cells in mental illnesses with the perspective that these cells may represent a new target for treatment.

**Keywords: psychiatric disorder, glia, astrocyte, oligodendrocyte, microglia, NG2 glia, mood, cognition**

## INTRODUCTION

Treatment of mental illnesses dates back to ancient times where imprisonment and confinement to chains were the mode of action to control what was perceived as influences of witchcraft and supernatural forces. With the introduction of Hippocratic medicine back in the 4th century B.C., mental illness had a physical attribute and the cause was linked to humoral imbalances. Though, the idea of demons and supernatural forces still persisted. Towards the end of the 18th century, the idea of mental illness as a disease of the mind rather than the body began to develop and it was towards the mid-19th century when it became viewed as a disease of the brain. Though, the term mental was coined to it till this day, mainly due to the lack of cerebral pathology at macroscopic and microscopic levels at the time (Kendell, 2001).

In the 1950s, psychopharmacology emerged. Following serendipitous clinical observations, chlorpromazine (dopamine antagonist) and iproniazid (monoamine oxidase inhibitor) were observed to have antipsychotic and antidepressant effects respectively (Deverteuil and Lehmann, 1958; Ban, 2007; Nestler and Hyman, 2010). These observations paved the way to the development of current psychotropic drugs whose pharmacology is essentially based on monoamine neurotransmission. Despite the availability of these psychoactive medicines, there remains however an increasing prevalence, undeniable disability, economic and social burden (Hyman, 2008). The reason for the lack of success is that these psychotherapeutic drugs were not founded on real evidence of underlying pathology. Instead, the reverse engineering of these drugs lead to the identification of molecular targets that are possibly not the actual culprit.

With the emergence of *in vivo* brain imaging techniques and improvement in the methods of microscopy, immunocytochemistry and stereology, interest in re-examining cerebral pathology at the macro- and micro-scopic level ensued (Rajkowska et al., 1999). The microscopic approach has notably brought glial cells to light with newly identified functions. With access to the right tools, findings of glia pathology in psychiatric disorders began to surface (Di Benedetto and Rupprecht, 2013). In this review, we will introduce the different types and functions of glia and then discuss findings implicating their involvement in the different types of mental illnesses.

## GLIA IN BRAIN FUNCTION AND HEALTH

While the legacy of the last century of research in psychiatry has centered on deciphering the role of neuronal systems in brain functions in health and disease, little attention has been paid to non-neuronal cells. Glial cells in fact outnumber neurons in several areas of the human brain (Kandel, 2000; Pelvig et al., 2008; Azevedo et al., 2009; Herculano-Houzel, 2011). Interestingly enough, this ratio is decreased in rodents (Nedergaard et al., 2003; Rajkowska and Miguel-Hidalgo, 2007; Herculano-Houzel, 2011) indicating that increased glial densities is associated with higher brain functions. The term neuroglia was initially coined by the German anatomist Rudolf Virchow in 1856 to refer to a scaffolding material. Traditionally seen as silent supportive cells, growing evidence suggest a more dynamic and active function. Glial cells provide a source of metabolic energy and growth/neurotrophic factors, are involved in regulating synaptic plasticity, modulating neuronal excitability, neurotransmitter modulation/reuptake and relay of information, among other functions. In short, they have emerged to be important players that alter neuronal state and connectivity.

Based on lineages, there are two types of Central Nervous System (CNS) glia: macroglia and microglia. Macroglia (astrocyte, oligodendrocyte) arise from ectoderm while microglia originate from monocyte-macrophage lineage (Ventura and Goldman, 2006; Rajkowska and Miguel-Hidalgo, 2007). Each type has a specialized function and a unique morphology (Ventura and Goldman, 2006; Rajkowska and Miguel-Hidalgo, 2007). While oligodendrocytes and microglia were long thought to have specialized functions, astrocytes proved to be the most complex and functionally diverse.

### Astrocytes

The term astrocyte was initially described by Von Lenhossek in 1893 based on its star-like morphology. It turns out that astrocytes are quite heterogeneous in cell morphology, a fact that also reflects inherent functional specialization. Astrocytes can be categorized into at least five different types: (1) white matter astrocytes which take on a star shape; (2) gray matter astrocytes, which have a less complex shape; (3) ependymal astrocytes, which are stained positive for a marker of astrocytes, GFAP, and are found in the stem cell niches of the brain; (4) radial glia found within ventricular zone which originally provide a scaffold for migrating neurons during brain development; and (5) perivascular, also GFAP+, whose end-feet are in close proximity to blood vessels (Claycomb et al., 2013). Novel discoveries on the diverse functions of astrocytes have challenged the long-time held dogma that astrocytes are merely passive cells. From an evolutionary point of view, the ratio of astrocytes to neurons and the morphology of astrocytes increase with the complexity of brain functions (Oberheim et al., 2009; Pereira and Furlan, 2010; Herculano-Houzel, 2011). The diversity of astrocytic roles are discussed below and range from local modulation of information processing within a synapse to brain large-scale integrative functions, and extend to interactions with the vasculature system and the immune system. Some of these functions support its involvement in cognitive and mood functions and the ones pertinent to psychiatric illnesses are discussed below.

#### Neurovascular Unit

Astrocytes form a bridging gap, coupling the vasculature system with neuronal circuits. The surface of intraparenchymal capillaries is covered at 99% by astrocytic end-feet (Kacem et al., 1998). Astrocytic end feet wrap around the endothelium of blood vessels and via this contact, they can influence cerebral blood flow (Takano et al., 2006; Magistretti and Allaman, 2015) and control the transport of substances in and out of the brain to ensure proper brain homeostasis (Abbott et al., 2006).

#### Metabolic Coupling

Astrocytes have been shown to support neurons metabolically. Astrocytes express glucose transporters of the GLUT1 type along their astrocytic end feet (Allaman and Magistretti, 2013). Upon increased neuronal activity and glutamate reuptake by astrocyte-specific glutamate transporters, a sequence of events is triggered resulting in the uptake of glucose from blood vessels and erobic glycolysis, a process also known as the Astrocyte Neuron Lactate Shuttle (for review, see Magistretti and Allaman, 2015). With Lactate being the end product, it is released into the interstitial space for neuronal uptake (Walz and Mukerji, 1988; Pellerin and Magistretti, 1994; Chuquet et al., 2010). Furthermore, astrocytes are the only cells to store energy in the form of glycogen in the adult brain. It was shown that this energy reserve can be mobilized by various neuroactive signals such as noradrenaline and vasoactive intestinal peptide (Magistretti et al., 1981; Sorg and Magistretti, 1991). Thus, there is an interplay between energy metabolism and neuronal activity with astrocytes being the mediators. Lactate released by astrocytes has been shown to exert additional important physiological functions such as induction of neuroplasticity and taking part in higher cognitive functions such as learning and memory (Suzuki et al., 2011; Yang et al., 2014).

#### Tripartite Synapse, Gliotransmission and Synaptic Function

Astrocytes express a range of receptors and ion channels that are similarly expressed in neurons (Verkhratsky et al., 1998). At most glutamatergic central synapses, the extremity of protoplasmic astrocyte process wraps the synaptic cleft, and communicates with pre- and post-synaptic neurons, forming what is called a tripartite synapse (Araque et al., 1999; Bezzi et al.,

2001). At those processes, they express glutamate transporters responsible for glutamate re-uptake and clearance from the synaptic cleft. With this feature, astrocytes can prevent the excitotoxic build-up of glutamate concentrations, and hence provide a form of neuroprotection (Choi, 1987; Rothstein et al., 1996; Tanaka et al., 1997). Furthermore, emerging data suggest that astrocytes are excitable cells able to release transmitters and thus regulate synaptic function. Some of the gliotransmitters released by astrocytes include ATP, D-serine, adenosine, glutamate and cytokines (Volterra and Meldolesi, 2005). Some of these gliotransmitters are involved in modulating synaptic function. For example, D-serine is one of the required coactivators of NMDA receptors at the glycine site. It is three times more potent than glycine (Miyazaki et al., 1999); both D-serine and glycine are released by astrocytes, hence enabling these cells to regulate N-Methyl-D-aspartate (NMDA) receptor activity (Schell et al., 1995; Wolosker et al., 1999a,b). To add another layer of complexity and heterogeneity of astrocyte specializations, distinct population of astrocytes contain exocytosis machinery such as vesicular glutamate transporter (vGluT) and are capable of initiating vesicular release of glutamate upon activation (Bezzi et al., 2004; Kreft et al., 2004; Montana et al., 2004; Zhang et al., 2004; Jourdain et al., 2007).

### Neurotrophic Function

Astrocytes can synthesize and release many neurotrophic factors such as fibroblast growth factor 2 (FGF2; Gonzalez et al., 1995), brain-derived neurotrophic factor (BDNF; Jean et al., 2008) and other growth factors involved in modulating synaptic transmission and plasticity (Levine et al., 1995; Lo, 1995; Zechel et al., 2010). These growth factors can ultimately impact cognition and mood associated behavior (Graham and Richardson, 2011; Elsayed et al., 2012; Quesseveur et al., 2013).

### Response to Injury and Pathogen

In response to injury, astrocytes become reactive, change their morphology and pattern of gene expression. They can also be induced to express major histocompatibility complex antigen to identify pathogen, modify Blood Brain Barrier permeability and secrete various cytokines to attract immune cells from the blood circulation (Sparacio et al., 1992; Farina et al., 2007; Burda and Sofroniew, 2014).

### Gap Junctions

The complexity of astrocytes is further enhanced by the expression of connexins which form gap junctions (Giaume et al., 2005; Orthmann-Murphy et al., 2008). This feature allows the formation of a syncytium whereby astroglia communicates intercellularly. Gap junction coupling is not static and is modulated by a number of signaling pathways (Anders et al., 2014). Mainly, sensory, cognitive and emotional patterns transmitted from spatially distributed neuronal and glial populations can result in the activation of astroglial calcium waves that can be transmitted across the astrocytic syncytium (Pereira and Furlan, 2010).

## Oligodendrocytes

Oligodendrocytes are smaller and less branched than astrocytes (Fawcett, 1994). Similarly to astrocytes, there are two types of oligodendrocyte residents in the cortex: (1) perineuronal oligodendrocytes, which are located in the gray matter and (2) interfascicular oligodendrocytes which are found in the white matter (Rajkowska and Miguel-Hidalgo, 2007). Myelin formation has been the classical function attributed to oligodendrocytes with the function of insulating axons hence enabling faster conduction speed of action of potential. White and gray matter myelinations are exceptionally high in humans when compared to other species including primates (Zhang and Sejnowski, 2000; Miller et al., 2012) pointing to a higher structural connectivity as part of an evolutionary mechanism.

All this comes at a high energetic cost, with a large proportion of brain energy metabolites being directed towards creating and supporting myelination along with maintenance of transmembrane ionic gradients to sustain excitability (Connor and Menzies, 1996; Attwell and Laughlin, 2001; Sanchez-Abarca et al., 2001; Alle et al., 2009; Rinholm et al., 2011).

While initially thought as static components of the nervous system, recent studies suggest that myelin formation by oligodendrocytes is a highly dynamic processes influenced by neuronal activity (Ishibashi et al., 2006), learning (Bengtsson et al., 2005) and environmental input (Markham and Greenough, 2004). Moreover, myelination is not restricted to a developmental program but can occur through adulthood suggesting contribution to brain plasticity (De Hoz and Simons, 2015). By enhancing speed and efficiency of action potential transmission, myelination enables synchronization of neural networks, which underlie the basis of our cognitive and behavioral repertoires and hence making this process a vital one for brain functioning (Haroutunian et al., 2014).

In addition to myelin formation, oligodendrocytes also express growth factors (Byravan et al., 1994), gap junctions (Orthmann-Murphy et al., 2008) and can supply energy in the form of Lactate to support axonal function (Funfschilling et al., 2012; Lee et al., 2012). Furthermore, they express glutamate receptors and are thus a target of neurotransmitters and glutamate excitotoxicity (Matute, 2006).

## NG2-Glia

The notion that the adult brain is a static organ has been disputed over at least the past 30 years. In fact, the brain is a dynamic organ with neuronal and non-neuronal cells undergoing cellular plastic events regulated by endogenous and exogenous cues (Dong and Greenough, 2004). It is accepted now that cell proliferation, one aspect of cellular plasticity, occurs during brain development and continues into adulthood. The areas and rates of cell proliferation vary depending on the cell type in question (i.e., neurons or glia), or on the conditions surrounding these cells. In healthy conditions, gliogenesis is a slow-turnover process that occurs in the white and gray matter of the adult brain. It involves the proliferation of NG2-glia, otherwise known as oligodendrocyte precursor cells (OPC). While, a generally agreed upon role of

NG2+ cells is to generate oligodendrocytes, they are also thought to generate neurons and astrocytes (Dayer et al., 2005). Though, the latter remains controversial (Clarke et al., 2012). They are one of the largest proliferative cells in the adult cortex (Dawson et al., 2003). Nevertheless, not all NG2+ cells are proliferating at rest (Butt et al., 2005). Furthermore, a subset of them also appears to be involved in some aspects of information processing in partnership with neurons (Bergles et al., 2000; Lin and Bergles, 2002; Hamilton et al., 2009; Richardson et al., 2011). The varied functional roles of NG2-glia are not yet completely understood and await further studies (Peters, 2004; Richardson et al., 2011).

Nevertheless, it is clear that these cells are influenced by different manipulations, environmental and pharmacological, triggering its proliferation. Gliogenesis has been shown to be influenced by stress (Banasr et al., 2007; Czeh et al., 2007), exercise (Mandyam et al., 2007), growth factors (Elsayed et al., 2012), pharmacological and non-pharmacological modes of antidepressant treatment (Kodama et al., 2004; Wennström et al., 2006; Czeh et al., 2007). Furthermore, formation of new myelin is speculated to contribute to motor learning in humans (Richardson et al., 2011) as indicated by studies reporting changes in white matter structure following extensive piano practice (Bengtsson et al., 2005) or juggling (Scholz et al., 2009).

### Microglia

Microglial cells are the resident macrophage cells of the CNS. Unlike the other glia, they are ontogenetically related to the mononuclear phagocyte lineage. They act as a warden (CNS surveillance) and cleaner (macrophage). Microglial cells have a distinct morphology, small soma with fine and short processes. In 2010, a fate mapping study shed new light on the period of microglia migration to the brain. The study demonstrates that migration occurs during early embryonic development, challenging the idea that it enters the brain after birth (Ginhoux et al., 2010). Hence, this study indicates that migration of microglia coincides with neuronal development. This realization led to the identification of new roles of microglia in neuronal development and wiring in the healthy brain (Tremblay et al., 2010; Schafer et al., 2012). In addition, microglia are involved in CNS surveillance and maintenance. They have constantly motile cellular processes canvassing the extracellular space (Kettenmann et al., 2011; Wu et al., 2013) and are involved in synaptic pruning and refinement of neuronal circuits (Chu et al., 2010). Furthermore, microglial cells are involved in neuroinflammation. In response to a pathogen or injury, microglial cells once activated change in morphology. They proliferate, migrate to the site of injury (or infection) and they phagocytose damaged neurons, myelin and degenerating cells (Ginhoux et al., 2013). They are also involved in activating the immune system by releasing factors (such as cytokines and chemo-attractive factors) to promote neuronal protection and survival.

## GLIA AND BEHAVIOR

The diverse functions of glia discussed above clearly indicate that they are not just structural fillers. Rather, they play an integral part of functional communication in the brain, see **Figure 1**. Thus, it is not surprising to come across studies demonstrating the impact of glia on behavior. While neurons have long received attention as the main and ultimate drivers in inducing a behavioral output, glia are emerging as equally important influencers in certain behavioral aspects. One supportive study demonstrates cognitive and mood deficits following glial damage. Upon infusion of the gliotoxin L-alpha-aminoadipic acid (L-AAA) into the prefrontal cortex (PFC), anhedonia- and despair-like behaviors were manifested. Moreover, the gliotoxin triggered morphological changes in the neurons. Interestingly, inducing neuronal loss by infusion of the neurotoxin ibotenate into the PFC did not replicate these results. This indicates that glial dysfunction is an important player with capability of inducing depressive symptoms possibly by contributing to neuronal adaptive changes responsible in eliciting the expression of symptoms of depression (Banasr and Duman, 2008). Behavioral impairments were also found when targeting specific astrocytic activities. Following impairment of astrocytic vesicular release through genetic manipulation, gamma oscillations were found to be impacted and this was accompanied by a deficit in novel object recognition test indicating memory impairment (Lee et al., 2014). Another study examined the behavioral impact following impairment of glycogenolysis in the rodent hippocampus. Glycogenolysis is a process that occurs uniquely in astrocytes and involves break down of glycogen and lactate formation. Inhibiting this astrocytic function interfered with long-term memory formation. A similar behavioral output also occurred following manipulation of astrocytic export or intra-neuronal uptake of lactate. These findings suggest that manipulating one aspect of astrocyte function can have a strong impact on important physiological functions, such as long-term memory formation (Suzuki et al., 2011). Additional evidence comes from a recent study suggesting that glial cells have computational and cognitive enhancement abilities. The authors engrafted human glial progenitor cells into neonatal immune-deficient mice. At adulthood and upon maturation, these chimeric mice contain both mice and human astroglia. What was puzzling about these mice is that they exhibited enhanced learning and LTP when compared to mice allografted with murine glial progenitor cells (Han et al., 2013). This study alludes to the notion of astrocytic evolution geared towards the enhancement of our cognitive abilities. In sum, these studies are some of many emerging findings that strongly highlight the importance and impact of glia on modulating cognition and emotions. Since impairments in cognition and mood are features of mental illnesses, it makes sense to draw our attention to glia and the pathological findings reported in these cell types.

## MENTAL ILLNESSES

According to Center for Disease Control and Prevention (CDC), mental illnesses refer to disorders generally characterized by dysregulation of mood, thought, and/or behavior, as recognized by the Diagnostic and Statistical Manual DSM-IV. Unlike neurodegenerative disorders, mental illness is not characterized

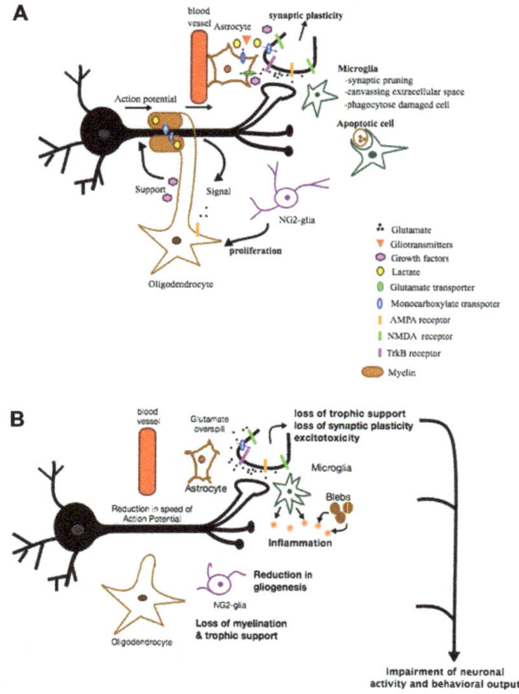


**FIGURE 1 | Role of glia in health and disease.** This is a figure depicting some of the various roles glial cells can play under normal and pathological conditions. **(A)** In healthy conditions, astrocytes provide protective and metabolic support to neurons via the supply of trophic factors and metabolic products and via the reuptake of synaptic glutamate. In addition, some of the factors and gliotransmitters released are involved in inducing synaptic plasticity. Microglia are involved in synaptic pruning, canvassing extracellular space and phagocytosing apoptotic cells. NG2-glia act mainly as oligodendrocyte progenitor cells. When activated, they proliferate and differentiate into oligodendrocytes. Oligodendrocytes, on the other hand, support neurons metabolically, are neuroprotective, and provide a source of myelin necessary for proper propagation of action potential. These various functions of glia are all crucial for maintaining proper neuronal functioning and communication. **(B)** In pathological conditions, loss of different types of glia can result in loss of trophic support, loss of synaptic plasticity, excitotoxicity, inflammation, loss of myelination, etc. All of these effects can impair neuronal activity and function and ultimately behavior.

by significant loss of neurons but rather by a prominent glial pathology (Rajkowska, 2002b; Rajkowska and Miguel-Hidalgo, 2007).

## MAJOR DEPRESSIVE DISORDER

### Clinical Studies

Major depressive disorder (MDD) is characterized by depressed mood, anhedonia and altered cognitive function. The experience of some of these symptoms can be disabling, interfering with one's daily activities and function. In some cases, these disabling symptoms are recurrent; they may reappear several times in the lifetime of MDD patients.

MDD is a multifactorial brain disorder with both genetic and environmental components. Brain imaging and molecular pathology studies have identified alterations in key structures involved in the regulation of mood and cognitive functions. Functional neuroimaging studies measuring changes in glucose metabolism (Positron Emission Tomography), blood perfusion (functional Magnetic Resonance Imaging) and volumetric studies (Magnetic Resonance Imaging) show structural and functional alterations in the PFC, hippocampus, striatum and amygdala (Drevets, 1999, 2000, 2001; Zhu et al., 1999). More specifically, reports indicate a decrease in metabolism of dorsolateral PFC (dlPFC), subgenual anterior cingulate, and an increase in orbital cortex/ventrolateral PFC, posterior cingulate cortex (Drevets et al., 2002a) and amygdala (Drevets et al., 2002b). Though, normal and hyperfrontal normal activities have also been reported (Mayberg, 2003; Fales et al., 2008) indicating some inconsistencies. The decrease in some of the cortical activity in depressed patients is restored following antidepressant treatment (Mayberg et al., 2000; Liotti and Mayberg, 2001). Amygdala activity is generally under negative control by PFC; the general decrease in PFC function and increased amygdala activity point to a disrupted circuitry. Indeed, studies have reported decreased prefrontal-amygdala functional connectivity (Matthews et al., 2008; Almeida et al., 2009). This is consistent with impaired cognitive regulation of negative emotions, a commonly experienced symptom by depressed subjects. The disruption of this circuitry is further substantiated by anatomical studies indicating cellular and myelination changes in many of these brain regions (Zhu et al., 1999; Manji et al., 2001).

One of the earliest reports of glia pathology dates back to 1998, when a preliminary histopathological assessment of subgenual part of Brodmann's are (BA24) indicated reduction in gray matter volume and diminution in glial density with no changes in neuronal density in familial forms of MDD and bipolar disorder (BPD; Ongur et al., 1998). Further cellular characterization was conducted indicating changes in different glial cell types (Rajkowska et al., 1999). Glia pathology in MDD has become well documented. **Table 1** lists some of these quantitative studies. Although there are numerous reports substantiating glial reductions in different limbic brain regions, there are some studies indicating otherwise. For a more detailed review, please refer to Sanacora and Banasr (2013).

Studies on specific markers for oligodendrocytes have shown a decrease in frontal cortex (Honer et al., 1999), in middle temporal gyrus (Aston et al., 2005), in deep white matter of the dlPFC (Regenold et al., 2007) and in white matter volume of genual and splenial portions of corpus callosum (Brambilla et al., 2004). The greatest changes were observed in layers III, V, and VI (Rajkowska et al., 1999; Cotter et al., 2001, 2002; Rajkowska, 2002b; Uranova et al., 2004; Banasr et al., 2007). Given the presence of a large component of myelinated fibers in these deeper layers, these findings support the hypothesis that myelinating oligodendrocyte's function is reduced in MDD. Reductions in limbic regions such as the amygdala (Hamidi et al., 2004) were also observed. Furthermore, white matter alterations in the anterior cingulate, dlPFC and central white matter regions were observed with Diffusion Tensor imaging and results suggest that disconnections of cortical and subcortical regions occur with depression (Bae et al., 2006).

In addition, changes in expression of astrocytic markers critical to the function and regulatory mechanisms of astrocytes have been reported in dlPFC, anterior cingulate cortex, orbitofrontal cortex and locus coeruleus. A number of postmortem brain studies of depressed subjects have consistently shown reductions in the expression of GFAP (Miguel-Hidalgo et al., 2000), AQP4 (Rajkowska et al., 2013), connexins (Miguel-Hidalgo et al., 2014), S100B (Gos et al., 2013), glutamate transporters and glutamine synthase expression (Choudary et al., 2005; Medina et al., 2013) and TrkB.1, an isoform specifically expressed in astrocytes (Ernst et al., 2009). One study identified a significant reduction (by 50%) in the coverage of blood vessels by astrocytic end feet in the gray matter of the orbitofrontal cortex (Rajkowska et al., 2013). Being an active participant in the neuro-vascular unit and a metabolic coupler of neuronal activity with blood glucose uptake, this suggests that there is a strong impairment in this particular metabolic astrocytic activity. Hence, it is not surprising that these cellular changes, particularly the coverage of blood vessels are accompanied with metabolic changes in this particular brain region when examined in anxious depressed subjects (Townsend et al., 2010). To identify the etiological mechanism of astrocytic pathology in depression, changes in DNA methylation patterns were reported in astrocytes that were specifically altered in the brain of depressed subjects (Nagy et al., 2015). Reductions of astrocyte related marker GFAP was however, not observed in the older MDD subjects (46-86 years of age; Miguel-Hidalgo et al., 2000). The lack of effect in the older MDD population is thought to be due to age-related astrocyte reactivity.

With regards to microglia, clinical evidence implicating microglial dysregulation in MDD is limited. While no studies to date have reported a loss of microglia, one study found significant microgliosis in dlPFC, anterior cingulate cortex and mediodorsal thalamus of suicidal subjects (Steiner et al., 2008). Furthermore, quinolinic acid and pro-inflammatory cytokines, whose main source of production and release is microglia are elevated in areas within anterior cingulate cortex and in the cerebrospinal fluid respectively in a subgroup of depressed subjects (Howren et al., 2009; Steiner et al., 2011). Readers are referred to a recent review that thoroughly discusses the findings and the potential role of activated microglia in the pathophysiology of MDD and other neuropsychiatric disorders (Beumer et al., 2012).

These cellular alterations are thought to be the underlying mechanism for the structural changes and volumetric reductions observed in specific brain regions of MDD subjects. Dysfunction of glial cells, glial loss and/or reduced gliogenesis (Rajkowska et al., 1999; Cotter et al., 2001, 2002), are possible mechanisms that could lead to the reported neuronal atrophy and impairment in neuronal functioning and output.

## Preclinical Studies of Depression

The importance of glia in mood modulation has been highlighted recently in animal models of depression. An increase in cell proliferation in the PFC of adult rats at baseline levels occurs after 3 weeks of antidepressant treatment (Kodama et al., 2004). Chronic stress and chronic corticosterone administration result in at least 30% decrease of cell proliferation in the medial PFC and cerebral cortex of adult rats (Alonso, 2000; Banasr et al., 2007; Czeh et al., 2007) and mice (Elsayed et al., 2012). Some of these changes are reversed by chronic fluoxetine treatment (Banasr et al., 2007; Czeh et al., 2007). Furthermore, the nature of the proliferative cells decreased by stress in the PFC was identified as NG2+ cells and endothelial cells

**TABLE 1 | Summary of the findings of glial cell reductions within the brain of depressed.**

| Cortical region | Glial density | Neuronal size | Reference |
|---|---|---|---|
| DLPFC | Decrease in glia | 20% | Cotter et al. (2002) |
| Supra and infragranular layers of DLPFC and OrbitoFrontal Cortex (OFC) | Dec. glia | 5–7% | Rajkowska et al. (1999) |
| Subgenual Anterior Cingulate changes in neuronal size/shape | Dec. in Glia (Area 24) across all layers | Selective decrease in layer Vb and | Gittins and Harrison (2011) |
| Anterior cingulate cortex | Dec. in Glia density layer 6 (22%) | 23% layer 6 | Cotter et al. (2001) |
| Hippocampus (CA1 region) | Dec. in astrocytes | Not reported | Gos et al. (2013) |
| Amygdala | Dec. in glia and oligodendrocytes | Not reported | Bowley et al. (2002) and Hamidi et al. (2004) |

(RECA-1+ marker; Banasr et al., 2007; Elsayed et al., 2012). This decrease in cell proliferation following chronic stress was accompanied by a reduction in the number of newly generated oligodendrocytes (RIP+; Banasr et al., 2007; Elsayed et al., 2012). These studies suggest that reductions in cortical cell proliferation could contribute to the glial alterations observed in depressed patients and that antidepressants might act in part by blocking or reversing these effects. In addition, rodent chronic stress and maternal deprivation models of depression also resulted in reduced astrocyte numbers and density in the hippocampus (Leventopoulos et al., 2007; Araya-Callis et al., 2012) and PFC (Banasr et al., 2010).

Factors that may contribute to a loss of glia include the alterations in glucocorticoid secretion and glutamatergic transmission evident during depression. Elevated glucocorticoid concentration, as a result of repeated stress, can decrease the proliferation of OPC (Alonso, 2000) and astrocyte density (Nichols et al., 1990). Furthermore, the early loss of glia in the initial stages of depression may lead to a reduction in glutamate clearance from the synaptic cleft. As a result, extracellular glutamate levels rise and can contribute to further glial damage (Rajkowska and Miguel-Hidalgo, 2007). Indeed, astrocytes, OPC and mature oligodendrocytes express glutamate receptors making them responsive to glutamate signaling and susceptible to excitotoxic damage from excess glutamate (Matute et al., 1997; McDonald et al., 1998; De Biase et al., 2011; Vielkind et al., 1990).

Astrocytes are functionally diverse and can exert a significant impact on cognitive and emotion-related behaviors. One study has shown that by interfering with astrocytic gliotransmission and vesicular ATP release, animals exhibit depressive-like symptoms (Cao et al., 2013). Furthermore, mice with knock-out of the gene encoding for Aquaporin-4, a protein predominantly expressed in astrocytes, show loss of astrocytes and exacerbated depressive-like behaviors when subjected to chronic corticosterone treatment (Kong et al., 2014). Together, these studies suggest that astrocytic pathology is implicated in the pathogenesis of depression.

Preclinical studies also suggest the involvement of microglial activity in the expression of depressive symptoms. Upon challenging the immune system and activating microglia, rodents express depressive-like symptoms that can be reversed with chronic antidepressant treatment (Yirmiya, 1996; Yirmiya et al., 2001). Furthermore, microglial activity is sensitive to antidepressant treatment and chronic stress (Hashioka et al., 2007; Goshen and Yirmiya, 2009). Chronic stress increases microglia activation in the rat PFC, an effect reversed by minocycline, an antibiotic that blocks microglial function (Hinwood et al., 2012) and exerts antidepressant effects (Arakawa et al., 2012). Further evidence implicating this cell type comes from studies on mice deficient in the fractalkine receptor CX3CR1 which is exclusively expressed by microglia; these mice exhibit depressive-like behaviors following activation of microglia by lipopolysaccharide treatment (Corona et al., 2010).

Interestingly, *in vitro* studies of pure glial cell cultures indicate a direct action of antidepressants on glia, in addition to their classical effects on monoaminergic neurons. Studies show that antidepressants can enhance astrocytic metabolism (Zhang et al., 1993; Kong et al., 2002; Allaman et al., 2011), increase growth factors expression (Allaman et al., 2011; Kajitani et al., 2012), and reduce the production of inflammatory cytokines (Obuchowicz et al., 2014). These *in vitro* studies point to a variety of glial-mediated mechanisms that could underlie therapeutic effects of antidepressants. The metabolic effects of antidepressants observed in culture could also explain the clinical findings indicating a recovery in glucose metabolism in affected brain regions following antidepressant treatment (Mayberg et al., 2000; Drevets et al., 2002a).

## BIPOLAR DISORDER

BPD, also known as manic-depressive illness is another classification of mood disorders. It is characterized by fluctuating moods between depression and mania, and both phases can occur with psychotic features. Moreover, unlike MDD it has a significant genetic component.

Structural and functional neuroimaging studies have indicated volumetric changes in cortico-limbic brain regions (Ongur et al., 1998; Rajkowska, 2002a) and compromised white matter integrity in BPD (Hercher et al., 2014). In addition to alterations in density/size of specific types of cortical neurons, glia loss has been reported to occur in postmortem brain studies of BPD subjects. Loss of glia is up to 40% in mPFC (area 24) as indicated by a study of a small cohort of familial BPD, and was consistent with the neuroimaging findings (Drevets et al., 1997; Ongur et al., 1998). Furthermore, unlike MDD, these glial reductions are lamina-specific within the dlPFC (Rajkowska et al., 2001) and are accompanied by glial hypertrophy (Rajkowska et al., 2001). Glial reductions also extend to subcortical regions such as the amygdala (Bowley et al., 2002) but do not appear to be widespread (i.e., there is no change in glia density in the supracallosal part of anterior cingulate cortex; Cotter et al., 2001). Hence, these results suggest reductions in glia density within regions of the cortico-limbic structures, particularly within the ventrally located regions and more subtle changes within dlPFC.

Studies delineating the specific types of glia involved suggest a severe loss of oligodendrocytes and myelin with some mixed results concerning astrocytes. In a microarray and qPCR study, markers for oligodendrocytes which include myelination related genes such as PLP1, MAG, CLDN11, MBP, MOG, GALC and Transferrin were decreased in the PFC of BPD subjects (Tkachev et al., 2003). Abnormalities in satellite oligodendrocytes were also evidenced by electron microscopic analysis of PFC in BPD (Uranova et al., 2001; Vostrikov et al., 2007; Drevets et al., 2008) suggesting oligodendrocyte dysfunction. On the other hand, decreased Glycogen Synthase Kinase 3 (GSK3) activity, as a result of lithium treatment or variation in the promoter of GSK3 gene seen in some patients, is associated with enhancement in white matter integrity and improvement in clinical feature of BDP (Benedetti et al., 2013). These results suggest the involvement of oligodendrocyte/myelin integrity in the development and treatment of BPD symptoms.

There are some mixed results when it comes to astrocytic reductions. One study reported a decrease in GFAP immunostaining across all layers of the orbitofrontal cortex while another study found no changes in the subgenual cingulate cortex (Toro et al., 2006; Williams et al., 2013) despite a decrease in GFAP mRNA expression in the dorsal portion (Webster et al., 2005). Furthermore, the expression of another astrocytic marker, glutamine synthase, was not changed in the dorsolateral and in the orbitofrontal cortex (Toro et al., 2006).

## Preclinical Studies of Bipolar Disorder

To date, there is no established animal model of BPD that exhibit mania-like symptoms, particularly alternating episodes of mania and depression-like behaviors. Hence, the field has relied mostly on genetic studies and/or examining the effects of two commonly used and oldest therapeutic drugs, Lithium and Valproate. One study found that chronic lithium treatment decreases NG2 cell proliferation within the hippocampus (Orre et al., 2009), and reduces glycogen synthesis in astrocytes (Souza Ade et al., 2010). Furthermore, lithium within therapeutic concentrations was found to inhibit GSK3 activity (Bain et al., 2007). One of the numerous effects of GSK3 is to regulate oligodendrocyte differentiation and myelination (Azim and Butt, 2011). As such, this can represent a mechanism by which lithium can exert therapeutic effects via possible regulation of oligodendrocyte differentiation and function. Additional targets include neuregulin and its receptor, erbB4 that are genetically linked to BPD and are implicated in oligodendrocyte development (Roy et al., 2007).

These findings suggest that treatment of BPD could be exerted via modulation of different pathways that regulate the activities and functioning of different glial cell types. Nevertheless, more preclinical studies would need to be carried out to further establish this link.

# ANXIETY DISORDERS

Anxiety disorders have a high degree of comorbidity with MDD. While anxiety is a natural response to a life threatening situation, it becomes a disorder when it disrupts one's daily activities. There are six subtypes of anxiety disorders defined by specific symptoms: generalized anxiety disorder (GAD), panic disorder (PD), obsessive-compulsive disorder (OCD), post-traumatic stress disorder (PTSD) and agora- or socio-phobias. All have a common feature which is a lack of correct processing of fear stimuli.

Imaging and magnetic resonance studies report brain structural alterations, (Li et al., 2014) and glial metabolite changes in different subtypes of anxiety disorders (Seedat et al., 2005; Kitamura et al., 2006). Furthermore, disruption in myelin integrity and structure has been observed particularly in OCD subjects within fronto-striato-thalamo cortical circuit. These structural changes were associated with a functional polymorphism in the myelin oligodendrocyte glycoprotein (MOG; Atmaca et al., 2010). White matter contains fiber tracts, surrounded by myelin sheaths and fibrous astrocytes. These studies indicate that disturbed myelination/oligodendrocyte function and/or astrocytic function are implicated in anxiety disorders. Additional studies showed an association between the polymorphisms in oligodendrocyte lineage transcription factor OLIG2 and OCD, further supporting white matter and oligodendrocyte abnormalities in this disorder (Stewart et al., 2007).

In addition, Riluzole, a drug used in the management of ALS has been shown to exert beneficial effects in patients with OCD (Coric et al., 2003) and GAD (Mathew et al., 2005; Pittenger et al., 2008). Riluzole can act on astrocytes and enhance astrocytic uptake of extracellular glutamate in addition to other effects. Given the numerous mechanisms it can exert, it is remains to be determined whether its therapeutic effect is via enhancement of astrocytic uptake of glutamate *per se*.

## Preclinical Studies

While the most consistent pathological findings in postmortem studies were disruptions in myelination, few preclinical studies have been carried out to examine a causal link between oligodendrocytes and anxiety. Rodents exposed to cuprizone, a demyelinating drug, exhibit anxiety related behavioral responses (Serra-De-Oliveira et al., 2015) thus providing a potential link between impairment in myelin/oligodendrocyte functioning and anxiety.

The association between astrocyte activation and different behavioral forms of anxiety has been explored to some extent. In one study, the metabolic and metabolite effects of antidepressant/antipanic drug phenelzine in rat cortex was examined using H1[13C]magnetic resonance spectroscopy. The rate of glutamate-glutamine cycling flux between neurons and glia was significantly reduced following treatment (Yang and Shen, 2005). A transcriptome analysis performed in the amygdala of rats exposed to fear learning, a behavioral model of Posttraumatic Stress Disorder (PTSD), showed induction of 84-astrocyte-enriched genes following shock exposure (Ponomarev et al., 2010). This indicates a possible involvement of astrocytes within the amygdala in stress-associated behavioral response. Expression of FGF2, predominantly expressed in astrocytes, is decreased in rats selectively bred for high anxiety. Treatment with FGF2, on the other hand, has anxiolytic effects. In addition, this treatment regimen results in increased hippocampal neurogenesis and gliogenesis pointing to the possible involvement of these cellular processes in anxiety modulation (Perez et al., 2009). In another model of PTSD that involves single prolonged stress (SPS), FGF2 administration was shown to inhibit SPS-induced hyperarousal and anxiety behavior, symptoms resembling PTSD. This was accompanied by a specific upregulation of GFAP expression in the hippocampus indicating that the anxiolytic effects of FGF2 could involve astrocyte-based mechanisms (Xia et al., 2013). Furthermore, riluzole administration in the medial PFC has been shown to block anxiety-like behavior indicating the possible involvement of astrocytic function in modulating anxiety via enhanced uptake of extracellular glutamate (Ohashi et al., 2015).

With regards to microglial involvement, knock-out mice for the Hoxb3 gene, a homeobox developmental patterning gene expressed prominently in the macrophage-lineage of hematopoietic cells and expressed by a subset of microglia, exhibit OCD-like behaviors which can be normalized following repopulation of the brain with wild-type microglia (Chen et al., 2010).

## SCHIZOPHRENIA

Schizophrenia is a chronic and disabling neurodevelopmental disorder with polygenic and environmental factors playing a role. It is characterized by positive symptoms such as delusions, hallucinations, disordered thoughts, and negative symptoms such as deficits of normal emotional responses and thought processes. While the positive symptoms are in general better controlled with antipsychotics, negative symptoms are not.

Schizophrenia is regarded as a syndrome of inter- and intra-hemispheric disconnectivity particularly that of reduced cortical connectivity, for which the underlying biological and genetic cause remains unclear. While cell biology studies have predominantly focused on neurons, multiple lines of evidence from neuroimaging, postmortem brains and genome-wide associations implicate oligodendrocyte abnormalities and compromised white matter/myelin integrity (Dwork et al., 2007; Bernstein et al., 2015). Genetic and protein expression studies in schizophrenia indicate abnormalities in Myelin associated markers (Flynn et al., 2003; Iwamoto et al., 2005) within the cortex (Aston et al., 2004; Aberg et al., 2006; Tkachev et al., 2007) and within subcortical brain regions (Dracheva et al., 2006; Barley et al., 2009) with the most profoundly affected brain regions being the hippocampal formation, cingulate and temporal cortices (Katsel et al., 2005a,b). One mechanism contributing to this oligodendrocyte/myelin abnormality could be linked to disrupted-in-schizophrenia-1 (DISC1) gene. DISC-1 disruption as a result of chromosomal translocation reduces expression of Neuregulin and its receptor ErbB3. These are some of several altered genes associated with the development of Schizophrenia (Millar et al., 2000; Blackwood et al., 2001; Hakak et al., 2001; Corfas et al., 2004; Silberberg et al., 2006). Being expressed by different cell types including oligodendrocytes (Deadwyler et al., 2000; Osbun et al., 2011), these proteins exert a variety of functions including regulating oligodendrocyte development, differentiation and CNS myelination (Vartanian et al., 1999; Taveggia et al., 2005; Chen et al., 2006; Hattori et al., 2014). Furthermore, postmortem histology studies indicate reductions in glial cells in anterior cingulate cortex (Stark et al., 2004) including decreases in oligodendrocyte density (Uranova et al., 2004) in hippocampus (Schmitt et al., 2009), in the perineuronal PFC (Vostrikov et al., 2007) as well as layer specific oligodendrocyte reductions in the dlPFC (Hof et al., 2003). This is accompanied with volumetric reductions, abnormalities in adulthood myelination in the frontal lobes, association areas (Bartzokis et al., 2003) and temporal lobes (Chambers and Perrone-Bizzozero, 2004) and in white matter fiber tracts interconnecting brain regions, particularly the frontal and temporal lobes (Breier et al., 1992; Paillere-Martinot et al., 2001). It was hypothesized that the abnormalities in oligodendrocyte/myelin are possibly due to alterations in proliferation and differentiation of oligodendrocyte progenitor cells, NG2. Indeed, a microarray study carried out on the brains of schizophrenic patients revealed changes in gene expression associated with the regulation of G1/S phase transition and oligodendrocyte differentiation (Katsel et al., 2008). In support of a cell cycle impairment, variation in OLIG2, a gene strongly implicated in the control of oligodendrocyte development, was identified as a susceptibility gene in schizophrenia (reviewed in Georgieva et al., 2006). In addition, the reduction of perineuronal non-myelinating oligodendrocytes suggests impairments in oligodendrocyte functions that are beyond myelination. Together, these studies indicate that inadequate myelination or myelin function, abnormalities in oligodendrocyte development, density and functions could contribute to the pathophysiology and expression of schizophrenia symptoms.

Findings of abnormalities of astrocytes were less consistent and not as well surveyed. Examination of the astrocytic GFAP marker yielded differential results when examining it in various affected brain regions. Studies examining GFAP expression in cortical gray matter have identified no changes (Falkai et al., 1999; Katsel et al., 2011a), decreased expression (Johnston-Wilson et al., 2000; Steffek et al., 2008) or increased expression (Pennington et al., 2008; Feresten et al., 2013). Furthermore, some studies reported specific changes restricted to subgroups of schizophrenic subjects (Arnold et al., 1996). In sum, studies using GFAP as an astrocyte marker have yielded inconsistent results. Since GFAP may not represent a direct link to astrocyte density, other astrocytic markers were examined. The expressions of a few selected markers were found altered implying possible changes in specific astrocytic functions and/or astrocytic subsets (Owen et al., 1987; Katsel et al., 2011a; Feresten et al., 2013). These changes in astrocytic markers were glutamate-related, an observation consistent with the view that schizophrenia is associated with a hypofunction of glutamatergic transmission. Supporting this, the expression of astrocytic glutamate transporter was found increased in the PFC of schizophrenic subjects (Matute et al., 2005; Lauriat et al., 2006) and normalized following antipsychotic treatment (Matute et al., 2005), while that of glutamine synthase was decreased in the deep layers of the anterior cingulate (Steffek et al., 2008).

Microglial cells are also altered in the brain of schizophrenic patients. Cytology and imaging studies report increased number of activated microglia in the frontal and temporal lobes of schizophrenic patients (Bayer et al., 1999; Radewicz et al., 2000; Wierzba-Bobrowicz et al., 2005; Van Berckel et al., 2008). Activation of microglia can result in the release of proinflammatory cytokines and free radicals that can lead to abnormalities in white matter and neurons and thus in the expression of schizophrenia symptoms. Interestingly, minocycline, an inhibitor of microglial activation was found to have therapeutic benefit when used as an adjunctive treatment (Miyaoka et al., 2007; Levkovitz et al., 2010; Chaudhry et al., 2012). These findings indicate overactive microglia may play an important role in the pathophysiology of schizophrenia.

### Preclinical Studies

Animal models of schizophrenia face serious and vexing challenges given the complexity and difficulty to recapitulate the symptoms of schizophrenia. Nevertheless, preclinical studies have shed light and provided key insights into the involvement of the different glial cells in the pathophysiology of schizophrenia. For instance, demyelination and downregulation of oligodendrocyte-associated genes in PFC was shown to induce behavioral deficits associated with schizophrenia (a deficit in the ability to shift between perceptual dimensions in the attentional set-shifting task; Gregg et al., 2009). Mice with selective ErbB3 receptor deletion in oligodendrocytes exhibit deficits in social interaction and working memory (Makinodan et al., 2012). Transgenic mice expressing mutant human DISC1 specifically in the forebrain also show behavioral deficits similar to schizophrenia. In addition, these mice were found to exhibit premature oligodendrocyte differentiation and increased proliferation of their progenitors (Katsel et al., 2011b). These studies indicate that oligodendrocyte functional impairment via ErbB3 signaling or alterations in DISC1 function can contribute to schizophrenia pathogenesis and symptoms. Furthermore, transgenic mice with a deficiency of DISC1 expression in astrocytes have impaired D-serine production which in turn can affect NMDAR activity. These mice also display schizophrenia like-behaviors (prepupulse inhibition in the acoustic startle tests) consistent with hypofunction of glutamatergic transmission via NMDA receptors (Ma et al., 2013). Furthermore, pharmacological upregulation of the astrocytic glutamate transporter Glt-1 expression result in impairment of information processing, mimicking what occurs in schizophrenia (Bellesi et al., 2009). In an animal model of schizophrenia based on maternal infection during pregnancy, microglia activation in brain regions involved in the pathogenesis of schizophrenia i.e., hippocampus and striatum was observed (Juckel et al., 2011; Mattei et al., 2014). The behavioral deficits triggered in this animal model of schizophrenia were rescued following treatment with minocycline (Mattei et al., 2014). Lastly, antipsychotics have been shown to modulate microglial activity promoting anti-inflammatory effects (Labuzek et al., 2005; Kato et al., 2007). In sum, these findings support the involvement of microglia, oligodendrocyte and astrocytes in the pathophysiology and treatment of schizophrenia.

## ATTENTION DEFICIT HYPERACTIVITY DISORDER

Attention deficit hyperactivity disorder (ADHD) is a highly heritable disorder characterized by a heterogeneous set of symptoms that include problems in attention, impulsivity and hyperactivity. Compelling lines of evidence indicate that symptoms of ADHD are associated with hypofunctionality of catecholaminergic pathways projecting to prefrontal cortical areas (Biederman and Spencer, 2000; Semrud-Clikeman et al., 2000; Todd and Botteron, 2001). For instance, unmedicated ADHD subjects exhibit increased dopamine transporter concentrations (Dougherty et al., 1999; Krause et al., 2000) that are normalized following treatment (Krause et al., 2000). It is well known that catecholamines can trigger glycogenolysis in astrocytes followed by lactate release (Magistretti, 1988; Sorg and Magistretti, 1991; Magistretti et al., 1993). It is hypothesized as such that catecholamine hypofunction could result in diminished activation of astrocytic energy metabolism and supply to prefrontal cortical neurons (Semrud-Clikeman et al., 2000; Russell et al., 2006; Killeen et al., 2013). In turn, rapid synchronized neuronal firing can be impaired, which might result in disturbances in neurotransmission (Todd and Botteron, 2001). This is supported by some imaging studies indicating changes in cerebral blood flow and glucose metabolism in ADHD subjects (Zametkin et al., 1990, 1993; Ernst et al., 1994; Gustafsson et al., 2000; Hart et al., 2012) though these findings were not always reproducible in other cohorts (Ernst et al., 1997). The inconsistencies in these imaging studies might be related to the phenotyping heterogeneity of the disease. In addition, ADHD individuals exhibit altered myelination and disrupted network connectivity (Fair et al., 2010; Nagel et al., 2011). Since Lactate is involved in myelin production (Rinholm et al., 2011), it is conceivable that this deficit in energy supply in the form of Lactate could also interfere with myelin production and hence neuronal transmission.

### Preclinical Studies

Spontaneously hypertensive rats (SHR) display hyperactivity, impulsivity and poor performance in tasks that require sustained attention. Thus, they represent a model of ADHD. These rats show reductions in proteins involved in energy metabolism and myelination (Dimatelis et al., 2015). Given that glia particularly astrocytes are key players in brain energy metabolism, this finding further support a role of astrocytic energy metabolism deficit in ADHD genesis. Further evidence supporting glial contribution to the pathophysiology of this disorder is provided by a study showing that mutant mice with a disrupted SynCam1 specifically in astrocytes result in behavioral deficits related to ADHD symptoms (Sandau et al., 2012).

## SUBSTANCE USE DISORDERS

Substance use disorders (SUD) is a chronic brain disorder with profound effects on our society. Addicted individuals untiringly seek substance of abuse despite the negative consequences associated with it. Apart from the huge economic burden it carries, SUD have devastating consequences on society and quality of life. Vulnerability to addiction is influenced by genetics, environmental factors and developmental stages (Volkow et al., 2011). Chronic drug abuse impairs many aspects of behavior necessary for proper functioning in social environment. For example, alcohol dependance leads to impairments in executive function and episodic memory (Bernardin et al., 2014). These impairments are seen as a result of structural and functional changes in limbic circuits and frontal brain regions. Indeed, imaging studies indicate volumetric changes in the frontal lobe in cocaine-, alcohol- and heroin-dependent subjects (Goldstein and Volkow, 2002). While neuronal dysfunction particularly dopaminergic, glutamatergic and opioidergic transmissions are the underlying pathophysiological mechanisms, pathological changes in glial cells are also observed (Miguel-Hidalgo, 2009).

Alcohol dependent subjects exhibit reductions in glial densities in dlPFC (Miguel-Hidalgo et al., 2002), orbitofrontal cortex (Miguel-Hidalgo et al., 2006) and hippocampus (Korbo, 1999). Glial loss includes astrocytes and oligodendrocytes. While there are also some neuronal losses, the deficit is not as widespread. Unlike glia, there is no loss of neurons in the hippocampus (Korbo, 1999) and it is limited to specific cortical layers of the orbitofrontal cortex (Miguel-Hidalgo et al., 2006). Several findings based on examination of a number of glial markers substantiate glial pathology in alcoholic subjects. For example, connexin 43, an astrocytic gap junction, is significantly reduced in the orbitofrontal cortex of alcoholics indicating impairment in astrocytic communication (Miguel-Hidalgo et al., 2014). Furthermore, a mutation in a glutamate transporter specifically expressed in astrocytes, GLT-1, was found to increase vulnerability to alcohol dependance (Sander et al., 2000). In addition to astrocytic pathologies, postmortem studies of the brains of alcohol dependent subjects indicate increased expression of microglial markers in specific brain regions (He and Crews, 2008) and altered oligodendrocyte/myelin gene expression indicating white matter dysfunction (Lewohl et al., 2000; Pfefferbaum et al., 2000; Mayfield et al., 2002; Liu et al., 2004). Some of these changes in oligodendrocyte markers and the expression of several myelination related genes were also observed in cocaine abusers (Albertson et al., 2004; Bannon et al., 2005).

### Preclinical Studies

Preclinical studies helped dissect the role of these pathologies play in addiction. Studies demonstrating impairment in astrocyte density/function particularly those pertaining to glutamate homeostasis are of particular interest. Chronic exposure to both cocaine and nicotine in rodents resulted in reduced expression of a catalytic subunit of cysteine glutamate antiporter expressed predominantly in glia (Kalivas et al., 2003; Kalivas, 2009). Exposure to other forms of substances of abuse (i.e., alcohol, heroin, etc.) was also shown to result in reduced expression levels of GLT-1 in the nucleus accumbens (Kalivas, 2009; Sari and Sreemantula, 2012; Gipson et al., 2013). While gene expression levels of GLAST, another glutamate transporter subtype, were found increased in the frontal cortex in alcohol-dependent rodents (Rimondini et al., 2002), GLT-1 mediated functions seem to be disrupted in this brain region (Mulholland et al., 2009). The reduction in glutamate re-uptake particularly in nucleus accumbens seems to be a consistent maladaptive response to these different drugs of abuse. This pathology may result in potentiation of glutamatergic transmission and in activation of non-synaptic glutamatergic compartment which is associated with drug seeking behavior (Kalivas, 2009; Scofield and Kalivas, 2014). Additional aspects of astrocytic functions seem to also be implicated. Alcohol preferring rats show increased GFAP-immunoreactive cells following few weeks of exposure (Miguel-Hidalgo, 2005) while longer duration resulted in reduction in perineuronal glial cell densities (Khokhrina et al., 1991). Furthermore, alcohol self-administration is increased following infusion of the gliotoxin L-AAA or astrocytic gap junction blockers into the prelimbic cortex (Miguel-Hidalgo et al., 2009). In addition to the astrocytic pathologies and consistent with clinical findings, chronic exposure to alcohol also results in a decrease in oligodendrocyte/myelin gene expression (Okamoto et al., 2006). Interestingly, the identification of a glial modulator, ibudilast was shown to exert therapeutic effects in rodent models of addiction (Snider et al., 2013; Bell et al., 2015).

Taken together, these studies suggest that alcohol and additional substances of abuse can have profound effects on glial density and function in relevant brain regions. Furthermore, interfering with glial density and/or function seems to affect vulnerability for addiction. Thus targeting specific functions of glia could represent a new therapeutic avenue.

## ALEXANDER DISEASE

Alexander disease is a rare and fatal disease of the CNS, predominantly affecting infants and children. Affected patients suffer from cognitive and motor impairments in the form of mental retardation, seizures, megaloencephaly and progressive deterioration (Prust et al., 2011; Verkhratsky et al., 2014). The pathology is a glial one associated with sporadic mutations in the non-conservative coding region of GFAP (Brenner et al., 2001; Rodriguez et al., 2001). These mutations are thought to result in cytotoxicity. Indeed, histological analysis has indicated cytoplasmic inclusions in astrocytes that contain the intermediate filament GFAP, otherwise referred as Rosenthal fibers. It is thought that these fibers, represent the hallmark of this disease (Sawaishi, 2009). Furthermore, variable degrees of cerebral white matter degeneration, referred as leukodystrophies, have been observed prominently in the frontal lobes (Messing et al., 2012) and in close apposition to Rosenthal fibers. Since astrocytes can release factors involved in myelination (Ishibashi et al., 2006; Sawaishi, 2009), it is thus speculated that white matter abnormalities are a consequence to astrocytic pathology.

### Preclinical Studies

To further cement the involvement of this astrocytic genetic defect in Alexander disease pathology, mouse models of Alexander Disease overexpressing human GFAP mutation were generated. A similar astrocytic pathology with inclusions of Rosenthal fibers was observed (Eng et al., 1998). In addition, decreased glutamate transporter levels that were also reported in human subjects (Tian et al., 2010) were demonstrated along with cognitive impairments (Hagemann et al., 2013).

In sum, these findings present Alexander disease as a primary astrocytic genetic disorder. Impairment in astrocytic function via decreased glutamate uptake and/or release of factors involved in myelin formation, can trigger the pathogenesis of neuronal and oligodendrocyte injury/death and ultimately manifesting symptoms of Alexander disease.

**TABLE 2 | Summary of the therapeutic drugs that target glial cells.**

| Neuropsychiatric disorder | Glial cells affected | Therapeutics targeting glial cells | Glial cells responsive to therapeutics |
|---|---|---|---|
| Major depressive disorder | Astrocytes<br>Microglia<br>Oligodendrocytes | Riluzole (Yoshizumi et al., 2012)<br>Fluoxetine, Paroxetine (Allaman et al., 2011)<br>Ceftriaxone (Li et al., 2012)<br>Minocycline (Hinwood et al. 2012) | -Astrocytes<br>-Oligodendrocyte progenitors<br>-Microglia |
| Bipolar disorder | Oligodendrocytes<br>Astrocytes<br>Microglia | Lithium (Orre et al., 2009; Souza Ade et al., 2010) | -Astrocytes<br>-Oligodendrocyte progenitors |
| Anxiety disorders | Oligodendrocytes<br>Astrocytes | Riluzole (Pittenger et al., 2008)<br>Benzodiazepines (Patte et al., 1999) | -Astrocytes |
| Schizophrenia | Astrocytes<br>Microglia<br>Oligodendrocytes | Minocycline (Chaudhry et al., 2012)<br>Risperidone (Kato et al., 2007)<br>Chlorpromazine and loxapine (Labuzek et al., 2005) | -Microglia |
| Substance use disorders | Astrocytes<br>Microglia<br>Oligodendrocytes | Ibudilast, AV1013, minocycline (Snider et al., 2013) | -Microglia |
| Alexander disease | Astrocytes | | |

## CONCLUSION

Converging lines of evidence from clinical and preclinical studies suggest that different types of glial cells can play a substantial role in the pathology of mental illnesses. Furthermore, there appears to be an overlap in glial pathologies in some of the mental illnesses pointing to the multi-functional impact of these cells in the expression of diverse symptoms. For example, reports of reductions in glial density within the dorsolateral PFC are indicated in subjects diagnosed with depression (Rajkowska et al., 1999) and alcoholism (Miguel-Hidalgo et al., 2002). A direct cause effect is further demonstrated in preclinical studies whereby injection of a gliotoxin into the PFC results in behavioral effects associated with depression (Banasr and Duman, 2008) and alcohol preference (Miguel-Hidalgo et al., 2009). These overwhelming findings implicating glial cells in the pathophysiology of mental illnesses should alter our perception of mental illnesses. It should also promote interest towards targeting glial cells as a new avenue of treatment. **Table 2** below is a summary of the glial pathological findings reported among the different types of mental illnesses and a list of compounds with therapeutic benefits that target different types of glial cells, in hope to shed light on these cast-aside cells that seem to hold more potential than we think.

## FUNDING

This work was supported by the National Center of Competence in Research (NNCR) "SYNAPSY" (n° 51AU40-125759), by FNRS grant 310030B-148169/1, and by the Préfargier and Panacée Foundations.

## ACKNOWLEDGMENTS

Research in P.J.M.'s laboratory has been supported over the years by the Swiss National Science Foundation and by the University of Lausanne, EPFL, CHUV, the NCCR Synapsy, the Biaggi and Panacée foundations, and by KAUST.

## REFERENCES

Abbott, N. J., Rönnbäck, L., and Hansson, E. (2006). Astrocyte-endothelial interactions at the blood-brain barrier. *Nat. Rev. Neurosci.* 7, 41–53. doi: 10.1038/nrn1824

Aberg, K., Saetre, P., Lindholm, E., Ekholm, B., Pettersson, U., Adolfsson, R., et al. (2006). Human QKI, a new candidate gene for schizophrenia involved in myelination. *Am. J. Med. Genet. B Neuropsychiatr. Genet.* 141B, 84–90. doi: 10.1002/ajmg.b.30243

Albertson, D. N., Pruetz, B., Schmidt, C. J., Kuhn, D. M., Kapatos, G., and Bannon, M. J. (2004). Gene expression profile of the nucleus accumbens of human cocaine abusers: evidence for dysregulation of myelin. *J. Neurochem.* 88, 1211–1219. doi: 10.1046/j.1471-4159.2003.02247.x

Allaman, I., Fiumelli, H., Magistretti, P. J., and Martin, J. L. (2011). Fluoxetine regulates the expression of neurotrophic/growth factors and glucose metabolism in astrocytes. *Psychopharmacology (Berl)* 216, 75–84. doi: 10.1007/s00213-011-2190-y

Allaman, I., and Magistretti, P. J. (2013). "Brain energy metabolism," in *Fundamental Neuroscience*, 4th Edn. ed. D. W. Pfaff (New York: Springer Science+Business Media), 1591–1620.

Alle, H., Roth, A., and Geiger, J. R. (2009). Energy-efficient action potentials in hippocampal mossy fibers. *Science* 325, 1405–1408. doi: 10.1126/science.1174331

Almeida, J. R., Versace, A., Mechelli, A., Hassel, S., Quevedo, K., Kupfer, D. J., et al. (2009). Abnormal amygdala-prefrontal effective connectivity to happy faces differentiates bipolar from major depression. *Biol. Psychiatry* 66, 451–459. doi: 10.1016/j.biopsych.2009.03.024

Alonso, G. (2000). Prolonged corticosterone treatment of adult rats inhibits the proliferation of oligodendrocyte progenitors present throughout white and gray matter regions of the brain. *Glia* 31, 219–231. doi: 10.1002/1098-1136(200009)31:3<219::aid-glia30>3.0.co;2-r

Anders, S., Minge, D., Griemsmann, S., Herde, M. K., Steinhäuser, C., and Henneberger, C. (2014). Spatial properties of astrocyte gap junction coupling in the rat hippocampus. *Philos. Trans. R. Soc. Lond. B Biol. Sci.* 369:20130600. doi: 10.1098/rstb.2013.0600

Arakawa, S., Shirayama, Y., Fujita, Y., Ishima, T., Horio, M., Muneoka, K., et al. (2012). Minocycline produced antidepressant-like effects on the learned helplessness rats with alterations in levels of monoamine in the amygdala and no changes in BDNF levels in the hippocampus at baseline. *Pharmacol. Biochem. Behav.* 100, 601–606. doi: 10.1016/j.pbb.2011.09.008

Araque, A., Parpura, V., Sanzgiri, R. P., and Haydon, P. G. (1999). Tripartite synapses: glia, the unacknowledged partner. *Trends Neurosci.* 22, 208–215. doi: 10.1016/s0166-2236(98)01349-6

Araya-Callis, C., Hiemke, C., Abumaria, N., and Flugge, G. (2012). Chronic psychosocial stress and citalopram modulate the expression of the glial proteins GFAP and NDRG2 in the hippocampus. *Psychopharmacology (Berl)* 224, 209–222. doi: 10.1007/s00213-012-2741-x

Arnold, S. E., Franz, B. R., Trojanowski, J. Q., Moberg, P. J., and Gur, R. E. (1996). Glial fibrillary acidic protein-immunoreactive astrocytosis in elderly patients with schizophrenia and dementia. *Acta Neuropathol.* 91, 269–277. doi: 10.1007/s004010050425

Aston, C., Jiang, L., and Sokolov, B. P. (2004). Microarray analysis of postmortem temporal cortex from patients with schizophrenia. *J. Neurosci. Res.* 77, 858–866. doi: 10.1002/jnr.20208

Aston, C., Jiang, L., and Sokolov, B. P. (2005). Transcriptional profiling reveals evidence for signaling and oligodendroglial abnormalities in the temporal cortex from patients with major depressive disorder. *Mol. Psychiatry* 10, 309–322. doi: 10.1038/sj.mp.4001565

Atmaca, M., Onalan, E., Yildirim, H., Yuce, H., Koc, M., and Korkmaz, S. (2010). The association of myelin oligodendrocyte glycoprotein gene and white matter volume in obsessive-compulsive disorder. *J. Affect. Disord.* 124, 309–313. doi: 10.1016/j.jad.2010.03.027

Attwell, D., and Laughlin, S. B. (2001). An energy budget for signaling in the grey matter of the brain. *J. Cereb. Blood Flow Metab.* 21, 1133–1145. doi: 10.1097/00004647-200110000-00001

Azevedo, F. A., Carvalho, L. R., Grinberg, L. T., Farfel, J. M., Ferretti, R. E., Leite, R. E., et al. (2009). Equal numbers of neuronal and nonneuronal cells make the human brain an isometrically scaled-up primate brain. *J. Comp. Neurol.* 513, 532–541. doi: 10.1002/cne.21974

Azim, K., and Butt, A. M. (2011). GSK3beta negatively regulates oligodendrocyte differentiation and myelination *in vivo*. *Glia* 59, 540–553. doi: 10.1002/glia.21122

Bae, J. N., MacFall, J. R., Krishnan, K. R., Payne, M. E., Steffens, D. C., and Taylor, W. D. (2006). Dorsolateral prefrontal cortex and anterior cingulate cortex white matter alterations in late-life depression. *Biol. Psychiatry* 60, 1356–1363. doi: 10.1016/j.biopsych.2006.03.052

Bain, J., Plater, L., Elliott, M., Shpiro, N., Hastie, C. J., McLauchlan, H., et al. (2007). The selectivity of protein kinase inhibitors: a further update. *Biochem. J.* 408, 297–315. doi: 10.1042/bj20070797

Ban, T. A. (2007). Fifty years chlorpromazine: a historical perspective. *Neuropsychiatr. Dis. Treat.* 3, 495–500.

Banasr, M., and Duman, R. S. (2008). Glial loss in the prefrontal cortex is sufficient to induce depressive-like behaviors. *Biol. Psychiatry* 64, 863–870. doi: 10.1016/j.biopsych.2008.06.008

Banasr, M., Chowdhury, G. M., Terwilliger, R., Newton, S. S., Duman, R. S., Behar, K. L., et al. (2010). Glial pathology in an animal model of depression: reversal of stress-induced cellular, metabolic and behavioral deficits by the glutamate-modulating drug riluzole. *Mol. Psychiatry* 15, 501–511. doi: 10.1038/mp.2008.106

Banasr, M., Valentine, G. W., Li, X. Y., Gourley, S. L., Taylor, J. R., and Duman, R. S. (2007). Chronic unpredictable stress decreases cell proliferation in the cerebral cortex of the adult rat. *Biol. Psychiatry* 62, 496–504. doi: 10.1016/j.biopsych.2007.02.006

Bannon, M., Kapatos, G., and Albertson, D. (2005). Gene expression profiling in the brains of human cocaine abusers. *Addict. Biol.* 10, 119–126. doi: 10.1080/13556210412331308921

Barley, K., Dracheva, S., and Byne, W. (2009). Subcortical oligodendrocyte- and astrocyte-associated gene expression in subjects with schizophrenia, major depression and bipolar disorder. *Schizophr. Res.* 112, 54–64. doi: 10.1016/j.schres.2009.04.019

Bartzokis, G., Nuechterlein, K. H., Lu, P. H., Gitlin, M., Rogers, S., and Mintz, J. (2003). Dysregulated brain development in adult men with schizophrenia: a magnetic resonance imaging study. *Biol. Psychiatry* 53, 412–421. doi: 10.1016/s0006-3223(02)01835-8

Bayer, T. A., Buslei, R., Havas, L., and Falkai, P. (1999). Evidence for activation of microglia in patients with psychiatric illnesses. *Neurosci. Lett.* 271, 126–128. doi: 10.1016/s0304-3940(99)00545-5

Bell, R. L., Lopez, M. F., Cui, C., Egli, M., Johnson, K. W., Franklin, K. M., et al. (2015). Ibudilast reduces alcohol drinking in multiple animal models of alcohol dependence. *Addict. Biol.* 20, 38–42. doi: 10.1111/adb.12106

Bellesi, M., Melone, M., Gubbini, A., Battistacci, S., and Conti, F. (2009). GLT-1 upregulation impairs prepulse inhibition of the startle reflex in adult rats. *Glia* 57, 703–713. doi: 10.1002/glia.20798

Benedetti, F., Bollettini, I., Barberi, I., Radaelli, D., Poletti, S., Locatelli, C., et al. (2013). Lithium and GSK3-beta promoter gene variants influence white matter microstructure in bipolar disorder. *Neuropsychopharmacology* 38, 313–327. doi: 10.1038/npp.2012.172

Bengtsson, S. L., Nagy, Z., Skare, S., Forsman, L., Forssberg, H., and Ullen, F. (2005). Extensive piano practicing has regionally specific effects on white matter development. *Nat. Neurosci.* 8, 1148–1150. doi: 10.1038/nn1516

Bergles, D. E., Roberts, J. D., Somogyi, P., and Jahr, C. E. (2000). Glutamatergic synapses on oligodendrocyte precursor cells in the hippocampus. *Nature* 405, 187–191. doi: 10.1038/35012083

Bernardin, F., Maheut-Bosser, A., and Paille, F. (2014). Cognitive impairments in alcohol-dependent subjects. *Front. Psychiatry* 5:78. doi: 10.3389/fpsyt.2014.00078

Bernstein, H. G., Steiner, J., Guest, P. C., Dobrowolny, H., and Bogerts, B. (2015). Glial cells as key players in schizophrenia pathology: recent insights and concepts of therapy. *Schizophr. Res.* 161, 4–18. doi: 10.1016/j.schres.2014.03.035

Beumer, W., Gibney, S. M., Drexhage, R. C., Pont-Lezica, L., Doorduin, J., Klein, H. C., et al. (2012). The immune theory of psychiatric diseases: a key role for activated microglia and circulating monocytes. *J. Leukoc. Biol.* 92, 959–975. doi: 10.1189/jlb.0212100

Bezzi, P., Domercq, M., Vesce, S., and Volterra, A. (2001). Neuron-astrocyte cross-talk during synaptic transmission: physiological and neuropathological implications. *Prog. Brain Res.* 132, 255–265. doi: 10.1016/s0079-6123(01)32081-2

Bezzi, P., Gundersen, V., Galbete, J. L., Seifert, G., Steinhauser, C., Pilati, E., et al. (2004). Astrocytes contain a vesicular compartment that is competent for regulated exocytosis of glutamate. *Nat. Neurosci.* 7, 613–620. doi: 10.1038/nn1246

Biederman, J., and Spencer, T. J. (2000). Genetics of childhood disorders: XIX. ADHD, part 3: is ADHD a noradrenergic disorder? *J. Am. Acad. Child Adolesc. Psychiatry* 39, 1330–1333. doi: 10.1097/00004583-200010000-00024

Blackwood, D. H., Fordyce, A., Walker, M. T., St Clair, D. M., Porteous, D. J., and Muir, W. J. (2001). Schizophrenia and affective disorders–cosegregation with a translocation at chromosome 1q32 that directly disrupts brain-expressed genes: clinical and P300 findings in a family. *Am. J. Hum. Genet.* 69, 428–433. doi: 10.1086/321969

Bowley, M. P., Drevets, W. C., Ongür, D., and Price, J. L. (2002). Low glial numbers in the amygdala in major depressive disorder. *Biol. Psychiatry* 52, 404–412. doi: 10.1016/s0006-3223(02)01404-x

Brambilla, P., Nicoletti, M., Sassi, R. B., Mallinger, A. G., Frank, E., Keshavan, M. S., et al. (2004). Corpus callosum signal intensity in patients with bipolar and unipolar disorder. *J. Neurol. Neurosurg. Psychiatry* 75, 221–225.

Breier, A., Buchanan, R. W., Elkashef, A., Munson, R. C., Kirkpatrick, B., and Gellad, F. (1992). Brain morphology and schizophrenia. A magnetic resonance imaging study of limbic, prefrontal cortex and caudate structures. *Arch. Gen. Psychiatry* 49, 921–926. doi: 10.1001/archpsyc.1992.01820120009003

Brenner, M., Johnson, A. B., Boespflug-Tanguy, O., Rodriguez, D., Goldman, J. E., and Messing, A. (2001). Mutations in GFAP, encoding glial fibrillary acidic protein, are associated with Alexander disease. *Nat. Genet.* 27, 117–120. doi: 10.1038/83679

Burda, J. E., and Sofroniew, M. V. (2014). Reactive gliosis and the multicellular response to CNS damage and disease. *Neuron* 81, 229–248. doi: 10.1016/j.neuron.2013.12.034

Butt, A. M., Hamilton, N., Hubbard, P., Pugh, M., and Ibrahim, M. (2005). Synantocytes: the fifth element. *J. Anat.* 207, 695–706. doi: 10.1111/j.1469-7580.2005.00458.x

Byravan, S., Foster, L. M., Phan, T., Verity, A. N., and Campagnoni, A. T. (1994). Murine oligodendroglial cells express nerve growth factor. *Proc. Natl. Acad. Sci. U S A* 91, 8812–8816. doi: 10.1073/pnas.91.19.8812

Cao, X., Li, L. P., Wang, Q., Wu, Q., Hu, H. H., Zhang, M., et al. (2013). Astrocyte-derived ATP modulates depressive-like behaviors. *Nat. Med.* 19, 773–777. doi: 10.1038/nm.3162

Chambers, J. S., and Perrone-Bizzozero, N. I. (2004). Altered myelination of the hippocampal formation in subjects with schizophrenia and bipolar disorder. *Neurochem. Res.* 29, 2293–2302. doi: 10.1007/s11064-004-7039-x

Chaudhry, I. B., Hallak, J., Husain, N., Minhas, F., Stirling, J., Richardson, P., et al. (2012). Minocycline benefits negative symptoms in early schizophrenia: a randomised double-blind placebo-controlled clinical trial in patients on standard treatment. *J. Psychopharmacol.* 26, 1185–1193. doi: 10.1177/0269881112444941

Chen, S. K., Tvrdik, P., Peden, E., Cho, S., Wu, S., Spangrude, G., et al. (2010). Hematopoietic origin of pathological grooming in Hoxb8 mutant mice. *Cell* 141, 775–785. doi: 10.1016/j.cell.2010.03.055

Chen, S., Velardez, M. O., Warot, X., Yu, Z. X., Miller, S. J., Cros, D., et al. (2006). Neuregulin 1-erbB signaling is necessary for normal myelination and sensory function. *J. Neurosci.* 26, 3079–3086. doi: 10.1523/jneurosci.3785-05.2006

Choi, D. W. (1987). Ionic dependence of glutamate neurotoxicity. *J. Neurosci.* 7, 369–379.

Choudary, P. V., Molnar, M., Evans, S. J., Tomita, H., Li, J. Z., Vawter, M. P., et al. (2005). Altered cortical glutamatergic and GABAergic signal transmission with glial involvement in depression. *Proc. Natl. Acad. Sci. U S A* 102, 15653–15658. doi: 10.1073/pnas.0507901102

Chu, Y., Jin, X., Parada, I., Pesic, A., Stevens, B., Barres, B., et al. (2010). Enhanced synaptic connectivity and epilepsy in C1q knockout mice. *Proc. Natl. Acad. Sci. U S A* 107, 7975–7980. doi: 10.1073/pnas.0913449107

Chuquet, J., Quilichini, P., Nimchinsky, E. A., and Buzsáki, G. (2010). Predominant enhancement of glucose uptake in astrocytes versus neurons during activation of the somatosensory cortex. *J. Neurosci.* 30, 15298–15303. doi: 10.1523/JNEUROSCI.0762-10.2010

Clarke, L. E., Young, K. M., Hamilton, N. B., Li, H., Richardson, W. D., and Attwell, D. (2012). Properties and fate of oligodendrocyte progenitor cells in the corpus callosum, motor cortex and piriform cortex of the mouse. *J. Neurosci.* 32, 8173–8185. doi: 10.1523/JNEUROSCI.0928-12.2012

Claycomb, K. I., Johnson, K. M., Winokur, P. N., Sacino, A. V., and Crocker, S. J. (2013). Astrocyte regulation of CNS inflammation and remyelination. *Brain Sci.* 3, 1109–11027. doi: 10.3390/brainsci3031109

Connor, J. R., and Menzies, S. L. (1996). Relationship of iron to oligodendrocytes and myelination. *Glia* 17, 83–93. doi: 10.1002/(sici)1098-1136(199606)17:2<83::aid-glia1>3.0.co;2-7

Corfas, G., Roy, K., and Buxbaum, J. D. (2004). Neuregulin 1-erbB signaling and the molecular/cellular basis of schizophrenia. *Nat. Neurosci.* 7, 575–580. doi: 10.1038/nn1258

Coric, V., Milanovic, S., Wasylink, S., Patel, P., Malison, R., and Krystal, J. H. (2003). Beneficial effects of the antiglutamatergic agent riluzole in a patient diagnosed with obsessive-compulsive disorder and major depressive disorder. *Psychopharmacology (Berl)* 167, 219–220.

Corona, A. W., Huang, Y., O'Connor, J. C., Dantzer, R., Kelley, K. W., Popovich, P. G., et al. (2010). Fractalkine receptor (CX3CR1) deficiency sensitizes mice to the behavioral changes induced by lipopolysaccharide. *J. Neuroinflammation* 7:93. doi: 10.1186/1742-2094-7-93

Cotter, D., Mackay, D., Chana, G., Beasley, C., Landau, S., and Everall, I. P. (2002). Reduced neuronal size and glial cell density in area 9 of the dorsolateral prefrontal cortex in subjects with major depressive disorder. *Cereb. Cortex* 12, 386–394. doi: 10.1093/cercor/12.4.386

Cotter, D., Mackay, D., Landau, S., Kerwin, R., and Everall, I. (2001). Reduced glial cell density and neuronal size in the anterior cingulate cortex in major depressive disorder. *Arch. Gen. Psychiatry* 58, 545–553. doi: 10.1001/archpsyc.58.6.545

Czeh, B., Muller-Keuker, J. I., Rygula, R., Abumaria, N., Hiemke, C., Domenici, E., et al. (2007). Chronic social stress inhibits cell proliferation in the adult medial prefrontal cortex: hemispheric asymmetry and reversal by fluoxetine treatment. *Neuropsychopharmacology* 32, 1490–1503. doi: 10.1038/sj.npp.1301275

Dawson, M. R., Polito, A., Levine, J. M., and Reynolds, R. (2003). NG2-expressing glial progenitor cells: an abundant and widespread population of cycling cells in the adult rat CNS. *Mol. Cell. Neurosci.* 24, 476–488. doi: 10.1016/s1044-7431(03)00210-0

Dayer, A. G., Cleaver, K. M., Abouantoun, T., and Cameron, H. A. (2005). New GABAergic interneurons in the adult neocortex and striatum are generated from different precursors. *J. Cell Biol.* 168, 415–427. doi: 10.1083/jcb.200407053

De Biase, L. M., Kang, S. H., Baxi, E. G., Fukaya, M., Pucak, M. L., Mishina, M., et al. (2011). NMDA receptor signaling in oligodendrocyte progenitors is not required for oligodendrogenesis and myelination. *J. Neurosci.* 31, 12650–12662. doi: 10.1523/JNEUROSCI.2455-11.2011

De Hoz, L., and Simons, M. (2015). The emerging functions of oligodendrocytes in regulating neuronal network behaviour. *Bioessays* 37, 60–69. doi: 10.1002/bies.201400127

Deadwyler, G. D., Pouly, S., Antel, J. P., and Devries, G. H. (2000). Neuregulins and erbB receptor expression in adult human oligodendrocytes. *Glia* 32, 304–312. doi: 10.1002/1098-1136(200012)32:3<304::aid-glia90>3.0.co;2-z

Deverteuil, R. L., and Lehmann, H. E. (1958). Therapeutic trial of iproniazid (marsilid) in depressed and apathetic patients. *Can. Med. Assoc. J.* 78, 131–133.

Di Benedetto, B., and Rupprecht, R. (2013). Targeting glia cells: novel perspectives for the treatment of neuropsychiatric diseases. *Curr. Neuropharmacol.* 11, 171–185. doi: 10.2174/1570159x11311020004

Dimatelis, J. J., Hsieh, J. H., Sterley, T. L., Marais, L., Womersley, J. S., Vlok, M., et al. (2015). Impaired energy metabolism and disturbed dopamine and glutamate signalling in the striatum and prefrontal cortex of the spontaneously hypertensive rat model of attention-deficit hyperactivity disorder. *J. Mol. Neurosci.* 56, 696–707. doi: 10.1007/s12031-015-0491-z

Dong, W. K., and Greenough, W. T. (2004). Plasticity of nonneuronal brain tissue: roles in developmental disorders. *Ment Retard. Dev. Disabil. Res. Rev.* 10, 85–90. doi: 10.1002/mrdd.20016

Dougherty, D. D., Bonab, A. A., Spencer, T. J., Rauch, S. L., Madras, B. K., and Fischman, A. J. (1999). Dopamine transporter density in patients with attention deficit hyperactivity disorder. *Lancet* 354, 2132–2133. doi: 10.1016/s0140-6736(99)04030-1

Dracheva, S., Davis, K. L., Chin, B., Woo, D. A., Schmeidler, J., and Haroutunian, V. (2006). Myelin-associated mRNA and protein expression deficits in the anterior cingulate cortex and hippocampus in elderly schizophrenia patients. *Neurobiol. Dis.* 21, 531–540. doi: 10.1016/j.nbd.2005.08.012

Drevets, W. C. (1999). Prefrontal cortical-amygdalar metabolism in major depression. *Ann. N Y Acad. Sci.* 877, 614–637. doi: 10.1111/j.1749-6632.1999.tb09292.x

Drevets, W. C. (2000). Functional anatomical abnormalities in limbic and prefrontal cortical structures in major depression. *Prog. Brain Res.* 126, 413–431. doi: 10 1016/s0079-6123(00)26027-5

Drevets, W. C. (2001). Neuroimaging and neuropathological studies of depression: implications for the cognitive-emotional features of mood disorders. *Curr. Opin. Neurobiol.* 11, 240–249. doi: 10.1016/s0959-4388(00)00203-8

Drevets, W. C., Price, J. L., and Furey, M. L. (2008). Brain structural and functional abnormalities in mood disorders: implications for neurocircuitry models of depression. *Brain Struct. Funct.* 213, 93–118. doi: 10.1007/s00429-008-0189-x

Drevets, W. C., Bogers, W., and Raichle, M. E. (2002a). Functional anatomical correlates of antidepressant drug treatment assessed using PET measures of regional glucose metabolism. *Eur. Neuropsychopharmacol.* 12, 527–544. doi: 10.1016/s0924-977x(02)00102-5

Drevets, W. C., Price, J. L., Bardgett, M. E., Reich, T., Todd, R. D., and Raichle, M. E. (2002b). Glucose metabolism in the amygdala in depression: relationship to diagnostic subtype and plasma cortisol levels. *Pharmacol. Biochem. Behav.* 71, 431–447. doi: 10.1016/s0091-3057(01)00687-6

Drevets, W. C., Price, J. L., Simpson, J. R. Jr., Todd, R. D., Reich, T., Vannier, M., et al. (1997). Subgenual prefrontal cortex abnormalities in mood disorders. *Nature* 386, 824–827. doi: 10.1038/386824a0

Dwork, A. J., Mancevski, B., and Rosoklija, G. (2007). White matter and cognitive function in schizophrenia. *Int. J. Neuropsychopharmacol.* 10, 513–536. doi: 10.1017/s1461145707007638

Elsayed, M., Banasr, M., Duric, V., Fournier, N. M., Licznerski, P., and Duman, R. S. (2012). Antidepressant effects of fibroblast growth factor-2 in behavioral and cellular models of depression. *Biol. Psychiatry* 72, 258–265. doi: 10.1016/j.biopsych.2012.03.003

Eng, L. F., Lee, Y. L., Kwan, H., Brenner, M., and Messing, A. (1998). Astrocytes cultured from transgenic mice carrying the added human glial fibrillary acidic protein gene contain Rosenthal fibers. *J. Neurosci. Res.* 53, 353–360. doi: 10.1002/(sici)1097-4547(19980801)53:3<353::aid-jnr9>3.3.co;2-o

Ernst, C., Chen, E. S., and Turecki, G. (2009). Histone methylation and decreased expression of TrkB.T1 in orbital frontal cortex of suicide completers. *Mol. Psychiatry* 14, 830–832. doi: 10.1038/mp.2009.35

Ernst, M., Cohen, R. M., Liebenauer, L. L., Jons, P. H., and Zametkin, A. J. (1997). Cerebral glucose metabolism in adolescent girls with attention-deficit/hyperactivity disorder. *J. Am. Acad. Child Adolesc. Psychiatry* 36, 1399–1406. doi: 10.1097/00004583-199710000-00022

Ernst, M., Liebenauer, L. L., King, A. C., Fitzgerald, G. A., Cohen, R. M., and Zametkin, A. J. (1994). Reduced brain metabolism in hyperactive girls. *J. Am. Acad. Child Adolesc. Psychiatry* 33, 858–868. doi: 10.1097/00004583-199407000-00012

Fair, D. A., Posner, J., Nagel, B. J., Bathula, D., Dias, T. G., Mills, K. L., et al. (2010). Atypical default network connectivity in youth with attention-deficit/hyperactivity disorder. *Biol. Psychiatry* 68, 1084–1091. doi: 10.1016/j.biopsych.2010.07.003

Fales, C. L., Barch, D. M., Rundle, M. M., Mintun, M. A., Snyder, A. Z., Cohen, J. D., et al. (2008). Altered emotional interference processing in affective and cognitive-control brain circuitry in major depression. *Biol. Psychiatry* 63, 377–384. doi: 10.1016/j.biopsych.2007.06.012

Falkai, P., Honer, W. G., David, S., Bogerts, B., Majtenyi, C., and Bayer, T. A. (1999). No evidence for astrogliosis in brains of schizophrenic patients. A post-mortem study. *Neuropathol. Appl. Neurobiol.* 25, 48–53. doi: 10.1046/j.1365-2990.1999.00162.x

Farina, C., Aloisi, F., and Meinl, E. (2007). Astrocytes are active players in cerebral innate immunity. *Trends Immunol.* 28, 138–145. doi: 10.1016/j.it.2007.01.005

Fawcett, F. D. B. A. (1994). *A Textbook of Histology.* New York: Chapman and Hall.

Feresten, A. H., Barakauskas, V., Ypsilanti, A., Barr, A. M., and Beasley, C. L. (2013). Increased expression of glial fibrillary acidic protein in prefrontal cortex in psychotic illness. *Schizophr. Res.* 150, 252–257. doi: 10.1016/j.schres.2013.07.024

Flynn, S. W., Lang, D. J., Mackay, A. L., Goghari, V., Vavasour, I. M., Whittall, K. P., et al. (2003). Abnormalities of myelination in schizophrenia detected *in vivo* with MRI and post-mortem with analysis of oligodendrocyte proteins. *Mol. Psychiatry* 8, 811–820. doi: 10.1038/sj.mp.4001337

Funfschilling, U., Supplie, L. M., Mahad, D., Boretius, S., Saab, A. S., Edgar, J., et al. (2012). Glycolytic oligodendrocytes maintain myelin and long-term axonal integrity. *Nature* 485, 517–521. doi: 10.1038/nature11007

Georgieva, L., Moskvina, V., Peirce, T., Norton, N., Bray, N. J., Jones, L., et al. (2006). Convergent evidence that oligodendrocyte lineage transcription factor 2 (OLIG2) and interacting genes influence susceptibility to schizophrenia. *Proc. Natl. Acad. Sci. U S A* 103, 12469–12474. doi: 10.1073/pnas.0603029103

Giaume, C., Froger, N., and Koulakoff, A. (2005). [Gap junction-mediated intercellular communication in astrocytes and neuroprotection]. *Ann. Fr. Anesth. Reanim.* 24, 695–696. doi: 10.1016/j.annfar.2005.03.014

Ginhoux, F., Greter, M., Leboeuf, M., Nandi, S., See, P., Gokhan, S., et al. (2010). Fate mapping analysis reveals that adult microglia derive from primitive macrophages. *Science* 330, 841–845. doi: 10.1126/science.1194637

Ginhoux, F., Lim, S., Hoeffel, G., Low, D., and Huber, T. (2013). Origin and differentiation of microglia. *Front. Cell. Neurosci.* 7:45. doi: 10.3389/fncel.2013.00045

Gipson, C. D., Reissner, K. J., Kupchik, Y. M., Smith, A. C., Stankeviciute, N., Hensley-Simon, M. E., et al. (2013). Reinstatement of nicotine seeking is mediated by glutamatergic plasticity. *Proc. Natl. Acad. Sci. U S A* 110, 9124–9129. doi: 10.1073/pnas.1220591110

Gittins, R. A., and Harrison, P. J. (2011). A morphometric study of glia and neurons in the anterior cingulate cortex in mood disorder. *J. Affect. Disord.* 133, 328–332. doi: 10.1016/j.jad.2011.03.042

Goldstein, R. Z., and Volkow, N. D. (2002). Drug addiction and its underlying neurobiological basis: neuroimaging evidence for the involvement of the frontal cortex. *Am. J. Psychiatry* 159, 1642–1652. doi: 10.1176/appi.ajp.159.10.1642

Gonzalez, A. M., Berry, M., Maher, P. A., Logan, A., and Baird, A. (1995). A comprehensive analysis of the distribution of FGF-2 and FGFR1 in the rat brain. *Brain Res.* 701, 201–226. doi: 10.1016/0006-8993(95)01002-x

Gos, T., Schroeter, M. L., Lessel, W., Bernstein, H. G., Dobrowolny, H., Schiltz, K., et al. (2013). S100B-immunopositive astrocytes and oligodendrocytes in the hippocampus are differentially afflicted in unipolar and bipolar depression: a postmortem study. *J. Psychiatr. Res.* 47, 1694–1699. doi: 10.1016/j.jpsychires.2013.07.005

Goshen, I., and Yirmiya, R. (2009). Interleukin-1 (IL-1): a central regulator of stress responses. *Front. Neuroendocrinol.* 30, 30–45. doi: 10.1016/j.yfrne.2008.10.001

Graham, B. M., and Richardson, R. (2011). Fibroblast growth factor-2 alters the nature of extinction. *Learn. Mem.* 18, 80–84. doi: 10.1101/lm.2006511

Gregg, J. R., Herring, N. R., Naydenov, A. V., Hanlin, R. P., and Konradi, C. (2009). Downregulation of oligodendrocyte transcripts is associated with impaired prefrontal cortex function in rats. *Schizophr. Res.* 113, 277–287. doi: 10.1016/j.schres.2009.05.023

Gustafsson, P., Thernlund, G., Ryding, E., Rosen, I., and Cederblad, M. (2000). Associations between cerebral blood-flow measured by single photon emission computed tomography (SPECT), electro-encephalogram (EEG), behaviour symptoms, cognition and neurological soft signs in children with attention-deficit hyperactivity disorder (ADHD). *Acta Paediatr.* 89, 830–835. doi: 10.1111/j.1651-2227.2000.tb00391.x

Hagemann, T. L., Paylor, R., and Messing, A. (2013). Deficits in adult neurogenesis, contextual fear conditioning and spatial learning in a Gfap mutant mouse model of Alexander disease. *J. Neurosci.* 33, 18698–18706. doi: 10.1523/JNEUROSCI.3693-13.2013

Hakak, Y., Walker, J. R., Li, C., Wong, W. H., Davis, K. L., Buxbaum, J. D., et al. (2001). Genome-wide expression analysis reveals dysregulation of myelination-related genes in chronic schizophrenia. *Proc. Natl. Acad. Sci. U S A* 98, 4746–4751. doi: 10.1073/pnas.081071198

Hamidi, M., Drevets, W. C., and Price, J. L. (2004). Glial reduction in amygdala in major depressive disorder is due to oligodendrocytes. *Biol. Psychiatry* 55, 563–569. doi: 10.1016/j.biopsych.2003.11.006

Hamilton, N., Hubbard, P. S., and Butt, A. M. (2009). Effects of glutamate receptor activation on NG2-glia in the rat optic nerve. *J. Anat.* 214, 208–218. doi: 10.1111/j.1469-7580.2008.01017.x

Han, X., Chen, M., Wang, F., Windrem, M., Wang, S., Shanz, S., et al. (2013). Forebrain engraftment by human glial progenitor cells enhances synaptic plasticity and learning in adult mice. *Cell Stem Cell* 12, 342–353. doi: 10.1016/j.stem.2012.12.015

Haroutunian, V., Katsel, P., Roussos, P., Davis, K. L., Altshuler, L. L., and Bartzokis, G. (2014). Myelination, oligodendrocytes and serious mental illness. *Glia* 62, 1856–1877. doi: 10.1002/glia.22716

Hart, H., Radua, J., Mataix-Cols, D., and Rubia, K. (2012). Meta-analysis of fMRI studies of timing in attention-deficit hyperactivity disorder (ADHD). *Neurosci. Biobehav. Rev.* 36, 2248–2256. doi: 10.1016/j.neubiorev.2012.08.003

Hashioka, S., Klegeris, A., Monji, A., Kato, T., Sawada, M., Mcgeer, P. L., et al. (2007). Antidepressants inhibit interferon-gamma-induced microglial production of IL-6 and nitric oxide. *Exp. Neurol.* 206, 33–42. doi: 10.1016/j.expneurol.2007.03.022

Hattori, T., Shimizu, S., Koyama, Y., Emoto, H., Matsumoto, Y., Kumamoto, N., et al. (2014). DISC1 (disrupted-in-schizophrenia-1) regulates differentiation of oligodendrocytes. *PLoS One* 9:e88506. doi: 10.1371/journal.pone.0088506

He, J., and Crews, F. T. (2008). Increased MCP-1 and microglia in various regions of the human alcoholic brain. *Exp. Neurol.* 210, 349–358. doi: 10.1016/j.expneurol.2007.11.017

Hercher, C., Chopra, V., and Beasley, C. L. (2014). Evidence for morphological alterations in prefrontal white matter glia in schizophrenia and bipolar disorder. *J. Psychiatry Neurosci.* 39, 376–385. doi: 10.1503/jpn.130277

Herculano-Houzel, S. (2011). Scaling of brain metabolism with a fixed energy budget per neuron: implications for neuronal activity, plasticity and evolution. *PLoS One* 6:e17514. doi: 10.1371/journal.pone.0017514

Hinwood, M., Morandini, J., Day, T. A., and Walker, F. R. (2012). Evidence that microglia mediate the neurobiological effects of chronic psychological stress on the medial prefrontal cortex. *Cereb. Cortex* 22, 1442–1454. doi: 10.1093/cercor/bhr229

Hof, P. R., Haroutunian, V., Friedrich, V. L. Jr., Byne, W., Buitron, C., Perl, D. P., et al. (2003). Loss and altered spatial distribution of oligodendrocytes in the superior frontal gyrus in schizophrenia. *Biol. Psychiatry* 53, 1075–1085. doi: 10.1016/s0006-3223(03)00237-3

Honer, W. G., Falkai, P., Chen, C., Arango, V., Mann, J. J., and Dwork, A. J. (1999). Synaptic and plasticity-associated proteins in anterior frontal cortex in severe mental illness. *Neuroscience* 91, 1247–1255. doi: 10.1016/s0306-4522(98)00679-4

Howren, M. B., Lamkin, D. M., and Suls, J. (2009). Associations of depression with C-reactive protein, IL-1 and IL-6: a meta-analysis. *Psychosom. Med.* 71, 171–186. doi: 10.1097/PSY.0b013e3181907c1b

Hyman, S. E. (2008). A glimmer of light for neuropsychiatric disorders. *Nature* 455, 890–893. doi: 10.1038/nature07454

Ishibashi, T., Dakin, K. A., Stevens, B., Lee, P. R., Kozlov, S. V., Stewart, C. L., et al. (2006). Astrocytes promote myelination in response to electrical impulses. *Neuron* 49, 823–832. doi: 10.1016/j.neuron.2006.02.006

Iwamoto, K., Bundo, M., Yamada, K., Takao, H., Iwayama-Shigeno, Y., Yoshikawa, T., et al. (2005). DNA methylation status of SOX10 correlates with its downregulation and oligodendrocyte dysfunction in schizophrenia. *J. Neurosci.* 25, 5376–5381. doi: 10.1523/jneurosci.0766-05.2005

Jean, Y. Y., Lercher, L. D., and Dreyfus, C. F. (2008). Glutamate elicits release of BDNF from basal forebrain astrocytes in a process dependent on metabotropic receptors and the PLC pathway. *Neuron Glia Biol.* 4, 35–42. doi: 10.1017/S1740925x09000052

Johnston-Wilson, N. L., Sims, C. D., Hofmann, J. P., Anderson, L., Shore, A. D., Torrey, E. F., et al. (2000). Disease-specific alterations in frontal cortex brain proteins in schizophrenia, bipolar disorder and major depressive disorder. The stanley neuropathology consortium. *Mol. Psychiatry* 5, 142–149. doi: 10.1038/sj.mp.4000696

Jourdain, P., Bergersen, L. H., Bhaukaurally, K., Bezzi, P., Santello, M., Domercq, M., et al. (2007). Glutamate exocytosis from astrocytes controls synaptic strength. *Nat. Neurosci.* 10, 331–339. doi: 10.1038/nn1849

Juckel, G., Manitz, M. P., Brüne, M., Friebe, A., Heneka, M. T., and Wolf, R. J. (2011). Microglial activation in a neuroinflammational animal model of schizophrenia-a pilot study. *Schizophr. Res.* 131, 96–100. doi: 10.1016/j.schres.2011.06.018

Kacem, K., Lacombe, P., Seylaz, J., and Bonvento, G. (1998). Structural organization of the perivascular astrocyte endfeet and their relationship with the endothelial glucose transporter: a confocal microscopy study. *Glia* 23, 1–10. doi: 10.1002/(sici)1098-1136(199805)23:1<1::aid-glia1>3.0.co;2-b

Kajitani, N., Hisaoka-Nakashima, K., Morioka, N., Okada-Tsuchioka, M., Kaneko, M., Kasai, M., et al. (2012). Antidepressant acts on astrocytes leading to an increase in the expression of neurotrophic/growth factors: differential regulation of FGF-2 by noradrenaline. *PLoS One* 7:e51197. doi: 10.1371/journal.pone.0051197

Kalivas, P. W. (2009). The glutamate homeostasis hypothesis of addiction. *Nat. Rev. Neurosci.* 10, 561–572. doi: 10.1038/nrn2515

Kalivas, P. W., McFarland, K., Bowers, S., Szumlinski, K., Xi, Z. X., and Baker, D. (2003). Glutamate transmission and addiction to cocaine. *Ann. N Y Acad. Sci.* 1003, 169–175. doi: 10.1196/annals.1300.009

Kandel, E. R. (2000). *Principles of Neuronal Science.* New York: McGraw-Hill.

Kato, T., Monji, A., Hashioka, S., and Kanba, S. (2007). Risperidone significantly inhibits interferon-gamma-induced microglial activation *in vitro*. *Schizophr. Res.* 92, 108–115. doi: 10.1016/j.schres.2007.01.019

Katsel, P., Byne, W., Roussos, P., Tan, W., Siever, L., and Haroutunian, V. (2011a). Astrocyte and glutamate markers in the superficial, deep and white matter layers of the anterior cingulate gyrus in schizophrenia. *Neuropsychopharmacology* 36, 1171–1177. doi: 10.1038/npp.2010.252

Katsel, P., Tan, W., Abazyan, B., Davis, K. L., Ross, C., Pletnikov, M. V., et al. (2011b). Expression of mutant human DISC1 in mice supports abnormalities in differentiation of oligodendrocytes. *Schizophr. Res.* 130, 238–249. doi: 10.1016/j.schres.2011.04.021

Katsel, P., Davis, K. L., Gorman, J. M., and Haroutunian, V. (2005a). Variations in differential gene expression patterns across multiple brain regions in schizophrenia. *Schizophr. Res.* 77, 241–252. doi: 10.1016/j.schres.2005.03.020

Katsel, P., Davis, K. L., and Haroutunian, V. (2005b). Variations in myelin and oligodendrocyte-related gene expression across multiple brain regions in schizophrenia: a gene ontology study. *Schizophr. Res.* 79, 157–173. doi: 10.1016/j.schres.2005.06.007

Katsel, P., Davis, K. L., Li, C., Tan, W., Greenstein, E., Kleiner Hoffman, L. B., et al. (2008). Abnormal indices of cell cycle activity in schizophrenia and their potential association with oligodendrocytes. *Neuropsychopharmacology* 33, 2993–3009. doi: 10.1038/npp.2008.19

Kendell, R. E. (2001). The distinction between mental and physical illness. *Br. J. Psychiatry* 178, 490–493. doi: 10.1192/bjp.178.6.490

Kettenmann, H., Hanisch, U. K., Noda, M., and Verkhratsky, A. (2011). Physiology of microglia. *Physiol. Rev.* 91, 461–553. doi: 10.1152/physrev.00011.2010

Khokhrina, N. T., Kazakova, P. B., and Rakhmanova, V. I. (1991). [Morphometric analysis of the changes in the cerebral cortex of rats after long-term administration of alcohol]. *Zh. Nevropatol. Psikhiatr. Im. S S Korsakova* 91, 66–77.

Killeen, P. R., Russell, V. A., and Sergeant, J. A. (2013). A behavioral neuroenergetics theory of ADHD. *Neurosci. Biobehav. Rev.* 37, 625–657. doi: 10.1016/j.neubiorev.2013.02.011

Kitamura, H., Shioiri, T., Kimura, T., Ohkubo, M., Nakada, T., and Someya, T. (2006). Parietal white matter abnormalities in obsessive-compulsive disorder: a magnetic resonance spectroscopy study at 3-Tesla. *Acta Psychiatr. Scand.* 114, 101–108. doi: 10.1111/j.1600-0447.2006.00858.x

Kodama, M., Fujioka, T., and Duman, R. S. (2004). Chronic olanzapine or fluoxetine administration increases cell proliferation in hippocampus and prefrontal cortex of adult rat. *Biol. Psychiatry* 56, 570–580. doi: 10.1016/j.biopsych.2004.07.008

Kong, E. K., Peng, L., Chen, Y., Yu, A. C., and Hertz, L. (2002). Up-regulation of 5-HT2B receptor density and receptor-mediated glycogenolysis in mouse astrocytes by long-term fluoxetine administration. *Neurochem. Res.* 27, 113–120. doi: 10.1023/A:1014862808126

Kong, H., Zeng, X. N., Fan, Y., Yuan, S. T., Ge, S., Xie, W. P., et al. (2014). Aquaporin-4 knockout exacerbates corticosterone-induced depression by inhibiting astrocyte function and hippocampal neurogenesis. *CNS Neurosci. Ther.* 20, 391–402. doi: 10.1111/cns.12222

Korbo, L. (1999). Glial cell loss in the hippocampus of alcoholics. *Alcohol. Clin. Exp. Res.* 23, 164–168. doi: 10.1111/j.1530-0277.1999.tb04039.x

Krause, K. H., Dresel, S. H., Krause, J., Kung, H. F., and Tatsch, K. (2000). Increased striatal dopamine transporter in adult patients with attention deficit hyperactivity disorder: effects of methylphenidate as measured by single photon emission computed tomography. *Neurosci. Lett.* 285, 107–110. doi: 10.1016/s0304-3940(00)01040-5

Kreft, M., Stenovec, M., Rupnik, M., Grilc, S., Krzan, M., Potokar, M., et al. (2004). Properties of Ca(2+)-dependent exocytosis in cultured astrocytes. *Glia* 46, 437–445. doi: 10.1002/glia.20018

Labuzek, K., Kowalski, J., Gabryel, B., and Herman, Z. S. (2005). Chlorpromazine and loxapine reduce interleukin-1beta and interleukin-2 release by rat mixed glial and microglial cell cultures. *Eur. Neuropsychopharmacol.* 15, 23–30. doi: 10.1016/j.euroneuro.2004.04.002

Lauriat, T. L., Dracheva, S., Chin, B., Schmeidler, J., McInnes, L. A., and Haroutunian, V. (2006). Quantitative analysis of glutamate transporter mRNA expression in prefrontal and primary visual cortex in normal and schizophrenic brain. *Neuroscience* 137, 843–851. doi: 10.1016/j.neuroscience.2005.10.003

Lee, H. S., Ghetti, A., Pinto-Duarte, A., Wang, X., Dziewczapolski, G., Galimi, F., et al. (2014). Astrocytes contribute to gamma oscillations and recognition memory. *Proc. Natl. Acad. Sci. U S A* 111, E3343–E3352. doi: 10.1073/pnas.1410893111

Lee, Y., Morrison, B. M., Li, Y., Lengacher, S., Farah, M. H., Hoffman, P. N., et al. (2012). Oligodendroglia metabolically support axons and contribute to neurodegeneration. *Nature* 487, 443–448. doi: 10.1038/nature11314

Leventopoulos, M., Rüedi-Bettschen, D., Knuesel, I., Feldon, J., Pryce, C. R., and Opacka-Juffry, J. (2007). Long-term effects of early life deprivation on brain glia in Fischer rats. *Brain Res.* 1142, 119–126. doi: 10.1016/j.brainres.2007.01.039

Levine, E. S., Dreyfus, C. F., Black, I. B., and Plummer, M. R. (1995). Brain-derived neurotrophic factor rapidly enhances synaptic transmission in hippocampal neurons via postsynaptic tyrosine kinase receptors. *Proc. Natl. Acad. Sci. U S A* 92, 8074–8077. doi: 10.1073/pnas.92.17.8074

Levkovitz, Y., Mendlovich, S., Riwkes, S., Braw, Y., Levkovitch-Verbin, H., Gal, G., et al. (2010). A double-blind, randomized study of minocycline for the treatment of negative and cognitive symptoms in early-phase schizophrenia. *J. Clin. Psychiatry* 71, 138–149. doi: 10.4088/JCP.08m04666yel

Lewohl, J. M., Wang, L., Miles, M. F., Zhang, L., Dodd, P. R., and Harris, R. A. (2000). Gene expression in human alcoholism: microarray analysis of frontal cortex. *Alcohol Clin. Exp. Res.* 24, 1873–1882. doi: 10.1111/j.1530-0277.2000.tb01993.x

Li, Y. K., Wang, F., Wang, W., Luo, Y., Wu, P. F., Xiao, J. L., et al. (2012). Aquaporin-4 deficiency impairs synaptic plasticity and associative fear memory in the lateral amygdala: involvement of downregulation of glutamate transporter-1 expression. *Neuropsychopharmacology* 37, 1867–1878. doi: 10.1038/npp.2012.34

Li, L., Wu, M., Liao, Y., Ouyang, L., Du, M., Lei, D., et al. (2014). Grey matter reduction associated with posttraumatic stress disorder and traumatic stress. *Neurosci. Biobehav. Rev.* 43, 163–172. doi: 10.1016/j.neubiorev.2014.04.003

Lin, S. C., and Bergles, D. E. (2002). Physiological characteristics of NG2-expressing glial cells. *J. Neurocytol.* 31, 537–549. doi: 10.1023/A:1025799816285

Liotti, M., and Mayberg, H. S. (2001). The role of functional neuroimaging in the neuropsychology of depression. *J. Clin. Exp. Neuropsychol.* 23, 121–136. doi: 10.1076/jcen.23.1.121.1223

Liu, J., Lewohl, J. M., Dodd, P. R., Randall, P. K., Harris, R. A., and Mayfield, R. D. (2004). Gene expression profiling of individual cases reveals consistent transcriptional changes in alcoholic human brain. *J. Neurochem.* 90, 1050–1058. doi: 10.1111/j.1471-4159.2004.02570.x

Lo, D. C. (1995). Neurotrophic factors and synaptic plasticity. *Neuron* 15, 979–981. doi: 10.1016/0896-6273(95)90085-3

Ma, T. M., Abazyan, S., Abazyan, B., Nomura, J., Yang, C., Seshadri, S., et al. (2013). Pathogenic disruption of DISC1-serine racemase binding elicits schizophrenia-like behavior via D-serine depletion. *Mol. Psychiatry* 18, 557–567. doi: 10.1038/mp.2012.97

Magistretti, P. J. (1988). Regulation of glycogenolysis by neurotransmitters in the central nervous system. *Diabete Metab.* 14, 237–246.

Magistretti, P. J., and Allaman, I. (2015). A cellular perspective on brain energy metabolism and functional imaging. *Neuron* 86, 883–901. doi: 10.1016/j.neuron.2015.03.035

Magistretti, P. J., Morrison, J. H., Shoemaker, W. J., Sapin, V., and Bloom, F. E. (1981). Vasoactive intestinal polypeptide induces glycogenolysis in mouse cortical slices: a possible regulatory mechanism for the local control of energy metabolism. *Proc. Natl. Acad. Sci. U S A* 78, 6535–6539. doi: 10.1073/pnas.78.10.6535

Magistretti, P. J., Sorg, O., Yu, N., Martin, J. L., and Pellerin, L. (1993). Neurotransmitters regulate energy metabolism in astrocytes: implications for the metabolic trafficking between neural cells. *Dev. Neurosci.* 15, 306–312. doi: 10.1159/000111349

Makinodan, M., Rosen, K. M., Ito, S., and Corfas, G. (2012). A critical period for social experience-dependent oligodendrocyte maturation and myelination. *Science* 337, 1357–1360. doi: 10.1126/science.1220845

Mandyam, C. D., Wee, S., Eisch, A. J., Richardson, H. N., and Koob, G. F. (2007). Methamphetamine self-administration and voluntary exercise have opposing effects on medial prefrontal cortex gliogenesis. *J. Neurosci.* 27, 11442–11450. doi: 10.1523/jneurosci.2505-07.2007

Manji, H. K., Drevets, W. C., and Charney, D. S. (2001). The cellular neurobiology of depression. *Nat. Med.* 7, 541–547. doi: 10.1038/87865

Markham, J. A., and Greenough, W. T. (2004). Experience-driven brain plasticity: beyond the synapse. *Neuron Glia Biol.* 1, 351–363. doi: 10.1017/s1740925x05000219

Mathew, S. J., Amiel, J. M., Coplan, J. D., Fitterling, H. A., Sackeim, H. A., and Gorman, J. M. (2005). Open-label trial of riluzole in generalized anxiety disorder. *Am. J. Psychiatry* 162, 2379–2381. doi: 10.1176/appi.ajp.162.12.2379

Mattei, D., Djodari-Irani, A., Hadar, R., Pelz, A., De Cossio, L. F., Goetz, T., et al. (2014). Minocycline rescues decrease in neurogenesis, increase in microglia cytokines and deficits in sensorimotor gating in an animal model of schizophrenia. *Brain Behav. Immun.* 38, 175–184. doi: 10.1016/j.bbi.2014.01.019

Matthews, S. C., Strigo, I. A., Simmons, A. N., Yang, T. T., and Paulus, M. P. (2008). Decreased functional coupling of the amygdala and supragenual cingulate is related to increased depression in unmedicated individuals with current major depressive disorder. *J. Affect. Disord.* 111, 13–20. doi: 10.1016/j.jad.2008.05.022

Matute, C. (2006). Oligodendrocyte NMDA receptors: a novel therapeutic target. *Trends Mol. Med.* 12, 289–292. doi: 10.1016/j.molmed.2006.05.004

Matute, C., Melone, M., Vallejo-Illarramendi, A., and Conti, F. (2005). Increased expression of the astrocytic glutamate transporter GLT-1 in the prefrontal cortex of schizophrenics. *Glia* 49, 451–455. doi: 10.1002/glia.20119

Matute, C., Sánchez-Gómez, M. V., Martínez-Millán, L., and Miledi, R. (1997). Glutamate receptor-mediated toxicity in optic nerve oligodendrocytes. *Proc. Natl. Acad. Sci. U S A* 94, 8830–8835. doi: 10.1073/pnas.94.16.8830

Mayberg, H. S. (2003). Modulating dysfunctional limbic-cortical circuits in depression: towards development of brain-based algorithms for diagnosis and optimised treatment. *Br. Med. Bull.* 65, 193–207. doi: 10.1093/bmb/65.1.193

Mayberg, H. S., Brannan, S. K., Tekell, J. L., Silva, J. A., Mahurin, R. K., McGinnis, S., et al. (2000). Regional metabolic effects of fluoxetine in major depression: serial changes and relationship to clinical response. *Biol. Psychiatry* 48, 830–843. doi: 10.1016/s0006-3223(00)01036-2

Mayfield, R. D., Lewohl, J. M., Dodd, P. R., Herlihy, A., Liu, J., and Harris, R. A. (2002). Patterns of gene expression are altered in the frontal and motor cortices of human alcoholics. *J. Neurochem.* 81, 802–813. doi: 10.1046/j.1471-4159.2002.00860.x

McDonald, J. W., Levine, J. M., and Qu, Y. (1998). Multiple classes of the oligodendrocyte lineage are highly vulnerable to excitotoxicity. *Neuroreport* 9, 2757–2762. doi: 10.1097/00001756-199808240-00014

Medina, A., Burke, S., Thompson, R. C., Bunney, W. Jr., Myers, R. M., Schatzberg, A., et al. (2013). Glutamate transporters: a key piece in the glutamate puzzle of major depressive disorder. *J. Psychiatr. Res.* 47, 1150–1156. doi: 10.1016/j.jpsychires.2013.04.007

Messing, A., Brenner, M., Feany, M. B., Nedergaard, M., and Goldman, J. E. (2012). Alexander disease. *J. Neurosci.* 32, 5017–5023. doi: 10.1523/JNEUROSCI.5384-11.2012

Miguel-Hidalgo, J. J. (2005). Lower packing density of glial fibrillary acidic protein-immunoreactive astrocytes in the prelimbic cortex of alcohol-naive and alcohol-drinking alcohol-preferring rats as compared with alcohol-nonpreferring and Wistar rats. *Alcohol. Clin. Exp. Res.* 29, 766–772. doi: 10.1097/01.alc.0000164378.92680.fa

Miguel-Hidalgo, J. J. (2009). The role of Glial cells in drug abuse. *Curr. Drug Abuse Rev.* 2, 76–82. doi: 10.2174/1874473710902010076

Miguel-Hidalgo, J. J., Baucom, C., Dilley, G., Overholser, J. C., Meltzer, H. Y., Stockmeier, C. A., et al. (2000). Glial fibrillary acidic protein immunoreactivity in the prefrontal cortex distinguishes younger from older adults in major depressive disorder. *Biol. Psychiatry* 48, 861–873. doi: 10.1016/s0006-3223(00)00999-9

Miguel-Hidalgo, J. J., Overholser, J. C., Meltzer, H. Y., Stockmeier, C. A., and Rajkowska, G. (2006). Reduced glial and neuronal packing density in the orbitofrontal cortex in alcohol dependence and its relationship with suicide and duration of alcohol dependence. *Alcohol. Clin. Exp. Res.* 30, 1845–1855. doi: 10.1111/j.1530-0277.2006.00221.x

Miguel-Hidalgo, J., Shoyama, Y., and Wanzo, V. (2009). Infusion of gliotoxins or a gap junction blocker in the prelimbic cortex increases alcohol preference in Wistar rats. *J. Psychopharmacol.* 23, 550–557. doi: 10.1177/0269881108091074

Miguel-Hidalgo, J. J., Wei, J., Andrew, M., Overholser, J. C., Jurjus, G., Stockmeier, C. A., et al. (2002). Glia pathology in the prefrontal cortex in alcohol dependence with and without depressive symptoms. *Biol. Psychiatry* 52, 1121–1133. doi: 10.1016/s0006-3223(02)01439-7

Miguel-Hidalgo, J. J., Wilson, B. A., Hussain, S., Meshram, A., Rajkowska, G., and Stockmeier, C. A. (2014). Reduced connexin 43 immunolabeling in the orbitofrontal cortex in alcohol dependence and depression. *J. Psychiatr. Res.* 55, 101–109. doi: 10.1016/j.jpsychires.2014.04.007

Miller, D. J., Duka, T., Stimpson, C. D., Schapiro, S. J., Baze, W. B., Mcarthur, M. J., et al. (2012). Prolonged myelination in human neocortical evolution. *Proc. Natl. Acad. Sci. U S A* 109, 16480–16485. doi: 10.1073/pnas.1117943109

Millar, J. K., Wilson-Annan, J. C., Anderson, S., Christie, S., Taylor, M. S., Semple, C. A., et al. (2000). Disruption of two novel genes by a translocation co-segregating with schizophrenia. *Hum. Mol. Genet.* 9, 1415–1423. doi: 10.1093/hmg/9.9.1415

Miyaoka, T., Yasukawa, R., Yasuda, H., Hayashida, M., Inagaki, T., and Horiguchi, J. (2007). Possible antipsychotic effects of minocycline in patients with schizophrenia. *Prog. Neuropsychopharmacol. Biol. Psychiatry* 31, 304–307. doi: 10.1016/j.pnpbp.2006.08.013

Miyazaki, J., Nakanishi, S., and Jingami, H. (1999). Expression and characterization of a glycine-binding fragment of the N-methyl-D-aspartate receptor subunit NR1. *Biochem. J.* 340(Pt. 3), 687–692. doi: 10.1042/0264-6021:3400687

Montana, V., Ni, Y., Sunjara, V., Hua, X., and Parpura, V. (2004). Vesicular glutamate transporter-dependent glutamate release from astrocytes. *J. Neurosci.* 24, 2633–2642. doi: 10.1523/jneurosci.3770-03.2004

Mulholland, P. J., Carpenter-Hyland, E. P., Woodward, J. J., and Chandler, L. J. (2009). Ethanol disrupts NMDA receptor and astroglial EAAT2 modulation of Kv2.1 potassium channels in hippocampus. *Alcohol* 43, 45–50. doi: 10.1016/j.alcohol.2008.10.001

Nagel, B. J., Bathula, D., Herting, M., Schmitt, C., Kroenke, C. D., Fair, D., et al. (2011). Altered white matter microstructure in children with attention-deficit/hyperactivity disorder. *J. Am. Acad. Child Adolesc. Psychiatry* 50, 283–292. doi: 10.1016/j.jaac.2010.12.003

Nagy, C., Suderman, M., Yang, J., Szyf, M., Mechawar, N., Ernst, C., et al. (2015). Astrocytic abnormalities and global DNA methylation patterns in depression and suicide. *Mol. Psychiatry* 20, 320–328. doi: 10.1038/mp.2014.21

Nedergaard, M., Ransom, B., and Goldman, S. A. (2003). New roles for astrocytes: redefining the functional architecture of the brain. *Trends Neurosci.* 26, 523–530. doi: 10.1016/j.tins.2003.08.008

Nestler, E. J., and Hyman, S. E. (2010). Animal models of neuropsychiatric disorders. *Nat. Neurosci.* 13, 1161–1169. doi: 10.1038/nn.2647

Nichols, N. R., Osterburg, H. H., Masters, J. N., Millar, S. L., and Finch, C. E. (1990). Messenger RNA for glial fibrillary acidic protein is decreased in rat brain following acute and chronic corticosterone treatment. *Brain Res. Mol. Brain Res.* 7, 1–7. doi: 10.1016/0169-328x(90)90066-m

Oberheim, N. A., Takano, T., Han, X., He, W., Lin, J. H., Wang, F., et al. (2009). Uniquely hominid features of adult human astrocytes. *J. Neurosci.* 29, 3276–3287. doi: 10.1523/JNEUROSCI.4707-08.2009

Obuchowicz, E., Bielecka, A. M., Paul-Samojedny, M., Pudelko, A., and Kowalski, J. (2014). Imipramine and fluoxetine inhibit LPS-induced activation and affect morphology of microglial cells in the rat glial culture. *Pharmacol. Rep.* 66, 34–43. doi: 10.1016/j.pharep.2013.08.002

Ohashi, M., Saitoh, A., Yamada, M., Oka, J., and Yamada, M. (2015). Riluzole in the prelimbic medial prefrontal cortex attenuates veratrine-induced anxiety-like behaviors in mice. *Psychopharmacology (Berl)* 232, 391–398. doi: 10.1007/s00213-014-3676-1

Okamoto, H., Miki, T., Lee, K. Y., Yokoyama, T., Kuma, H., Wang, Z. Y., et al. (2006). Oligodendrocyte myelin glycoprotein (OMgp) in rat hippocampus is depleted by chronic ethanol consumption. *Neurosci. Lett.* 406, 76–80. doi: 10.1016/j.neulet.2006.07.023

Ongur, D., Drevets, W. C., and Price, J. L. (1998). Glial reduction in the subgenual prefrontal cortex in mood disorders. *Proc. Natl. Acad. Sci. U S A* 95, 13290–13295. doi: 10.1073/pnas.95.22.13290

Orre, K., Wennström, M., and Tingström, A. (2009). Chronic lithium treatment decreases NG2 cell proliferation in rat dentate hilus, amygdala and corpus callosum. *Prog. Neuropsychopharmacol. Biol. Psychiatry* 33, 503–510. doi: 10.1016/j.pnpbp.2009.01.015

Orthmann-Murphy, J. L., Abrams, C. K., and Scherer, S. S. (2008). Gap junctions couple astrocytes and oligodendrocytes. *J. Mol. Neurosci.* 35, 101–116. doi: 10.1007/s12031-007-9027-5

Osbun, N., Li, J., O'Driscoll, M. C., Strominger, Z., Wakahiro, M., Rider, E., et al. (2011). Genetic and functional analyses identify DISC1 as a novel callosal agenesis candidate gene. *Am. J. Med. Genet. A* 155A, 1865–1876. doi: 10.1002/ajmg.a.34081

Owen, F., Crow, T. J., Frith, C. D., Johnson, J. A., Johnstone, E. C., Lofthouse, R., et al. (1987). Selective decreases in MAO-B activity in post-mortem brains from schizophrenic patients with type II syndrome. *Br. J. Psychiatry* 151, 514–519. doi: 10.1192/bjp.151.4.514

Paillere-Martinot, M., Caclin, A., Artiges, E., Poline, J. B., Joliot, M., Mallet, L., et al. (2001). Cerebral gray and white matter reductions and clinical correlates in patients with early onset schizophrenia. *Schizophr. Res.* 50, 19–26. doi: 10.1016/s0920-9964(00)00137-7

Patte, C., Gandolfo, P., Leprince, J., Thoumas, J. L., Fontaine, M., Vaudry, H., et al. (1999). GABA inhibits endozepine release from cultured rat astrocytes. *Glia* 25, 404–411. doi: 10.1002/(sici)1098-1136(19990215)25:4<404::aid-glia9>3.0.co;2-q

Pellerin, L., and Magistretti, P. J. (1994). Glutamate uptake into astrocytes stimulates aerobic glycolysis: a mechanism coupling neuronal activity to glucose utilization. *Proc. Natl. Acad. Sci. U S A* 91, 10625–10629. doi: 10.1073/pnas.91.22.10625

Pelvig, D. P., Pakkenberg, H., Stark, A. K., and Pakkenberg, B. (2008). Neocortical glial cell numbers in human brains. *Neurobiol. Aging* 29, 1754–1762. doi: 10.1016/j.neurobiolaging.2007.04.013

Pennington, K., Beasley, C. L., Dicker, P., Fagan, A., English, J., Pariante, C. M., et al. (2008). Prominent synaptic and metabolic abnormalities revealed by proteomic analysis of the dorsolateral prefrontal cortex in schizophrenia and bipolar disorder. *Mol. Psychiatry* 13, 1102–1117. doi: 10.1038/sj.mp.4002098

Pereira, A. Jr., and Furlan, F. A. (2010). Astrocytes and human cognition: modeling information integration and modulation of neuronal activity. *Prog. Neurobiol.* 92, 405–420. doi: 10.1016/j.pneurobio.2010.07.001

Perez, J. A., Clinton, S. M., Turner, C. A., Watson, S. J., and Akil, H. (2009). A new role for FGF2 as an endogenous inhibitor of anxiety. *J. Neurosci.* 29, 6379–6387. doi: 10.1523/JNEUROSCI.4829-08.2009

Peters, A. (2004). A fourth type of neuroglial cell in the adult central nervous system. *J. Neurocytol.* 33, 345–357. doi: 10.1023/b:neur.0000044195.64009.27

Pfefferbaum, A., Sullivan, E. V., Hedehus, M., Adalsteinsson, E., Lim, K. O., and Moseley, M. (2000). *In vivo* detection and functional correlates of white matter microstructural disruption in chronic alcoholism. *Alcohol. Clin. Exp. Res.* 24, 1214–1221. doi: 10.1111/j.1530-0277.2000.tb02086.x

Pittenger, C., Coric, V., Banasr, M., Bloch, M., Krystal, J. H., and Sanacora, G. (2008). Riluzole in the treatment of mood and anxiety disorders. *CNS Drugs* 22, 761–786. doi: 10.2165/00023210-200822090-00004

Ponomarev, I., Rau, V., Eger, E. I., Harris, R. A., and Fanselow, M. S. (2010). Amygdala transcriptome and cellular mechanisms underlying stress-enhanced fear learning in a rat model of posttraumatic stress disorder. *Neuropsychopharmacology* 35, 1402–1411. doi: 10.1038/npp.2010.10

Prust, M., Wang, J., Morizono, H., Messing, A., Brenner, M., Gordon, E., et al. (2011). GFAP mutations, age at onset and clinical subtypes in Alexander disease. *Neurology* 77, 1287–1294. doi: 10.1212/WNL.0b013e3182309f72

Quesseveur, G., David, D. J., Gaillard, M. C., Pla, P., Wu, M. V., Nguyen, H. T., et al. (2013). BDNF overexpression in mouse hippocampal astrocytes promotes local neurogenesis and elicits anxiolytic-like activities. *Transl. Psychiatry* 3:e253. doi: 10.1038/tp.2013.30

Radewicz, K., Garey, L. J., Gentleman, S. M., and Reynolds, R. (2000). Increase in HLA-DR immunoreactive microglia in frontal and temporal cortex of chronic schizophrenics. *J. Neuropathol. Exp. Neurol.* 59, 137–150.

Rajkowska, G. (2002a). Cell pathology in bipolar disorder. *Bipolar Disord.* 4, 105–116. doi: 10.1034/j.1399-5618.2002.01149.x

Rajkowska, G. (2002b). Cell pathology in mood disorders. *Semin. Clin. Neuropsychiatry* 7, 281–292. doi: 10.1053/scnp.2002.35228

Rajkowska, G., Halaris, A., and Selemon, L. D. (2001). Reductions in neuronal and glial density characterize the dorsolateral prefrontal cortex in bipolar disorder. *Biol. Psychiatry* 49, 741–752. doi: 10.1016/s0006-3223(01)01080-0

Rajkowska, G., Hughes, J., Stockmeier, C. A., Javier Miguel-Hidalgo, J., and Maciag, D. (2013). Coverage of blood vessels by astrocytic endfeet is reduced in major depressive disorder. *Biol. Psychiatry* 73, 613–621. doi: 10.1016/j.biopsych.2012.09.024

Rajkowska, G., and Miguel-Hidalgo, J. J. (2007). Gliogenesis and glial pathology in depression. *CNS Neurol. Disord. Drug Targets* 6, 219–233. doi: 10.2174/187152707780619326

Rajkowska, G., Miguel-Hidalgo, J. J., Wei, J., Dilley, G., Pittman, S. D., Meltzer, H. Y., et al. (1999). Morphometric evidence for neuronal and glial prefrontal cell pathology in major depression. *Biol. Psychiatry* 45, 1085–1098. doi: 10.1016/s0006-3223(99)00041-4

Regenold, W. T., Phatak, P., Marano, C. M., Gearhart, L., Viens, C. H., and Hisley, K. C. (2007). Myelin staining of deep white matter in the dorsolateral prefrontal cortex in schizophrenia, bipolar disorder and unipolar major depression. *Psychiatry Res.* 151, 179–188. doi: 10.1016/j.psychres.2006.12.019

Richardson, W. D., Young, K. M., Tripathi, R. B., and McKenzie, I. (2011). NG2-glia as multipotent neural stem cells: fact or fantasy? *Neuron* 70, 661–673. doi: 10.1016/j.neuron.2011.05.013

Rimondini, R., Arlinde, C., Sommer, W., and Heilig, M. (2002). Long-lasting increase in voluntary ethanol consumption and transcriptional regulation in the rat brain after intermittent exposure to alcohol. *FASEB J.* 16, 27–35. doi: 10.1096/fj.01-0593com

Rinholm, J. E., Hamilton, N. B., Kessaris, N., Richardson, W. D., Bergersen, L. H., and Attwell, D. (2011). Regulation of oligodendrocyte development and myelination by glucose and lactate. *J. Neurosci.* 31, 538–548. doi: 10.1523/JNEUROSCI.3516-10.2011

Rodriguez, D., Gauthier, F., Bertini, E., Bugiani, M., Brenner, M., N'Guyen, S., et al. (2001). Infantile Alexander disease: spectrum of GFAP mutations and genotype-phenotype correlation. *Am. J. Hum. Genet.* 69, 1134–1140. doi: 10.1086/323799

Rothstein, J. D., Dykes-Hoberg, M., Pardo, C. A., Bristol, L. A., Jin, L., Kuncl, R. W., et al. (1996). Knockout of glutamate transporters reveals a major role for astroglial transport in excitotoxicity and clearance of glutamate. *Neuron* 16, 675–686. doi: 10.1016/s0896-6273(00)80086-0

Roy, K., Murtie, J. C., El-Khodor, B. F., Edgar, N., Sardi, S. P., Hooks, B. M., et al. (2007). Loss of erbB signaling in oligodendrocytes alters myelin and dopaminergic function, a potential mechanism for neuropsychiatric disorders. *Proc. Natl. Acad. Sci. U S A* 104, 8131–8136. doi: 10.1073/pnas.0702157104

Russell, V. A., Oades, R. D., Tannock, R., Killeen, P. R., Auerbach, J. G., Johansen, E. B., et al. (2006). Response variability in attention-deficit/hyperactivity disorder: a neuronal and glial energetics hypothesis. *Behav. Brain Funct.* 2:30. doi: 10.1186/1744-9081-2-30

Sanacora, G., and Banasr, M. (2013). From pathophysiology to novel antidepressant drugs: glial contributions to the pathology and treatment of mood disorders. *Biol. Psychiatry* 73, 1172–1179. doi: 10.1016/j.biopsych.2013.03.032

Sanchez-Abarca, L. I., Tabernero, A., and Medina, J. M. (2001). Oligodendrocytes use lactate as a source of energy and as a precursor of lipids. *Glia* 36, 321–329. doi: 10.1002/glia.1119

Sandau, U. S., Alderman, Z., Corfas, G., Ojeda, S. R., and Raber, J. (2012). Astrocyte-specific disruption of SynCAM1 signaling results in ADHD-like behavioral manifestations. *PLoS One* 7:e36424. doi: 10.1371/journal.pone.0036424

Sander, T., Ostapowicz, A., Samochowiec, J., Smolka, M., Winterer, G., and Schmidt, L. G. (2000). Genetic variation of the glutamate transporter EAAT2 gene and vulnerability to alcohol dependence. *Psychiatr. Genet.* 10, 103–107. doi: 10.1097/00041444-200010030-00001

Sari, Y., and Sreemantula, S. N. (2012). Neuroimmunophilin GPI-1046 reduces ethanol consumption in part through activation of GLT1 in alcohol-preferring rats. *Neuroscience* 227, 327–335. doi: 10.1016/j.neuroscience.2012.10.007

Sawaishi, Y. (2009). Review of Alexander disease: beyond the classical concept of leukodystrophy. *Brain Dev.* 31, 493–498. doi: 10.1016/j.braindev.2009.03.006

Schafer, D. P., Lehrman, E. K., Kautzman, A. G., Koyama, R., Mardinly, A. R., Yamasaki, R., et al. (2012). Microglia sculpt postnatal neural circuits in an activity and complement-dependent manner. *Neuron* 74, 691–705. doi: 10.1016/j.neuron.2012.03.026

Schell, M. J., Molliver, M. E., and Snyder, S. H. (1995). D-serine, an endogenous synaptic modulator: localization to astrocytes and glutamate-stimulated release. *Proc. Natl. Acad. Sci. U S A* 92, 3948–3952. doi: 10.1073/pnas.92.9.3948

Schmitt, A., Steyskal, C., Bernstein, H. G., Schneider-Axmann, T., Parlapani, E., Schaeffer, E. L., et al. (2009). Stereologic investigation of the posterior part of the hippocampus in schizophrenia. *Acta Neuropathol.* 117, 395–407. doi: 10.1007/s00401-008-0430-y

Scholz, J., Klein, M. C., Behrens, T. E., and Johansen-Berg, H. (2009). Training induces changes in white-matter architecture. *Nat. Neurosci.* 12, 1370–1371. doi: 10.1038/nn.2412

Scofield, M. D., and Kalivas, P. W. (2014). Astrocytic dysfunction and addiction: consequences of impaired glutamate homeostasis. *Neuroscientist* 20, 610–622. doi: 10.1177/1073858413520347

Seedat, S., Videen, J. S., Kennedy, C. M., and Stein, M. B. (2005). Single voxel proton magnetic resonance spectroscopy in women with and without intimate partner violence-related posttraumatic stress disorder. *Psychiatry Res.* 139, 249–258. doi: 10.1016/j.pscychresns.2005.06.001

Semrud-Clikeman, M., Steingard, R. J., Filipek, P., Biederman, J., Bekken, K., and Renshaw, P. F. (2000). Using MRI to examine brain-behavior relationships in males with attention deficit disorder with hyperactivity. *J. Am. Acad. Child Adolesc. Psychiatry* 39, 477–484. doi: 10.1097/00004583-200004000-00017

Serra-De-Oliveira, N., Boilesen, S. N., Prado De Franca Carvalho, C., LeSueur-Maluf, L., Zollner, R. L., Spadari, R. C., et al. (2015). Behavioural changes observed in demyelination model shares similarities with white matter abnormalities in humans. *Behav. Brain Res.* 287, 265–275. doi: 10.1016/j.bbr.2015.03.038

Silberberg, G., Darvasi, A., Pinkas-Kramarski, R., and Navon, R. (2006). The involvement of ErbB4 with schizophrenia: association and expression studies. *Am. J. Med. Genet. B Neuropsychiatr. Genet.* 141B, 142–148. doi: 10.1002/ajmg.b.30275

Snider, S. E., Hendrick, E. S., and Beardsley, P. M. (2013). Glial cell modulators attenuate methamphetamine self-administration in the rat. *Eur. J. Pharmacol.* 701, 124–130. doi: 10.1016/j.ejphar.2013.01.016

Sorg, O., and Magistretti, P. J. (1991). Characterization of the glycogenolysis elicited by vasoactive intestinal peptide, noradrenaline and adenosine in primary cultures of mouse cerebral cortical astrocytes. *Brain Res.* 563, 227–233. doi: 10.1016/0006-8993(91)91538-c

Souza Ade, A., Da Silva, G. S., Velez, B. S., Santoro, A. B., and Montero-Lomeli, M. (2010). Glycogen synthesis in brain and astrocytes is inhibited by chronic lithium treatment. *Neurosci. Lett.* 482, 128–132. doi: 10.1016/j.neulet.2010.07.016

Sparacio, S. M., Zhang, Y., Vilcek, J., and Benveniste, E. N. (1992). Cytokine regulation of interleukin-6 gene expression in astrocytes involves activation of an NF-$\kappa$ B-like nuclear protein. *J. Neuroimmunol.* 39, 231–242. doi: 10.1016/0165-5728(92)90257-l

Stark, A. K., Uylings, H. B., Sanz-Arigita, E., and Pakkenberg, B. (2004). Glial cell loss in the anterior cingulate cortex, a subregion of the prefrontal cortex, in subjects with schizophrenia. *Am. J. Psychiatry* 161, 882–888. doi: 10.1176/appi.ajp.161.5.882

Steffek, A. E., McCullumsmith, R. E., Haroutunian, V., and Meador-Woodruff, J. H. (2008). Cortical expression of glial fibrillary acidic protein and glutamine synthetase is decreased in schizophrenia. *Schizophr. Res.* 103, 71–82. doi: 10.1016/j.schres.2008.04.032

Steiner, J., Bielau, H., Brisch, R., Danos, P., Ullrich, O., Mawrin, C., et al. (2008). Immunological aspects in the neurobiology of suicide: elevated microglial density in schizophrenia and depression is associated with suicide. *J. Psychiatr. Res.* 42, 151–157. doi: 10.1016/j.jpsychires.2006.10.013

Steiner, J., Walter, M., Gos, T., Guillemin, G. J., Bernstein, H. G., Sarnyai, Z., et al. (2011). Severe depression is associated with increased microglial quinolinic acid in subregions of the anterior cingulate gyrus: evidence for an immune-modulated glutamatergic neurotransmission? *J. Neuroinflammation* 8:94. doi: 10.1186/1742-2094-8-94

Stewart, S. E., Platko, J., Fagerness, J., Birns, J., Jenike, E., Smoller, J. W., et al. (2007). A genetic family-based association study of OLIG2 in obsessive-compulsive disorder. *Arch. Gen. Psychiatry* 64, 209–214. doi: 10.1001/archpsyc.64.2.209

Suzuki, A., Stern, S. A., Bozdagi, O., Huntley, G. W., Walker, R. H., Magistretti, P. J., et al. (2011). Astrocyte-neuron lactate transport is required for long-term memory formation. *Cell* 144, 810–823. doi: 10.1016/j.cell.2011.02.018

Takano, T., Tian, G. F., Peng, W., Lou, N., Libionka, W., Han, X., et al. (2006). Astrocyte-mediated control of cerebral blood flow. *Nat. Neurosci.* 9, 260–267. doi: 10.1038/nn1623

Tanaka, K., Watase, K., Manabe, T., Yamada, K., Watanabe, M., Takahashi, K., et al. (1997). Epilepsy and exacerbation of brain injury in mice lacking the glutamate transporter GLT-1. *Science* 276, 1699–1702. doi: 10.1126/science.276.5319.1699

Taveggia, C., Zanazzi, G., Petrylak, A., Yano, H., Rosenbluth, J., Einheber, S., et al. (2005). Neuregulin-1 type III determines the ensheathment fate of axons. *Neuron* 47, 681–694. doi: 10.1016/j.neuron.2005.08.017

Tian, R., Wu, X., Hagemann, T. L., Sosunov, A. A., Messing, A., McKhann, G. M., et al. (2010). Alexander disease mutant glial fibrillary acidic protein compromises glutamate transport in astrocytes. *J. Neuropathol. Exp. Neurol.* 69, 335–345. doi: 10.1097/NEN.0b013e3181d3cb52

Tkachev, D., Mimmack, M. L., Huffaker, S. J., Ryan, M., and Bahn, S. (2007). Further evidence for altered myelin biosynthesis and glutamatergic dysfunction in schizophrenia. *Int. J. Neuropsychopharmacol.* 10, 557–563. doi: 10.1017/s1461145706007334

Tkachev, D., Mimmack, M. L., Ryan, M. M., Wayland, M., Freeman, T., Jones, P. B., et al. (2003). Oligodendrocyte dysfunction in schizophrenia and bipolar disorder. *Lancet* 362, 798–805. doi: 10.1016/s0140-6736(03)14297-3

Todd, R. D., and Botteron, K. N. (2001). Is attention-deficit/hyperactivity disorder an energy deficiency syndrome? *Biol. Psychiatry* 50, 151–158. doi: 10.1016/S0006-3223(01)01173-8

Toro, C. T., Hallak, J. E., Dunham, J. S., and Deakin, J. F. (2006). Glial fibrillary acidic protein and glutamine synthetase in subregions of prefrontal cortex in schizophrenia and mood disorder. *Neurosci. Lett.* 404, 276–281. doi: 10.1016/j.neulet.2006.05.067

Townsend, J. D., Eberhart, N. K., Bookheimer, S. Y., Eisenberger, N. I., Foland-Ross, L. C., Cook, I. A., et al. (2010). fMRI activation in the amygdala and the orbitofrontal cortex in unmedicated subjects with major depressive disorder. *Psychiatry Res.* 183, 209–217. doi: 10.1016/j.pscychresns.2010.06.001

Tremblay, M. E., Lowery, R. L., and Majewska, A. K. (2010). Microglial interactions with synapses are modulated by visual experience. *PLoS Biol.* 8:e1000527. doi: 10.1371/journal.pbio.1000527

Uranova, N. A., Vostrikov, V. M., Orlovskaya, D. D., and Rachmanova, V. I. (2004). Oligodendroglial density in the prefrontal cortex in schizophrenia and mood disorders: a study from the stanley neuropathology consortium. *Schizophr. Res.* 67, 269–275. doi: 10.1016/s0920-9964(03)00181-6

Uranova, N., Orlovskaya, D., Vikhreva, O., Zimina, I., Kolomeets, N., Vostrikov, V., et al. (2001). Electron microscopy of oligodendroglia in severe mental illness. *Brain Res. Bull.* 55, 597–610. doi: 10.1016/s0361-9230(01)00528-7

Van Berckel, B. N., Bossong, M. G., Boellaard, R., Kloet, R., Schuitemaker, A., Caspers, E., et al. (2008). Microglia activation in recent-onset schizophrenia: a quantitative (R)-[11C]PK11195 positron emission tomography study. *Biol. Psychiatry* 64, 820–822. doi: 10.1016/j.biopsych.2008.04.025

Vartanian, T., Fischbach, G., and Miller, R. (1999). Failure of spinal cord oligodendrocyte development in mice lacking neuregulin. *Proc. Natl. Acad. Sci. U S A* 96, 731–735. doi: 10.1073/pnas.96.2.731

Ventura, R. E., and Goldman, J. E. (2006). Telencephalic oligodendrocytes battle it out. *Nat. Neurosci.* 9, 153–154. doi: 10.1038/nn0206-153

Verkhratsky, A., Orkand, R. K., and Kettenmann, H. (1998). Glial calcium: homeostasis and signaling function. *Physiol. Rev.* 78, 99–141.

Verkhratsky, A., Rodríguez, J. J., and Steardo, L. (2014). Astrogliopathology: a central element of neuropsychiatric diseases? *Neuroscientist* 20, 576–588. doi: 10.1177/1073858413510208

Vielkind, U., Walencewicz, A., Levine, J. M., and Bohn, M. C. (1990). Type II glucocorticoid receptors are expressed in oligodendrocytes and astrocytes. *J. Neurosci. Res.* 27, 360–373. doi: 10.1002/jnr.490270315

Volkow, N. D., Baler, R. D., and Goldstein, R. Z. (2011). Addiction: pulling at the neural threads of social behaviors. *Neuron* 69, 599–602. doi: 10.1016/j.neuron.2011.01.027

Volterra, A., and Meldolesi, J. (2005). Astrocytes, from brain glue to communication elements: the revolution continues. *Nat. Rev. Neurosci.* 6, 626–640. doi: 10.1038/nrn1722

Vostrikov, V. M., Uranova, N. A., and Orlovskaya, D. D. (2007). Deficit of perineuronal oligodendrocytes in the prefrontal cortex in schizophrenia and mood disorders. *Schizophr. Res.* 94, 273–280. doi: 10.1016/j.schres.2007.04.014

Walz, W., and Mukerji, S. (1988). Lactate release from cultured astrocytes and neurons: a comparison. *Glia* 1, 366–370. doi: 10.1002/glia.440010603

Webster, M. J., O'Grady, J., Kleinman, J. E., and Weickert, C. S. (2005). Glial fibrillary acidic protein mRNA levels in the cingulate cortex of individuals with depression, bipolar disorder and schizophrenia. *Neuroscience* 133, 453–461. doi: 10.1016/j.neuroscience.2005.02.037

Wennström, M., Hellsten, J., Ekstrand, J., Lindgren, H., and Tingström, A. (2006). Corticosterone-induced inhibition of gliogenesis in rat hippocampus is counteracted by electroconvulsive seizures. *Biol. Psychiatry* 59, 178–186. doi: 10.1016/j.biopsych.2005.08.032

Wierzba-Bobrowicz, T., Lewandowska, E., Lechowicz, W., Stepień, T., and Pasennik, E. (2005). Quantitative analysis of activated microglia, ramified and damage of processes in the frontal and temporal lobes of chronic schizophrenics. *Folia Neuropathol.* 43, 81–89.

Williams, M. R., Hampton, T., Pearce, R. K., Hirsch, S. R., Ansorge, O., Thom, M., et al. (2013). Astrocyte decrease in the subgenual cingulate and callosal genu in schizophrenia. *Eur. Arch. Psychiatry Clin. Neurosci.* 263, 41–52. doi: 10.1007/s00406-012-0328-5

Wolosker, H., Blackshaw, S., and Snyder, S. H. (1999a). Serine racemase: a glial enzyme synthesizing D-serine to regulate glutamate-N-methyl-D-aspartate neurotransmission. *Proc. Natl. Acad. Sci. U S A* 96, 13409–13414. doi: 10.1073/pnas.96.23.13409

Wolosker, H., Sheth, K. N., Takahashi, M., Mothet, J. P., Brady, R. O. Jr., Ferris, C. D., et al. (1999b). Purification of serine racemase: biosynthesis of the neuromodulator D-serine. *Proc. Natl. Acad. Sci. U S A* 96, 721–725. doi: 10.1073/pnas.96.2.721

Wu, L. J., Stevens, B., Duan, S., and MacVicar, B. A. (2013). Microglia in neuronal circuits. *Neural Plast.* 2013:586426. doi: 10.1155/2013/586426

Xia, L., Zhai, M., Wang, L., Miao, D., Zhu, X., and Wang, W. (2013). FGF2 blocks PTSD symptoms via an astrocyte-based mechanism. *Behav. Brain Res.* 256, 472–480. doi: 10.1016/j.bbr.2013.08.048

Yang, J., Ruchti, E., Petit, J. M., Jourdain, P., Grenningloh, G., Allaman, I., et al. (2014). Lactate promotes plasticity gene expression by potentiating NMDA signaling in neurons. *Proc. Natl. Acad. Sci. U S A* 111, 12228–12233. doi: 10.1073/pnas.1322912111

Yang, J., and Shen, J. (2005). *In vivo* evidence for reduced cortical glutamate-glutamine cycling in rats treated with the antidepressant/antipanic drug phenelzine. *Neuroscience* 135, 927–937. doi: 10.1016/j.neuroscience.2005.06.067

Yirmiya, R. (1996). Endotoxin produces a depressive-like episode in rats. *Brain Res.* 711, 163–174. doi: 10.1016/0006-8993(95)01415-2

Yirmiya, R., Pollak, Y., Barak, O., Avitsur, R., Ovadia, H., Bette, M., et al. (2001). Effects of antidepressant drugs on the behavioral and physiological responses to lipopolysaccharide (LPS) in rodents. *Neuropsychopharmacology* 24, 531–544. doi: 10.1016/s0893-133x(00)00226-8

Yoshizumi, M., Eisenach, J. C., and Hayashida, K. (2012). Riluzole and gabapentinoids activate glutamate transporters to facilitate glutamate-induced glutamate release from cultured astrocytes. *Eur. J. Pharmacol.* 677, 87–92. doi: 10.1016/j.ejphar.2011.12.015

Zametkin, A. J., Liebenauer, L. L., Fitzgerald, G. A., King, A. C., Minkunas, D. V., Herscovitch, P., et al. (1993). Brain metabolism in teenagers with attention-deficit hyperactivity disorder. *Arch. Gen. Psychiatry* 50, 333–340. doi: 10.1001/archpsyc.1993.01820170011002

Zametkin, A. J., Nordahl, T. E., Gross, M., King, A. C., Semple, W. E., Rumsey, J., et al. (1990). Cerebral glucose metabolism in adults with hyperactivity of childhood onset. *N. Engl. J. Med.* 323, 1361–1366. doi: 10.1056/nejm199011153232001

Zechel, S., Werner, S., Unsicker, K., and von Bohlen und Halbach, O. (2010). Expression and functions of fibroblast growth factor 2 (FGF-2) in hippocampal formation. *Neuroscientist* 16, 357–373. doi: 10.1177/1073858410371513

Zhang, Q., Pangrsic, T., Kreft, M., Krzan, M., Li, N., Sul, J. Y., et al. (2004). Fusion-related release of glutamate from astrocytes. *J. Biol. Chem.* 279, 12724–12733. doi: 10.1074/jbc.m312845200

Zhang, X., Peng, L., Chen, Y., and Hertz, L. (1993). Stimulation of glycogenolysis in astrocytes by fluoxetine, an antidepressant acting like 5-HT. *Neuroreport* 4, 1235–1238. doi: 10.1097/00001756-199309000-00006

Zhang, K., and Sejnowski, T. J. (2000). A universal scaling law between gray matter and white matter of cerebral cortex. *Proc. Natl. Acad. Sci. U S A* 97, 5621–5626. doi: 10.1073/pnas.090504197

Zhu, M. Y., Klimek, V., Dilley, G. E., Haycock, J. W., Stockmeier, C., Overholser, J. C., et al. (1999). Elevated levels of tyrosine hydroxylase in the locus coeruleus in major depression. *Biol. Psychiatry* 46, 1275–1286. doi: 10.1016/s0006-3223(99)00135-3

# 14

# Astrocytes and Microglia and their Potential Link with Autism Spectrum Disorders

***Francesco Petrelli, Luca Pucci and Paola Bezzi****

*Department of Fundamental Neurosciences, University of Lausanne, Lausanne, Switzerland*

***Correspondence:**
*Paola Bezzi*
*paola.bezzi@unil.ch*

The cellular mechanism(s) underlying autism spectrum disorders (ASDs) are not fully understood although it has been shown that various genetic and environmental factors contribute to their etiology. As increasing evidence indicates that astrocytes and microglial cells play a major role in synapse maturation and function, and there is evidence of deficits in glial cell functions in ASDs, one current hypothesis is that glial dysfunctions directly contribute to their pathophysiology. The aim of this review is to summarize microglia and astrocyte functions in synapse development and their contributions to ASDs.

**Keywords: astrocytes, microglia, neurosciences, autism spectrum disorders (ASD)**

## INTRODUCTION

Autism spectrum disorders (ASDs) have a worldwide prevalence of about 12-15% and are characterized by significant social, intellectual, behavioral impairment, and sometimes cognitive deficits (Abrahams and Geschwind, 2008; Geschwind, 2009; Quaak et al., 2013). They typically manifest early in development and are associated distinct neurodevelopmental syndromes.

The conceptualisation of autism and related disorders has undergone considerable changes over the last ten years, which are reflected in the fifth edition of the Diagnostic and Statistical Manual of Mental Disorders (DSM-V, www.dsm5.org). The proposed revisions of the preceding edition (DSM IV-TR) include combining specific DSM-IV-TR diagnoses into a single broad ASD, and identifying two domains of impairment (social communication and interactions, and restricted repetitive behavior) rather than three (social interaction, communication, and restricted repetitive and stereotyped patterns of behavior, interests, and activities). There are also considerable differences in clinical presentation and disease progression as ASD patient's present variously severe core symptoms and variable co-morbid conditions such as epilepsy, gastrointestinal problems, intellectual disability, anxiety, and depression (Kim and Lord, 2012). Early estimates that the heritability of ASDs is approximately 90% (Steffenburg et al., 1989; Bailey et al., 1995), and even recently revised estimates that it is about 45%, strongly suggest that genetic mutations are a major cause (Hallmayer et al., 2011; Sandin et al., 2014). However, ASDs are genetically very heterogeneous (State and Levitt, 2011) and seem to be associated with a large number of genetic mutations, including possibly 100s of rare causal variants and common variants with small effects (Murdoch and State, 2013). The genetic heterogeneity of ASD has made it challenging to identify specific genes associated with the disorder, which has thus hindered efforts to dissect disease mechanisms. Recent insights into the genetic pathways that are altered in ASDs have come from studies of syndromic disorders with a high incidence of ASDs caused by mutations of a single gene, including fragile X syndrome (fragile X mental retardation 1 protein, FMR1), Rett syndrome (methyl-CpG-binding protein 2 protein, MECP2), tuberous sclerosis (tuberous sclerosis 1 protein, TSC1), neurofibromatosis type 1 (neurofibromin 1 protein, NF1), and PTEN (phosphatase and tensin homologue) macrocephaly. Recent studies also implicate neurodevelopmental genes in ASDs through the identification of recurrent *de novo* loss of function mutations in affected individuals (Parikshak et al., 2013; Willsey et al., 2013). Neurodevelopmental genes are indeed an important factor to take into consideration since functional and anatomical insults associated to defects in these genes during brain development can trigger the appearance of ASDs in the childhood. Genome-wide association studies have identified susceptibility genes for ASDs such as forkhead box p2 (FOXP2) (Toma et al., 2013) or the MAM domain containing glycosylphosphatidylinositol anchor (MDGA) genes (Bucan et al., 2009; Pettem et al., 2013; Perez-Garcia and O'Leary, 2016) and have provided evidence supporting the idea that the large numbers of variants associated with ASDs converge toward a core set of dysregulated biological processes (Murdoch and State, 2013). The genes that have been linked to ASDs can be grouped into three broad categories: those involved in synapse structure and activity (Etherton et al., 2011a,b; Peca and Feng, 2012), those involved in protein synthesis (Kelleher and Bear, 2008), and those involved in regulating gene expression (van Bokhoven, 2011). Many of them encode for proteins that have a clear synaptic function, thus making the pathological features of ASDs mainly "neurocentric". However, as the usefulness of parsing neuronal mechanisms in order to investigate the etiology of ASDs has proved to be limited, alternative biological analyses may help to reveal previously unknown cellular and molecular mechanisms.

Extending the theory of purely genetic causes, it seems likely that genetics alone may not account for all cases of autism. In addition to a certain combination of autism-related genes, exposure to a number of non-heritable environmental factors may significantly affect susceptibility to, and the variable expression of autism and autism-related traits (Pessah and Lein, 2008; Rosenberg et al., 2009; Hallmayer et al., 2011; Estes and McAllister, 2015). In addition to exposure to chemicals or toxins, these include factors such as parental age at the time of conception, and maternal nutrition and infections (including autoimmune diseases) during pregnancy and prematurity (Grabrucker, 2012). One important area of research concerns the way in which environmental influences interact with genetic susceptibility: for example, recent studies have shown that glial cells in the brains of autistic subjects were constantly activated and their inflammation response genes were turned on (Voineagu et al., 2011; Edmonson et al., 2014; Gupta et al., 2014). It is still not clear what role inflammation plays in autism or whether it is beneficial or not, or what causes the activation of glial cells, but these findings and the recent discovery that glial cells may interact with synaptic activity by influencing synapse formation and maturation (Clarke and Barres, 2013; Sahlender et al., 2014; Petrelli and Bezzi, 2016), strongly suggest that glial cells may be involved in the pathogenesis of ASDs. Although some excellent reviews have recently discussed the involvement of glial cells in neuropsychiatric disorders (McGann et al., 2012; Molofsky et al., 2012; Chung et al., 2015), we will give our perspective on the role of microglia and astrocytes in the late step of synapse formation and maturation and in the pathophysiology of ASDs.

## ASTROCYTES AND MICROGLIA INFLUENCE SYNAPSE FORMATION AND FUNCTION

Over the last ten years, it has gradually emerged that glial cells (in particular microglia and astrocytes) influence synapse formation and function (Araque et al., 2014; Chung et al., 2015; Rossi, 2015). Neurons and glial cells are closely associated with each other from an early stage of development, and recent discoveries suggest that the appropriate assembly of neural circuits requires extensive neuron-glia signaling (Ullian et al., 2001; Christopherson et al., 2005; Eroglu, 2009; Allen et al., 2012). In addition to carrying out various homeostatic functions within the central nervous system (CNS), they can also engage in bi-directional communication with neurons by releasing neuroactive substances (Petrelli and Bezzi, 2016). In particular, astrocytes can make contact with multiple neurons and up to 100,000 synapses (Bushong et al., 2002; Halassa et al., 2007), and possess many receptors (mainly G-protein coupled receptors) and ion channels present in neurons, thus enabling them to sense and respond to an array of neuronal signals (Fiacco and McCarthy, 2006). The generation and expansion of astrocytes is largely completed before birth, but the elaboration and maturation of their fine peri-synaptic processes persists during the active period of synaptogenesis (Ullian et al., 2001) in the post-natal period. This suggests that they are in a crucial position to communicate actively with neurons during synaptogenesis and, thus, coordinate the development of neural circuits. The formation of synapses (Clarke and Barres, 2013) and the modulation of synaptic activity and plasticity by astrocytes (Araque et al., 2014) mainly take place as a result of the secretion of neuroactive substances now known as synaptogenic factors. Pfrieger and Barres (1997) were the first to demonstrate the key role of astrocyte-derived soluble molecules in synapse formation, and many subsequent studies by the same group and others have identified the nature of these synaptogenic factors, with the thrombospondins 1- 5, hevin, and glypicans seeming to be crucial substances for the formation of excitatory synapses (Ullian et al., 2001; Christopherson et al., 2005; Kucukdereli et al., 2011; Allen et al., 2012). Overall, these findings are seminally important as they have changed our "neurocentric" view of the astrocytic-dependent processes involved in the formation and maturation of functional synapses. However, we are still only beginning to understand the role of astrocyte-derived synaptogenic molecules in terms of cell biology, and our knowledge of the molecular and cell mechanisms regulating the active release of synaptogenic factors is very limited (Petrelli and Bezzi, 2016). Many of them have only been studied in cultured cells, and the cellular and molecular pathways governing their secretion are still unknown, including whether they are calcium-dependent or not. Interestingly, astrocytes also release many other factors, such as substances regulating metabolism, the energy supply (including cerebral blood flow) and inflammation, and substances regulating synaptic transmission, including neurotransmitters and neuromodulators (i.e., gliotransmitters) (Bezzi and Volterra, 2001; Petrelli and Bezzi, 2016). The cell mechanisms governing the release of gliotransmitters and their effects on synaptic activities have been extensively studied, and there is a large amount of experimental evidence indicating that gliotransmitters play an active role in synaptic physiology (Araque et al., 2014). For example, the tumor necrosis factor alpha (TNFα) released by astrocytes (and possibly also by microglial cells) is required for synaptic scaling (Stellwagen and Malenka, 2006), and can control glutamatergic gliotransmission under both physiological (Santello et al., 2011) and pathological conditions (Bezzi et al., 2001; Habbas et al., 2015). A recent study has shown that pathological concentrations of pro-inflammatory TNFα signal through astrocytes to alter synaptic transmission and impair cognition in a mouse model of multiple sclerosis (Habbas et al., 2015). As inflammation of the CNS is a common feature of nearly all neurological disorders and insults (including ASDs), and cognitive impairments are also common to many neuroinflammatory neurological conditions (including ASDs), it is likely that the activation of glial cells and pathological concentrations of cytokines (notably TNFα) can contribute to the cognitive and behavioral impairments characterizing ASDs.

Microglial cells are resident macrophages of the brain that form the innate defensive system (Hanisch and Kettenmann, 2007; Kettenmann, 2011) and, by acting as sentinels, can detect the first signs of pathogenic invasion or tissue damage. After their conversion from a resting (or surveillance) cell type to an activated form, they remove damaged synapses and their protective or detrimental functions have been extensively studied in various brain pathologies (Kettenmann et al., 2013). During the resting/surveillance phase, microglial processes constantly extend and retract to check the local environment (Nimmerjahn et al., 2005), which includes peri-synaptic astrocytes, pre-synaptic boutons, and post-synaptic spines (Tremblay et al., 2010). Many of their functions are still unclear and there has been much debate about whether they are beneficial or detrimental. Like astrocytes, microglial cells have heterogeneous functions within the brain (Carson et al., 2007; Bailey-Bucktrout et al., 2008; Bulloch et al., 2008; Gowing et al., 2008), and release a wide variety of molecules (e.g., brain-derived neurotrophic factor, BDNF) that can interact with synapses and play important physiological roles in learning and memory (Parkhurst et al., 2013).

In addition to affecting synaptic activity, astrocytes and microglial cells seem to play an important role in removing ('pruning') synaptic connections (Stanfield et al., 1982; Nakamura and O'Leary, 1989), a process of structural formation and elimination that is vital for controlling and refining the connectivity of mature neuronal circuits (Steven et al., 2007; Barres, 2008). For example, in the developing brain, astrocytes can physically eliminate synapses through the multiple EGF-like domains 10 (MEGF10) and c-mer proto-oncogene tyrosine kinase (MERTK) phagocytic pathways (Chung et al., 2013) and, in line with this, mice deficient in MEGF10 and MERTK receptors fail to refine their retino-geniculate connections and retain excess functional synapses. Interestingly, the rate of synaptic pruning decreases with age and is regulated by synaptic activity. Like astrocytes, microglia cells are also important in the structural elimination of synapses in developing brain. Microglia processes are highly motile and are well positioned to interact with boutons and spines. However, synaptic pruning particularly involves phagocytic microglial processes that, during the first weeks after birth, can engulf pre- and post-synaptic elements (Paolicelli et al., 2011; Schafer et al., 2012). This early post-natal process depends of different molecules such as CX3C chemokine receptor 1 (CX3CR1), also known as the fractalkine receptor or G-protein coupled receptor 13 (GPR13), and complement receptor 3 (CX3C) (Harrison et al., 1998; Stevens et al., 2007; Zhan et al., 2014; Wu et al., 2015). The importance of the CX3CR1-mediated mechanisms by means of which microglial cells remove synapses has been confirmed by studies of CX3CR1 knockout animals, which have aberrant long-range functional connectivity (Schafer et al., 2012) as well as a deficit in hippocampal LTP and aberrant social behavior (Zhan et al., 2014). Overall, these studies show that physiological interactions of astrocytes and microglia with synapses are crucial for synapse formation and network functioning, and point out that their loss, deviation or functional perturbation might contribute to autism pathogenesis and progression (**Figure 1**).

## THE ROLE OF GLIAL CELLS IN AUTISM SPECTRUM DISORDERS

The importance of glial cells in the pathophysiology of ASDs is primarily supported by a recent transcriptomic analysis of autistic brains. RNA sequencing revealed a close association between ASDs and the genes related to glial cell activation and genes belonging to immune and inflammatory categories (Voineagu et al., 2011). These transcriptional results are supported by immunohistochemistry data obtained from human post mortem brain samples showing increased reactive gliosis and glial cell proliferation (Purcell et al., 2001; Vargas et al., 2005; Fatemi et al., 2008; Morgan et al., 2012; Tetreault et al., 2012; Edmonson et al., 2014), and by a recent positron emission tomography (PET) functional imaging study showing microglial activation in multiple brain regions of young adults with ASDs (such in the cerebellum, midbrain, pons, fusiform gyri, and the anterior cingulate and orbitofrontal cortices; Suzuki et al., 2013). In line with this, high levels of various pro-inflammatory cytokines, such as interleukin (IL)-6, TNFα, and IL-1β have been reported in the post-mortem brain tissues, (Watkins et al., 2001; Vargas et al., 2005; Li et al., 2009; Wei et al., 2011) and blood of autistic subjects (Gupta et al., 1998; Jyonouchi et al., 2001).

It is now recognized that pro-inflammatory factors play an important role in the etiology of various neurological and neuropsychiatric disorders, including those such as ASDs whose pathogenetic onset occurs during early brain development (Meyer et al., 2011; Voineagu et al., 2011; Gupta et al., 2014; Estes and McAllister, 2015). The developing brain is highly vulnerable to environmental insults such as those associated with strong inflammatory reactions (Dammann and Leviton,

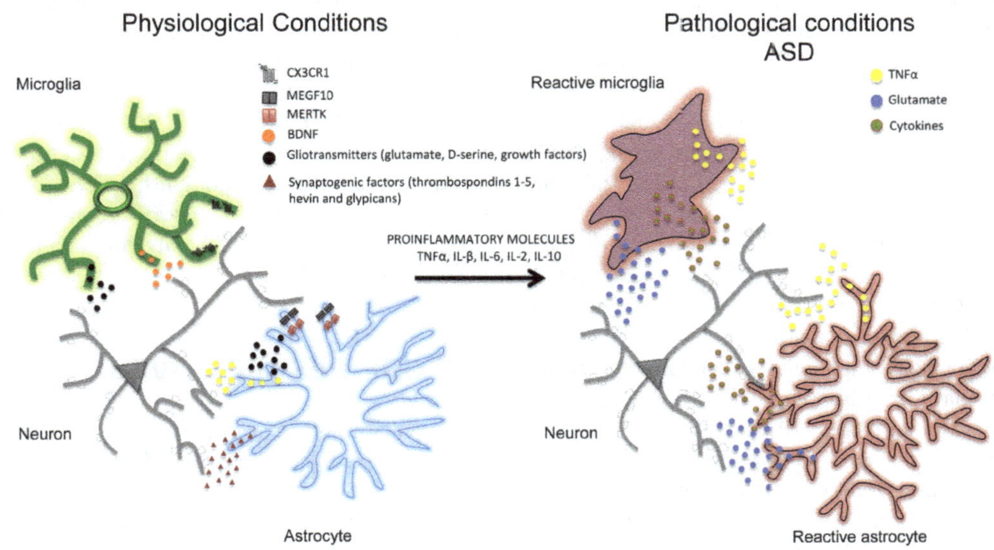


**FIGURE 1 | In physiological conditions and during postnatal development, neurons (gray) and glial cells (notably astrocytes -blue- and microglia -green-) are closely associated with each other.** Astrocytes and microglia release a number of neuroactive substances such as gliotransmitters together with growth factors (such as TNFα, BDNF, glutamate, D-serine; black dots) and synaptogenic factors (such as thrombospondins 1-5, hevin, and glypicans; red dots) that can promote the formation and maturation of synapses. Glial cells can also contribute to synapse remodeling and pruning through CX3CR1, multiple EGF-like domains 10 (MEGF10), c-mer proto-oncogene tyrosine kinase (MERTK) phagocytic pathways. In pathological conditions (i.e., in autistic brains) pro-inflammatory factors (including pro-inflammatory cytokines TNFα, IL-β, IL-6, IL-2, IL-10) may lead to a chronic neuroinflammation in which astrocytes and microglia become reactive (red), release pro-inflammatory mediators (such as TNFα, glutamate and pro-inflammatory cytokines) and may exacerbate the initial inflammatory condition. Although the specific contribution of aberrant glial cells (i.e., reactive gliosis) to the pathophysiology of autism has still to be determined, studies on animal models support a direct association between neuroinflammation and autism, suggesting that reactive gliosis may have a crucial role in many autism phenotypes including the structural and functional alterations of brain connectivity.

2004) and specific brain lesions (Hagberg et al., 2015). Under normal conditions, inflammatory processes in the developing brain are controlled by a number of homeostatic mechanisms that limit the inflammation induced by an environmental stimulus such as infection (Serhan and Savill, 2005). These surveillance mechanisms are mainly controlled by microglia and astrocytes, and are crucial in ensuring that inflammatory processes efficiently remove invading pathogens and contribute to tissue repair.

It is therefore likely that, under inflammatory conditions, any dysfunction in these mechanisms may lead to deleterious chronic inflammation, and this (together with reports of increased levels of pro-inflammatory cytokines in the post-mortem brains of subjects with ASDs) has led to the hypothesis that chronic neuroinflammation plays a role in the pathogenesis of ASDs, which is supported by the fact that chronic systemic inflammatory conditions such as those associated with autoimmune disorders or infections (together with acute immune activation) are often observed in the mothers of children with ASDs (Atladottir et al., 2009; Keil et al., 2010; Estes and McAllister, 2015). Although the specific contribution of maternal immune dysregulation to the onset of ASDs has yet to be determined in humans, animal models have shown a causal link between the activation of the maternal immune system and altered neurodevelopment. Studies of various animal models of maternal infection during pregnancy support the association between systemic inflammatory processes and ASDs phenotypes (Malkova et al., 2012; Knuesel et al., 2014; Missault et al., 2014), all of which seem to indicate that the ASD-like behavior in the offspring may be caused by altered levels of maternal cytokines, including TNFα, IL1β, IL-2, IL-6, and IL-10 (Ponzio et al., 2007; Smith et al., 2007). It is important to note that there is a specific temporal window in which cytokines confer a risk of developing ASD (i.e., the perinatal period), which suggests that the permeability of the developing blood brain barrier is crucial for the onset of ASD (Meyer et al., 2011). Pro-inflammatory cytokines in the developing brain classically lead to neuroinflammation, a condition in which microglia and astrocytes become reactive (gliosis), proliferate and, depending on the entity of the gliosis, recruit peripheral leukocytes and thus amplify the initial tissue damage (Sofroniew, 2015).

The idea that reactive gliosis may exacerbate the inflammatory conditions caused by immune activation and contribute to the pathogenesis of ASDs is intriguing, but it is still not clear what the changes in glial cell activation tell us about the molecular and cellular mechanisms underlying the disorders. One possibility is that reactive gliosis may perturb the ability of microglia and astrocytes to modulate the maturation, elimination (phagocytosis), or functioning of developing synapses because developing neural networks are highly vulnerable to insults affecting the glial pathways governing the pruning of synapses (Chung et al., 2015). For example, CX3CR1 knockout mice show impaired synaptic pruning, social behavior and functional connectivity (Zhan et al., 2014), all of which are features of ASDs. It can therefore be expected that the inflammatory processes targeting the developing brain have a long-lasting impact on brain and behavioral functions throughout life.

The use of animal models of ASDs has led to substantial advances in our understanding of the role of glial cells, which have been found to be abnormal in mouse models of Rett syndrome (RTT; Maezawa et al., 2009; Yasui et al., 2013), fragile X syndrome (Yuskaitis et al., 2010), and tuberous sclerosis (Uhlmann et al., 2002). In particular, a study of a mouse model of RTT, a devastating neurodevelopmental disorder caused by loss-of-function mutations in the X-linked MECP2 encoding methyl-CpG-binding protein 2 (MeCP2) (Chahrour and Zoghbi, 2007), has shown that MeCP2-deficient microglia cells release an abnormally high level of glutamate, causing excitotoxicity that may contribute to dendritic and synaptic abnormalities (Maezawa and Jin, 2010). MECP2 is a well-known transcription factor that is important in controlling gene expression by interpreting and regulating epigenetic markers (Chao and Zoghbi, 2012). MECP2 is expressed in many tissues but, although the disease is generally attributed to a primary neuronal dysfunction, glial MECP2 seems to play a pathophysiological role as it has been recently shown that MECP2-null astrocytes are unable to support the normal dendritic ramification of wild-type neurons growing in culture (Ballas et al., 2009), and two remarkable studies have found that the expression of wild-type MECP2 protein in the astrocytes or microglia of MECP2-null hosts dramatically improves the pathology (Lioy et al., 2011; Derecki et al., 2012).

Finally, it is interesting to note that a recent RNA-Seq transcriptome and splicing database of glia and neurons (Cahoy et al., 2008) indicates that many of the ASD candidate genes are enriched in glial cells. For example, some genes, such as Homer1 (HOMER1) (Ronesi et al., 2012), 4-aminobutyrate aminotransferase (ABAT; Barnby et al., 2005), fatty acid binding protein 7 (FABP7; Maekawa et al., 2010), and glutathione *S*-transferase 1 (GSTM1; Ming et al., 2010), are not specific for neurons but, instead, are highly enriched in astrocytes; other genes are equally present in astrocytes and neurons (such as MeCP2), and some are highly enriched in both astrocytes and microglial cells (such as dual-specificity tyrosine-(*Y*)-phosphorylation- regulated kinase 1A or DYRK1A). Mutations in the genes encoding a number of members of the IL-1 cytokine receptor family are also associated with ASDs, and glial cells are the major contributors to the response of IL-1 signaling pathways to neuroinflammation (Moynagh et al., 1993; Zhang et al., 1996; Molina-Holgado et al., 2000). For example, recent exome-sequencing studies of ASD patients have found a single-nucleotide polymorphism in the gene encoding IL-1 receptor type 2 (IL-1R2) (O'Roak et al., 2011; Sanders et al., 2012) that is highly enriched in microglial cells (Cahoy et al., 2008), and a rare ASD-associated mutation has been identified in the gene encoding IL-1 receptor accessory protein –like 1 (IL-1RAPL1; Bhat et al., 2008), which is highly enriched in astrocytes (Cahoy et al., 2008).

## FUTURE PERSPECTIVES

Until very recently, the role of glial cells in the onset of ASDs was almost completely overlooked, and so neuropharmacological strategies for treating the symptoms were almost exclusively aimed at neuronal activity and synaptic transmission. However, as accumulating evidence supports the view that astrocytes and microglia are significantly involved in the regulation of synapse formation, function, plasticity, and elimination, the role of astrocyte-derived factors in regulating synapse formation and the role of microglia in synaptic pruning during postnatal development (a period that coincides with the onset of many ASDs) are particularly relevant. These findings may change our "neurocentric" view of the mechanisms involved in the onset and progression of ASDs because that it is unlikely that research solely concentrated on neurons will fully reveal their underlying pathophysiological mechanisms. Recent data suggest that many ASDs are at least partially due to disorders affecting glial cells or neuron-glial interactions, and future pharmacological research should consider the possibility of improving glial cell functions.

## AUTHOR CONTRIBUTIONS

PB wrote the review together with FP and LP.

## ACKNOWLEDGMENT

This review was supported by grants from the Swiss National Foundation NCCR "Synapsy" and "Transcure" to PB.

## REFERENCES

Abrahams, B. S., and Geschwind, D. H. (2008). Advances in autism genetics: on the threshold of a new neurobiology. *Nat. Rev. Genet.* 9, 341–355. doi: 10.1038/nrg2346

Allen, N. J., Bennett, M. L., Foo, L. C., Wang, G. X., Chakraborty, C., Smith, S. J., et al. (2012). Astrocyte glypicans 4 and 6 promote formation of excitatory synapses via GluA1 AMPA receptors. *Nature* 486, 410–414. doi: 10.1038/nature11059

Araque, A., Carmignoto, G., Haydon, P. G., Oliet, S. H. R., Robitaille, R., and Volterra, A. (2014). Gliotransmitters travel in time and space. *Neuron* 81, 728–739. doi: 10.1016/j.neuron.2014.02.007

Atladottir, H. O., Pedersen, M. G., Thorsen, P., Mortensen, P. B., Deleuran, B., Eaton, W. W., et al. (2009). Association of family history of autoimmune diseases and autism spectrum disorders. *Pediatrics* 124, 687–694. doi: 10.1542/peds.2008-2445

Bailey, A., Lecouteur, A., Gottesman, I., Bolton, P., Simonoff, E., Yuzda, E., et al. (1995). Autism as a strongly genetic disorder - evidence from a british twin study. *Psychol. Med.* 25, 63–77. doi: 10.1017/S0033291700028099

Bailey-Bucktrout, S. L., Caulkins, S. C., Goings, G., Fischer, J. A. A., Dzionek, A., and Miller, S. D. (2008). Central nervous system plasmacytoid dendritic cells regulate the severity of relapsing experimental autoimmune encephalomyelitis. *J. Immunol.* 180, 6457–6461. doi: 10.4049/jimmunol.180.10.6457

Ballas, N., Lioy, D. T., Grunseich, C., and Mandel, G. (2009). Non-cell autonomous influence of MeCP2-deficient glia on neuronal dendritic morphology. *Nat. Neurosci.* 12, 311–317. doi: 10.1038/nn.2275

Barnby, G., Abbott, A., Sykes, N., Morris, A., Weeks, D. E., Mott, R., et al. (2005). Candidate-gene screening and association analysis at the autism-susceptibility locus on chromosome 16p: evidence of association at GRIN2A and ABAT. *Am. J. Hum. Genet.* 76, 950–966. doi: 10.1086/430454

Barres, B. A. (2008). The mystery and magic of glia: a perspective on their roles in health and disease. *Neuron* 60, 430–440. doi: 10.1016/j.neuron.2008.10.013

Bezzi, P., Domercq, M., Brambilla, L., Galli, R., Schols, D., De Clercq, E., et al. (2001). CXCR4-activated astrocyte glutamate release via TNFa: amplification by microglia triggers neurotoxicity. *Nat. Neurosci.* 4, 702–710. doi: 10.1038/89490

Bezzi, P., and Volterra, A. (2001). A neuron-glia signalling network in the active brain. *Curr. Opin. Neurobiol.* 11, 387–394. doi: 10.1016/S0959-4388(00)00223-3

Bhat, S. S., Ladd, S., Grass, F., Spence, J. E., Brasington, C. K., Simensen, R. J., et al. (2008). Disruption of the IL1RAPL1 gene associated with a pericentromeric inversion of the X chromosome in a patient with mental retardation and autism. *Clin. Genet.* 73, 94–96. doi: 10.1111/j.1399-0004.2007.00920.x

Bucan, M., Abrahams, B. S., Wang, K., Glessner, J. T., Herman, E. I., Sonnenblick, L. I., et al. (2009). Genome-wide analyses of exonic copy number variants in a family-based study point to novel autism susceptibility genes. *PLoS Genet.* 5:e1000536. doi: 10.1371/journal.pgen.1000536

Bulloch, K., Miller, M. M., Gal-Toth, J., Milner, T. A., Gottfried-Blackmore, A., Waters, E. M., et al. (2008). CD11c/EYFP transgene illuminates a discrete network of dendritic cells within the embryonic, neonatal, adult, and injured mouse brain. *J. Compar. Neurol.* 508, 687–710. doi: 10.1002/cne.21668

Bushong, E. A., Martone, M. E., Jones, Y. Z., and Ellisman, M. H. (2002). Protoplasmic astrocytes in CA1 stratum radiatum occupy separate anatomical domains. *J. Neurosci.* 22, 183–192.

Cahoy, J. D., Emery, B., Kaushal, A., Foo, L. C., Zamanian, J. L., Christopherson, K. S., et al. (2008). A transcriptome database for astrocytes, neurons, and oligodendrocytes: a new resource for understanding brain development and function. *J. Neurosci.* 28, 264–278. doi: 10.1523/JNEUROSCI.4178-07.2008

Carson, M. J., Bilousova, T. V., Puntambekar, S. S., Melchior, B., Doose, J. M., and Ethell, I. M. (2007). A rose by any other name? The potential consequences of microglial heterogeneity during CNS health and disease. *Neurotherapeutics* 4, 571–579. doi: 10.1016/j.nurt.2007.07.002

Chahrour, M., and Zoghbi, H. Y. (2007). The story of rett syndrome: from clinic to neurobiology. *Neuron* 56, 422–437. doi: 10.1016/j.neuron.2007.10.001

Chao, H. T., and Zoghbi, H. Y. (2012). MeCP2: only 100% will do. *Nat. Neurosci.* 15, 176–177. doi: 10.1038/nn.3027

Christopherson, K. S., Ullian, E. M., Stokes, C. C. A., Mullowney, C. E., Hell, J. W., Agah, A., et al. (2005). Thrombospondins are astrocyte-secreted proteins that promote CNS synaptogenesis. *Cell* 120, 421–433. doi: 10.1016/j.cell.2004.12.020

Chung, W., Choi, S. Y., Lee, E., Park, H., Kang, J., Choi, Y., et al. (2015). Social deficits in IRSp53 mutant mice improved by NMDAR and mGluR5 suppression. *Nat. Neurosci.* 18, 435–443. doi: 10.1038/nn.3927

Chung, W. S., Clarke, L. E., Wang, G. X., Stafford, B. K., Sher, A., Chakraborty, C., et al. (2013). Astrocytes mediate synapse elimination through MEGF10 and MERTK pathways. *Nature* 504, 394–400. doi: 10.1038/nature12776

Clarke, L. E., and Barres, B. A. (2013). Emerging roles of astrocytes in neural circuit development. *Nat. Rev. Neurosci.* 14, 311–321. doi: 10.1038/nrn3484

Dammann, O., and Leviton, A. (2004). Inflammatory brain damage in preterm newborns - dry numbers, wet lab, and causal inferences. *Early Hum. Dev.* 79, 1–15. doi: 10.1016/j.earlhumdev.2004.04.009

Derecki, N. C., Cronk, J. C., Lu, Z. J., Xu, E., Abbott, S. B. G., Guyenet, P. G., et al. (2012). Wild-type microglia arrest pathology in a mouse model of Rett syndrome. *Nature* 484, 105–109. doi: 10.1038/nature10907

Edmonson, C., Ziats, M. N., and Rennert, O. M. (2014). Altered glial marker expression in autistic post-mortem prefrontal cortex and cerebellum. *Mol. Autism* 5:9. doi: 10.1186/2040-2392-5-3

Eroglu, C. (2009). The role of astrocyte-secreted matricellular proteins in central nervous system development and function. *J. Cell Commun. Signal.* 3, 167–176. doi: 10.1007/s12079-009-0078-y

Estes, M. L., and McAllister, A. K. (2015). Immune mediators in the brain and peripheral tissues in autism spectrum disorder. *Nat. Rev. Neurosci.* 16, 469–486. doi: 10.1038/nrn3978

Etherton, M., Foldy, C., Sharma, M., Tabuchi, K., Liu, X. R., Shamloo, M., et al. (2011a). Autism-linked neuroligin-3 R451C mutation differentially alters hippocampal and cortical synaptic function. *Proc. Natl. Acad. Sci. U.S.A.* 108, 13764–13769. doi: 10.1073/pnas.1111093108

Etherton, M. R., Tabuchi, K., Sharma, M., Ko, J., and Sudhof, T. C. (2011b). An autism-associated point mutation in the neuroligin cytoplasmic tail selectively impairs AMPA receptor-mediated synaptic transmission in hippocampus. *Embo J.* 30, 2908–2919. doi: 10.1038/emboj.2011.182

Fatemi, S. H., Folsom, T. D., Reutiman, T. J., and Lee, S. (2008). Expression of astrocytic markers aquaporin 4 and connexin 43 is altered in brains of subjects with autism. *Synapse* 62, 501–507. doi: 10.1002/syn.20519

Fiacco, T. A., and McCarthy, K. D. (2006). Astrocyte calcium elevations: properties, propagation, and effects on brain signaling. *Glia* 54, 676–690. doi: 10.1002/glia.20395

Geschwind, D. H. (2009). *Advances in Autism. In: Annual Review of Medicine.* Palo Alto, CA: Annual Reviews, 367–380.

Gowing, G., Philips, T., Van Wijmeersch, B., Audet, J. N., Dewil, M., Van Den Bosch, L., et al. (2008). Ablation of proliferating microglia does not affect motor neuron degeneration in amyotrophic lateral sclerosis caused by mutant superoxide dismutase. *J. Neurosci.* 28, 10234–10244. doi: 10.1523/JNEUROSCI.3494-08.2008

Grabrucker, A. M. (2012). Environmental factors in autism. *Front. Psychiatry* 2012:118.

Gupta, S., Aggarwal, S., Rashanravan, B., and Lee, T. (1998). Th1- and Th2-like cytokines in CD4(+) and CD8(+) T cells in autism. *J. Neuroimmunol.* 85, 106–109. doi: 10.1016/S0165-5728(98)00021-6

Gupta, S., Ellis, S. E., Ashar, F. N., Moes, A., Bader, J. S., Zhan, J. N., et al. (2014). Transcriptome analysis reveals dysregulation of innate immune response genes and neuronal activity-dependent genes in autism. *Nat. Commun.* 5:5748. doi: 10.1038/ncomms5748

Habbas, S., Santello, M., Becker, D., Stubbe, H., Zappia, G., Liaudet, N., et al. (2015). Neuroinflammatory TNF alpha impairs memory via astrocyte signaling. *Cell* 163, 1730–1741. doi: 10.1016/j.cell.2015.11.023

Hagberg, H., Mallard, C., Ferriero, D. M., Vannucci, S. J., Levison, S. W., Vexler, Z. S., et al. (2015). The role of inflammation in perinatal brain injury. *Nat. Rev. Neurol.* 11, 192–208. doi: 10.1038/nrneurol.2015.13

Halassa, M. M., Fellin, T., Takano, H., Dong, J. H., and Haydon, P. G. (2007). Synaptic islands defined by the territory of a single astrocyte. *J. Neurosci.* 27, 6473–6477. doi: 10.1523/JNEUROSCI.1419-07.2007

Hallmayer, J., Cleveland, S., Torres, A., Phillips, J., Cohen, B., Torigoe, T., et al. (2011). Genetic heritability and shared environmental factors among twin Pairs with autism. *Arch. Genet. Psychiatry* 68, 1095–1102. doi: 10.1001/archgenpsychiatry.2011.76

Hanisch, U. K., and Kettenmann, H. (2007). Microglia: active sensor and versatile effector cells in the normal and pathologic brain. *Nat. Neurosci.* 10, 1387–1394. doi: 10.1038/nn1997

Harrison, J. K., Jiang, Y., Chen, S. Z., Xia, Y. Y., Maciejewski, D., McNamara, R. K., et al. (1998). Role for neuronally derived fractalkine in mediating interactions between neurons and CX3CR1-expressing microglia. *Proc. Natl. Acad. Sci. U.S.A.* 95, 10896–10901. doi: 10.1073/pnas.95.18.10896

Jyonouchi, H., Sun, S. N., and Le, H. (2001). Proinflammatory and regulatory cytokine production associated with innate and adaptive immune responses in children with autism spectrum disorders and developmental regression. *J. Neuroimmunol.* 120, 170–179. doi: 10.1016/S0165-5728(01)00421-0

Keil, A., Daniels, J. L., Forssen, U., Hultman, C., Cnattingius, S., Soderberg, K. C., et al. (2010). Parental autoimmune diseases associated with autism spectrum disorders in offspring. *Epidemiology* 21, 805–808. doi: 10.1097/EDE.0b013e3181f26e3f

Kelleher, R. J., and Bear, M. F. (2008). The autistic neuron: troubled translation? *Cell* 135, 401–405. doi: 10.1016/j.cell.2008.10.017

Kettenmann, H. (2011). MICROGLIA. *Glia* 59, S2–S3.

Kettenmann, H., Kirchhoff, F., and Verkhratsky, A. (2013). Microglia: new roles for the synaptic stripper. *Neuron* 77, 10–18. doi: 10.1016/j.neuron.2012.12.023

Kim, S. H., and Lord, C. (2012). New autism diagnostic interview-revised algorithms for toddlers and young preschoolers from 12 to 47 months of age. *J. Autism Dev. Disord.* 42, 82–93. doi: 10.1007/s10803-011-1213-1

Knuesel, I., Chicha, L., Britschgi, M., Schobel, S. A., Bodmer, M., Hellings, J. A., et al. (2014). Maternal immune activation and abnormal brain development across CNS disorders. *Nat. Rev. Neurol.* 10, 643–660. doi: 10.1038/nrneurol.2014.187

Kucukdereli, H., Allen, N. J., Lee, A. T., Feng, A., Ozlu, M. I., Conatser, L. M., et al. (2011). Control of excitatory CNS synaptogenesis by astrocyte-secreted proteins hevin and SPARC. *Proc. Natl. Acad. Sci. U.S.A.* 108, E440–E449. doi: 10.1073/pnas.1104977108

Li, X. H., Chauhan, A., Sheikh, A. M., Patil, S., Chauhan, V., Li, X. M., et al. (2009). Elevated immune response in the brain of autistic patients. *J. Neuroimmunol.* 207, 111–116. doi: 10.1016/j.jneuroim.2008.12.002

Lioy, D. T., Garg, S. K., Monaghan, C. E., Raber, J., Foust, K. D., Kaspar, B. K., et al. (2011). A role for glia in the progression of Rett's syndrome. *Nature* 475, 497–500. doi: 10.1038/nature10214

Maekawa, M., Iwayama, Y., Arai, R., Nakamura, K., Ohnishi, T., Toyota, T., et al. (2010). Polymorphism screening of brain-expressed FABP7, 5 and 3 genes and association studies in autism and schizophrenia in Japanese subjects. *J. Hum. Genet.* 55, 127–130. doi: 10.1038/jhg.2009.133

Maezawa, I., and Jin, L. W. (2010). Rett syndrome microglia damage dendrites and synapses by the elevated release of glutamate. *J. Neurosci.* 30, 5346–5356. doi: 10.1523/JNEUROSCI.5966-09.2010

Maezawa, I., Swanberg, S., Harvey, D., LaSalle, J. M., and Jin, L. W. (2009). Rett Syndrome astrocytes are abnormal and spread MeCP2 deficiency through gap junctions. *J. Neurosci.* 29, 5051–5061. doi: 10.1523/JNEUROSCI.0324-09.2009

Malkova, N. V., Yu, C. Z., Hsiao, E. Y., Moore, M. J., and Patterson, P. H. (2012). Maternal immune activation yields offspring displaying mouse versions of the three core symptoms of autism. *Brain Behav. Immun.* 26, 607–616. doi: 10.1016/j.bbi.2012.01.011

McGann, J. C., Lioy, D. T., and Mandel, G. (2012). Astrocytes conspire with neurons during progression of neurological disease. *Curr. Opin. Neurobiol.* 22, 850–858. doi: 10.1016/j.conb.2012.03.009

Meyer, K. A., Ingersoll, B., and Hambrick, D. Z. (2011). Factors influencing adjustment in siblings of children with autism spectrum disorders. *Res. Autism Spect. Disord.* 5, 1413–1420. doi: 10.1016/j.rasd.2011.01.027

Ming, X., Johnson, W. G., Stenroos, E. S., Mars, A., Lambert, G. H., and Buyske, S. (2010). Genetic variant of glutathione peroxidase 1 in autism. *Brain Dev.* 32, 105–109. doi: 10.1016/j.braindev.2008.12.017

Missault, S., Van den Eynde, K., Berghe, W. V., Fransen, E., Weeren, A., Timmermans, J. P., et al. (2014). The risk for behavioural deficits is determined by the maternal immune response to prenatal immune challenge in a neurodevelopmental model. *Brain Behav. Immun.* 42, 138–146. doi: 10.1016/j.bbi.2014.06.013

Molina-Holgado, F., Toulmond, S., and Rothwell, N. J. (2000). Involvement of interleukin-1 in glial responses to lipopolysaccharide: endogenous versus exogenous interleukin-1 actions. *J. Neuroimmunol.* 111, 1–9. doi: 10.1016/S0165-5728(00)00344-1

Molofsky, A. V., Krenick, R., Ullian, E., Tsai, H. H., Deneen, B., Richardson, W. D., et al. (2012). Astrocytes and disease: a neurodevelopmental perspective. *Genes Dev.* 26, 891–907. doi: 10.1101/gad.188326.112

Morgan, J. T., Chana, G., Abramson, I., Semendeferi, K., Courchesne, E., and Everall, I. P. (2012). Abnormal microglial-neuronal spatial organization in the dorsolateral prefrontal cortex in autism. *Brain Res.* 1456, 72–81. doi: 10.1016/j.brainres.2012.03.036

Moynagh, P. N., Williams, D. C., and Oneill, L. A. J. (1993). Interleukin-1 activates transcription factor nf-kappa-b in glial-cells. *Biochem. J.* 294, 343–347. doi: 10.1042/bj2940343

Murdoch, J. D., and State, M. W. (2013). Recent developments in the genetics of autism spectrum disorders. *Curr. Opin. Genet. Dev.* 23, 310–315. doi: 10.1016/j.gde.2013.02.003

Nakamura, H., and O'Leary, D. D. M. (1989). Inaccuracies in initial growth and arborization of chick retinotectal axons followed by course corrections and axon remodeling to develop topographic order. *J. Neurosci.* 9, 3776–3795.

Nimmerjahn, A., Kirchhoff, F., and Helmchen, F. (2005). Resting microglial cells are highly dynamic surveillants of brain parenchyma in vivo. *Science* 308, 1314–1318. doi: 10.1126/science.1110647

O'Roak, B. J., Deriziotis, P., Lee, C., Vives, L., Schwartz, J. J., Girirajan, S., et al. (2011). Exome sequencing in sporadic autism spectrum disorders identifies severe de novo mutations. *Nat. Genet.* 43, 585–589. doi: 10.1038/ng.835

Paolicelli, R. C., Bolasco, G., Pagani, F., Maggi, L., Scianni, M., Panzanelli, P., et al. (2011). Synaptic pruning by microglia is necessary for normal brain development. *Science* 333, 1456–1458. doi: 10.1126/science.1202529

Parikshak, N. N., Luo, R., Zhang, A., Won, H., Lowe, J. K., Chandran, V., et al. (2013). Integrative functional genomic analyses implicate specific molecular pathways and circuits in autism. *Cell* 155, 1008–1021. doi: 10.1016/j.cell.2013.10.031

Parkhurst, C. N., Yang, G., Ninan, I., Savas, J. N., Yates, J. R., Lafaille, J. J., et al. (2013). Microglia promote learning-dependent synapse formation through brain-derived neurotrophic factor. *Cell* 155, 1596–1609. doi: 10.1016/j.cell.2013.11.030

Peca, J., and Feng, G. P. (2012). Cellular and synaptic network defects in autism. *Curr. Opin. Neurobiol.* 22, 866–872. doi: 10.1016/j.conb.2012.02.015

Perez-Garcia, C. G., and O'Leary, D. D. M. (2016). Formation of the cortical subventricular zone requires MDGA1-mediated aggregation of basal progenitors. *Cell Rep.* doi: 10.1016/j.celrep.2015.12.066 [Epub ahead of print].

Pessah, I. N., and Lein, P. J. (2008). "Evidence for environmental susceptibility in autism what we need to know about gene x environment interactions," in *Autism: Current Theories and Evidence*, ed. A. W. Zimmerman (Totowa, NJ: Humana Press Inc.), 409–428.

Petrelli, F., and Bezzi, P. (2016). Novel insights into gliotransmitters. *Curr. Opin. Pharmacol.* 26, 138–145. doi: 10.1016/j.coph.2015.11.010

Pettem, K. L., Yokomaku, D., Takahashi, H., Ge, Y., and Craig, A. M. (2013). Interaction between autism-linked MDGAs and neuroligins suppresses inhibitory synapse development. *J. Cell Biol.* 200, 321–336. doi: 10.1083/jcb.201206028

Pfrieger, F. W., and Barres, B. A. (1997). Synaptic efficacy enhanced by glia cells *in vitro*. *Science* 277, 1684–1687. doi: 10.1126/science.277.5332.1684

Ponzio, N. M., Servatius, R., Beck, K., Marzouk, A., and Kreider, T. (2007). Cytokine levels during pregnancy influence immunological profiles and neurobehavioral patterns of the offspring. *Ann. N. Y. Acad. Sci.* 1107, 118–128.

Purcell, A. E., Jeon, O. H., Zimmerman, A. W., and Pevsner, J. (2001). Postmortem brain abnormalities of the glutamate neurotransmitter system in autism. *Neurology* 57, 1618–1628. doi: 10.1212/WNL.57.9.1618

Quaak, I., Brouns, M. R., and Van de Bor, M. (2013). The dynamics of autism spectrum disorders: how neurotoxic compounds and neurotransmitters interact. *Int. J. Environ. Res. Public Health* 10, 3384–3408. doi: 10.3390/ijerph10083384

Ronesi, J. A., Collins, K. A., Hays, S. A., Tsai, N. P., Guo, W. R., Birnbaum, S. G., et al. (2012). Disrupted Homer scaffolds mediate abnormal mGluR5 function in a mouse model of fragile X syndrome. *Nat. Neurosci.* 15, 431–440. doi: 10.1038/nn.3033

Rosenberg, R. E., Daniels, A. M., Law, J. K., Law, P. A., and Kaufmann, W. E. (2009). Trends in autism spectrum disorder diagnoses: 1994-2007. *J. Autism Dev. Disord.* 39, 1099–1111. doi: 10.1007/s10803-009-0723-6

Rossi, D. (2015). Astrocyte physiopathology: at the crossroads of intercellular networking, inflammation and cell death. *Prog. Neurobiol.* 130, 86–120. doi: 10.1016/j.pneurobio.2015.04.003

Sahlender, D. A., Savtchouk, I., and Volterra, A. (2014). What do we know about gliotransmitter release from astrocytes? *Philos. Trans. R. Soc. B Biol. Sci.* 369:20130592. doi: 10.1098/rstb.2013.0592

Sanders, S. J., Murtha, M. T., Gupta, A. R., Murdoch, J. D., Raubeson, M. J., Willsey, A. J., et al. (2012). De novo mutations revealed by whole-exome sequencing are strongly associated with autism. *Nature* 485, 237–241. doi: 10.1038/nature 10945

Sandin, S., Lichtenstein, P., Kuja-Halkola, R., Larsson, H., Hultman, C. M., and Reichenberg, A. (2014). The familial risk of autism. *JAMA* 311, 1770–1777. doi: 10.1001/jama.2014.4144

Santello, M., Bezzi, P., and Volterra, A. (2011). TNF alpha controls glutamatergic gliotransmission in the hippocampal dentate gyrus. *Neuron* 69, 988–1001. doi: 10.1016/j.neuron.2011.02.003

Schafer, D. P., Lehrman, E. K., Kautzman, A. G., Koyama, R., Mardinly, A. R., Yamasaki, R., et al. (2012). Microglia sculpt postnatal neural circuits in an activity and complement-dependent manner. *Neuron* 74, 691–705. doi: 10.1016/j.neuron.2012.03.026

Serhan, C. N., and Savill, J. (2005). Resolution of inflammation: the beginning programs the end. *Nat. Immunol.* 6, 1191–1197. doi: 10.1038/ni1276

Smith, S. E. P., Li, J., Garbett, K., Mirnics, K., and Patterson, P. H. (2007). Maternal immune activation alters fetal brain development through interleukin-6. *J. Neurosci.* 27, 10695–10702. doi: 10.1523/JNEUROSCI.2178-07.2007

Sofroniew, M. V. (2015). Astrocyte barriers to neurotoxic inflammation. *Nat. Rev. Neurosci.* 16, 249–263. doi: 10.1038/nrn3898

Stanfield, B. B., Oleary, D. D. M., and Fricks, C. (1982). Selective collateral elimination in early postnatal-development restricts cortical distribution of rat pyramidal tract neurons. *Nature* 298, 371–373. doi: 10.1038/298371a0

State, M. W., and Levitt, P. (2011). The conundrums of understanding genetic risks for autism spectrum disorders. *Nat. Neurosci.* 14, 1499–1506. doi: 10.1038/nn.2924

Steffenburg, S., Gillberg, C., Hellgren, L., Andersson, L., Gillberg, I. C., Jakobsson, G., et al. (1989). A twin study of autism in denmark, finland, iceland, norway and sweden. *J. Child Psychol. Psychiatry.* 30, 405–416. doi: 10.1111/j.1469-7610.1989.tb00254.x

Stellwagen, D., and Malenka, R. C. (2006). Synaptic scaling mediated by glial TNF-alpha. *Nature* 440, 1054–1059. doi: 10.1038/nature04671

Steven, M. C., Kiehl, K. A., Pearlson, G. D., and Calhoun, V. D. (2007). Functional neural networks underlying response inhibition in adolescents and adults. *Behav. Brain Res.* 181, 12–22. doi: 10.1016/j.bbr.2007.03.023

Stevens, B., Allen, N. J., Vazquez, L. E., Howell, G. R., Christopherson, K. S., Nouri, N., et al. (2007). The classical complement cascade mediates CNS synapse elimination. *Cell* 131, 1164–1178. doi: 10.1016/j.cell.2007.10.036

Suzuki, K., Sugihara, G., Ouchi, Y., Nakamura, K., Futatsubashi, M., Takebayashi, K., et al. (2013). Microglial activation in young adults with autism spectrum disorder. *JAMA Psychiatry* 70, 49–58. doi: 10.1001/jamapsychiatry.2013.272

Tetreault, N. A., Hakeem, A. Y., Jiang, S., Williams, B. A., Allman, E., Wold, B. J., et al. (2012). Microglia in the cerebral cortex in autism. *J. Autism Dev. Disord.* 42, 2569–2584. doi: 10.1007/s10803-012-1513-0

Toma, C., Hervas, A., Torrico, B., Balmana, N., Salgado, M., Maristany, M., et al. (2013). Analysis of two language-related genes in autism: a case-control association study of FOXP2 and CNTNAP2. *Psychiatr. Genet.* 23, 82–85. doi: 10.1097/YPG.0b013e32835d6fc6

Tremblay, M. E., Lowery, R. L., and Majewska, A. K. (2010). Microglial interactions with synapses are modulated by visual experience. *PLoS Biol.* 8:e1000527. doi: 10.1371/journal.pbio.1000527

Uhlmann, E. J., Wong, M., Baldwin, R. L., Bajenaru, M. L., Onda, H., Kwiatkowski, D. J., et al. (2002). Astrocyte-specific TSC1 conditional knockout mice exhibit abnormal neuronal organization and seizures. *Ann. Neurol.* 52, 285–296. doi: 10.1002/ana.10283

Ullian, E. M., Sapperstein, S. K., Christopherson, K. S., and Barres, B. A. (2001). Control of synapse number by glia. *Science* 291, 657–661. doi: 10.1126/science.291.5504.657

van Bokhoven, H. (2011). *Genetic and Epigenetic Networks in Intellectual Disabilities. In: Annual Review Genetics*, Vol. 45. Palo Alto, CA: Annual Reviews, 81–104.

Vargas, D. L., Nascimbene, C., Krishnan, C., Zimmerman, A. W., and Pardo, C. A. (2005). Neuroglial activation and neuroinflammation in the brain of patients with autism. *Ann. Neurol.* 57, 67–81. doi: 10.1002/ana.20315

Voineagu, I., Wang, X. C., Johnston, P., Lowe, J. K., Tian, Y., Horvath, S., et al. (2011). Transcriptomic analysis of autistic brain reveals convergent molecular pathology. *Nature* 474, 380–384. doi: 10.1038/nature10110

Watkins, L. R., Milligan, E. D., and Maier, S. F. (2001). Glial activation: a driving force for pathological pain. *Trends Neurosci.* 24, 450–455. doi: 10.1016/S0166-2236(00)01854-3

Wei, H. G., Zou, H., Sheikh, A. M., Malik, M., Dobkin, C., Brown, W. T., et al. (2011). IL-6 is increased in the cerebellum of autistic brain and alters neural cell adhesion, migration and synaptic formation. *J. Neuroinflamm.* 8:52. doi: 10.1186/1742-2094-8-52

Willsey, A. J., Sanders, S. J., Li, M. F., Dong, S., Tebbenkamp, A. T., Muhle, R. A., et al. (2013). Coexpression networks implicate human midfetal deep cortical projection neurons in the pathogenesis of autism. *Cell* 155, 997–1007. doi: 10.1016/j.cell.2013.10.020

Wu, Y. W., Dissing-Olesen, L., MacVicar, B. A., and Stevens, B. (2015). Microglia: dynamic mediators of synapse development and plasticity. *Trends Immunol.* 36, 605–613. doi: 10.1016/j.it.2015.08.008

Yasui, D. H., Xu, H. C., Dunaway, K. W., LaSalle, J. M., Jin, L. W., and Maezawa, I. (2013). MeCP2 modulates gene expression pathways in astrocytes. *Mol. Autism* 4:3. doi: 10.1186/2040-2392-4-3

Yuskaitis, C. J., Beurel, E., and Jope, R. S. (2010). Evidence of reactive astrocytes but not peripheral immune system activation in a mouse model of Fragile X syndrome. *Biochim. Biophys. Acta Mol. Basis Dis.* 1802, 1006–1012. doi: 10.1016/j.bbadis.2010.06.015

Zhan, Y., Paolicelli, R. C., Sforazzini, F., Weinhard, L., Bolasco, G., Pagani, F., et al. (2014). Deficient neuron-microglia signaling results in impaired functional brain connectivity and social behavior. *Nat. Neurosci.* 17, 400–406. doi: 10.1038/nn.3641

Zhang, P. S., Miller, B. S., Rosenzweig, S. A., and Bhat, N. R. (1996). Activation of c-Jun N-terminal kinase stress-activated protein kinase in primary glial cultures. *J. Neurosci. Res.* 46, 114–121. doi: 10.1002/(SICI)1097-4547(19961001)46:1<114::AID-JNR14>3.0.CO;2-5

# 15

# MK-801 Treatment Affects Glycolysis in Oligodendrocytes More than in Astrocytes and Neuronal Cells: Insights for Schizophrenia

*Paul C. Guest[1†], Keiko Iwata[2,3†], Takahiro A. Kato[4,5†], Johann Steiner[6], Andrea Schmitt[7,8], Christoph W. Turck[9]* and Daniel Martins-de-Souza[1,8,10]**

*[1] Laboratory of Neuroproteomics, Department of Biochemistry and Tissue Biology, Institute of Biology, University of Campinas, Campinas, Brazil, [2] Research Center for Child Mental Development, University of Fukui, Fukui, Japan, [3] Department of Development of Functional Brain Activities, United Graduate School of Child Development, Osaka University–Kanazawa University–Hamamatsu University School of Medicine–Chiba University–University of Fukui, Fukui, Japan, [4] Department of Neuropsychiatry, Graduate School of Medical Sciences, Kyushu University, Fukuoka, Japan, [5] Innovation Center for Medical Redox Navigation, Kyushu University, Fukuoka, Japan, [6] Department of Psychiatry and Psychotherapy–Center for Behavioral Brain Sciences, University of Magdeburg, Magdeburg, Germany, [7] Department of Psychiatry and Psychotherapy, Ludwig-Maximilians University, Munich, Germany, [8] Laboratory of Neurosciences (LIM-27), Institute of Psychiatry, University of São Paulo, São Paulo, Brazil, [9] Department of Translational Research in Psychiatry Proteomics and Biomarkers, Max Planck Institute of Psychiatry, Munich, Germany, [10] UNICAMP's Neurobiology Center, Campinas, Brazil*

***Correspondence:***
*Daniel Martins-de-Souza, Laboratory of Neuroproteomics, Department of Biochemistry and Tissue Biology, Institute of Biology, University of Campinas, Rua Monteiro Lobato, 255, 13083-862 Campinas, São Paulo, Brazil dmsouza@unicamp.br; Christoph W. Turck, Department of Translational Research in Psychiatry Proteomics and Biomarkers, Max Planck Institute of Psychiatry, Kraepelinstraße 2-10, 80804 Munich, Germany turck@psych.mpg.de*

*† These authors have contributed equally to this work.*

Schizophrenia is a debilitating mental disorder, affecting more than 30 million people worldwide. As a multifactorial disease, the underlying causes of schizophrenia require analysis by multiplex methods such as proteomics to allow identification of whole protein networks. Previous post-mortem proteomic studies on brain tissues from schizophrenia patients have demonstrated changes in activation of glycolytic and energy metabolism pathways. However, it is not known whether these changes occur in neurons or in glial cells. To address this question, we treated neuronal, astrocyte, and oligodendrocyte cell lines with the NMDA receptor antagonist MK-801 and measured the levels of six glycolytic enzymes by Western blot analysis. MK-801 acts on the glutamatergic system and has been proposed as a pharmacological means of modeling schizophrenia. Treatment with MK-801 resulted in significant changes in the levels of glycolytic enzymes in all cell types. Most of the differences were found in oligodendrocytes, which had altered levels of hexokinase 1 (HK1), enolase 2 (ENO2), phosphoglycerate kinase (PGK), and phosphoglycerate mutase 1 after acute MK-801 treatment (8 h), and HK1, ENO2, PGK, and triosephosphate isomerase (TPI) following long term treatment (72 h). Addition of the antipsychotic clozapine to the cultures resulted in counter-regulatory effects to the MK-801 treatment by normalizing the levels of ENO2 and PGK in both the acute and long term cultures. In astrocytes, MK-801 affected only aldolase C (ALDOC) under both acute conditions and HK1 and ALDOC following long term treatment, and TPI was the only enzyme affected under long term conditions in the neuronal cells. In conclusion, MK-801 affects glycolysis in oligodendrocytes to a larger extent than neuronal cells and this may be modulated by antipsychotic treatment. Although cell culture studies do not necessarily reflect the *in vivo* pathophysiology and drug effects within the brain, these results suggest that neurons, astrocytes, and oligodendrocytes are affected differently in schizophrenia. Employing in vitro models using neurotransmitter agonists and antagonists may provide new insights about the pathophysiology of schizophrenia which could lead to a novel system for drug discovery.

**Keywords: schizophrenia, MK-801, clozapine, neurons, astrocytes, oligodendrocytes, Western blot, glycolysis**

## Introduction

Schizophrenia is a severe, debilitating mental disorder that directly affects more than 30 million people worldwide (van Os and Kapur, 2009). It is manifested in various forms with symptoms ranging from delusions, hallucinations, and disorganized thoughts to anhedonia, lack of motivation, social withdrawal, and cognitive impairments. The current diagnosis is interview-based and involves communication of subjective symptoms, emotions, and histories between the patient and physician, and categorization of patients is performed using the Diagnostic and Statistical Manual of Mental Disorders 5 (DSM-5) or the International Statistical Classification of Diseases and Related Health Problems 10th revision (WHO, 2010; American Psychiatric Association, 2013). However, these manuals only provide descriptions and qualify the symptoms of psychiatric disorders without providing any neurobiological correlates of the disease (Möller et al., 2015). Therefore, knowledge of the molecular pathways affected in these conditions is still lacking. Furthermore, frequent misdiagnosis occurs since multiple psychiatric disorders can exhibit similar symptoms. For example, symptoms of delusions and depression can occur in schizophrenia, major depressive disorder, and bipolar disorder (WHO, 2010; American Psychiatric Association, 2013). Since it is now recognized as a multifactorial disease with an insidious onset, increasing our understanding of the underlying causes of schizophrenia requires analysis by multiplex methods such as proteomics to allow identification of whole protein networks (Turck et al., 2008). Over the past decade, a number of proteomic studies of *post mortem* brain tissues from schizophrenia patients have been carried out using techniques such as two-dimensional gel electrophoresis and shotgun mass spectrometry. These have resulted in identification of changes in proteins mostly involved in energy metabolism (English et al., 2009, 2011; Martins-de-Souza et al., 2011a), and this is likely to be linked to other observed effects on proteins associated with oxidative stress (English et al., 2009, 2011; Martins-de-Souza et al., 2011a), neuronal structure and transport (Carlino et al., 2011; Chan et al., 2011; English et al., 2011), and cell trafficking and signal transduction (Pennington et al., 2008; English et al., 2011; Föcking et al., 2011; Martins-de-Souza et al., 2011a). Taken together, the changes in these proteins suggest that there is net effect on loss of myelination and synaptic function, leading to dysfunction of specific brain areas, and perturbed networking across distal brain regions (Stephan et al., 2009; Martins-de-Souza, 2010).

Despite these advances in understanding different pathways affected in schizophrenia, it is still not known whether such changes are more prominent in neurons or in specific glial cells. In particular, oligodendrocyte pathology has been reported in several brain regions, whereas no astrocytosis has been detected, leading to the concept that schizophrenia is not a classical neurodegenerative disease (Schmitt et al., 2009). One of the most affected neurotransmitters is the glutamatergic system. A hypofunction of the glutamatergic *N*-methyl-D-aspartate (NMDA) receptor has been proposed to play an important role in the pathophysiology of schizophrenia and recently this receptor became a target of new treatment strategies (Hashimoto et al., 2013; Zink et al., 2014). Dizocilpine (MK-801) is a non-competitive antagonist at the NMDA receptor and has been used as pharmacological model of schizophrenia (Zink et al., 2014). Here, we have addressed this question of cell-specific alterations by acute and long term treatment of neuronal, oligodendrocyte, and astrocyte cell lines with MK-801 and measuring the effects on energy metabolism (Meltzer et al., 2011). This was achieved by Western blot analysis of six enzymes involved in the glycolysis pathway, which we found consistently different in schizophrenia brain tissue (Martins-de-Souza et al., 2011a). It was also of interest to evaluate the potential use of these cell lines and associated biomarker signatures as a novel system for drug discovery in schizophrenia research by investigating the effects of add-on treatment with the antipsychotic drug clozapine on the levels of glycolytic enzymes, since clozapine is known to counteract symptoms produced by MK-801 (Feinstein and Kritzer, 2013).

## Materials and Methods

### Materials

Biochemical reagents were from Sigma–Aldrich (St Louis, MO, USA), unless specified otherwise. The immortalized mouse hippocampal neuronal cell line, HT22 (Li et al., 1997), was a generous gift from Dr. David Schubert (The Salk Institute; La Jolla, CA, USA). The cells were cultured in Dulbecco's Modified Eagle Medium (DMEM) containing 10% fetal bovine serum (FBS) and differentiated in modified serum-free DMEM, containing 1X N2 supplement, 50 ng/mL nerve growth factor-β, 100 μM phorbol 12,13-dibutyrate, and 100 μM dibutyryl cAMP for 24–48 h before treatment. All treatments were performed in differentiation medium containing 5 ng/mL nerve growth factor-β. Astrocytes (cell line 1321N1; Haedicke et al., 2009) were cultured in DMEM, containing Nutrient Mixture F-12, penicillin (100 units/mL), streptomycin (100 μg/ml) and L-glutamine (2 mM), and 5% FBS. The MO3.13 cell line (Cellutions Incorporated; Burlington, ON, Canada) is an immortalized human cell line with phenotypic characteristics of oligodendrocyte precursor cells (McLaurin et al., 1995; Buntinx et al., 2003). MO3.13 cells were cultured in DMEM containing 10% FBS, penicillin (100 U/mL) and streptomycin (100 μg/mL). To induce an oligodendrocyte phenotype, the cells were treated with 100 nM Phorbol 12-myristate 13-acetate (PMA) for 4 days. All cell lines were cultured at 37°C in 5% $CO_2$.

### Cell Culture Treatments with MK-801 and Clozapine

The HT22, 1321N1, and MO3.13 cells were treated with MK-801 and/or clozapine under acute (8 h) and long term (72 h) conditions. For the acute treatment, all cells were treated for 8 h with either vehicle (water), 50 μM MK-801, or 50 μM clozapine. For the combined acute treatment, cells were treated first for 4 h with 50 μM MK-801 and then 50 μM clozapine was added and the incubation continued for another 4 h. The cells were collected and stored at −80°C. In the long-term treatment, cells were treated with either vehicle, 10 μM MK-801, or 10 μM clozapine at 0, 24, and 48 h. For the combined chronic treatment, the cells were incubated as above with 10 μM MK-801 and then 10 μM clozapine was added at 8, 32, and 52 h. Concentrations were chosen based on those of previous studies (Kondziella et al., 2006; Paulson et al., 2007; Martins-de-Souza et al., 2011b). The cells were collected after a total of 72 h and stored at −80°C. All incubations in all experiments were performed three times.

### Western Blot Analysis

Western blot analysis was carried out essentially as described previously (Krishnamurthy et al., 2013). Frozen cell pellets were homogenized in 100 μL of 7 M urea, 2 M thiourea, 4% CHAPS, 2% ASB-14, and 70 mM dithiothreitol (DTT) using a kit for sample grinding (GE Healthcare; Munich, Germany). Protein lysates were centrifuged at 14,000 × *g* for 10 min. The resulting supernatants were collected and protein concentrations determined using the Bradford assay (BioRad; Munich, Germany). The protein extracts (20 μg) from each cell sample were electrophoresed on 12% sodium dodecyl sulphate (SDS) minigels (BioRad; Hercules, CA, USA). The proteins were then transferred electrophoretically to Immobilon-FL polyvinyldiphenyl fluoride (PVDF) membranes (Millipore; Bedford, MA, USA) at 100 V for 1 h using a cooling system. PVDF membranes containing the transferred proteins were treated with 5% Carnation instant non-fat dry milk powder in Tris buffered saline (pH 7.4) containing 0.1% Tween −20 (TBS-T) for 4 h, rinsed in TBS-T three times for a total of 20 min and incubated with hexokinase 1 (HK1), aldolase C (ALDOC), and enolase 2 (ENO2) antibodies at a 1:2000 dilution and with phosphoglycerate kinase (PGK), phosphoglycerate mutase 1 (PGAM1), and triosephosphate isomerase (TPI) antibodies at a dilution of 1:000 in TBS-T overnight at 4°C (all antibodies were from Abcam; Cambridge, UK). Following the overnight incubation, the membranes were washed twice with TBS-T for 15 min per wash. Next, the membranes were incubated with anti-c-MYC-peroxidase antibody (GE Healthcare; Uppsala, Sweden) for 40 min at room temperature, washed with water and TBS-T, and incubated with Enhanced Chemiluminescence (ECL) solution (GE Healthcare) for 1 min. The membranes were scanned using a Gel Doc$^{TM}$ XR+ System (Silk Scientific Incorporated; Orem, UT, USA) and the optical densities of the immunoreactive bands were measured using Quantity One software (Bio-Rad). Protein loading was determined by staining PVDF membranes with Coomassie Blue R-250 to ensure equal loading in each gel lane.

### Statistical Analysis

In preliminary analyses, Kolmogorov–Smirnov tests were used for all dependent variables to analyze whether there were significant deviations from the normality assumption, which was not the case. Significant differences across groups were determined by analysis of variance (ANOVA) using GraphPad Prism (La Jolla, CA, USA). Differences between groups were determined by *post hoc* analyses using unpaired two-tailed *t*-tests with Welch's correction. Bonferroni adjustment of the type I error probability was not applied since an adjustment of the error probability would decrease the test power. Due to the explorative study design the findings presented here are not conclusive for a causal relationship.

## Results

### Effects of Treatment of Cultured Cells with MK-801 and Clozapine

#### HT22 Neuronal Cells

Acute treatment of HT22 cells led to significantly increased levels of HK1 and PGAM1, as determined by ANOVA (**Table 1**; see Supplementary Figure S1 for Western blot images of the immunoreactive protein bands for each enzyme under acute and long term conditions in the three cell types). None of the other enzymes showed significant changes. Long term treatment led to a significant increase in the levels of only one enzyme, TPI (**Table 2**). *Post hoc* analysis using unpaired two-tailed *t*-tests with Welch's correction showed that acute clozapine treatment of the HT22 cells resulted in a marked 2.35-fold increase in HK1 ($P = 0.001$) and a smaller 1.17-fold increase in PGAM1 levels ($P = 0.050$). In addition, acute MK-801 treatment led to a significant 1.24-fold increase in PGAM1 levels ($P = 0.026$). Finally, separate long term treatments with clozapine and MK-801 resulted in respective small but significant increases of 1.04-fold ($P = 0.032$) and 1.11-fold ($P = 0.003$) in the levels of TPI (**Figure 1**).

#### 1321N1 Astrocyte Cells

Analysis of variance showed that the acute treatment had significant effects on the levels of different enzymes in 1321N1 cells compared with those altered in HT22 cells. In the 1321N1 astrocyte line, ALDOC and PGK were significantly altered (**Table 1**). None of the other enzymes showed significant changes. *Post hoc* testing (unpaired two-tailed *t*-test with Welch's correction) showed that ALDOC was increased 1.62-fold by acute MK-801 treatment ($P = 0.001$; **Figure 2**). In addition, ENO2 and TPI were increased 1.09-fold ($P = 0.018$) and 1.57-fold ($P = 0.048$), respectively, following the combined MK-801/clozapine treatment in comparison to the treatment with MK-801 alone, and PGK levels were increased 1.08-fold by the clozapine treatment ($P = 0.001$).

Long term treatment of 1321N1 cells resulted in significantly altered levels of five (HK1, ALDOC, PGK, PGAM1, and TPI) out of the six glycolytic enzymes (**Table 2**), as determined by ANOVA. The only enzyme which did not show a change was EN02, which had a non-significant *P*-value of 0.3191. *Post hoc* analysis showed that HK1 was significantly decreased 1.30-fold

**TABLE 1 | Acute treatment of neuronal, astrocyte, and oligodendrocyte cells.**

| Enzyme | CLOZ | CTRL | MK-801 | MK-801/ CLOZ | *P*-value |
|---|---|---|---|---|---|
| **HT22 cells (neurons)** | | | | | |
| HK1 | 78.09 ± 0.07 | 33.29 ± 1.95 | 42.66 ± 5.57 | 77.45 ± 15.37 | **0.0237** |
| ALDOC | 45.82 ± 1.26 | 45.87 ± 3.08 | 46.85 ± 3.42 | 47.27 ± 0.11 | 0.4965 |
| ENO2 | 45.87 ± 0.86 | 46.48 ± 1.14 | 47.06 ± 0.96 | 47.38 ± 0.83 | 0.1540 |
| PGK | 44.82 ± 13.41 | 51.00 ± 10.60 | 59.15 ± 2.13 | 61.08 ± 3.20 | 0.2875 |
| PGAM1 | 50.10 ± 0.52 | 42.81 ± 2.88 | 53.16 ± 0.73 | 50.75 ± 4.69 | **0.0444** |
| TPI | 43.53 ± 4.05 | 40.13 ± 8.03 | 43.15 ± 0.75 | 46.31 ± 2.31 | 0.3611 |
| **1321N1 cells (astrocytes)** | | | | | |
| HK1 | 49.63 ± 2.42 | 51.25 ± 2.30 | 49.38 ± 1.67 | 52.44 ± 1.71 | 0.3061 |
| ALDOC | 52.62 ± 6.90 | 41.50 ± 2.74 | 67.30 ± 1.96 | 62.77 ± 2.41 | **0.0156** |
| ENO2 | 210.1 ± 1.79 | 208.3 ± 15.58 | 200.7 ± 4.16 | 218.9 ± 0.93 | 0.1234 |
| PGK | 53.74 ± 0.29 | 49.67 ± 0.40 | 46.83 ± 1.36 | 46.50 ± 0.02 | **0.0237** |
| PGAM1 | 75.92 ± 3.64 | 76.03 ± 0.89 | 72.86 ± 3.15 | 76.04 ± 0.42 | 0.4415 |
| TPI | 214.3 ± 18.13 | 214.2 ± 45.22 | 178.0 ± 15.60 | 278.9 ± 36.73 | 0.0586 |
| **MO3.13 cells (oligodendrocytes)** | | | | | |
| HK1 | 55.94 ± 0.09 | 43.63 ± 1.31 | 59.90 ± 2.85 | 51.51 ± 0.25 | **0.0156** |
| ALDOC | 51.84 ± 3.87 | 49.40 ± 2.87 | 54.32 ± 3.35 | 60.29 ± 2.60 | 0.0572 |
| ENO2 | 337.4 ± 72.78 | 373.4 ± 13.08 | 594.4 ± 64.33 | 235.3 ± 37.45 | **0.0307** |
| PGK | 157.4 ± 6.37 | 155.5 ± 13.11 | 265.6 ± 7.82 | 164.4 ± 10.66 | 0.0770 |
| PGAM1 | 58.94 ± 0.45 | 62.17 ± 2.40 | 55.01 ± 0.02 | 51.79 ± 1.33 | **0.0156** |
| TPI | 76.15 ± 4.95 | 78.65 ± 6.15 | 84.60 ± 0.40 | 80.60 ± 1.40 | 0.1441 |

*All cells were treated for 4 h with 50 μM MK-801. After this, 50 mM clozapine (CLOZ) was added and the incubation continued for another 4 h. Cells treated with CLOZ alone were incubated for 8 h. The cells were analyzed by Western blot and densitometric scanning of the immunoreactive bands for the glycolytic enzymes hexokinase 1 (HK1), aldolase C (ALDOC), enolase 2 (ENO2) phosphoglycerate kinase (PGK), phosphoglyceratemutase 1 (PGAM1), and triosphosphateisomerase (TPI). Significantly different treatment groups were detected by ANOVA and post hoc analysis was carried out using unpaired two-tailed t-tests with Welch's correction to identify differences between specific groups. P-values in bold were significant.*

**TABLE 2 | Chronic treatment of neuronal, astrocyte, and oligodendrocyte cells.**

| Enzyme | CLOZ | CTRL | MK-801 | MK-801/ CLOZ | *P*-value |
|---|---|---|---|---|---|
| **HT22 cells (neurons)** | | | | | |
| HK1 | 43.53 ± 4.05 | 43.71 ± 4.44 | 43.48 ± 0.95 | 47.12 ± 3.62 | 0.5666 |
| ALDOC | 53.28 ± 7.39 | 55.97 ± 4.85 | 56.70 ± 10.55 | 51.71 ± 8.59 | 0.7888 |
| ENO2 | 36.69 ± 5.44 | 42.62 ± 3.98 | 30.74 ± 13.40 | 27.84 ± 15.11 | 0.4243 |
| PGK | 59.20 ± 1.78 | 57.08 ± 0.25 | 58.91 ± 1.32 | 59.58 ± 3.26 | 0.2815 |
| PGAM1 | 51.03 ± 2.43 | 54.04 ± 3.08 | 49.26 ± 2.79 | 45.36 ± 4.18 | 0.1129 |
| TPI | 45.49 ± 0.73 | 43.66 ± 0.41 | 48.42 ± 0.16 | 48.95 ± 4.03 | **0.0434** |
| **1321N1 cells (astrocytes)** | | | | | |
| HK1 | 52.91 ± 0.10 | 52.17 ± 1.08 | 39.98 ± 0.79 | 45.33 ± 3.67 | **0.0237** |
| ALDOC | 60.98 ± 3.71 | 59.00 ± 0.71 | 70.73 ± 3.57 | 72.09 ± 1.92 | **0.0378** |
| ENO2 | 180.2 ± 15.30 | 184.7 ± 16.48 | 161.5 ± 31.66 | 151.1 ± 32.02 | 0.3191 |
| PGK | 43.71 ± 0.75 | 48.56 ± 0.79 | 48.65 ± 3.50 | 37.70 ± 2.27 | **0.0249** |
| PGAM1 | 71.52 ± 0.84 | 73.14 ± 0.03 | 72.80 ± 3.50 | 61.77 ± 3.95 | **0.0444** |
| TPI | 186.2 ± 31.83 | 221.8 ± 45.36 | 165.6 ± 8.69 | 322.7 ± 44.19 | **0.0378** |
| **MO3.13 oligodendrocytes** | | | | | |
| HK1 | 54.67 ± 1.39 | 50.03 ± 0.08 | 48.24 ± 0.64 | 61.73 ± 1.26 | **0.0156** |
| ALDOC | 50.92 ± 1.42 | 52.78 ± 7.10 | 54.33 ± 0.88 | 62.63 ± 0.66 | **0.0444** |
| ENO2 | 409.5 ± 78.89 | 221.9 ± 10.61 | 617.6 ± 53.2 | 229.7 ± 13.22 | **0.0237** |
| PGK | 259.0 ± 14.26 | 158.5 ± 12.36 | 513.0 ± 13.32 | 132.0 ± 31.06 | **0.0216** |
| PGAM1 | 45.32 ± 2.80 | 45.85 ± 2.07 | 44.45 ± 4.31 | 43.00 ± 2.59 | 0.7152 |
| TPI | 78.85 ± 1.25 | 71.10 ± 0.30 | 87.95 ± 2.35 | 92.90 ± 10.20 | **0.0237** |

*Cells were treated with 10 μM MK-801 at 0, 24, and 48 h and then with 10 μM CLOZ at 8, 32, and 52 h. The cells were collected after a total of 72 h and analyzed by Western blot and densitometric scanning of the immunoreactive bands for the HK1, ALDOC, ENO2, PGK, PGAM1, and TPI. Significantly different treatment groups were detected by ANOVA and post hoc analysis was carried out using unpaired two-tailed t-tests with Welch's correction to identify differences between specific groups. P-values in bold were significant.*

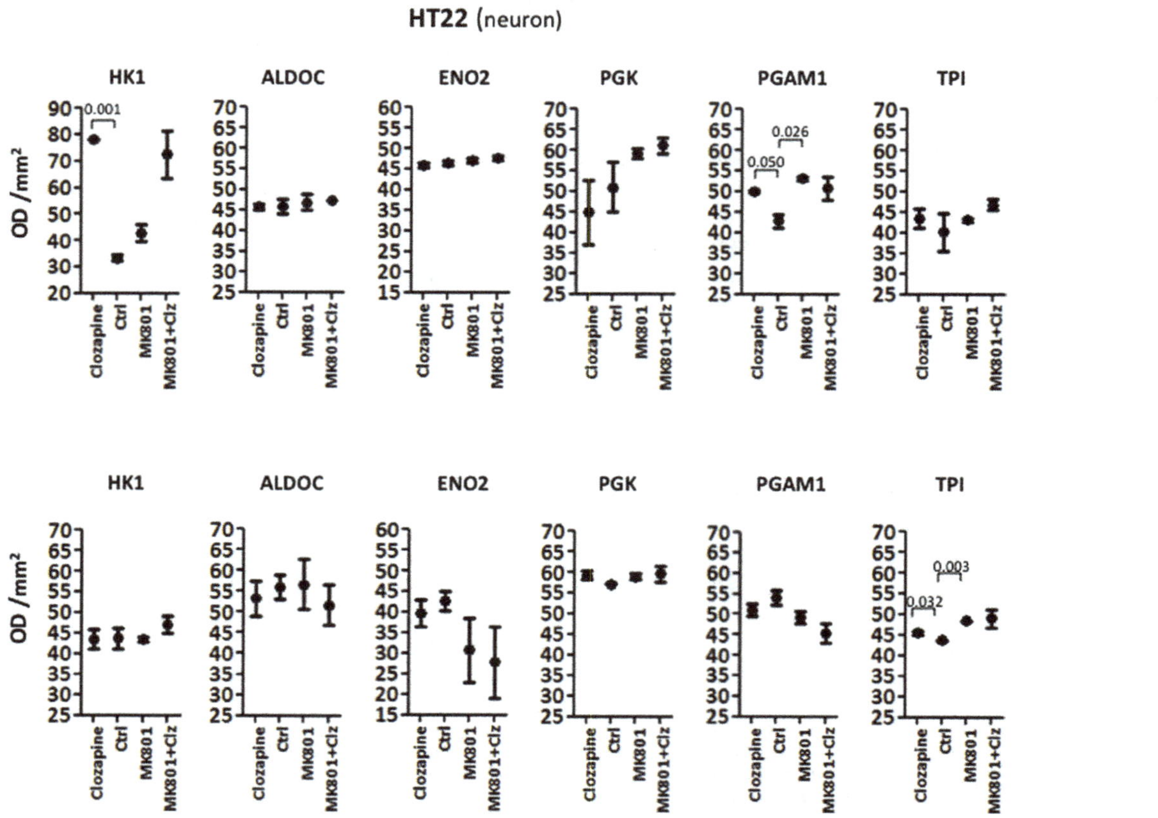


**FIGURE 1 | Levels of glycolytic enzymes in a neuronal cell line (HT22) determined by Western Blot analysis.** The upper panel shows acute effects of MK-801 and Clozapine, and the lower panel shows long-term effects.

($P$ = 0.001) and ALDOC increased 1.20-fold ($P$ = 0.031) by the long term MK-801 treatment (**Figure 2**). Also, PGK levels were decreased 1.11-fold ($P$ = 0.004) by clozapine and 1.29-fold ($P$ = 0.012) by the combined MK-801/clozapine treatments compared with the separate MK-801 treatment. Also, PGAM1 levels were significantly decreased 1.18-fold ($P$ = 0.036) and TPI levels increased markedly 1.95-fold ($P$ = 0.026) by the combined MK-801/clozapine treatment, compared to the MK-801 mono-treatment. Thus, MK-801 had consistent effects on increasing ALDOC levels and the MK-801/clozapine combination led to consistently increased TPI levels relative to the MK-801 treatment alone in both the acute and long term treatment protocols. However, the long term MK-801 treatment led to decreased levels of HK1 and the combined chonic MK-801/clozapine treatment led to decreased PGK and PGAM1, although none of these molecules were affected by the same treatments under acute conditions.

## MO3.13 Oligodendrocyte Cells

Analysis of variance NOVA analysis showed that the M03.13 cells were affected the greatest by the both the acute and long term treatments, with the highest number of changes in the levels of the glycolytic enzymes tested.

The acute treatment resulted in significantly altered levels of HK1, ENO2, and PGAM1. Furthermore ALDOC and PGK showed borderline changes with $P$-values of 0.057 and 0.077, respectively (**Table 1**). Only TPI showed no significant effects ($P$ = 0.1441). *Post hoc t*-test analysis, as carried out above, showed that HK1 levels were increased 1.28-fold ($P$ = 0.004) by clozapine and 1.38-fold by the MK-801 ($P$ = 0.012) treatments, and decreased 1.16-fold by the combined MK-801/clozapine treatment ($P$ = 0.037) in comparison to the MK-801 mono-treatment (**Figure 3**). The levels of both ENO2 and PGK were increased markedly by the MK-801 treatment at 1.59-fold ($P$ = 0.028) and 1.71-fold and ($P$ = 0.001), respectively, and these were decreased to approximately control levels by the combined MK-801/clozapine treatment ($P$ = 0.004 and $P$ = 0.001, respectively). Finally, PGAM1 levels showed a 1.13-fold decrease ($P$ = 0.038) by MK-801 treatment and TPI was decreased 1.05-fold ($P$ = 0.041) by the combined MK-801/clozapine treatment compared with the MK-801 mono-treatment.

Long term treatment of M03.13 cells resulted in altered levels of five (HK1, ALDOC, ENO2, PGK, and TPI) out of the six enzymes, as determined by ANOVA (**Table 2**). Four of these (HK1, ALDOC, PGK, and TPI) were changed in common with the 1321N1 astrocyte cells above. PGAM1 was the only enzyme which did not show a significant response to any of the treatments ($P$ = 0.7152). *Post hoc* testing showed that HK1 was increased (1.09-fold, $P$ = 0.029) by clozapine as found in the acute treatment. However, HK1 levels were affected oppositely

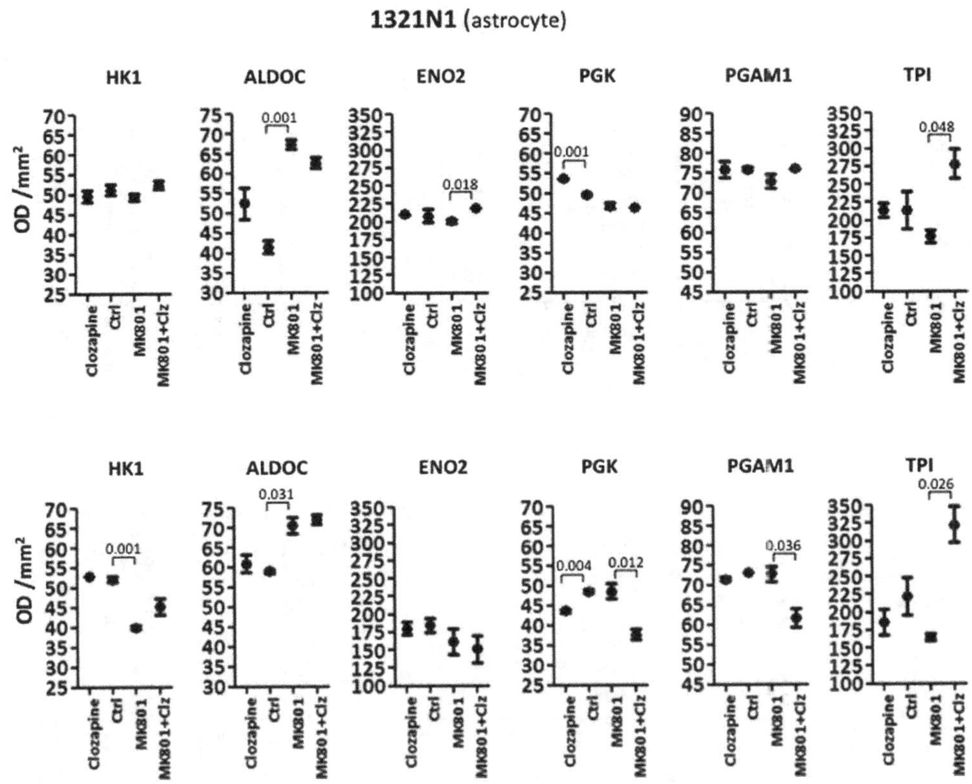


**FIGURE 2 | Levels of glycolytic enzymes in an astrocyte cell line (1321N1) analyzed by Western Blot.** The upper panel represents acute effects of MK-801 and Clozapine, while the lower panel shows long term effects.

in the long term compared to the acute treatment group with a small decrease of 1.04-fold ($P = 0.041$) induced by the MK-801 treatment and a 1.13-fold ($P = 0.004$) increase following the combined MK-801/clozapine treatment compared with MK-801 treatment alone (**Figure 3**). ALDOC was also increased (1.15-fold, $P = 0.001$) by the combined treatment compared to the MK-801 mono-treatment. ENO2 and PGK showed the same pattern as found after the acute treatment with robust increases of 2.78-fold ($P = 0.006$) and 3.24-fold ($P = 0.001$), respectively, following long term treatment with MK-801 and treatment with the MK-801/clozapine combination again led to a decrease approximating the control levels ($P = 0.007$ and 0.003, respectively). However, PGK levels also showed a 1.63-fold increase following the chronic clozapine treatment ($P = 0.003$). Lastly, TPI levels were increased 1.11-fold ($P = 0.009$) by the long-term clozapine treatment and 1.24-fold ($P = 0.007$) by the MK-801 mono-treatment.

## Discussion

This is the first study to show that the main effects on energy metabolism pathways are likely to occur in astrocytes and oligodendrocytes, rather than in neurons, using MK-801 treated cellular models of schizophrenia. Treatment with MK-801 resulted in significant changes in the levels of glycolytic enzymes in all cell types although MO3.13 oligodendrocytes appeared to be the most strongly affected. These cells showed altered levels of four of the enzymes (HK1, ENO2, PGK, and PGAM1) after acute 8 h MK-801 treatment, and the long term 72 h treatment led to similar changes in four of the enzymes (HK1, ENO2, PGK, and TPI). In contrast, the same analysis of the 1321N astrocyte cells showed that MK-801 treatment affected only one enzyme (ALDOC) under acute conditions and two enzymes (HK1 and ALDOC) following long term treatment, and HT22 neuronal cells showed changes in only one enzyme (TPI) following the long term MK-801 treatment protocol. This suggests that astrocytes and neuronal cells are either more resistant to the stresses induced by MK-801 treatment or that oligodendrocytes are more susceptible to treatment with this reagent. It is not clear how these effects are mediated but the findings or recent studies suggest that this could occur through MK-801-induced disruption of glutamate transporters which are associated with mitochondria and energy metabolism enzymes, as found in glial cells and neurons (Domercq et al., 2007; Jackson et al., 2014; Roberts et al., 2014). Considering both the acute and long term treatment protocols, clozapine treatment also had greater effects on the MO3.13 oligodendrocyte cells with changes seen in five out of the six enzymes, 1321N1 cells showed a similar response with changes in four of the enzymes and HT22 cells again showed the lowest response with changes found in only two of the enzymes. Therefore, treatment with the antipsychotic clozapine may have a greater effect on

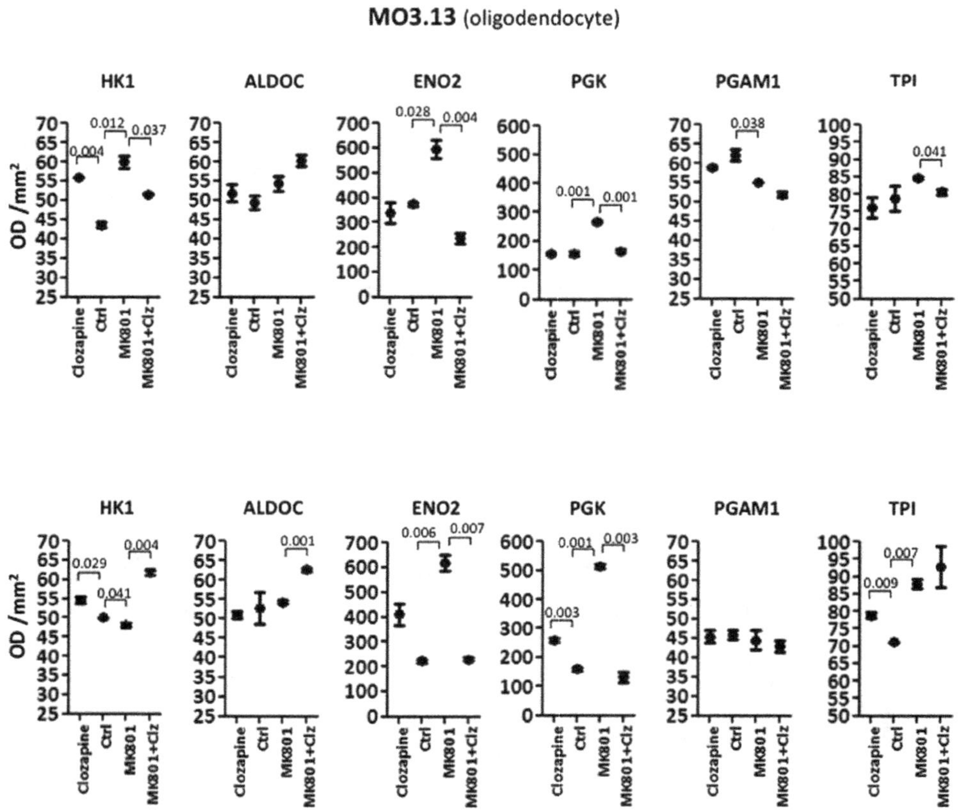


**FIGURE 3 | Levels of glycolytic enzymes in oligodendrocyte cell line (MO3.13) measured by Western Blot analysis.** The upper panel represents acute effects of MK-801 and clozapine treatment, while the lower panel shows long term treatment effects.

both oligodendrocytes and astrocytes as opposed to neurons. Since all of these cell types possess NMDA receptors which should be susceptible to MK-801 blockade as well as other receptors which are known to mediate the effects of clozapine, the observed differential responses suggest that other systems may be involved. Therefore, further studies aimed at elucidating these differences may lead to identification of novel biomarkers and targets for use in future drug discovery efforts in schizophrenia research.

A previous study using cultured OLN-93 oligodendrocyte cells showed that clozapine treatment improved glucose uptake, as well as the production and release of lactate (Steiner et al., 2014). Under acute conditions in the present study, the MK-801 treatment had only a small effect on the HT22 neuronal cell line in terms of the number of glycolytic enzymes affected. However acute clozapine treatment of these cells led to increased levels of PGAM1. In addition, under chronic conditions, both the MK-801 and clozapine treatments resulted in increased levels of TPI in the neuronal cell line. This suggested that effects on TPI are not likely to be involved in the response to antipsychotic treatment in neurons. It is possible that the observed effect of clozapine on TPI in the neuronal cells is associated with the widely reported metabolic side effects of antipsychotic treatment, such as weight gain and insulin resistance (Deng, 2013). Perturbations of glycolysis are known to be linked with impaired insulin signaling (Belfiore et al., 1979).

Previous studies have found changes in the levels of enzymes involved in glycolysis in brain tissues from rodent models of schizophrenia and from *post mortem* schizophrenia patients. A study of the chronic MK-801 rat model using $^{13}$C-glucose labeling, found reduced glycolysis along with lower glutamate and γ-aminobutyric acid (GABA) levels in multiple brain regions (Eyjolfsson et al., 2011). This demonstrated how reduced supply of glucose or perturbed glycolysis can have effects on the neurotransmitter systems which have been implicated in schizophrenia (Lang et al., 2007). In addition, a proteomic study found that glycolysis was one of the major pathways affected in both gray and white matter areas of *post mortem* brain tissues from schizophrenia patients (Martins-de-Souza et al., 2012a). This is consistent with our finding of effects on the levels of glycolytic enzyme in all three cell types, albeit with more numerous effects in glial cells. One study showed a decrease in HK1 attachment to mitochondria in *post mortem* parietal cortex brain tissue of individuals with schizophrenia which is thought to result in uncoupling of glycolysis with oxidative phosphorylation and, therefore, reduced adenosine triphosphate (ATP) generation (Regenold et al., 2012). HK1 mitochondrial attachment is also thought be important for survival of neuronal cells through prevention of apoptosis and oxidative damage (Saraiva et al., 2010). Again, we found that HK1 levels were affected only in the oligodendrocyte and astrocyte cells after treatment with MK-801. We also found that TPI levels were decreased only in the astrocyte cell line. Martins-de-Souza et al. (2012b) found that the levels of TPI were also decreased in frontal cortex tissue from an acute treatment phencyclidine (PCP) rat model, using selective reaction monitoring (SRM) mass spectrometry in the analysis. The same study also showed that a multivariate signal composed of HK1, ALDOC, ENO2, PGK, PGAM1, TPI, and glyceraldehyde 3-phosphate dehydrogenase (GAPDH) could distinguish the PCP-treated from vehicle-treated control rats using partial least squares discriminant analysis (PLS-DA).

The finding that the oligodendrocyte cells showed a higher number of glycolytic enzyme changes is interesting considering the important role of these cells in myelination of neurons (Nave and Werner, 2014). Numerous lines of evidence have implicated myelin and oligodendrocyte function as critical factors affecting neuronal connectivity, which has also been implicated widely in schizophrenia (Lee et al., 2012; Bernstein et al., 2015; Mighdoll et al., 2015). Therefore, our finding that the MO3.13 cells showed the greatest number of glycolytic enzyme changes in response to the MK-801 treatment is consistent with the possibility that oligodendrocyte pathology and disturbances in white matter tracts may contribute to the pathophysiology of schizophrenia (Schmitt et al., 2009; Yao et al., 2013). Our results suggest that an NMDA receptor hypofunction is associated with oligodendrocyte dysfunction by inducing deficits in glycolysis. However, it remains to be determined whether the effects on glycolysis in these cells are a causative factor or simply a consequence of these processes. Nevertheless, the effects on the glycolytic enzymes in these cells may provide useful biomarkers in drug discovery efforts. In this regard, it is interesting that ENO2 and PGK levels were increased strongly by the MK-801 treatment in the oligodendrocyte cell line and both enzymes were normalized to approximately control levels following treatment with clozapine. Therefore, further studies are warranted to test these two enzymes as antipsychotic treatment response markers in the MO3.13 oligodendrocytes and related cell lines.

### Limitations

Although cell culture studies do not necessarily reflect the *in vivo* pathophysiology and drug effects within the brain, these results suggest that neurons, astrocytes, and oligodendrocytes are affected differently in schizophrenia. Both the acute and long term treatment protocols showed that MK-801 treatment affects glycolysis more in oligodendrocytes than in the other cell types and in some cases these effects could be reversed by antipsychotic treatment. It is not clear whether some of the effects of the antipsychotic treatment are associated with therapeutic efficacy or with the metabolic side-effect profile of these drugs. Further studies are required to address this question. It will also be important to validate the findings by looking for direct changes on mitochondrial structure in the three cell lines. Another set of validation studies will explore if similar changes in glycolysis can be identified in other neuronal or glial cell lines. As a means of validation of these findings, it will also be important to explore if similar changes in glycolysis can be identified in other neuronal or glial cell lines. It will also be important to validate the findings by looking for direct changes on mitochondrial structure in the three cell lines. Finally, the time scale over which the cellular effects occurred in this study is most likely more rapid than that of the disease pathology. We suggest that this is likely to be the case *in vivo* considering that effects at the cellular level precede the systemic effects that eventually lead to the disease and manifestation of symptoms.

## Conclusion

The translation of academic findings to the clinic is now a major objective of biomarker validation studies, especially in support of drug discovery (Owens, 2006; Marson, 2007). We suggest that assays for glycolytic enzymes such as ENO2 and PGK could be implemented on high throughput platforms such as SRM mass spectrometry instruments, considering that this method is robust and user friendly for use in clinical studies. SRM mass spectrometry has already been used in clinical investigations, including screening the levels of dihydroartemisinin (DHA) in plasma of malaria patients (Wiesner et al., 2011), measuring the levels of apolipoproteins in human plasma (Agger et al., 2010) and in cancer biomarker screening studies (Ang and Nice, 2010; Welinder et al., 2014). Finally, the results of the current study indicate that MK-801 treated oligodendrocyte cells may be a useful model for some aspects of metabolic dysfunction and for biomarker screening in schizophrenia studies, considering the known effects on glycolysis-related enzymes in brain tissues from schizophrenia patients. In addition, we propose the use of glycolytic enzymes such as ENO2 and PGK as companion biomarkers for use with this model.

## Author Contributions

PG analyzed the data, researched, wrote, and edited the manuscript. KI carried out the experiments, analyzed the data, wrote, and edited the manuscript. TK conceived experiments, analyzed the data, wrote, and edited the manuscript. JS carried out the experiments, wrote, and edited the manuscript. AS carried out the experiments, wrote, and edited the manuscript. CT researched, wrote, and edited the manuscript. DM conceived and researched the project, analyzed the data, wrote, and edited the manuscript.

## Acknowledgments

This research was supported by FAPESP (São Paulo Research Foundation) grant number 13/08711-3 and FAEPEX UNICAMP grant number 519.292.

## References

Agger, S. A., Marney, L. C., and Hoofnagle, A. N. (2010). Simultaneous quantification of apolipoprotein A-I and apolipoprotein B by liquid-chromatography-multiple-reaction-monitoring mass spectrometry. *Clin. Chem.* 56, 1804–1813. doi: 10.1373/clinchem.2010.152264

American Psychiatric Association. (2013). *Diagnostic and Statistical Manual of Mental Disorders*, 5th Edn. Arlington, VA: American Psychiatric Publishing.

Ang, C. S., and Nice, E. C. (2010). Targeted in-gel MRM: a hypothesis driven approach for colorectal cancer biomarker discovery in human feces. *J. Proteome Res.* 9, 4346–4355. doi: 10.1021/pr100509e

Belfiore, F., Iannello, S., and Rabuazzo, A. M. (1979). Insulin resistance in obesity: a critical analysis at enzyme level. A review. *Int. J. Obes.* 3, 301–323.

Bernstein, H. G., Steiner, J., Guest, P. C., Dobrowolny, H., and Bogerts, B. (2015). Glial cells as key players in schizophrenia pathology: recent insights and concepts of therapy. *Schizophr. Res.* 161, 4–18. doi: 10.1016/j.schres.2014.03.035

Buntinx, M., Vanderlocht, J., Hellings, N., Vandenabeele, F., Lambrichts, I., Raus, J., et al. (2003). Characterization of three human oligodendroglial cell lines as a model to study oligodendrocyte injury: morphology and oligodendrocyte-specific gene expression. *J. Neurocytol.* 32, 25–38. doi: 10.1023/A:1027324230923

Carlino, D., Leone, E., Di Cola, F., Baj, G., Marin, R., Dinelli, G., et al. (2011). Low serum truncated-BDNF isoform correlates with higher cognitive impairment in schizophrenia. *J. Psychiatr. Res.* 45, 273–279. doi: 10.1016/j.jpsychires.2010.06.012

Chan, M. K., Tsang, T. M., Harris, L. W., Guest, P. C., Holmes, E., and Bahn, S. (2011). Evidence for disease and antipsychotic medication effects in post-mortem brain from schizophrenia patients. *Mol. Psychiatry* 16, 1189–1202. doi: 10.1038/mp.2010.100

Deng, C. (2013). Effects of antipsychotic medications on appetite, weight, and insulin resistance. *Endocrinol. Metab. Clin. North Am.* 42, 545–563. doi: 10.1016/j.ecl.2013.05.006

Domercq, M., Sánchez-Gómez, M. V., Sherwin, C., Etxebarria, E., Fern, R., and Matute, C. (2007). System xc- and glutamate transporter inhibition mediates microglial toxicity to oligodendrocytes. *J. Immunol.* 178, 6549–6556. doi: 10.4049/jimmunol.178.10.6549

English, J. A., Dicker, P., Föcking, M., Dunn, M. J., and Cotter, D. R. (2009). 2-D DIGE analysis implicates cytoskeletal abnormalities in psychiatric disease. *Proteomics* 9, 3368–3382. doi: 10.1002/pmic.200900015

English, J. A., Pennington, K., Dunn, M. J., and Cotter, D. R. (2011). The neuroproteomics of schizophrenia. *Biol. Psychiatry* 69, 163–172. doi: 10.1016/j.biopsych.2010.06.031

Eyjolfsson, E. M., Nilsen, L. H., Kondziella, D., Brenner, E., Håberg, A., and Sonnewald, U. (2011). Altered 13C glucose metabolism in the cortico-striato-thalamo-cortical loop in the MK-801 rat model of schizophrenia. *J. Cereb. Blood Flow Metab.* 31, 976–985. doi: 10.1038/jcbfm.2010.193

Feinstein, I., and Kritzer, M. F. (2013). Acute N-methyl-D-aspartate receptor hypofunction induced by MK801 evokes sex-specific changes in behaviors observed in open-field testing in adult male and proestrus female rats. *Neuroscience* 228, 200–214. doi: 10.1016/j.neuroscience.2012.10.026

Föcking, M., Dicker, P., English, J. A., Schubert, K. O., Dunn, M. J., and Cotter, D. R. (2011). Common proteomic changes in the hippocampus in schizophrenia and bipolar disorder and particular evidence for involvement of cornuammonis regions 2 and 3. *Arch. Gen. Psychiatry* 68, 477–488. doi: 10.1001/archgenpsychiatry.2011.43

Haedicke, J., Brown, C., and Naghavi, M. H. (2009). The brain-specific factor FEZ1 is a determinant of neuronal susceptibility to HIV-1 infection. *Proc. Natl. Acad. Sci. U.S.A.* 106, 14040–14045. doi: 10.1073/pnas.0900502106

Hashimoto, K., Malchow, B., Falkai, P., and Schmitt, A. (2013). Glutamate modulators as potential therapeutic drugs in schizophrenia and affective disorders. *Eur. Arch. Psychiatry Clin. Neurosci.* 263, 367–377. doi: 10.1007/s00406-013-0399-y

Jackson, J. G., O'Donnell, J. C., Krizman, E., and Robinson, M. B. (2014). Displacing hexokinase from mitochondrial voltage-dependent anion channel impairs GLT-1-mediated glutamate uptake but does not disrupt interactions between GLT-1 and mitochondrial proteins. *J. Neurosci. Res.* doi: 10.1002/jnr.23533 [Epub ahead of print].

Kondziella, D., Brenner, E., Eyjolfsson, E. M., Markinhuhta, K. R., Carlsson, M. L., and Sonnewald, U. (2006). Glial-neuronal interactions are impaired in the schizophrenia model of repeated MK801 exposure. *Neuropsychopharmacology* 31, 1880–1887. doi: 10.1038/sj.npp.1300993

Krishnamurthy, D., Harris, L. W., Levin, Y., Koutroukides, T. A., Rahmoune, H., Pietsch, S., et al. (2013). Metabolic, hormonal and stress-related molecular changes in post-mortem pituitary glands from schizophrenia subjects. *World J. Biol. Psychiatry* 14, 478–489. doi: 10.3109/15622975.2011.601759

Lang, U. E., Puls, I., Muller, D. J., Strutz-Seebohm, N., and Gallinat, J. (2007). Molecular mechanisms of schizophrenia. *Cell. Physiol. Biochem.* 20, 687–702. doi: 10.1159/000110430

Lee, Y., Morrison, B. M., Li, Y., Lengacher, S., Farah, M. H., Hoffman, P. N., et al. (2012). Oligodendroglia metabolically support axons and contribute to neurodegeneration. *Nature* 487, 443–448. doi: 10.1038/nature11314

Li, Y., Maher, P., and Schubert, D. (1997). A role for 12-lipoxygenase in nerve cell death caused by glutathione depletion. *Neuron* 19, 453–463. doi: 10.1016/S0896-6273(00)80953-8

Marson, B. (2007). "Critical Path" is on the road forward; FDA reports industry activity is high. *The Pink Sheet* 69:29.

Martins-de-Souza, D. (2010). Proteome and transcriptome analysis suggests oligodendrocyte dysfunction in schizophrenia. *J. Psychiatr. Res.* 44, 149–156. doi: 10.1016/j.jpsychires.2009.07.007

Martins-de-Souza, D., Alsaif, M., Ernst, A., Harris, L. W., Aerts, N., Lenaerts, I., et al. (2012a). The application of selective reaction monitoring confirms dysregulation of glycolysis in a preclinical model of schizophrenia. *BMC Res. Notes* 5:146. doi: 10.1186/1756-0500-5-146

Martins-de-Souza, D., Guest, P. C., Rahmoune, H., and Bahn, S. (2012b). Proteomic approaches to unravel the complexity of schizophrenia. *Expert Rev. Proteomics* 9, 97–108. doi: 10.1586/epr.11.70

Martins-de-Souza, D., Harris, L. W., Guest, P. C., and Bahn, S. (2011a). The role of energy metabolism dysfunction and oxidative stress in schizophrenia revealed by proteomics. *Antioxid. Redox Signal.* 15, 2067–2079. doi: 10.1089/ars.2010.3459

Martins-de-Souza, D., Lebar, M., and Turck, C. W. (2011b). Proteome analyses of cultured astrocytes treated with MK-801 and clozapine: similarities with schizophrenia. *Eur. Arch. Psychiatry Clin. Neurosci.* 261, 217–228. doi: 10.1007/s00406-010-0166-2

McLaurin, J., Trudel, G. C., Shaw, I. T., Antel, J. P., and Cashman, N. R. (1995). A human glial hybrid cell line differentially expressing genes subservingoligodendrocyte and astrocyte phenotype. *J. Neurobiol.* 26, 283–293. doi: 10.1002/neu.480260212

Meltzer, H. Y., Horiguchi, M., and Massey, B. W. (2011). The role of serotonin in the NMDA receptor antagonist models of psychosis and cognitive impairment. *Psychopharmacology (Berl.)* 213, 289–305. doi: 10.1007/s00213-010-2137-8

Mighdoll, M. I., Tao, R., Kleinman, J. E., and Hyde, T. M. (2015). Myelin, myelin-related disorders, and psychosis. *Schizophr. Res.* 161, 85–93. doi: 10.1016/j.schres.2014.09.040

Möller, H. J., Bandelow, B., Bauer, M., Hampel, H., Herpertz, S. C., Soyka, M., et al. (2015). DSM-5 reviewed from different angles: goal attainment, rationality, use of evidence, consequences-part 2: bipolar disorders, schizophrenia spectrum disorders, anxiety disorders, obsessive-compulsive disorders, trauma- and stressor-related disorders, personality disorders, substance-related and addictive disorders, neurocognitive disorders. *Eur. Arch. Psychiatry Clin. Neurosci.* 265, 87–106. doi: 10.1007/s00406-014-0521-9

Nave, K. A., and Werner, H. B. (2014). Myelination of the nervous system: mechanisms and functions. *Annu. Rev. Cell Dev. Biol.* 30, 503–533. doi: 10.1146/annurev-cellbio-100913-013101

Owens, J. (2006). Funding for accelerating drug development initiative critical. *Nat. Rev. Drug Discov.* 5:271. doi: 10.1038/nrd2015

Paulson, L., Martin, P., Ljung, E., Blennow, K., and Davidsson, P. (2007). Proteome analysis after co-administration of clozapine or haloperidol to MK-801-treated rats. *J. Neural. Transm.* 114, 885–891. doi: 10.1007/s00702-007-0626-7

Pennington, K., Beasley, C. L., Dicker, P., Fagan, A., English, J., Pariante, C. M., et al. (2008). Prominent synaptic and metabolic abnormalities revealed by proteomic analysis of the dorsolateral prefrontal cortex in schizophrenia and bipolar disorder. *Mol. Psychiatry* 13, 1102–1117. doi: 10.1038/sj.mp.4002098

Regenold, W. T., Pratt, M., Nekkalapu, S., Shapiro, P. S., Kristian, T., and Fiskum, G. (2012). Mitochondrial detachment of hexokinase 1 in mood and psychotic disorders: implications for brain energy metabolism and neurotrophic signaling. *J. Psychiatr. Res.* 46, 95–104. doi: 10.1016/j.jpsychires.2011.09.018

Roberts, R. C., Roche, J. K., and McCullumsmith, R. E. (2014). Localization of excitatory amino acid transporters EAAT1 and EAAT2 in human postmortem cortex: a light and electron microscopic study. *Neuroscience* 277, 522–540. doi: 10.1016/j.neuroscience.2014.07.019

Saraiva, L. M., Seixas da Silva, G. S., Galina, A., da-Silva, W. S., Klein, W. L., Ferreira, S. T., et al. (2010). Amyloid-β triggers the release of neuronal hexokinase 1 from mitochondria. *PLoS ONE* 5:e15230. doi: 10.1371/journal.pone.0015230

Schmitt, A., Steyskal, C., Bernstein, H. G., Parlapani, E., Schaeffer, E. L., Gattaz, W. F., et al. (2009). Stereologic investigation of the posterior part of the hippocampus in schizophrenia. *Acta Neuropathologica* 117, 395–407. doi: 10.1007/s00401-008-0430-y

Steiner, J., Martins-de-Souza, D., Schiltz, K., Sarnyai, Z., Westphal, S., Isermann, B., et al. (2014). Clozapine promotes glycolysis and myelin lipid synthesis in cultured oligodendrocytes. *Front. Cell. Neurosci.* 8:384. doi: 10.3389/fncel.2014.00384

Stephan, K. E., Friston, K. J., and Frith, C. D. (2009). Dysconnection in schizophrenia: from abnormal synaptic plasticity to failures of self-monitoring. *Schizophr. Bull.* 35, 509–527. doi: 10.1093/schbul/sbn176

Turck, C. W., Ditzen, C., and Sayan-Ayata, E. (2008). "Proteomic strategies for biomarker discovery: from differential expression to isoforms to pathways," in, *Biomarkers for Psychiatric Disorders*, ed. C. W. Turck (New York, NY: Springer), 57–74.

van Os, J., and Kapur, S. (2009). Schizophrenia. *Lancet* 374, 635–645. doi: 10.1016/S0140-6736(09)60995-8

Welinder, C., Jönsson, G. B., Ingvar, C., Lundgren, L., Baldetorp, B., Olsson, H., et al. (2014). Analysis of alpha-synuclein in malignant melanoma – Development of a SRM quantification assay. *PLoS ONE* 9:e110804. doi: 10.1371/journal.pone.0110804

WHO. (2010). *International Statistical Classification of Diseases and Related Health Problems*, 10th revision, 4th Edn. Geneva: WHO.

Wiesner, L., Govender, K., Meredith, S. A., Norman, J., and Smith, P. J. (2011). A liquid-liquid LC/MS/MS assay for the determination of artemether and DHA in malaria patient samples. *J. Pharm. Biomed. Anal.* 55, 373–378. doi: 10.1016/j.jpba.2011.01.036

Yao, L., Lui, S., Liao, Y., Du, M. Y., Hu, N., Thomas, J. A., et al. (2013). White matter deficits in first episode schizophrenia: an activation likelihood meta-analysis. *Prog. Neuropsychopharmacol. Biol. Psychiatry* 45, 100–106. doi: 10.1016/j.pnpbp.2013.04.019

Zink, M., Englisch, S., and Schmitt, A. (2014). Antipsychotic treatment modulates glutamate transport and NMDA receptor expression. *Eur. Arch. Psychiatry Clin. Neurosci.* 264(Suppl. 1), S67–S82. doi: 10.1007/s00406-014-0534-4

# 16

# Exploring the Role of Microglia in Mood Disorders Associated with Experimental Multiple Sclerosis

*Antonietta Gentile*[1,2], *Francesca De Vito*[1,2], *Diego Fresegna*[1,2], *Alessandra Musella*[1], *Fabio Buttari*[2,3], *Silvia Bullitta*[1], *Georgia Mandolesi*[1] *and Diego Centonze*[2,3]*

[1] *Fondazione Santa Lucia/Centro Europeo per la Ricerca sul Cervello (CERC), Rome, Italy,* [2] *Clinica Neurologica, Dipartimento di Medicina dei Sistemi, Università Tor Vergata, Rome, Italy,* [3] *IRCCS Istituto Neurologico Mediterraneo (INM) Neuromed, Pozzilli, Italy*

***Correspondence:***
*Diego Centonze,*
*Clinica Neurologica, Dipartimento di Medicina dei Sistemi, Università Tor Vergata, Via Montpellier 1, Rome 00133, Italy*
*centonze@uniroma2.it*

Microglia is increasingly recognized to play a crucial role in the pathogenesis of psychiatric diseases. In particular, microglia may be the cellular link between inflammation and behavioral alterations: by releasing a number of soluble factors, among which pro-inflammatory cytokines, that can regulate synaptic activity, thereby leading to perturbation of behavior. In multiple sclerosis (MS), the most common neuroinflammatory disorder affecting young adults, microglia activation and dysfunction may account for mood symptoms, like depression and anxiety, that are often diagnosed in patients even in the absence of motor disability. Behavioral studies in experimental autoimmune encephalomyelitis (EAE), the animal model of MS, have shown that emotional changes occur early in the disease and in correlation to inflammatory mediator and neurotransmitter level alterations. However, such studies lack a full and comprehensive analysis of the role played by microglia in EAE-behavioral syndrome. We review the experimental studies addressing behavioral symptoms in EAE, and propose the study of neuron-glia interaction as a powerful but still poorly explored tool to investigate the burden of microglia in mood alterations associated to MS.

**Keywords: microglia, experimental autoimmune encephalomyelitis, multiple sclerosis, behavioral syndrome, neuron-microglia interaction, depression, anxiety**

## Introduction

Multiple Sclerosis (MS) is a chronic inflammatory demyelinating and neurodegenerative disease of the central nervous system (CNS), which represents the leading cause of non-traumatic disability in young adults in Western countries (Compston and Coles, 2008). In addition to physical impairment, MS is frequently associated to mood disorders, like anxiety and depression even in non-disabled patients (Marrie et al., 2009). Structural and functional brain changes, induced by inflammation, seem to be implicated in MS psychiatric symptoms (Feinstein et al., 2014). In fact, T-lymphocytes peripherally primed against myelin-like components infiltrate the brain and initiate a chain of inflammatory events, including both gray and white matter microgliosis (Centonze et al., 2010). Interestingly, recent studies in MS animal model, the experimental autoimmune encephalomyelitis (EAE), have shown that activated microglia, by releasing pro-inflammatory cytokines, can alter brain synaptic transmission also before the appearance of motor symptoms (Centonze et al., 2009, 2010). Notably, changes in neuronal compartment and abnormalities in microglial physiology have been related to several psychopathological conditions in both humans and animal models (Price and Drevets, 2010; Frick et al., 2013), raising the possibility that microglia may have a crucial role in mediating mood disorders in MS.

This paper briefly discusses the current studies about anxious- and depressive-like behaviors in the EAE model and proposes the contribution of microglia to EAE mood disorders, as an important but quite unexplored field for future research.

## Microglia in Mood Disorders

Microglia derive from macrophage lineage and represent 10–20% of the glial cells in the CNS (Lynch, 2009). Exposure to foreign antigens or cellular debris induces microglial cytotoxic activation required for brain immune surveillance. Such activated microglia release a variety of proinflammatory mediators, like interleukin-1β (IL-1β) and tumor necrosis factor (TNF; Lynch, 2009; Kettenmann et al., 2011).

However, cytokines, such as interleukin-4 (IL-4) or interleukin-25 (IL-25), can shift microglial state from the resting to the neuroprotective one (Zhou et al., 2012; Maiorino et al., 2013). Activated microglia can switch from the characteristic ramified morphology to the hyperramified or amoeboid/phagocytic one with upregulation of several markers, including the ionized calcium-binding adapter molecule 1 (Iba1) and CD11b (Kettenmann et al., 2011).

Microglia mutually interact by contact or via mediators with several cells, like T cells, astrocytes and even neurons and such interactions can induce changes in microglial state (Lynch, 2009). The direct and indirect communication between microglia and neurons reveals microglia synaptic functions in addition to the well-established immune ones. In fact, it has been demonstrated that microglia participate in neurogenesis (Butovsky et al., 2006), neuronal transmission (Graeber, 2010) and synaptic pruning in memory and neuronal plasticity (Schafer et al., 2012).

Both abnormalities in microglial physiology and dysfunction of neuron-microglia cross-talk have been involved in psychiatric diseases. For example, several *postmortem* studies have reported abundant activated microglia surrounding neurons (Vargas et al., 2005) and a switch to amoeboid morphology (Morgan et al., 2010; Tetreault et al., 2012) in multiple brain regions from patient with autism spectrum disorders. Moreover, positron emission tomography (PET) imaging has confirmed *postmortem* findings about microglial activation in autism patients (Suzuki et al., 2013). Similar results have been observed in different animal models of autism (Zerrate et al., 2007; Heo et al., 2011; MacFabe et al., 2011). Furthermore, a recent work in MECP2-null mice, which model Rett syndrome, an X-linked autism spectrum disorder, has provided one of the first causal links between microglial alterations and psychiatric disturbances: the authors succeeded in the mitigation of Rett syndrome-like symptoms by supplying wild-type microglia through bone marrow transplantation or genetic rescue in MECP2-null mice (Derecki et al., 2012).

A role for microglia in anxiety and depression is also emerging on the basis of several observations. First, IL-1β and TNF, which are proinflammatory cytokines released during peripheral infection as well as by activated microglia, can induce sickness behavior, resulting in decreased motor activity, fatigue, reduced food intake, anhedonia and social withdrawal in both rodents and humans. Many of these symptoms are commonly observed in depressed patients (Dantzer et al., 2008), whose levels of proinflammatory cytokines have been found increased in both peripheral blood and cerebrospinal fluid (CSF; Zorrilla et al., 2001). Second, *postmortem* studies have revealed consistent microgliosis in suicide-attempters compared to controls (Steiner et al., 2008). Moreover, both activation state of microglia and proinflammatory cytokine levels have been suggested to predict depression relapse and, even, to evaluate the therapeutic response (Miller et al., 2009; Munkholm et al., 2013; Watkins et al., 2014).

Studies on animal models have provided further evidence for involvement of microglia in the pathogenesis of anxious- and depressive-like behaviors. Rodent paradigms of chronic stress, such as repeated constrain or repeated social defeat, have been reported to induce anxious- and depressive-like symptoms, associated to changes in both microglial activation state and morphology in several brain regions (Tynan et al., 2010; Wohleb et al., 2011; Hinwood et al., 2013). Notably, the treatment of stressed animals with the antibiotic minocycline is able to recover microglial homeostasis together with mood dysfunctions (Hinwood et al., 2013).

Both preclinical and clinical data support the theory of the inflammatory etiology for anxious and depressive behavior, and implicate microglia as possible cellular mediators of these mental disorders (Eyre and Baune, 2012).

## EAE Models Behavioral Symptoms of MS

Although it is reasonable to expect that mood alterations in MS patients are a consequence of their physical progressive disability, the prevalence of anxiety and depression, is generally higher in persons with MS with respect to both the general population (Patten et al., 2003) and patients with other neurological disorders (Schiffer and Babigian, 1984; Schubert and Foliart, 1993; Thielscher et al., 2013). In some cases, psychiatric symptoms may occur at the onset of the disease and independently of physical disability (Haussleiter et al., 2009; Lo Fermo et al., 2010; Suh et al., 2010; Rietberg et al., 2011).

While physical disability is the primary target of pharmacological treatment, mood disorders are currently undervalued and undertreated in clinical practice (Marrie et al., 2009), although they can dramatically worsen the quality of life of MS patients. The scarce attention paid to the psychiatric aspects of MS symptomatology is in part due to the lack of knowledge of their pathological basis. In this respect, studies in animal models of MS may represent the unique opportunity to address this critical issue. Although many of the clinical features of mental illness generally cannot be modeled in rodents, some animal models of depression and anxiety provide reliable and measurable correlate of human behavior and allow the study of their molecular underpinnings. Most of MS clinical and histopathological features are well shaped by EAE, in particular the myelin oligodendrocyte glycoprotein $p_{35-55}$ ($MOG_{35-55}$)-induced "chronic" EAE in C57BL/6 mice (Furlan et al., 2009). In such model different phases of the disease can be distinguished: the pre-symptomatic phase with absence of motor deficits, the acute phase starting from the onset to the peak of clinical symptoms and the following chronic phase, in which motor symptoms become milder. Several studies have reported both anxiety- and depression-like behaviors in all EAE clinical phases in correlation with a number of cellular and molecular players (**Table 1**).

Former studies by Pollak and colleagues characterized the so-called "sickness behavior" in EAE mice (Pollak et al., 2000, 2003a,b). All the hallmarks of sickness behavior, observed in acute-phase-EAE mice, were recovered in later phases of the disease, with the exception of the body weight. Notably, such behavior affected EAE mice from the day before the onset of neurological symptoms, demonstrating that emotional changes in EAE are not the mere consequence of motor disability (Pollak et al., 2000). Also, chronic treatment with anti-depressant imipramine prevented body-weight loss in EAE mice (Pollak et al., 2002).

Next, they found that the onset of behavioral syndrome coincided with elevation of TNF and IL-1β in the brain and prostaglandin E2 (PGE2) in the hypothalamus (Pollak et al., 2003a). Interestingly, pro-inflammatory cytokines reached their peak expression in the sickness-behavior phase and decreased along with behavioral recovery, which correlated with worsening of motor symptoms, confirming the hypothesis that cytokines sustain the initial process leading to neurological symptoms but their role dampens with time. Moreover, mice showing sickness behavior but lacking neurological deficits had cerebellar levels of cytokines comparable to motor impaired and behaviorally sick mice, corroborating previous observations (Pollak et al., 2000) and linking for the first time behavioral alterations and inflammation in EAE. However, neither the cellular source of cytokines nor the cytokine levels in EAE mice prior to the behavioral depression were investigated. By using different anti-inflammatory approaches aimed at blocking IL-1β, TNF and PGE2 signaling, they further demonstrated the correlation between inflammation and sickness behavior (Pollak et al., 2003b). Notably, the treatment against TNF signaling was ineffective if administered alone, but when associated to IL-1β antagonist (IL-1ra) improved the effect of IL-1ra on behavior, suggesting a synergistic interaction between the two cytokines.

The picture herein described is limited to sickness behavior, which is a phenotypic trait of depression- and anxiety-like behaviors in both humans and rodents (Dantzer et al., 2008). Several ethological paradigms have been developed to assess such behaviors in rodents and some of them have been used to characterize EAE-linked behavioral syndrome. Peruga and colleagues demonstrated both anxiety- and depressive-like behaviors in mice with mild-EAE phenotype (only with tail weakness) during the acute and chronic phases, through well-established behavioral paradigms requiring regular motor abilities, like open field test (OFT), light-dark test (LDT), startle response test (SR) for anxious-like behavior, pre-pulse inhibition (PPI) and learned helpless test (LH) for depressive-like behavior (Peruga et al., 2011). The emotional changes observed in EAE mice were associated with inflammation (lymphocyte infiltration, microglia activation and TNF expression) in peri-hippocampal regions and a significant and progressive neuronal loss in CA1 hippocampal region. Also, although monoaminergic neurotransmitters were not significantly changed in EAE hippocampus, amytriptiline treatment significantly increased norepinephrine levels and attenuated behavioral response. Musgrave and colleagues also addressed a role for catecholamine in EAE-behavioral syndrome: the anti-depressant phenelzine (PLZ) improved EAE motor disability and behavioral performance in the OFT and corrected altered monoamine levels in several brain areas, without affecting microgliosis in the spinal cord (Musgrave et al., 2011). Therefore, they suggested that the behavioral response to PLZ observed in EAE is likely due to normalization of serotonin levels in ventral horn of spinal cord. Although valid, such interpretation lacks information about microgliosis and inflammation in brain areas more likely involved in mood control.

In a study published in 2012, we showed anxiety-like behavior in pre-symptomatic EAE mice (Haji et al., 2012) by OFT and elevated plus maze (EPM) behavioral tasks. Interestingly, such behavior was associated with strong microglia activation, increased TNF levels and potentiated glutamatergic transmission in the striatum of EAE mice. Preventive intracerebroventricular blockade of TNF had anxiolytic-like effect on EAE mice and normalized glutamatergic transmission. Notably, the striatum is a subcortical area involved in MS and EAE (Bermel et al., 2003; Centonze et al., 2009) as well as in mood control (Báez-Mendoza and Schultz, 2013) and striatal glutamatergic transmission alterations already occurs in pre-symptomatic phase (Centonze et al., 2009), suggesting that synaptic dysregulation in this area may account for EAE behavioral changes.

In contrast, others did not detect any signs of anxiety-like behavior in both pre-symptomatic and acute EAE mice at the EPM (Rodrigues et al., 2011). Conversely, Acharjee and colleagues confirmed our findings and showed for the first time depressive-like behavior in pre-symptomatic EAE mice, through classical paradigms for depressive-like behavior in rodents, the tail suspension (TST) and the forced swimming tests (FST; Acharjee et al., 2013). The authors correlated emotional impairment in EAE mice with increased expression of IL-1β and TNF in the hypothalamus. They did detect neither astro-nor microgliosis in the hypothalamus, the amygdala and the hippocampus of EAE brains, concluding that EAE emotional changes were linked to alteration of hypothalamic-pituitary-adrenal axis (HPA), as already suggested for the acute phase of EAE (Pollak et al., 2003a).

**TABLE 1 | Summary of studies about EAE behavioral syndrome.**

| Reference | EAE protocol | Behavioral tests | Time (dpi) | Treatment | Behavioral results | Molecular and cellular link |
|---|---|---|---|---|---|---|
| Pollak et al. (2000) | ♀ *SJL/J mice*: adoptive transfer PLP-lymph node cells | Sickness behavior (body weight; food and water intake; sucrose-preference; SI) | Acute phase (5–12 dpi); recovery (13–22 dpi); chronic (23–53 dpi) | None | The onset (acute phase) and recovery of the sickness behavior preceded the onset and recovery of the neurological signs | None |
| Pollak et al. (2003a) | See Pollak et al. (2000) | Sickness behavior (body weight; food intake; sucrose-preference; SI) | Pre-symptomatic phase; acute phase; recovery | None | See Pollak et al. (2000) | *Onset of the behavioral syndrome*:<br>↑ brain infiltration<br>↑ IL-1β and TNF mRNAs<br>↑ IL1β protein and PGE2<br>*Behavioral recovery*:<br>↓ cytokine expression |
| Pollak et al. (2003b) | ♀ *SJL/J mice*:<br>see Pollak et al. (2000);<br>♀ *C57BL/6 mice*:<br>$MOG_{35-55}$ 300 μg; M. tub. (8 mg/ml); PTX 500 ng. | See Pollak et al. (2003a) | Disease onset | Dexamethasone (3 mg/kg ip); IL-1ra (100 mg/kg i.p.); indomethacin (10 mg/kg s.c.); pentoxifylline (100 mg/kg i.p.); at disease onset and for 2–3 days | *Dexamethasone or IL-1ra or indomethacin*:<br>↓ behavioral symptoms<br>*Pentoxifylline or TNFR1 (–/–)*<br>No behavioral effects<br>*Pentoxifylline + IL-1ra*:<br>↓↓ behavioral depression. | None |
| Peruga et al. (2011) | ♀*C57BL/6 mice*:<br>$MOG_{35-55}$ 50 μg; M. tub. (500 μg/ml); PTX 100 ng (mild EAE) | Exploratory and anxiety-like behavior (LDT, OFT, SR); depressive-like behavior (PPI, LH) | Late acute and chronic phase (30–80 dpi) | Amitriptyline (10 mg/kg i.p.) start at 20 dpi and stop 40 dpi | *Mild EAE*:<br>↑ anxiety-like behavior (LDT and SR)<br>↑ depressive-like behavior (LH);<br>*Amitriptyline*:<br>↓ Mild EAE depressive-like behavior (SR) | *Mild EAE (hip)*:<br>↑ CD3+ infiltrates<br>↑ **microglia activation**<br>↑ neuronal loss<br>Behavior correlates with ↑ TNF levels and neuronal loss.<br>*Amitriptyline (hip)*:<br>↑ norepinephrine levels |
| Musgrave et al. (2011) | ♀ C57BL/6 mice;<br>$MOG_{35-55}$ 50 μg; M. tub. (1 mg/ml); PTX 300 ng | Exploratory and anxiety-like behavior (OFT) | 0–35 dpi | Phenelzine (PLZ, 15 mg/kg/day i.p.) starting at 7 dpi and lasted 28 days | *PLZ*:<br>↑ explorative behavior (from the onset of clinical signs) | *Chronic PLZ treatment*:<br>No reduction of **microgliosis** (scr)<br>↑ catecholamine (in scr, cb, crb and bs) |
| Rodrigues et al. (2011) | ♀ C57BL/6 mice;<br>$MOG_{35-55}$ 100 μg; M. tub. (ns); PTX 300 ng | Anxiety-like behavior (EPM) | Pre-symptomatic phase (9 dpi) | None | No difference in the EPM performance | None |

*(Continued)*

**TABLE 1 | Continued**

| Reference | EAE protocol | Behavioral tests | Time (dpi) | Treatment | Behavioral results | Molecular and cellular link |
|---|---|---|---|---|---|---|
| Haji et al. (2012) | ♀ C57BL/6 mice; $MOG_{35-55}$ 300 μg; M. tub. (8 mg/ml); PTX 500 ng | Anxiety-like behavior (OFT, EPM) | Pre-symptomatic phase (7, 9 dpi) | Etanercept (10 μg/μl, 4 week i.c.v. minipump) starting 1 week before immunization | *EAE*:<br>↑ anxiety-like behavior (OFT, EPM) in EAE mice<br>*Etanercept*:<br>↓ EAE-anxiety like-behavior | *EAE (str)*:↑ **Microglia activation**<br>↑ TNF protein<br>↑ sEPSC duration<br>*Etanercept*:<br>↓ sEPSC duration *(str)* |
| Acharjee et al. (2013) | ♀ C57BL/6 mice; $MOG_{35-55}$ 100 μg; M. tub. (4 mg/ml); PTX 800 ng | Exploratory and anxiety-like behavior (OFT, EPM); depression-like behavior (TST, FST, SI) | Pre-symptomatic phase (9 dpi) | None | *EAE*:<br>↑ increased anxiety-like behavior (EPM)<br>↑ depression-like behavior (TST, FST, SI) | *EAE*:<br>No demyelination, **microglial activation** or astrogliosis<br>↑ IL-1β and TNF mRNAs in hyp (no in amy or hip)<br>↑ plasma corticosterone levels |
| Piras et al. (2013) | ♂ C57BL/6 mice; $MOG_{35-55}$ 300 μg; M. tub. (2 mg/ml); PTX 500 ng | Anxiety-like behavior (OFT) | Pre-symptomatic phase (0–8 dpi) | Glatiramer acetate (GA, 150 μg/100 μl, s.c.) every day for 7 days before the immunization | *EAE (2, 4, 6 dpi)*:<br>↑ (n of squares, central squares and latency to rearing)<br>*GA*:<br>↓ latency to rearing | *EAE*:<br>↑ blood circulating T cells (from 4 dpi, before CNS infiltration)<br>= kinetic of T cell entry in the blood and of behavioral changes (OFT)<br>*GA*:<br>↓ behavioral changes<br>T cell retaining in lymph nodes. |
| Gentile et al. (2015) | See Haji et al. (2012) | Depression-like (TST, FST) and motivation-based behavior (NB) | Pre-symptomatic phase (9 dpi); Acute phase of mice with mild clinical score and preserved motor skills (20 dpi mild-EAE) | IL-1ra (150 ng/day, 4 week i.c.v. minipump) starting 1 week before immunization | *EAE (9 and 20 dpi)*:<br>↑ depressive-like behavior (TST, FST)<br>↓ motivation-based behavior (NB)<br>*IL-1ra*<br>↓ EAE-behavioral alterations (FST) | *EAE (str)*:<br>↑ IL-1β mRNA<br>↑ **microgliosis**<br>↓ DA release<br>Alteration in DA signaling through DA D1- and D2-like receptors<br>*IL-1ra*<br>↑ *DA release*<br>↓ **microgliosis**<br>Recovery of DA signaling |

*Abbreviations: EAE, Experimental Autoimmune Encephalomyelitis; dpi, day post immunization; PLP, Proteolipid protein peptide; SI, Social Interaction; IL-1β, interleukin-1β; TNF, Tumor Necrosis Factor; PGE2, Prostaglandin E2; $MOG_{35-55}$, Myelin oligodendrocyte glycoprotein $p_{35-55}$; M. tub., Mycobacterium tuberculosis; PTX, Pertussis toxin; i.p., intraperitoneal injection; IL-1ra, interleukin-1 receptor antagonist; s.c., subcutaneous injection; TNFR1, TNF receptor type 1; LDT, Light Dark Test; OFT, Open Field Test; SR, Startle-Response test; PPI, pre-pulse inhibition; LH, Learned Helplessness test; hip, hippocampus; scr, spinal cord; cb, cerebrum; crb, cerebellum; bs, brainstem; EPM, Elevated Plus Maze; i.c.v., intracerebroventricular; str, striatum; sEPSC, spontaneous excitatory postsynaptic currents; TST, Tail Suspention Test; FST, Forced Swimming Test; hyp, hypothalamus; amy, amygdala; NB, Nest Building; DA, Dopamine.*

Accordingly, we recently linked EAE depressive-like behavior to striatal IL-1β expression and dopaminergic system alterations in the acute phase (Gentile et al., 2015). By studying mice with mild-EAE phenotype, we demonstrated the occurrence of depressive-like (TST and FST) and motivation-based behaviors (nest building test-NB test) in the acute phase of the disease in correlation with striatal and hippocampal microgliosis. Since IL-1β was expressed by microglia in such areas but the cytokine expression raised significantly in EAE striatum, we hypothesized that IL-1β released by microglia in this area may affect the dopaminergic system thus contributing to EAE depressive-like behavior. Accordingly, the preventive central treatment with IL-1ra corrected emotional changes as well as defective striatal dopaminergic neurotransmission, thus linking inflammation-induced neurotransmission alteration and behavior.

Summarizing, TNF and IL1-β alter EAE behavior likely by affecting catecholamine and glutamatergic neurotransmission in several brain areas, pointing to microglia as possible cellular mediator.

## The Impact of MS Drugs on Behavioral Outcomes: The Example of Glatiramer Acetate and Interferon-1 Beta

Most of the drugs approved for MS therapy are immunomodulatory or immunosuppressive agents, providing to variable extent functional recovery. However, they may have a strong impact on mood control, making necessary *ad hoc* pharmacological interventions. Among the currently available therapeutic approaches for MS treatment, interferon-1β (IFNB) and glatiramer acetate (GA) are first-line disease-modifying drugs. Unfortunately, there is some evidence that IFNB treatment exacerbates depressive symptoms more likely than GA (Pandya and Patten, 2002; Goëb et al., 2003; Arnett and Randolph, 2006), therefore in patients with a history of depression GA treatment is often preferred (Wilken and Sullivan, 2007). However, this issue seems not entirely solved, with some studies reporting no differences between IFNB and GA (Kirzinger et al., 2013) or no significant beneficial effect of GA on mood-related outcomes (Jongen et al., 2010).

Due to the restricted literature about EAE-linked behavioral changes, it is clear that animal studies are far from succeeding in clarifying this matter. Only one paper examined MS drug impact on EAE anxiety-like behavior (Piras et al., 2013; **Table 1**), correlating EAE emotional changes with time-dependent increased peripheral lymphocytosis. The authors observed that GA attenuated lymphocytosis and behavioral impairment in a very early phase of the disease. Consistently, we found that GA reduced anxiety-like behavior in pre-symptomatic EAE mice (7 dpi) by OFT (**Figures 1A,B**). We previously demonstrated that GA treatment protected against the TNF-induced synaptotoxic effect on striatal glutamatergic transmission by reducing microgliosis and microglia expression of TNF in the striatum of acute-phase EAE mice (Gentile et al., 2013). Interestingly, activated microglia stimulated with GA *in vitro* mimicked the electrophysiological effect of GA treatment in EAE mice. It has been supposed that GA interacts with microglial surface proteins, involved in microglia activation, like MHC-II complex (Fridkis-Hareli et al., 1997) and P2X7 receptor (Caragnano et al., 2012).

Therefore, we examined GA effect on striatal microglia activation of pre-symptomatic mice. In accordance to our previous findings (Haji et al., 2012), a strong microgliosis was observed in pre-symptomatic EAE striatum (**Figure 1C**), while GA induced additional proliferation of microglial cells with a resting phenotype, suggesting reduced inflammation. The microglial changes induced by GA may abolish the potentiated glutamatergic transmission in the pre-symptomatic striatum, through mechanisms similar to those described in the acute phase. Also, in GA striatum we could occasionally observe amoeboid-like microglial cells, resembling cells in phagocytic activity (not shown): *in vitro* studies on primary murine microglia and human monocytes have shown that GA promotes phagocytosis in those cells (Pul et al., 2011, 2012), likely with protective effects.

Lastly, PET studies in MS patients treated with GA corroborate the effect of GA on microglial activation (Ratchford et al., 2012).

## Conclusions and Perspectives

The investigation of the role of microglia in MS pathogenesis is flourishing, but the contribution of these cells to MS mood disturbances has been only partially addressed. The analysis of pre-symptomatic or non-disabled EAE mice allows dissecting the different contribution of microglia to behavior and motor symptoms.

From the above overview, several elements have emerged: inflammation and microglia activation are involved in EAE-behavioral syndrome and impaired neurotransmission is likely the final outcome of the overactive microglia-immune-neuronal interaction, leading to behavioral alterations. The interplay between microglia and neurons is still poorly explored, but promising and therapeutically attractive. Therefore, we propose to further study the interaction between microglia activation and neurotransmission in brain areas involved in mood control: for example by investigating microglia contribution to EAE/MS hippocampal synaptic dysfunctions (Dutta et al., 2013; Nisticò et al., 2013; Michailidou et al., 2015), and by extending studies in EAE striatum from glutamate and catecholamine to other compromised neurotransmitter systems, such as GABA or cannabinoids (Musumeci et al., 2011; Rossi et al., 2011; Musella et al., 2014). Targeting microglia to limit synaptic damage and behavioral distortion by using immunomodulatory agents, such as GA, or the antibiotic minocycline, known to reduce microgliosis and depressive symptoms (Hinwood et al., 2013), may represent an alternative therapeutic strategy to conventional anti-depressants.

The study of microglia should be fostered in experimental as well as in human investigations and with regard to mood etiology, by using novel *in vivo* imaging techniques. Interestingly, the recent introduction of second-generation PET

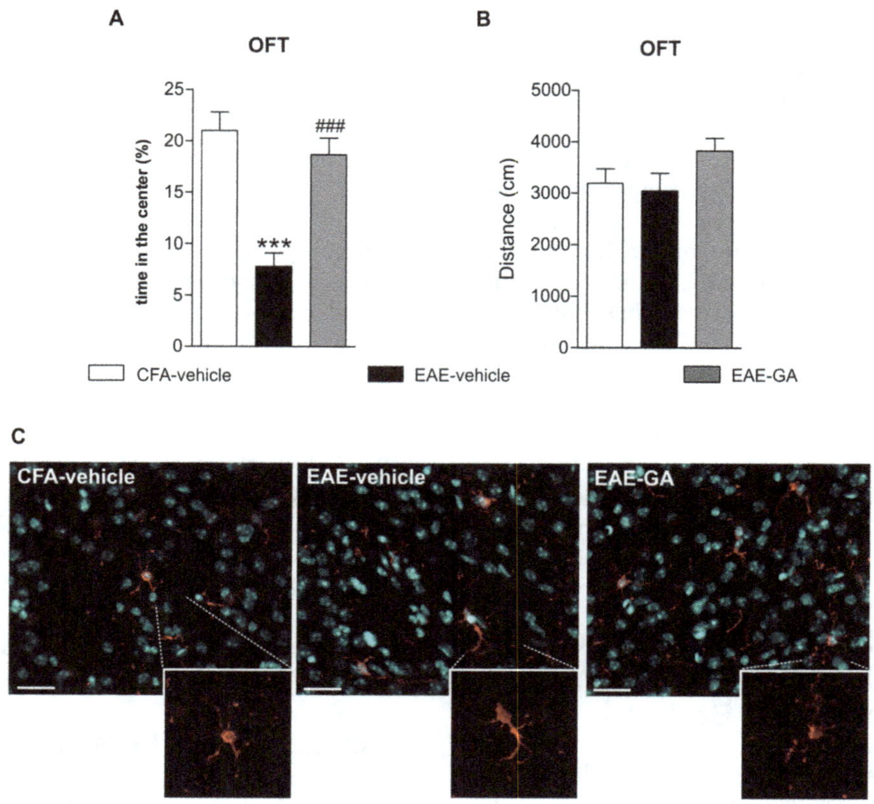


| Microglia analysis | CFA-vehicle | EAE-vehicle | EAE-GA |
|---|---|---|---|
| Microglial density (1/mm^2) | 34.18±3.509 | 139.3±6.703 *** | 203.8±12.60 *** ### |
| Microglial total surface (%) | 0.085±0.016 | 0.585±0.070 *** | 0.590±0.062 *** |
| Mean microglial cell surface (μm^2/cell) | 30.68±2.999 | 51.34±5.734 ** | 34.12±2.053 # |

**FIGURE 1 | Glatiramer acetate (GA) treatment protects from EAE-induced anxiety-like behavior and attenuates microglia activation.** **(A)** Anxiety-like behavior was assessed in pre-symptomatic EAE mice (7 days post immunization, dpi) by means of open field test (OFT). The time in the center of the arena is reduced in EAE-vehicle mice compared to control CFA-vehicle mice and significantly increased in GA-treated mice. CFA-vehicle mice are the experimental control of EAE, receiving the same treatment of EAE mice with the exception of the immunogen $MOG_{35-55}$. Data are expressed as mean ± S.E.M. One-way ANOVA analysis, Tukey's *post hoc* test: EAE-GA vs. EAE-vehicle $^{###}p < 0.001$, EAE-vehicle vs. CFA-vehicle $^{***}p < 0.001$. **(B)** The total distance traveled in the arena was unchanged among the groups, confirming the absence of motor dysfunction in 7 dpi EAE mice. Data are expressed as mean ± S.E.M. One-way ANOVA analysis, Tukey's *post hoc* test: EAE-vehicle vs. CFA-vehicle $p > 0.05$; EAE-GA vs. EAE-vehicle $p > 0.05$; CFA-vehicle vs. EAE-GA $p > 0.05$. **(C)** GA treatment affects microglia proliferation and activation in the striatum of pre-symptomatic (7 dpi) EAE mice. The microphotographs are low magnification confocal images showing microglial cell density in the striatum of control CFA-vehicle, EAE-vehicle and EAE-GA mice: Iba1 staining for microglia (red; counter-staining with DAPI–blue), reveals increase in microglial cell density in EAE-vehicle vs. CFA-vehicle striatum with further enhancement in EAE-GA striatum. Insets show different morphologies of microglial cells among the groups: microglia from EAE striatum is visibly hypertrophic if compared to both microglia from CFA-vehicle and EAE-GA striatum. Scale bar: 25 μm. Quantitative and qualitative analysis of microglia, based on IBA1 immunofluorescence, is reported down the immunofluorescence images: GA increases microglia density and restores resting state of microglial cells. The morphological analysis of microglial cells, based on the area covered by IBA1 positive cells inside the striatum, shows the effect of GA in reducing microglial hypertrophy observed in EAE-vehicle, expressed as mean cell area, while the total microglial area is similar to EAE-vehicle microglia. For image acquisition and analysis method, refer to Gentile et al., 2013. Data are expressed as mean ± S.E.M. One-way ANOVA analysis, Tukey's *post hoc* test: EAE-vehicle and EAE-GA vs. CFA-vehicle: $^{***}p < 0.001$, $^{**}p < 0.01$; EAE-GA vs. EAE-vehicle: $^{###}p < 0.001$, $^{\#}p < 0.05$.

radioligands has been found able to reveal the extent of microglial activation by quantifying the increased expression of the 18-kDa translocator protein (TSPO) in EAE (Mattner et al., 2013) and MS (Giannetti et al., 2014, 2015) brains. The use of this technique is not yet widespread for economic and safety reasons, but it is viewed as highly promising for EAE/MS pathogenesis studies (Politis et al., 2012b), as well as to monitor and to distinguish drug effects on microgliosis (Airas et al., 2015) and to predict clinical outcomes (Politis et al., 2012a). Increased TSPO binding was observed in normal-appearing gray and white matters in MS remitting patients (Versijpt et al., 2005), corroborating the hypothesis that microglia activation occurs early in the disease and can affect the neuronal compartment (Centonze et al., 2010). The application of such technique to behavioral disorders is embryonic (Kenk et al., 2015): microglial metabolite PET measurements could be correlated to data from psychological assessment in MS or behavioral testing and electrophysiological recordings in EAE.

To conclude, we are confident that the integration of data from clinical and preclinical studies and the combined use of different techniques for monitoring microglia state and action are a fruitful strategy to find novel diagnostic and therapeutic tools for MS mood-related disorders.

## Acknowledgments

This investigation was supported by the Italian National Ministero della Università to DC (grant No. 2010BN3MXM_007), by the Italian National Ministero della Salute to AM (grant No. GR-2011-02351422) and to DC (grant No. RF-2011-02347280), and by Fondazione Italiana Sclerosi Multipla (grant No. 2012/S/2) to DC. DF is supported by a Fondazione Italiana Sclerosi Multipla fellowship.

## References

Acharjee, S., Nayani, N., Tsutsui, M., Hill, M. N., Ousman, S. S., and Pittman, Q. J. (2013). Altered cognitive-emotional behavior in early experimental autoimmune encephalitis-cytokine and hormonal correlates. *Brain Behav. Immun.* 33, 164–172. doi: 10.1016/j.bbi.2013.07.003

Airas, L., Dickens, A. M., Elo, P., Marjamäki, P., Johansson, J., Eskola, O., et al. (2015). *In vivo* PET imaging demonstrates diminished microglial activation after fingolimod treatment in an animal model of multiple sclerosis. *J. Nucl. Med.* 56, 305–310. doi: 10.2967/jnumed.114.149955

Arnett, P. A., and Randolph, J. J. (2006). Longitudinal course of depression symptoms in multiple sclerosis. *J. Neurol. Neurosurg. Psychiatry.* 77, 606–610. doi: 10.1136/jnnp.2004.047712

Báez-Mendoza, R., and Schultz, W. (2013). The role of the striatum in social behavior. *Front. Neurosci.* 7:233. doi: 10.3389/fnins.2013.00233

Bermel, R. A., Innus, M. D., Tjoa, C. W., and Bakshi, R. (2003). Selective caudate atrophy in multiple sclerosis: a 3D MRI parcellation study. *Neuroreport.* 14, 335–339. doi: 10.1097/00001756-200303030-00008

Butovsky, O., Ziv, Y., Schwartz, A., Landa, G., Talpalar, A. E., Pluchino, S., et al. (2006). Microglia activated by IL-4 or IFN-gamma differentially induce neurogenesis and oligodendrogenesis from adult stem/progenitor cells. *Mol. Cell. Neurosci.* 31, 149–160. doi: 10.1016/j.mcn.2005.10.006

Caragnano, M., Tortorella, P., Bergami, A., Ruggieri, M., Livrea, P., Specchio, L. M., et al. (2012). Monocytes P2X7 purinergic receptor is modulated by glatiramer acetate in multiple sclerosis. *J. Neuroimmunol.* 245, 93–97. doi: 10.1016/j.jneuroim.2012.02.002

Centonze, D., Muzio, L., Rossi, S., Cavasinni, F., De Chiara, V., Bergami, A., et al. (2009). Inflammation triggers synaptic alteration and degeneration in experimental autoimmune encephalomyelitis. *J. Neurosci.* 29, 3442–3452. doi: 10.1523/JNEUROSCI.5804-08.2009

Centonze, D., Muzio, L., Rossi, S., Furlan, R., Bernardi, G., and Martino, G. (2010). The link between inflammation, synaptic transmission and neurodegeneration in multiple sclerosis. *Cell Death Differ.* 17, 1083–1091. doi: 10.1038/cdd.2009.179

Compston, A., and Coles, A. (2008). Multiple sclerosis. *Lancet* 372, 1502–1517. doi: 10.1016/S0140-6736(08)61620-7

Dantzer, R., O'Connor, J. C., Freund, G. G., Johnson, R. W., and Kelley, K. W. (2008). From inflammation to sickness and depression: when the immune system subjugates the brain. *Nat. Rev. Neurosci.* 9, 46–56. doi: 10.1038/nrn2297

Derecki, N. C., Cronk, J. C., Lu, Z., Xu, E., Abbott, S. B., Guyenet, P. G., et al. (2012). Wild-type microglia arrest pathology in a mouse model of Rett syndrome. *Nature* 484, 105–109. doi: 10.1038/nature10907

Dutta, R., Chomyk, A. M., Chang, A., Ribaudo, M. V., Deckard, S. A., Doud, M. K., et al. (2013). Hippocampal demyelination and memory dysfunction are associated with increased levels of the neuronal microRNA miR-124 and reduced AMPA receptors. *Ann. Neurol.* 73, 637–645. doi: 10.1002/ana.23860

Eyre, H., and Baune, B. T. (2012). Neuroplastic changes in depression: a role for the immune system. *Psychoneuroendocrinology* 37, 1397–1416. doi: 10.1016/j.psyneuen.2012.03.019

Feinstein, A., Magalhaes, S., Richard, J. F., Audet, B., and Moore, C. (2014). The link between multiple sclerosis and depression. *Nat. Rev. Neurol.* 10, 507–517. doi: 10.1038/nrneurol.2014.139

Frick, L. R., Williams, K., and Pittenger, C. (2013). Microglial dysregulation in psychiatric disease. *Clin. Dev. Immunol.* 2013:608654. doi: 10.1155/2013/608654

Fridkis-Hareli, M., Teitelbaum, D., Pecht, I., Arnon, R., and Sela, M. (1997). Binding of copolymer 1 and myelin basic protein leads to clustering of class II MHC molecules on antigen-presenting cells. *Int. Immunol.* 9, 925–934. doi: 10.1093/intimm/9.7.925

Furlan, R., Cuomo, C., and Martino, G. (2009). Animal models of multiple sclerosis. *Methods Mol. Biol.* 549, 157–173. doi: 10.1007/978-1-60327-931-4_11

Gentile, A., Fresegna, D., Federici, M., Musella, A., Rizzo, F. R., Sepman, H., et al. (2015). Dopaminergic dysfunction is associated with IL-1β-dependent mood alterations in experimental autoimmune encephalomyelitis. *Neurobiol. Dis.* 74, 347–358. doi: 10.1016/j.nbd.2014.11.022

Gentile, A., Rossi, S., Studer, V., Motta, C., De Chiara, V., Musella, A., et al. (2013). Glatiramer acetate protects against inflammatory synaptopathy in experimental autoimmune encephalomyelitis. *J. Neuroimmune Pharmacol.* 8, 651–663. doi: 10.1007/s11481-013-9436-x

Giannetti, P., Politis, M., Su, P., Turkheimer, F., Malik, O., Keihaninejad, S., et al. (2014). Microglia activation in multiple sclerosis black holes predicts outcome in progressive patients: an *in vivo* [(11)C](R)-PK11195-PET pilot study. *Neurobiol. Dis.* 65, 203–210. doi: 10.3410/f.718271295.793491239

Giannetti, P., Politis, M., Su, F., Turkheimer, F. E., Malik, O., Keihaninejad, S., et al. (2015). Increased PK11195-PET binding in normal-appearing white matter in clinically isolated syndrome. *Brain* 138, 110–119. doi: 10.1093/brain/awu331

Goëb, J. L., Cailleau, A., Lainé, P., Etcharry-Bouyx, F., Maugin, D., Duverger, P., et al. (2003). Acute delirium, delusion and depression during IFN-beta-1a therapy for multiple sclerosis: a case report. *Clin. Neuropharmacol.* 26, 5–7. doi: 10.1097/00002826-200301000-00002

Graeber, M. B. (2010). Changing face of microglia. *Science* 330, 783–788. doi: 10.1126/science.1190929

Haji, N., Mandolesi, G., Gentile, A., Sacchetti, L., Fresegna, D., Rossi, S., et al. (2012). TNF-α-mediated anxiety in a mouse model of multiple sclerosis. *Exp. Neurol.* 237, 296–303. doi: 10.1016/j.expneurol.2012.07.010

Haussleiter, I. S., Brüne, M., and Juckel, G. (2009). Psychopathology in multiple sclerosis: diagnosis, prevalence and treatment. *Ther. Adv. Neurol. Disord.* 2, 13–29. doi: 10.1177/1756285608100325

Heo, Y., Zhang, Y., Gao, D., Miller, V. M., and Lawrence, D. A. (2011). Aberrant immune responses in a mouse with behavioural disorders. *PLoS One* 6:e20912. doi: 10.1371/journal.pone.0020912

Hinwood, M., Tynan, R. J., Charnley, J. L., Beynon, S. B., Day, T. A., and Walker, F. R. (2013). Chronic stress induced remodeling of the prefrontal cortex: structural re-organization of microglia and the inhibitory effect of minocycline. *Cereb. Cortex* 23, 1784–1797. doi: 10.1093/cercor/bhs151

Jongen, P. J., Lehnick, D., Sanders, E., Seeldrayers, P., Fredrikson, S., Andersson, M., et al. (2010). Health-related quality of life in relapsing remitting multiple sclerosis patients during treatment with glatiramer acetate: a prospective, observational, international, multi-centre study. *Health Qual. Life Outcomes* 8:133. doi: 10.1186/1477-7525-8-133

Kenk, M., Selvanathan, T., Rao, N., Suridjan, I., Rusjan, P., Remington, G., et al. (2015). Imaging neuroinflammation in gray and white matter in schizophrenia: an *in vivo* PET study with [18F]-FEPPA. *Schizophr. Bull.* 41, 85–93. doi: 10.1093/schbul/sbu157

Kettenmann, H., Hanisch, U. K., Noda, M., and Verkhratsky, A. (2011). Physiology of microglia. *Physiol. Rev.* 91, 461–553. doi: 10.1152/physrev.00011.2010

Kirzinger, S. S., Jones, J., Siegwald, A., and Crush, A. B. (2013). Relationship between disease-modifying therapy and depression in multiple sclerosis. *Int. J. MS Care* 15, 107–112. doi: 10.7224/1537-2073.2012-036

Lo Fermo, S., Barone, R., Patti, F., Laisa, P., Cavallaro, T. L., Nicoletti, A., et al. (2010). Outcome of psychiatric symptoms presenting at onset of multiple sclerosis: a retrospective study. *Mult. Scler.* 16, 742–748. doi: 10.1177/1352458510365157

Lynch, M. A. (2009). The multifaceted profile of activated microglia. *Mol. Neurobiol.* 40, 139–156. doi: 10.1007/s12035-009-8077-9

MacFabe, D. F., Cain, N. E., Boon, F., Ossenkopp, K. P., and Cain, D. P. (2011). Effects of the enteric bacterial metabolic product propionic acid on object-directed behavior, social behavior, cognition and neuroinflammation in adolescent rats: relevance to autism spectrum disorder. *Behav. Brain Res.* 217, 47–54. doi: 10.1016/j.bbr.2010.10.005

Maiorino, C., Khorooshi, R., Ruffini, F., Løbner, M., Bergami, A., Garzetti, L., et al. (2013). Lentiviral-mediated administration of IL-25 in the CNS induces alternative activation of microglia. *Gene Ther.* 20, 487–496. doi: 10.1038/gt.2012.58

Marrie, R. A., Horwitz, R., Cutter, G., Tyry, T., Campagnolo, D., and Vollmer, T. (2009). The burden of mental comorbidity in multiple sclerosis: frequent, underdiagnosed and undertreated. *Mult. Scler.* 15, 385–392. doi: 10.1177/1352458508099477

Mattner, F., Staykova, M., Berghofer, P., Wong, H. J., Fordham, S., Callaghan, P., et al. (2013). Central nervous system expression and PET imaging of the translocator protein in relapsing-remitting experimental autoimmune encephalomyelitis. *J. Nucl. Med.* 54, 291–298. doi: 10.2967/jnumed.112.108894

Michailidou, I., Willems, J. G., Kooi, E. J., van Eden, C., Gold, S. M., Geurts, J. J., et al. (2015). Complement C1q-C3-associated synaptic changes in multiple sclerosis hippocampus. *Ann. Neurol.* 77, 1007–1026. doi: 10.1002/ana.24398

Miller, A. H., Maletic, V., and Raison, C. L. (2009). Inflammation and its discontents: the role of cytokines in the pathophysiology of major depression. *Biol. Psychiatry* 65, 732–741. doi: 10.1016/j.biopsych.2008.11.029

Morgan, J. T., Chana, G., Pardo, C. A., Achim, C., Semendeferi, K., Buckwalter, J., et al. (2010). Microglial activation and increased microglial density observed in the dorsolateral prefrontal cortex in autism. *Biol. Psychiatry* 68, 368–376. doi: 10.1016/j.biopsych.2010.05.024

Munkholm, K., Vinberg, M., and Vedel Kessing, L. (2013). Cytokines in bipolar disorder: a systematic review and meta-analysis. *J. Affect. Disord.* 144, 16–27. doi: 10.1016/j.jad.2012.06.010

Musella, A., Sepman, H., Mandolesi, G., Gentile, A., Fresegna, D., Haji, N., et al. (2014). Pre- and postsynaptic type-1 cannabinoid receptors control the alterations of glutamate transmission in experimental autoimmune encephalomyelitis. *Neuropharmacology* 79, 567–572. doi: 10.1016/j.neuropharm.2014.01.007

Musgrave, T., Benson, C., Wong, G., Browne, I., Tenorio, G., Rauw, G., et al. (2011). The MAO inhibitor phenelzine improves functional outcomes in mice with experimental autoimmune encephalomyelitis (EAE). *Brain Behav. Immun.* 25, 1677–1688. doi: 10.1016/j.bbi.2011.06.011

Musumeci, G., Grasselli, G., Rossi, S., De Chiara, V., Musella, A., Motta, C., et al. (2011). Transient receptor potential vanilloid 1 channels modulate the synaptic effects of TNF-α and of IL-1β in experimental autoimmune encephalomyelitis. *Neurobiol. Dis.* 43, 669–677. doi: 10.1016/j.nbd.2011.05.018

Nisticò, R., Mori, F., Feligioni, M., Nicoletti, F., and Centonze, D. (2013). Synaptic plasticity in multiple sclerosis and in experimental autoimmune encephalomyelitis. *Philos. Trans. R. Soc. Lond. B Biol. Sci.* 369:20130162. doi: 10.1098/rstb.2013.0162

Pandya, R., and Patten, S. (2002). Depression in multiple sclerosis associated with interferon beta-1a (Rebif). *Can. J. Psychiatry* 47, 686.

Patten, S. B., Beck, C. A., Williams, J. V., Barbui, C., and Metz, L. M. (2003). Major depression in multiple sclerosis: a population-based perspective. *Neurology* 61, 1524–1527. doi: 10.1212/01.wnl.0000095964.34294.b4

Peruga, I., Hartwig, S., Thöne, J., Hovemann, B., Gold, R., Juckel, G., et al. (2011). Inflammation modulates anxiety in an animal model of multiple sclerosis. *Behav. Brain Res.* 220, 20–29. doi: 10.1016/j.bbr.2011.01.018

Piras, G., Rattazzi, L., McDermott, A., Deacon, R., and D'Acquisto, F. (2013). Emotional change-associated T cell mobilization at the early stage of a mouse model of multiple sclerosis. *Front. Immunol.* 4:400. doi: 10.3389/fimmu.2013.00400

Politis, M., Giannetti, P., Su, P., Turkheimer, F., Keihaninejad, S., Wu, K., et al. (2012a). Increased PK11195 PET binding in the cortex of patients with MS correlates with disability. *Neurology* 79, 523–530. doi: 10.1212/WNL.0b013e3182635645

Politis, M., Su, P., and Piccini, P. (2012b). Imaging of microglia in patients with neurodegenerative disorders. *Front. Pharmacol.* 3:96. doi: 10.3389/fphar.2012.00096

Pollak, Y., Orion, E., Goshen, I., Ovadia, H., and Yirmiya, R. (2002). Experimental autoimmune encephalomyelitis-associated behavioral syndrome as a model of 'depression due to multiple sclerosis'. *Brain Behav. Immun.* 16, 533–543. doi: 10.1016/s0889-1591(02)00010-7

Pollak, Y., Ovadia, H., Goshen, I., Gurevich, R., Monsa, K., Avitsur, R., et al. (2000). Behavioral aspects of experimental autoimmune encephalomyelitis. *J. Neuroimmunol.* 104, 31–36. doi: 10.1016/s0165-5728(99)00257-x

Pollak, Y., Ovadia, H., Orion, E., Weidenfeld, J., and Yirmiya, R. (2003a). The EAE-associated behavioral syndrome: I. Temporal correlation with inflammatory mediators. *J. Neuroimmunol.* 137, 94–99. doi: 10.1016/s0165-5728(03)00075-4

Pollak, Y., Ovadia, H., Orion, E., and Yirmiya, R. (2003b). The EAE-associated behavioral syndrome: II. Modulation by anti-inflammatory treatments. *J. Neuroimmunol.* 137, 100–108. doi: 10.1016/s0165-5728(03)00073-0

Price, J. L., and Drevets, W. C. (2010). Neurocircuitry of mood disorders. *Neuropsychopharmacology* 35, 192–216. doi: 10.1038/npp.2009.104

Pul, R., Moharregh-Khiabani, D., Škuljec, J., Skripuletz, T., Garde, N., Voss, E. V., et al. (2011). Glatiramer acetate modulates TNF-α and IL-10 secretion in microglia and promotes their phagocytic activity. *J. Neuroimmune Pharmacol.* 6, 381–388. doi: 10.1007/s11481-010-9248-1

Pul, R., Morbiducci, F., Škuljec, J., Skripuletz, T., Singh, V., Diederichs, U., et al. (2012). Glatiramer acetate increases phagocytic activity of human monocytes *in vitro* and in multiple sclerosis patients. *PLoS One* 7:e51867. doi: 10.1371/journal.pone.0051867

Ratchford, J. N., Endres, C. J., Hammoud, D. A., Pomper, M. G., Shiee, N., McGready, J., et al. (2012). Decreased microglial activation in MS patients treated with glatiramer acetate. *J. Neurol.* 259, 1199–1205. doi: 10.1007/s00415-011-6337-x

Rietberg, M. B., van Wegen, E. E., Uitdehaag, B. M., and Kwakkel, G. (2011). The association between perceived fatigue and actual level of physical activity in multiple sclerosis. *Mult. Scler.* 17, 1231–1237. doi: 10.1177/1352458511407102

Rodrigues, D. H., Vilela Mde, C., Lacerda-Queiroz, N., Miranda, A. S., Sousa, L. F., Reis, H. J., et al. (2011). Behavioral investigation of mice with experimental autoimmune encephalomyelitis. *Arq. Neuropsiquiatr.* 69, 938–942. doi: 10.1590/s0004-282x2011000700018

Rossi, S., Muzio, L., De Chiara, V., Grasselli, G., Musella, A., Musumeci, G., et al. (2011). Impaired striatal GABA transmission in experimental autoimmune encephalomyelitis. *Brain Behav. Immun.* 25, 947–956. doi: 10.1016/j.bbi.2010.10.004

Schafer, D. P., Lehrman, E. K., Kautzman, A., Koyama, R., Mardinly, A. R., Yamasaki, R., et al. (2012). Microglia sculpt postnatal neural circuits in an activity and complement-dependent manner. *Neuron* 74, 691–705. doi: 10.1016/j.neuron.2012.03.026

Schiffer, R. B., and Babigian, H. M. (1984). Behavioral disorders in multiple sclerosis, temporal lobe epilepsy and amyotrophic lateral sclerosis. An epidemiologic study. *Arch. Neurol.* 41, 1067–1069. doi: 10.1001/archneur.1984.04050210065016

Schubert, D. S., and Foliart, R. H. (1993). Increased depression in multiple sclerosis: a meta-analysis. *Psychosomatics* 34, 124–130. doi: 10.1016/s0033-3182(93)71902-7

Steiner, J., Bielau, H., Brisch, R., Danos, P., Ullrich, O., Mawrin, C., et al. (2008). Immunological aspects in the neurobiology of suicide: elevated microglial density in schizophrenia and depression is associated with suicide. *J. Psychiatr. Res.* 42, 151–157. doi: 10.1016/j.jpsychires.2006.10.013

Suh, Y., Motl, R. W., and Mohr, D. C. (2010). Physical activity, disability and mood in the early stage of multiple sclerosis. *Disabil. Health J.* 3, 93–98. doi: 10.1016/j.dhjo.2009.09.002

Suzuki, K., Sugihara, G., Ouchi, Y., Nakamura, K., Futatsubashi, M., Takebayashi, K., et al. (2013). Microglial activation in young adults with autism spectrum disorder. *JAMA Psychiatry* 70, 49–58. doi: 10.1001/jamapsychiatry.2013.272

Tetreault, N. A., Hakeem, A. Y., Jiang, S., Williams, B. A., Allman, E., Wold, B. J., et al. (2012). Microglia in the cerebral cortex in autism. *J. Autism Dev. Disord.* 42, 2569–2584. doi: 10.1007/s10803-012-1513-0

Thielscher, C., Thielscher, S., and Kostev, K. (2013). The risk of developing depression when suffering from neurological diseases. *Ger. Med. Sci.* 11:Doc02. doi: 10.3205/000170

Tynan, R. J., Naicker, S., Hinwood, M., Nalivaiko, E., Buller, K. M., Pow, D. V., et al. (2010). Chronic stress alters the density and morphology of microglia in a subset of stress-responsive brain regions. *Brain Behav. Immun.* 24, 1058–1068. doi: 10.1016/j.bbi.2010.02.001

Vargas, D. L., Nascimbene, C., Krishnan, C., Zimmerman, A. W., and Pardo, C. A. (2005). Neuroglial activation and neuroinflammation in the brain of patients with autism. *Ann. Neurol.* 57, 67–81. doi: 10.1002/ana.20315

Versijpt, J., Debruyne, J. C., Van Laere, K. J., De Vos, F., Keppens, J., Strijckmans, K., et al. (2005). Microglial imaging with positron emission tomography and atrophy measurements with magnetic resonance imaging in multiple sclerosis: a correlative study. *Mult. Scler.* 11, 127–134. doi: 10.1191/1352458505ms1140oa

Watkins, C. C., Sawa, A., and Pomper, M. G. (2014). Glia and immune cell signaling in bipolar disorder: insights from neuropharmacology and molecular imaging to clinical application. *Transl. Psychiatry* 4:e350. doi: 10.1038/tp.2013.119

Wilken, J. A., and Sullivan, C. (2007). Recognizing and treating common psychiatric disorders in multiple sclerosis. *Neurologist* 13, 343–354. doi: 10.1097/nrl.0b013e31806dc2e8

Wohleb, E. S., Hanke, M. L., Corona, A. W., Powell, N. D., Stiner, L. M., Bailey, M. T., et al. (2011). β-adrenergic receptor antagonism prevents anxiety-like behaviour and microglial reactivity induced by repeated social defeat. *J. Neurosci.* 31, 6277–6288. doi: 10.1523/JNEUROSCI.0450-11.2011

Zerrate, M. C., Pletnikov, M., Connors, S. L., Vargas, D. L., Seidler, F. J., Zimmerman, A. W., et al. (2007). Neuroinflammation and behavioral abnormalities after neonatal terbutaline treatment in rats: implications for autism. *J. Pharmacol. Exp. Ther.* 322, 16–22. doi: 10.1124/jpet.107.121483

Zhou, X., Spittau, B., and Krieglstein, K. (2012). TGFβ signalling plays an important role in IL4-induced alternative activation of microglia. *J. Neuroinflammation* 9:210. doi: 10.1186/1742-2094-9-210

Zorrilla, E. P., Luborsky, L., McKay, J. R., Rosenthal, R., Houldin, A., Tax, A., et al. (2001). The relationship of depression and stressors to immunological assays: a meta-analytic review. *Brain Behav. Immun.* 15, 199–226. doi: 10.1006/brbi.2000.0597

# 17

# Understanding the Role of P2X7 in Affective Disorders—Are Glial Cells the Major Players?

*Leanne Stokes* [1,2]*, *Sarah J. Spencer* [3] *and Trisha A. Jenkins* [1]

[1] School of Medical Sciences, Health Innovations Research Institute, RMIT University, Melbourne, VIC, Australia, [2] School of Pharmacy, University of East Anglia, Norwich, UK, [3] School of Health Sciences, Health Innovations Research Institute, RMIT University, Melbourne, VIC, Australia

***Correspondence:***
*Leanne Stokes,*
*School of Pharmacy, University of East Anglia, Norwich Research Park, Norwich, NR4 7TJ, UK*
*l.stokes@uea.ac.uk*

Pathophysiology associated with several psychiatric disorders has been linked to inflammatory biomarkers. This has generated a theory of major depressive disorders as an inflammatory disease. The idea of pro-inflammatory cytokines altering behavior is now well accepted however many questions remain. Microglia can produce a plethora of inflammatory cytokines and these cells appear to be critical in the link between inflammatory changes and depressive disorders. Microglia play a known role in sickness behavior which has many components of depressive-like behavior such as social withdrawal, sleep alterations, and anorexia. Numerous candidate genes have been identified for psychiatric disorders in the last decade. Single nucleotide polymorphisms (SNPs) in the human P2X7 gene have been linked to bipolar disorder, depression, and to the severity of depressive symptoms. P2X7 is a ligand-gated cation channel expressed on microglia with lower levels found on astrocytes and on some neuronal populations. In microglia P2X7 is a major regulator of pro-inflammatory cytokines of the interleukin-1 family. Genetic deletion of P2X7 in mice is protective for depressive behavior in addition to inflammatory responses. P2X7$^{-/-}$ mice have been shown to demonstrate anti-depressive-like behavior in forced swim and tail suspension behavioral tests and stressor-induced behavioral responses were blunted. Both neurochemical (norepinephrine, serotonin, and dopamine) and inflammatory changes have been observed in the brains of P2X7$^{-/-}$ mice. This review will discuss the recent evidence for involvement of P2X7 in the pathophysiology of depressive disorders and propose mechanisms by which altered signaling through this ion channel may affect the inflammatory state of the brain.

**Keywords: P2X7, depression, microglia, inflammation, mouse models, SNP**

## Inflammation as a Theory for Pathogenesis of Mood-Related Behavioral Changes

Recent evidence suggests that activation of inflammatory responses may contribute to the pathogenesis of affective disorders such as depression, bipolar disorders and schizophrenia. Results from studies of clinical psychosis indicate high levels of pro-inflammatory macrophage-derived cytokines in both serum and plasma in psychotic relative to normal patients. Much of the available research to date has focused on circulating levels of pro-inflammatory agents, including the key interleukins (particularly IL-6, IL-2, IL-1β), tumor necrosis factor (TNF-α) and its receptors, and interferon gamma (IFN-γ) in schizophrenia (Gaughran, 2002; Drzyzga et al., 2006), bipolar disorder (O'Brien et al., 2006; Hope et al., 2009) and depression (Hiles et al., 2012; Liu et al., 2012; Dahl et al., 2014). However there is also increasing evidence of inflammatory cytokines and activation of microglia in the brains of affective disorder subjects. In schizophrenic patients elevated levels of IL-6 (Garver et al., 2003; Sasayama et al., 2013) and IL-1β cytokines (Miller et al., 2011) have been observed in cerebrospinal fluid (CSF); while in bipolar disorder an increase in IL-1β in the CSF of patients was recently found (Söderlund et al., 2011). Cytokines, in turn, promote detrimental neuronal consequences through activation of neuro-inflammatory cascades involving microglial release of oxidative species. Several post-mortem studies have reported an increased density of microglia in the hippocampus (Bayer et al., 1999) and regions of the prefrontal, cingulate and temporal cortices (Bayer et al., 1999; Radewicz et al., 2000; Steiner et al., 2008). Indeed, imaging and histological studies also report increased levels astrocyte and microglial markers (e.g., glial fibrillary acidic protein, GFAP, CD11b) in the prefrontal cortex (Rao et al., 2010) and hippocampus (Haarman et al., 2014) in bipolar patients and increased microglial priming and macrophage recruitment in the cingulate cortex of depressed brains (Torres-Platas et al., 2014). Moreover, in CSF collected from depressive patients, increases in inflammatory mediators, such as kynurenine and quinolinic acid released from microglia, are correlated with increased IFN-α, soluble TNF-α receptor 2 and the chemokine monocyte chemo-attractant protein (MCP-1) in CSF (Raison et al., 2010). While there should also be consideration of the external influence of medications (lithium, antidepressants antipsychotics), age, and patient health status (such as metabolic syndrome or chronic pain) which can all have their own inflammatory influences, it is still clear that elevated immune-inflammatory signaling activity is important in the etiology of mood disorders.

## Sickness Behavior; Inflammation-Related Behavioral Changes

The origin of pro-inflammatory cytokines found in the brain is yet to be clearly elucidated. While cytokines can be produced centrally, it is also of consideration that they are released by circulating immune cells and move to the brain through specific transport mechanisms such as via the circumventricular organs or across a dysfunctioning blood brain barrier. Evidence from animal studies indeed show that activation of the peripheral immune system influences brain pathology, cytokine levels, and behavior. Exposure to the bacterial endotoxin lipopolysaccharide (LPS) or the viral immunostimulant polyinosinic: polycytidylic acid (poly I:C) can induce sickness behavior, a depressive-like state where reductions in food consumption, body weight, social interaction and activity are observed (Yirmiya, 1996; Cunningham et al., 2007). This so-called sickness behavior is both a physical and psychological illness and is observed in humans, encompassing such complications as fatigue, lethargy, anhedonia, anorexia, and muscle and joint pain (Dantzer, 2009). Triggered by the production of pro-inflammatory cytokines by the immune system, it is thought to be part of a highly organized strategy to fight infections.

There are several glial (non-neuronal) cell populations in the brain, notably astrocytes, microglia and oligodendrocytes. The activation of brain microglia has been associated with depressive-like behavior in a number of recent studies (Tynan et al., 2010; Hinwood et al., 2012; Kreisel et al., 2014). In many cases psychological stress induced through prolonged restraint or unpredictable events, is demonstrated to alter microglial responses upregulating various cellular activation markers such as Iba-1, CD11b, and MHC Class II. The number and density of microglia in particular brain regions appears to be altered on the same time-scale as the behavioral changes. Dynamic changes in both number and activation status of microglia have been recently documented with acute increases in microglial number followed by a decline in number with more sustained (chronic) stress (Kreisel et al., 2014). Potentially, this early increased density of activated microglia could amplify pro-inflammatory signaling through the release of inflammatory and neurotoxic mediators such as cytokines. Blocking the initial activation with minocycline rescued the decline in microglial numbers and the behavioral change (Kreisel et al., 2014).

## P2X7 is an Ion Channel Regulating Inflammatory Signaling

P2X7 is a purinergic ion channel activated by the known danger signal molecule and neurotransmitter, ATP (Bartlett et al., 2014). Many immune cells express this purinergic ion channel including myeloid lineage cells such as macrophages and their brain-resident counterparts, microglia. P2X7 expression is not restricted to microglia in the brain, with astrocytes, oligodendrocytes and certain populations of neurons exhibiting low levels of expression (reviewed in Bartlett et al., 2014). Over the last decade research into understanding the role of this ion channel in immune cell responses has revealed a critical function in the regulation of cytokine secretion from macrophages and microglia. It is clear that activation of P2X7 is a major physiological stimulus for rapid secretion of IL-1 family cytokines from macrophages and microglia (Ferrari et al., 1997, 2006). Evidence for involvement of P2X7 activation in regulating other pro-inflammatory cytokine secretion is less robust although there is evidence for a role in IL-6 secretion from macrophages (Solle et al., 2001) and both TNF-α and IL-6 secretion from microglia (Shieh et al., 2014). In addition to cytokines P2X7 is involved in inflammatory prostaglandin secretion (Barberà-Cremades et al., 2012) and release of lysosomal proteases such as cathepsins (Lopez-Castejon et al., 2010).

Transgenic mice deficient in P2X7 (P2X7$^{-/-}$) were generated over a decade ago and have aided our understanding of the physiological and pathophysiological roles of this ion channel.

P2X7$^{-/-}$ mice were originally demonstrated to display reduced cytokine responses (Solle et al., 2001) and subsequent studies have documented reduced inflammatory-related disorders such as anti-collagen induced arthritis (Labasi et al., 2002). *Ex vivo* macrophages isolated from P2X7$^{-/-}$ mice display no secretion of IL-1β, IL-18 and IL-1α cytokines in response to *in vitro* priming and challenge with ATP (Pelegrin et al., 2008). Furthermore, intraperitoneal injection of LPS into P2X7$^{-/-}$ mice caused a reduced febrile response compared to wild-type mice, which was restored upon injection of recombinant IL-1β (Barberà-Cremades et al., 2012). This suggests that P2X7–induced IL-1β secretion plays a key pyrogenic role *in vivo*. The behavioral effects of injected LPS were not investigated by Barberà-Cremades et al. (2012), however a separate study by Csölle et al. (2013b) has demonstrated that LPS-induced anhedonia measured using a sucrose preference test is reduced in P2X7$^{-/-}$ mice. These studies suggest that inflammatory responses to LPS are reduced in P2X7 deficient mice.

## P2X7 and Microglial Responses

Early studies demonstrated that activation of P2X7 stimulated IL-1β cytokine release from mouse microglial cells (Ferrari et al., 1997). Experiments utilizing P2X7$^{-/-}$ mice demonstrated that P2X7 was crucial for ATP-mediated IL-1β release from microglia and that P2X7 deficiency attenuated LPS-induced expression of both IL-1β and TNFα (Mingam et al., 2008). In addition to control of cytokines, P2X7 on microglial cells has been linked to glial cytotoxicity, with the induction of apoptotic cell death following prolonged stimulation (Bartlett et al., 2013). P2X7 on microglia can also induce cortical neuron cell injury in a co-culture model system, using a process not requiring direct cellular contact (Skaper et al., 2006). Microglia deficient in P2X7 or treated with a P2X7 antagonist did not induce neuronal toxicity in this study highlighting a key role for this ion channel in secreting mediators capable of reducing neuronal viability (Skaper et al., 2006).

More recently P2X7 has been implicated in cellular proliferative responses in microglia amongst other cell types, with a study reporting that overexpression of P2X7 was sufficient to drive proliferation and activation of microglia (Monif et al., 2009). These observations are complemented by a study investigating basal and TNFα cytokine-induced proliferation in hippocampal-entorhinal slices where P2X7 was demonstrated to play a key role in proliferation (Zou et al., 2012). The involvement of P2X7 in microglial responses is summarized in **Figure 1**.

## P2X7 Deficient Mice are Resilient to Depressive-like Behavior

Four studies by different groups have so far investigated the effect of genetic deletion of P2X7 on behavior using standard depression tests in mice, namely the forced swim test and tail suspension test. All four studies demonstrated

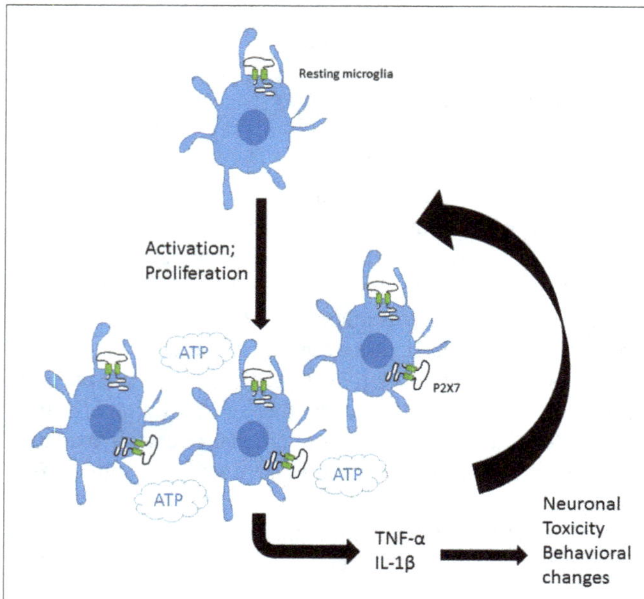


**FIGURE 1 | P2X7 on central glial cells may drive inflammation.** Resting microglia express purinergic receptors including P2X7. Induction of microglial activation and proliferation increases microglial density in the brain. P2X7 is involved in both activation and proliferation of microglia. The presence of ATP, the major agonist for P2X7 channels would drive release of pro-inflammatory mediators from central microlia. These could amplify activation and proliferation of glia and induce toxic damage to neurons and neuronal signaling pathways potentially driving behavioral changes.

a significant reduction in immobility time in P2X7$^{-/-}$ mice, a feature associated with anti-depressive behavior (Basso et al., 2009; Boucher et al., 2011; Csölle et al., 2013a,b). Differences between genotypes were more obvious after repeated challenge or stress suggesting that the demonstrated resilience is more pronounced to stressor-induced behavioral changes. Pharmacological blockade of P2X7 was also effective in altering depressive-like behavior and LPS-induced sickness behavior in mice (Csölle et al., 2013a,b). Selective, centrally penetrating P2X7 modulators may have potential for further development as therapies for CNS disorders including affective disorders. Three P2X7 antagonists A-438079, JNJ-47965567, and JNJ-42253432, have recently been demonstrated to attenuate amphetamine-induced behavioral sensitization in rodents (Bhattacharya et al., 2013; Gubert et al., 2014; Lord et al., 2014), a key process underlying motivational behavior. Moreover antidepressant and anxiolytic like behavior is observed after P2X7 antagonism in animal models exhibiting depressive-like symptomatology in forced swim and social interaction paradigms (Pereira et al., 2013; Lord et al., 2014; Wilkinson et al., 2014).

A major finding from the work by Csölle et al. (2013a) was that peripheral immune cells such as infiltrating monocytes or macrophages do not appear to be involved in protection from depressive behavior associated with P2X7 deficiency. To demonstrate this they used bone marrow chimera experiments. Here mice were irradiated to destroy circulating immune cells and underwent a bone marrow transplant from donor mice which were either wild-type (P2X7+) or knockout (P2X7−).

Reconstituted mice with both P2X7 expressing and P2X7 deficient bone marrow demonstrated no difference in immobility time in the tail suspension test. The study concluded that deficiency of P2X7 only in peripheral immune cells gave no protection from depressive-like behavior (Csölle et al., 2013a). Whilst this study also suggested central microglia were not involved through the same bone marrow chimera approach, more data would be helpful to strengthen this particular conclusion. For example, does central injection of IL-1β restore depressive-like behavior in the P2X7$^{-/-}$ mouse? This would indicate whether cytokines were driving depressive behavior. In addition, these behavioral studies use C57BL/6 mice which are known to carry a single nucleotide polymorphism (SNP) in the C-terminus of P2X7 affecting downstream signaling pathways including cytokine secretion (Adriouch et al., 2002). It would be interesting and relevant to determine if this effect is maintained in mouse strains carrying a high functioning P2X7.

Significant differences in expression (both up- and down-regulation) of genes involved in synaptic signaling were found by whole genome microarrays in the amygdala of P2X7$^{-/-}$ mice (Csölle et al., 2013a). Moreover, exposure to restraint stress caused an acute elevation in adrenocorticotropic hormone (ACTH) and corticosterone levels in wild-type C57BL/6 mice but this was reduced in P2X7$^{-/-}$ mice (Csölle et al., 2013a). This suggests that P2X7 deficiency may blunt the stress hormone response. The anterior pituitary, which is responsible for the production of stress hormones amongst others, expresses P2X channels (Koshimizu et al., 2000; Zemkova et al., 2006) and ATP is known to modulate ACTH secretion. Therefore it is possible P2X7 may play a role in the amplification of secretagogue signals from the hypothalamus.

## A Mutant P2X7 Allele Linked to Depression and Bipolar Disorder in Human Studies

There have been a number of genetic studies over the last decade linking a SNP in the human *P2RX7* gene to depression, anxiety, and bipolar disorder (Barden et al., 2006; Lucae et al., 2006; McQuillin et al., 2009; Soronen et al., 2011). Inheritance of the minor allele of this SNP (rs2230912-G) has also been correlated to severity of depression in diabetic and psychiatric patients (Hejjas et al., 2009; Nagy et al., 2008; Halmai et al., 2013). In contrast there are several genetic studies that do not find an association with *P2RX7* genotype at this polymorphic site and bipolar disorder, major depression or schizophrenia (Green et al., 2009; Viikki et al., 2011). A recent meta-analysis also suggested no association (Feng et al., 2014). Addressing the functional relevance of this SNP *in vitro* studies on circulating immune cells isolated from humans carrying the rs2230912-G allele have demonstrated that this genetic variant of P2X7 is inherited on a gain-of-function allele (Stokes et al., 2010). Importantly human monocytes expressing this rs2230912-G variant secreted more IL-1β in response to activation of P2X7 than monocytes expressing a wild-type variant (Stokes et al., 2010). Therefore one could speculate that microglia in the brain may also display enhanced cytokine secretion in response to P2X7 ion channel activation. Whilst this is difficult to demonstrate in the human system, a transgenic mouse approach knocking-in this human variant of P2X7 could begin to address this question.

In transgenic mouse studies genetic deletion of P2X7 eliminates a full-length P2X7 protein and protects against depressive learned helplessness behavior (Basso et al., 2009; Boucher et al., 2011; Csölle et al., 2013a). Could this also be true for humans? There are numerous loss-of-function SNPs in the human P2X7 gene which are demonstrated to have dramatic effects on receptor trafficking or receptor function (Sluyter and Stokes, 2011). Several studies have included some (but not all) loss-of-function P2X7 SNPs in their analysis but no difference in genotype frequency has so far been documented (Barden et al., 2006; Hansen et al., 2008).

## The Gliotransmitter ATP and Depressive Behavior

The purinergic signaling system is extensive in the body involving many receptors, ion channels and enzymes. ATP is a known co-transmitter released at synapses and extra-synaptic sites modulating the responses of glial and neurons (Burnstock, 2008). A recent study by Cao et al. presents a novel case for astrocyte-derived ATP as a rapid anti-depressant neurotransmitter (Cao et al., 2013). But how does this idea fit with a role for P2X7 (and potentially other purinergic receptors) in depressive disorders? Cao et al. (2013) suggest that astrocytes release ATP in the medial prefrontal cortex where the P2X2 receptor seems to be the downstream target for this anti-depressant action of ATP as evidenced by shRNA experiments. Astrocytes and microglia both express P2X7, which can be activated by relatively high concentrations of ATP (>100 μM); levels that may not be achieved in the brain where nucleotidases are widely expressed (Robson et al., 2006). Thus astrocyte-derived ATP may not reach concentrations high enough to stimulate pro-inflammatory signaling through P2X7. In P2X7$^{-/-}$ mice, which demonstrate an antidepressant-like phenotype, Csölle et al. (2013a) demonstrated an up-regulation of a number of genes in the amygdala including *P2RX2* (11-fold change). Together with the evidence that immune cells (including microglia) do not affect the behavioral phenotype, perhaps this highlights a role for astrocytes, ATP, and P2X2, in the antidepressant effect of P2X7 deficiency? It is clear that more studies are required to understand the role of purinergic signaling in psychiatric disorders.

## Future Perspectives

In humans a correlation between high functioning P2X7 and affective disorders is often observed but this may be limited to patients with an inflammatory component, for example diabetic patients. Perhaps understanding more about the clinical features associated with affective disorders will lead to a useful stratification of these disorders and co-morbidity with other diseases. The evidence for involvement of P2X7 in depressive disorders from animal studies is promising but it is clear that more information about this ion channel and its role in inflammation and behavior is needed. Microglia are known to play a role in stress-induced depressive behavior but is P2X7 a major driver of inflammatory signaling in central microglia under conditions of chronic stress? P2X7 is not restricted to microglia and it is likely that astrocytes participate in regulation of microglial and neuronal responses. Future studies will hopefully address these issues and begin to determine whether this ion channel could be a novel drug target for affective disorders.

## References


Adriouch, S., Dox, C., Welge, V., Seman, M., Koch-Nolte, F., and Haag, F. (2002). Cutting edge: a natural P451L mutation in the cytoplasmic domain impairs the function of the mouse P2X7 receptor. *J. Immunol.* 169, 4108–4112. doi: 10.4049/jimmunol.169.8.4108

Barberà-Cremades, M., Baroja-Mazo, A., Gomez, A. I., Machado, F., Di Virgilio, F., and Pelegrin, P. (2012). P2X7 receptor-stimulation causes fever via PGE2 and IL-1beta release. *FASEB J.* 26, 2951–2962. doi: 10.1096/fj.12-205765

Barden, N., Harvey, M., Gagné, B., Shink, E., Tremblay, M., Raymond, C., et al. (2006). Analysis of single nucleotide polymorphisms in genes in the chromosome 12Q24.31 region points to P2RX7 as a susceptibility gene to bipolar affective disorder. *Am. J. Med. Genet. B Neuropsychiatr. Genet.* 141B, 374–382. doi: 10.1002/ajmg.b.30303

Bartlett, R., Stokes, L., and Sluyter, R. (2014). The P2X7 receptor channel: recent developments and the use of P2X7 antagonists in models of disease. *Pharmacol. Rev.* 66, 638–675. doi: 10.1124/pr.113.008003

Bartlett, R., Yerbury, J. J., and Sluyter, R. (2013). P2X7 receptor activation induces reactive oxygen species formation and cell death in murine EOC13 microglia. *Mediators Inflamm.* 2013:271813. doi: 10.1155/2013/271813

Basso, A., Bratcher, N., Harris, R., Jarvis, M., Decker, M., and Rueter, L. (2009). Behavioral profile of P2X7 receptor knockout mice in animal models of depression, anxiety: relevance for neuropsychiatric disorders. *Behav. Brain Res.* 198, 83–90. doi: 10.1016/j.bbr.2008.10.018

Bayer, T. A., Buslei, R., Havas, L., and Falkai, P. (1999). Evidence for activation of microglia in patients with psychiatric illnesses. *Neurosci. Lett.* 271, 126–128. doi: 10.1016/s0304-3940(99)00545-5

Bhattacharya, A., Wang, Q., Ao, H., Shoblock, J. R., Lord, B., Aluisio, L., et al. (2013). Pharmacological characterization of a novel centrally permeable P2X7 receptor antagonist: JNJ-47965567. *Br. J. Pharmacol.* 170, 624–640. doi: 10.1111/bph.12314

Boucher, A. A., Arnold, J. C., Hunt, G. E., Spiro, A., Spencer, J., Brown, C., et al. (2011). Resilience and reduced c-Fos expression in P2X7 receptor knockout mice exposed to repeated forced swim test. *Neuroscience* 189, 170–177. doi: 10.1016/j.neuroscience.2011.05.049

Burnstock, G. (2008). Purinergic signalling and disorders of the central nervous system. *Nat. Rev. Drug Discov.* 7, 575–590. doi: 10.1038/nrd2605

Cao, X., Li, L.-P., Wang, Q., Wu, Q., Hu, H.-H., Zhang, M., et al. (2013). Astrocyte-derived ATP modulates depressive-like behaviors. *Nat. Med.* 19, 773–777. doi: 10.1038/nm.3162

Csölle, C., Andó, R., Kittel, Å., Gölöncsér, F., Baranyi, M., Soproni, K., et al. (2013a). The absence of P2X7 receptors (P2rx7) on non-haematopoietic cells leads to selective alteration in mood-related behaviour with dysregulated gene expression and stress reactivity in mice. *Int. J. Neuropsychopharmacol.* 16, 213–233. doi: 10.1017/s1461145711001933

Csölle, C., Baranyi, M., Zsilla, G., Kittel, Á., Gölöncsér, F., Illes, P., et al. (2013b). Neurochemical changes in the mouse hippocampus underlying the antidepressant effect of genetic deletion of P2X7 receptors. *PLoS One* 8:e66547. doi: 10.1371/journal.pone.0066547

Cunningham, C., Campion, S., Teeling, J., Felton, L., and Perry, V. H. (2007). The sickness behaviour and CNS inflammatory mediator profile induced by systemic challenge of mice with synthetic double-stranded RNA (poly I:C). *Brain Behav. Immun.* 21, 490–502. doi: 10.1016/j.bbi.2006.12.007

Dahl, J., Ormstad, H., Aass, H. C., Malt, U. F., Bendz, L. T., Sandvik, L., et al. (2014). The plasma levels of various cytokines are increased during ongoing depression and are reduced to normal levels after recovery. *Psychoneuroendocrinology* 45, 77–86. doi: 10.1016/j.psyneuen.2014.03.019

Dantzer, R. (2009). Cytokine, sickness behavior and depression. *Immunol. Allergy Clin. North Am.* 29, 247–264. doi: 10.1016/j.iac.2009.02.002

Drzyzga, L., Obuchowicz, E., Marcinowska, A., and Herman, Z. S. (2006). Cytokines in schizophrenia and the effects of antipsychotic drugs. *Brain Behav. Immun.* 20, 532–545. doi: 10.1016/j.bbi.2006.02.002

Feng, W.-P., Zhang, B., Li, W., and Liu, J. (2014). Lack of association of P2RX7 gene rs2230912 polymorphism with mood disorders: a meta-analysis. *PLoS One* 9:e88575. doi: 10.1371/journal.pone.0088575

Ferrari, D., Chiozzi, P., Falzoni, S., Hanau, S., and Di Virgilio, F. (1997). Purinergic modulation of interleukin-1 beta release from microglial cells stimulated with bacterial endotoxin. *J. Exp. Med.* 185, 579–582. doi: 10.1084/jem.185.3.579

Ferrari, D., Pizzirani, C., Adinolfi, E., Lemoli, R. M., Curti, A., Idzko, M., et al. (2006). The P2X7 receptor: a key player in IL-1 processing and release. *J. Immunol.* 176, 3877–3883. doi: 10.4049/jimmunol.176.7.3877

Garver, D. L., Tamas, R. L., and Holcomb, J. A. (2003). Elevated interleukin-6 in the cerebrospinal fluid of a previously delineated schizophrenia subtype. *Neuropsychopharmacology* 28, 1515–1520. doi: 10.1038/sj.npp.1300217

Gaughran, F. (2002). Immunity and schizophrenia: autoimmunity, cytokines and immune responses. *Int. Rev. Neurobiol.* 52, 275–302. doi: 10.1016/s0074-7742(02)52013-4

Green, E. K., Grozeva, D., Raybould, R., Elvidge, G., Macgregor, S., Craig, I., et al. (2009). P2RX7: a bipolar and unipolar disorder candidate susceptibility gene? *Am. J. Med. Genet. B Neuropsychiatr. Genet.* 150B, 1063–1069. doi: 10.1002/ajmg.b.30931

Gubert, C., Fries, G., Pfaffenseller, B., Ferrari, P., Coutinho-Silva, R., Morrone, F., et al. (2014). Role of P2X7 receptor in an animal model of mania induced by D-Amphetamine. *Mol. Neurobiol.* doi: 10.1007/s12035-014-9031-z [Epub ahead of print].

Haarman, B., Doorduin, J., Riemersma-Van Der Lek, R. F., Zandstra, T. E., Drexhage, H. A., and Nolen, W. A. (2014). Neuroinflammation in bipolar disorder? An [11c] PK11195 PET study in euthymic patients. *Bipolar Disord.* 16, 42–42. doi: 10.1016/j.bbi.2014.03.016

Halmai, Z., Dome, P., Vereczkei, A., Abdul-Rahman, O., Szekely, A., Gonda, X., et al. (2013). Associations between depression severity and purinergic receptor P2RX7 gene polymorphisms. *J. Affect. Disord.* 150, 104–109. doi: 10.1016/j.jad.2013.02.033

Hansen, T., Jakobsen, K. D., Fenger, M., Nielsen, J., Krane, K., Fink-Jensen, A., et al. (2008). Variation in the purinergic P2RX7 receptor gene and schizophrenia. *Schizophr. Res.* 104, 146–152. doi: 10.1016/j.schres.2008.05.026

Hejjas, K., Szekely, A., Domotor, E., Halmai, Z., Balogh, G., Schilling, B., et al. (2009). Association between depression and the Gln460Arg polymorphism of P2RX7 gene: a dimensional approach. *Am. J. Med. Genet. B Neuropsychiatr. Genet.* 150B, 295–299. doi: 10.1002/ajmg.b.30799

Hiles, S. A., Baker, A. L., de Malmanche, T., and Attia, J. (2012). A meta-analysis of differences in IL-6 and IL-10 between people with and without depression: exploring the causes of heterogeneity. *Brain Behav. Immun.* 26, 1180–1188. doi: 10.1016/j.bbi.2012.06.001

Hinwood, M., Morandini, J., Day, T. A., and Walker, F. R. (2012). Evidence that microglia mediate the neurobiological effects of chronic psychological stress on the medial prefrontal cortex. *Cereb. Cortex* 22, 1442–1454. doi: 10.1093/cercor/bhr229

Hope, S., Melle, I., Aukrust, P., Steen, N. E., Birkenaes, A. B., Lorentzen, S., et al. (2009). Similar immune profile in bipolar disorder and schizophrenia: selective increase in soluble tumor necrosis factor receptor I and von Willebrand factor. *Bipolar Disord.* 11, 726–734. doi: 10.1111/j.1399-5618.2009.00757.x

Koshimizu, T.-A., Van Goor, F., Tomić, M., Wong, A. O.-L., Tanoue, A., Tsujimoto, G., et al. (2000). Characterization of calcium signaling by purinergic receptor-channels expressed in excitable cells. *Mol. Pharmacol.* 58, 936–945. doi: 10.1124/mol.58.5.936

Kreisel, T., Frank, M. G., Licht, T., Reshef, R., Ben-Menachem-Zidon, O., Baratta, M. V., et al. (2014). Dynamic microglial alterations underlie stress-induced depressive-like behavior and suppressed neurogenesis. *Mol. Psychiatry* 19, 699–709. doi: 10.1038/mp.2013.155

Labasi, J. M., Petrushova, N., Donovan, C., McCurdy, S., Lira, P., Payette, M. M., et al. (2002). Absence of the P2X7 receptor alters leukocyte function and attenuates an inflammatory response. *J. Immunol.* 168, 6436–6445. doi: 10.4049/jimmunol.168.12.6436

Liu, Y., Ho, R. C. M., and Mak, A. (2012). Interleukin (IL)-6, tumour necrosis factor alpha (TNF-α) and soluble interleukin-2 receptors (sIL-2R) are elevated in patients with major depressive disorder: a meta-analysis and meta-regression. *J. Affect. Disord.* 139, 230–239. doi: 10.1016/j.jad.2011.08.003

Lopez-Castejon, G., Theaker, J., Pelegrin, P., Clifton, A. D., Braddock, M., and Surprenant, A. (2010). P2X7 receptor-mediated release of cathepsins from macrophages is a cytokine-independent mechanism potentially involved in joint diseases. *J. Immunol.* 185, 2611–2619. doi: 10.4049/jimmunol.1000436

Lord, B., Aluisio, L., Shoblock, J. R., Neff, R. A., Varlinskaya, E. I., Ceusters, M., et al. (2014). Pharmacology of a novel central nervous system-penetrant P2X7 antagonist JNJ-42253432. *J. Pharmacol. Exp. Ther.* 351, 628–641. doi: 10.1124/jpet.114.218487

Lucae, S., Salyakina, D., Barden, N., Harvey, M., Gagné, B., Labbé, M., et al. (2006). P2RX7, a gene coding for a purinergic ligand-gated ion channel, is associated with major depressive disorder. *Hum. Mol. Genet.* 15, 2438–2445. doi: 10.1093/hmg/ddl166

McQuillin, A., Bass, N., Choudhury, K., Puri, V., Kosmin, M., Lawrence, J., et al. (2009). Case-control studies show that a non-conservative amino-acid change from a glutamine to arginine in the P2RX7 purinergic receptor protein is associated with both bipolar- and unipolar-affective disorders. *Mol. Psychiatry* 14, 614–620. doi: 10.1038/mp.2008.6

Miller, B. J., Buckley, P., Seabolt, W., Mellor, A., and Kirkpatrick, B. (2011). Meta-analysis of cytokine alterations in schizophrenia: clinical status and antipsychotic effects. *Biol. Psychiatry* 70, 663–671. doi: 10.1016/j.biopsych.2011.04.013

Mingam, R., De Smedt, V., Amédée, T., Bluthé, R.-M., Kelley, K. W., Dantzer, R., et al. (2008). *In vitro* and *in vivo* evidence for a role of the P2X7 receptor in the release of IL-1β in the murine brain. *Brain Behav. Immun.* 22, 234–244. doi: 10.1016/j.bbi.2007.08.007

Monif, M., Reid, C., Powell, K., Smart, M., and Williams, D. (2009). The P2X7 receptor drives microglial activation and proliferation: a trophic role for P2X7R pore. *J. Neurosci.* 29, 3781–3791. doi: 10.1523/JNEUROSCI.5512-08.2009

Nagy, G., Ronai, Z., Somogyi, A., Sasvari-Szekely, M., Rahman, O., Mate, A., et al. (2008). P2RX7 Gln460Arg polymorphism is associated with depression among diabetic patients. *Prog. Neuropsychopharmacol. Biol. Psychiatry* 32, 1884–1888. doi: 10.1016/j.pnpbp.2008.08.021

O'Brien, S. M., Scully, P., Scott, L. V., and Dinan, T. G. (2006). Cytokine profiles in bipolar affective disorder: focus on acutely ill patients. *J. Affect. Disord.* 90, 263–267. doi: 10.1016/j.jad.2005.11.015

Pelegrin, P., Barroso-Gutierrez, C., and Surprenant, A. (2008). P2X7 receptor differentially couples to distinct release pathways for IL-1β in mouse macrophage. *J. Immunol.* 180, 7147–7157. doi: 10.4049/jimmunol.180.11.7147

Pereira, V. S., Casarotto, P. C., Hiroaki-Sato, V. A., Sartim, A. G., Guimarães, F. S., and Joca, S. R. L. (2013). Antidepressant- and anticompulsive-like effects of purinergic receptor blockade: involvement of nitric oxide. *Eur. Neuropsychopharmacol.* 23, 1769–1778. doi: 10.1016/j.euroneuro.2013.01.008

Radewicz, K., Garey, L. J., Gentleman, S. M., and Reynolds, R. (2000). Increase in HLA-DR immunoreactive microglia in frontal and temporal cortex of chronic schizophrenics. *J. Neuropathol. Exp. Neurol.* 59, 137–150.

Raison, C. L., Dantzer, R., Kelley, K. W., Lawson, M. A., Woolwine, B. J., Vogt, G., et al. (2010). CSF concentrations of brain tryptophan and kynurenines during immune stimulation with IFN-alpha: relationship to CNS immune responses and depression. *Mol. Psychiatry* 15, 393–403. doi: 10.1038/mp.2009.116

Rao, J. S., Harry, G. J., Rapoport, S. I., and Kim, H. W. (2010). Increased excitotoxicity and neuroinflammatory markers in postmortem frontal cortex from bipolar disorder patients. *Mol. Psychiatry* 15, 384–392. doi: 10.1038/mp.2009.47

Robson, S. C., Sévigny, J., and Zimmermann, H. (2006). The E-NTPDase family of ectonucleotidases: structure function relationships and pathophysiological significance. *Purinergic Signal.* 2, 409–430. doi: 10.1007/s11302-006-9003-5

Sasayama, D., Hattori, K., Wakabayashi, C., Teraishi, T., Hori, H., Ota, M., et al. (2013). Increased cerebrospinal fluid interleukin-6 levels in patients with schizophrenia and those with major depressive disorder. *J. Psychiatr. Res.* 47, 401–406. doi: 10.1016/j.jpsychires.2012.12.001

Shieh, C.-H., Heinrich, A., Serchov, T., van Calker, D., and Biber, K. (2014). P2X7-dependent, but differentially regulated release of IL-6, CCL2 and TNF-α in cultured mouse microglia. *Glia* 62, 592–607. doi: 10.1002/glia.22628

Skaper, S. D., Facci, L., Culbert, A. A., Evans, N. A., Chessell, I., Davis, J. B., et al. (2006). P2X7 receptors on microglial cells mediate injury to cortical neurons *in vitro*. *Glia* 54, 234–242. doi: 10.1002/glia.20379

Sluyter, R., and Stokes, L. (2011). Significance of P2X7 receptor variants to human health and disease. *Recent Pat. DNA Gene Seq.* 5, 41–54. doi: 10.2174/187221511794839219

Söderlund, J., Olsson, S. K., Samuelsson, M., Walther-Jallow, L., Johansson, C., Erhardt, S., et al. (2011). Elevation of cerebrospinal fluid interleukin-1β in bipolar disorder. *J. Psychiatry Neurosci.* 36, 114–118. doi: 10.1503/jpn.100080

Solle, M., Labasi, J., Perregaux, D. G., Stam, E., Petrushova, N., Koller, B. H., et al. (2001). Altered cytokine production in mice lacking P2X(7) receptors. *J. Biol. Chem.* 276, 125–132. doi: 10.1074/jbc.m006781200

Soronen, P., Mantere, O., Melartin, T., Suominen, K., Vuorilehto, M., Rytsala, H., et al. (2011). P2RX7 gene is associated consistently with mood disorders and predicts clinical outcome in three clinical cohorts. *Am. J. Med. Genet. B Neuropsychiatr. Genet.* 156, 435–447. doi: 10.1002/ajmg.b.31179

Steiner, J., Bielau, H., Brisch, R., Danos, P., Ullrich, O., Mawrin, C., et al. (2008). Immunological aspects in the neurobiology of suicide: elevated microglial density in schizophrenia and depression is associated with suicide. *J. Psychiatr. Res.* 42, 151–157. doi: 10.1016/j.jpsychires.2006.10.013

Stokes, L., Fuller, S., Sluyter, R., Skarratt, K. K., Gu, B. J., and Wiley, J. S. (2010). Two haplotypes of the P2X(7) receptor containing the Ala-348 to Thr polymorphism exhibit a gain-of-function effect and enhanced interleukin-1beta secretion. *FASEB J.* 24, 2916–2927. doi: 10.1096/fj.09-150862

Torres-Platas, S. G., Cruceanu, C., Chen, G. G., Turecki, G., and Mechawar, N. (2014). Evidence for increased microglial priming and macrophage recruitment in the dorsal anterior cingulate white matter of depressed suicides. *Brain Behav. Immun.* 42, 50–59. doi: 10.1016/j.bbi.2014.05.007

Tynan, R. J., Naicker, S., Hinwood, M., Nalivaiko, E., Buller, K. M., Pow, D. V., et al. (2010). Chronic stress alters the density and morphology of microglia in a subset of stress-responsive brain regions. *Brain Behav. Immun.* 24, 1058–1068. doi: 10.1016/j.bbi.2010.02.001

Viikki, M., Kampman, O., Anttila, S., Illi, A., Setala-Soikkeli, E., Huhka, M., et al. (2011). P2RX7 polymorphisms Gln460Arg and His155Tyr are not associated with major depressive disorder or remission after SSRI or ECT. *Neurosci. Lett.* 493, 127–130. doi: 10.1016/j.neulet.2011.02.023

Wilkinson, S. M., Gunosewoyo, H., Barron, M. L., Boucher, A., Mcdonnell, M., Turner, P., et al. (2014). The first CNS-Active carborane: a novel P2X7 receptor antagonist with antidepressant activity. *ACS Chem. Neurosci.* 5, 335–339. doi: 10.1021/cn500054n

Yirmiya, R. (1996). Endotoxin produces a depressive-like episode in rats. *Brain Res.* 711, 163–174. doi: 10.1016/0006-8993(95)01415-2

Zemkova, H., Balik, A., Jiang, Y., Kretschmannova, K., and Stojilkovic, S. S. (2006). Roles of purinergic P2X receptors as pacemaking channels and modulators of calcium-mobilizing pathway in pituitary gonadotrophs. *Mol. Endocrinol.* 20, 1423–1436. doi: 10.1210/me.2005-0508

Zou, J., Vetreno, R. P., and Crews, F. T. (2012). ATP-P2X7 receptor signaling controls basal and TNFα-stimulated glial cell proliferation. *Glia* 60, 661–673. doi: 10.1002/glia.22302

# 18

# Potential Primary Roles of Glial Cells in the Mechanisms of Psychiatric Disorders

*Kazuhiko Yamamuro[1], Sohei Kimoto[1], Kenneth M. Rosen[2], Toshifumi Kishimoto[1] and Manabu Makinodan[1]**

[1] Department of Psychiatry, Faculty of Medicine, Nara Medical University, Kashihara, Japan, [2] BioAxone BioSciences Inc., Cambridge, MA, USA

***Correspondence:***
*Manabu Makinodan,*
*Department of Psychiatry, Faculty of Medicine, Nara Medical University, 840 Shijo-cho, Kashihara, Nara 634-8522, Japan*
*mmm@naramed-u.ac.jp*

While neurons have long been considered the major player in multiple brain functions such as perception, emotion, and memory, glial cells have been relegated to a far lesser position, acting as merely a "glue" to support neurons. Multiple lines of recent evidence, however, have revealed that glial cells such as oligodendrocytes, astrocytes, and microglia, substantially impact on neuronal function and activities and are significantly involved in the underlying pathobiology of psychiatric disorders. Indeed, a growing body of evidence indicates that glial cells interact extensively with neurons both chemically (e.g., through neurotransmitters, neurotrophic factors, and cytokines) and physically (e.g., through gap junctions), supporting a role for these cells as likely significant modifiers not only of neural function in brain development but also disease pathobiology. Since questions have lingered as to whether glial dysfunction plays a primary role in the biology of neuropsychiatric disorders or a role related solely to their support of neuronal physiology in these diseases, informative and predictive animal models have been developed over the last decade. In this article, we review recent findings uncovered using glia-specific genetically modified mice with which we can evaluate both the causation of glia dysfunction and its potential role in neuropsychiatric disorders such as autism and schizophrenia.

**Keywords: glia, schizophrenia, autism, mouse models, astrocytes, oligodenrocytes, microglia, MeCP2**

## Introduction

Glial cells are the non-excitable supporting cells of the central nervous system (CNS) and classified mainly as oligodendrocytes, astrocytes, and microglia. These cells are typically smaller in size, but can be far more numerous than neurons in certain brain regions such as the cerebral cortex. Overall, the ratio between neurons, and glial cells in the human CNS is approximately 4:1 (Azevedo et al., 2009), with oligodendrocytes being the most abundant type of glial cells (75.6%), followed by astrocytes (17.3%) and microglia (6.5%) in human male brains (Pelvig et al., 2008). Glial cells clearly provide "support" for both cells such as neurons and structures such as blood vessels, but also can function to increase action potential conduction velocity via saltatory conduction from one node of Ranvier to the next in myelinated axons, and also the response to damage in the CNS via gliosis, a non-specific reactive change in glial cells associated with their proliferation or hypertrophy. Convergent lines of evidence from multiple studies in neuroimaging, postmortem brains, and genome-wide association studies (GWAS) have revealed a wide range of white matter abnormalities in schizophrenia (Dwork et al., 2007; Bernstein et al., 2015). Indeed, the implication of oligodendrocytes and myelin in schizophrenia has come from analyses of postmortem brains using microarray gene expression (Iwamoto et al., 2005; Katsel et al., 2005), protein expression (Dracheva et al., 2006), electron microscopic studies (Uranova et al., 2011), and neuroimaging (Kubicki et al., 2007).

Astrocytes are regarded as neuronal partners since they hold concerted cross-talk with neighboring neurons, which is crucial for normal brain function. Astrocytes are able to sense neurogenesis, development, and maturation of brain circuits and neuronal activity leading to both homeostatic changes and increased cellular crosstalk (Wang and Bordey, 2008; Parpura et al., 2012). The homeostatic responses of astrocytes includes increases in metabolic activity, the synthesis of a neuronal preferred energy substrate lactate, clearance of neurotransmitters and buffering of extracellular $K^+$ ions to name but a few (Kimelberg, 2007; Wang and Bordey, 2008; Parpura and Verkhratsky, 2012). The existence of bidirectional communication between astrocytes and neurons during synaptic communication and function has been conceptualized as the "tripartite synapse" with its associated alterations in neuron–glia cross talk (Newman, 2003; Perea et al., 2009).

Oligodendrocytes, the myelin forming cells of the CNS, have a small round cell body and about 4–6 branching processes, which can myelinate up to 60 axons depending on the diameter (Miller, 2002). By ensheathing axons, mature oligodendrocytes provide critical insulation to facilitate axonal conduction by increasing the resistance and reducing the effective capacitance of the axonal membrane, resulting in faster conduction speed in myelinated axons compared to unmyelinated axons of the same diameter. In addition, recent studies have provided unique roles of oligodendrocytes, indicating that myelination of the axons cannot only influence neuronal properties in ways not previously considered, but also may be a key source of trophic and metabolic support for maintaining axonal integrity (Nave, 2010).

Microglia function as not only members of the innate immune system but also participate in synaptic modulation and maturation, learning, and memory processes. Importantly, they extend a broad network of ramified processes in the CNS parenchyma. After an injury to the brain, microglia rapidly extend highly active exploratory processes into the sites of injury without any corresponding cell body movement, potentially establishing a barrier between healthy and injured tissues in which microglia actively and constantly interact with neurons and astrocytes and survey the local environment (Davalos et al., 2005; Nimmerjahn et al., 2005). Moreover, microglia can directly regulate both synaptic function and synaptic maintenance in the absence of injury or neuroinflammation (Bessis et al., 2007; Wake et al., 2009).

The focus of this review is to examine what is known regarding the relationship between altered glial cell function and the pathobiology of psychiatric disorders, and whether glial dysfunction can play a causative role. First, we examine the monogenic disorder Rett syndrome (RTT) and examine the mouse model harboring a mutant *methyl-CpG binding protein 2* (MeCP2) gene where neuronal and glial biology have been extensively investigated (**Table 1**). Subsequently, we examine several other mouse models for schizophrenia (**Table 2**) and how glial cell function or dysfunction contributes both to the phenotype and pathophysiology.

**TABLE 1 | Summary of mutant MeCP2 mouse models.**

| Genotype | Phenotype | Reference |
|---|---|---|
| **MeCP2** | | |
| **MeCP2-deficiency astrocytes**<br>*MeCP2tm1.1Bird/+ mice* | Reduced BDNF<br>Reduced IL-1β and IL-6<br>Hyper-activated p38MARK pathways<br>Abnormal neuronal dendritic neurodevelopment | Maezawa et al. (2009) |
| **MeCP2-deficiency astrocyte *in vitro* co-culture** | MeCP2 is present in all glial cell types in normal brain<br>Abnormal neuronal dendritic neurodevelopment | Ballas et al. (2009) |
| **In globally MecP2 deficit mice, re-expression of MeCP2 preferentially in astrocytes** | Improved locomotion and anxiety level Restored respiratory abnormalities | Lioy et al. (2011) |
| **MeCP2-deficiency microglia**<br>*MeCP2tm1.1Bird/+ mice* | Increased glutamate release<br>Increased neurotoxicity<br>Glutamate inhibitor, gap channel hemichannel blocker, and glutamate receptor antagonist blocked the neurotoxicity | Maezawa and Jin (2010) |
| **Re-expression of MeCP2 in microglia in MeCP2 null mice**<br>*MeCP2tm1.1Bird/+ and MecP2tm1.1Jae mice* | Improved RTT-like phenotype<br>Related phagocytic activity | Derecki et al. (2012) |
| **Re-expression of MeCP2 in oligodendrocytes in MeCP2 null mice**<br>*MeCP2loxJ/y/NRG2Cre mice* | Milder RTT-like phenotype<br>Mildly prolonging their life span<br>Significantly improved the locomotor deficits and hindlimb clasping both in male and female<br>Fully restored the body weight<br>PLP and MBP remain reducing | Nguyen et al. (2013) |

**TABLE 2 | Summary of mutant DISC1, neuregulin-ErbB signaling mouse models, and others.**

| Genotype | Phenotype | Reference |
|---|---|---|
| **DISC1** | | |
| **DISC1-deficiency astrocyte** | Diminished production of D-serine | Ma et al. (2013) |
| *B6.Cg-Tg(GFAP-tTA) 110Pop/J mice* | Abnormal behavior similar to schizophrenia | |
| | Increased sensitivity to NMDA antagonist and he ameliorative effects of D-serine | |
| **DISC1-increased or decreased expression oligodendrocyte** | Knockdown of DISC1 increased oligodendrocytes differentiation<br>DISC1 overexpression decreased oligodendrocytes differentiation | Hattori et al. (2014) |
| **DBZ-decreased expression oligodendrocyte**<br>*DBZ KO mice* | Myelination in the corpus callosum was delayed but is mostly recovered by adulthood<br>Oligodendrocytes with immature structural features were more abundant | Shimizu et al. (2014) |
| **Neuregulin-ErbB signaling** | | |
| **Astrocyte specific disruption of synCAM1 signaling** | Increased locomotor activity in the dark period that are attenuated by the psychostimulant D,L-amphetamine | Sandau et al. (2012) |
| *GFAP-DNSynCAM1 mice* | Exhibited attenuation of changes in diurnal rhythm activity | |
| | Reduced anxiety levels | |
| | Reduced the acoustic startle paradigm | |
| **Neuregulin-ErbB4 receptor signaling-deficiency oligodendrocyte** | Myelin sheath is significantly thinner and<br>OLs morphology is less complex | Roy et al. (2007) |
| *CNP-DNErbB4 mice* | Heightened anxiety and had an abnormal behavior | |
| | Enhanced sensitization to amphetamine | |
| | Altered dopamine signaling including levels of DAT and D1-like receptor binding | |
| **Neuregulin-ErbB3 receptor Signaling-deficiency oligodendrocyte** | Deletion of selective ErbB3 receptor in oligodendrocytes | Makinodan et al. (2012) |
| *PLP/CreERT-ErbB3flox/flox mice* | Deficits in social interaction and working memory | |
| **Others** | | |
| **Mice with proteolipid protein overexpression**<br>*$plp^{tg/-}$ mice* | The myelin was intact at the 2 months of age, but developed demyelination<br>Reduced conduction velocity | Tanaka et al. (2009) |
| | Increased anxiety | |
| | Spatial learning deficits and working memory deficits | |
| **Nogo-A knock out mice** | Sensorimotor deficit | Willi et al. (2010) |
| *Nogo-$A^{-/-}$ mice* | Motor stimulant response to systemic amphetamine | |
| | Increased dopamine D2 receptor expression in the striatal and limbic regions | |
| **Selective overexpression of heme oxygenase-1 (HO-1) in astrocytes** | Hyperdopaminergic tone in the nigrostriatal and mesolimbic systems | Song et al. (2012) |
| *HMOX1 transgenic mice* | Sensorimotor deficit | |

## MeCP2

Rett syndrome is currently considered a severe neurodevelopmental disorder caused by sporadic mutations in the *X-chromosome-linked gene* MeCP2 (Amir et al., 1999). Females born with RTT develop normally for 6–18 months and then begin to regress, losing speech, motor skills, and purposeful hand motions and suffering other severe problems including mental retardation, epileptic seizures, and overall retarded growth (Hagberg, 2002). In fact, RTT brain shares certain features with regressive type autism including small neuronal size, as well as reduced dendritic branching and spines in selected regions (Zoghbi, 2003; Armstrong, 2005).

### MeCP2 Knockout Mice

In fact, male MeCP2 null mice show severe neurological symptoms at approximately 6 weeks of age, while heterozygous female mice also develop behavioral symptoms after several months (Guy et al., 2001). Loss of MeCP2 function in RTT mice leads to abnormalities in dendritic arborization (Armstrong, 2005), basal synaptic transmission (Moretti et al., 2006), excitatory synaptic plasticity (Asaka et al., 2006; Moretti et al., 2006; Chao et al., 2007) and reduced spontaneous cortical activity (Dani et al., 2005). Studies utilizing a mouse line with a conditional MeCP2 gene knockout specific to neural stem/progenitor cells, (*nestin*-Cre/*MeCP2-*/y) identified phenotypes that resemble some of the symptoms of RTT-like phenotypes (Chen et al., 2001; Guy et al., 2001). However, mice carrying a conditional knockout of MeCP2 in post-mitotic neurons driven by the *calcium/calmodulin-dependent protein kinase 2 (Camk2)-cre* transgene (*CamkII*-Cre/*MeCP2-*/y; Chen et al., 2001) exhibit milder and delayed RTT-like phenotypes compared with the *nestin-cre* driven transgenic mice (Chen et al., 2001). While the neurological symptoms of MeCP2 knockout mice are reversed by restoring MeCP2 expression (Guy et al., 2007), normal MeCP2 expression in neuronal cells is unable to prevent the phenotypes of the MeCP2 null mice (Alvarez-Saavedra et al., 2007), which implicates the specific loss of glial MeCP2 expression in the pathobiology of RTT. Thus, while MeCP2 is widely expressed throughout various cell types in the normal brain including neurons, and all types of glial cell such as astrocytes, oligodendrocytes, and microglia (Ballas et al., 2009), it appears plausible that while neuronal dysfunction was formerly viewed as a significant contributor to RTT causation, glial dysfunction actually may play a greater role in the development of RTT.

## MeCP2-Deficiency in Astrocytes

With the loss of MeCP2 expression in astrocytes, there are significant abnormalities in the expression of *brain-derived neurotrophic factor* (BDNF); an established target of MeCP2 binding (Chang et al., 2006). Interestingly, astrocytes are known to be involved in the initiation and regulation of nervous system immune responses through the release of proinflammatory cytokines (Farina et al., 2007), and it is noteworthy that the expression of interleukin (IL)-1β and IL-6 in response to administration of lipopolysaccharide is reduced in this model compared to that of controls. In addition, *p38 mitogen activated protein kinases* (MARK) pathways are hyper-activated in this model irrespective of exposure to lipopolysaccharide.

A prominent neuropathological feature associated with brains of RTT is small neuronal size and reduction in dendritic branching and spine density (Armstrong, 2005). Since neurons with more extensive contact with astrocytes promote more extensive dendritic growth (van den Pol and Spencer, 2000), co-culture experiments using intact neurons and astrocytes with MeCP2 deficiency were performed. In this study, neurons cultured in the presence of the MeCP2 deficient astrocytes displayed a much less developed dendritic arborization than did neurons cultured with wild type astrocytes (Ballas et al., 2009). Furthermore, the engineered re-expression of MeCP2 in astrocytes *in vivo* mouse model led to both significantly improved locomotion and anxiety levels as well as respiratory state (Maezawa et al., 2009; Lioy et al., 2011).

## MeCP2 Deficiency in Oligodendrocytes

When mice were engineered that lacked MeCP2 expression in oligodendrocytes, they showed a normal lifespan and the symptoms associated with the RTT-like phenotype commenced at ~10 weeks of age and were milder than those of MeCP2 null mice where the symptoms typically began at 4–5 weeks of age (Chen et al., 2001). With the observational phenotypic scoring system (score = 0–10) considering five typical RTT phenotypic traits such as mobility, gait, hindlimb clasping, tremors, and general conditions (Guy et al., 2007; Nguyen et al., 2012), while MeCP2 null mice reached a score of 6–10 between 9 and 15 weeks of age (Chen et al., 2001), oligodendrocyte MeCP2 knockout mice reached a score of 2 at 20 weeks of age. Additionally, these mice are more active and develop severe hindlimb clasping phenotypes. Restoration of MeCP2 expression solely in cells of the oligodendrocyte lineage in MeCP2 global null mice partially reverses the RTT-like phenotypes associated with loss of MeCP2 such as diminished life span, locomotor deficits, and hindlimb clasping both in male and female, and fully restored normal body weight. However, while MeCP2 expression in the oligodendrocyte lineage cells partially rescues the aberrant expression of MBP protein, it does not affect the expression of either *2′,3′-cyclic-nucleotide-3′-phosphodiesterase* (CNPase), *myelin oligodendrocyte glycoprotein* (MOG), or *myelin proteolipid protein* (PLP) (Nguyen et al., 2012).

## MeCP2-Deficiency in Microglia

Activated microglia release a large amount of glutamate and this microglial-associated neurotoxicity is mediated primarily by NMDA receptor signaling (Takeuchi et al., 2005). In addition to glutamate, activated microglia release pro-inflammatory cytokines such as IL-1β, IL-6, interferon (IFN)-γ, and tumor necrosis factor (TNF-α), which also promote neuronal damage (Sawada et al., 1989; Mizuno et al., 1994, 2003; Suzumura et al., 1996). TNF-α secreted from activated microglia is a major neurotoxic cytokine that induces neurodegeneration through silencing of cell survival signals and caspase-dependent cascades including promotion of signaling through Fas ligand (Greig et al., 2004; Block and Hong, 2005). Neurons treated with conditioned media from MeCP2 null microglia display damaged dendrites and the concentration of glutamate in the media is five time higher than that in control media. The blocking of both microglial glutamate synthesis by a glutaminase inhibitor and microglial glutamate release by a gap junction connexin32 (Cx32) hemichannel blocker abolishes the neurotoxic activity as well as the blocking of a glutamate receptor antagonist. These reports indicate that aberrant glutaminase activity or Cx32 expression in microglia is responsible for the increased production and release of glutamate, potentially implicating these modulators in the pathobiology of microglia-induced RTT-like symptoms (Maezawa and Jin, 2010).

## Introduction of Wild Type Microglia into the MeCP2 Null Mouse

Allogeneic transplantation of wild type bone marrow into irradiation-conditioned MeCP2 null mice led to the engraftment of wild type microglia into the MeCP2 null brain parenchyma. The lifespan of these mice was significantly extended as compared with MeCP2 null mice that received either an autologous bone marrow transplant or untreated MeCP2 null mice. Similarly, body and brain weights of MeCP2-null mice recipients of wild type bone marrow recovered approximately to the level seen in wild type mice. And while the overall appearance, tremor, and gait of MeCP2 null mice recipients of wild type bone marrow were improved, the hindlimb clasping phenotype was not changed. Additionally, these mice exhibited significantly reduced numbers of apneic episodes and greatly reduced respiratory irregularities. Interestingly, these benefits resulting from engraftment with wild-type microglia were diminished when phagocytic activity was inhibited pharmacologically by using annexin V which results in substantial blocking of phagocytic activities (Lu et al., 2011; Derecki et al., 2012).

Thus, the focus of RTT studies using animal models has begun to swing from only studying potential neuronal dysfunction to include interrogation of a role for glial dysfunction and the results of the above studies lends credence to the hypothesis that glial dysfunction may play a primary rather than a secondary role in the causation of RTT-like symptoms. Similarly, studies of DISC1 knockout mice and *neuregulin 1* (NRG1) knockout mice as models for schizophrenia initially focused on the role these proteins play in neurons, but more recently, their activities in glial cells have begun to be considered.

## Disrupted in Schizophrenia 1 (DISC1)

Schizophrenia, which affects ~1% of the worldwide population, is also known as a neurodevelopmental disorder (Weinberger, 1987). The clinical features of schizophrenia cluster in three domains, characterized by positive symptoms (e.g., delusions, hallucinations, thought disorder), negative symptoms (e.g., social withdrawal, blunted affect, reduced motivation) and cognitive symptoms (e.g., attention and working memory deficits). Although schizophrenia is a complex disorder with polygenic and environmental antecedents, multiple lines of evidence have proposed some putative susceptibility genes for schizophrenia (Harrison and Weinberger, 2005; Schizophrenia Working Group of the Psychiatric Genomics, 2014). For example, two overlapping and opposite strand genes on chromosome 1, DISC1 and DISC2, are specifically disrupted by a *t*(1;11; q42.1; q14.3) balanced translocation, in a large Scottish pedigree, resulting in a cohort with several major mental illnesses such as schizophrenia, bipolar affective disorder, and recurrent major depression (St Clair et al., 1990; Millar et al., 2000, 2001; Blackwood et al., 2001; Muir et al., 2008). DISC1 is expressed in neurons within various brain areas including the olfactory bulb, cortex, hippocampus, hypothalamus, cerebellum, and brain stem, especially during development (Schurov et al., 2004). DISC1 has been shown to be involved in several neurodevelopmental processes including progenitor cell proliferation (Mao et al., 2009), radial migration (Tomita et al., 2011), dendritic arborization (Kamiya et al., 2006; Duan et al., 2007), and synapse formation (Camargo et al., 2007; Duan et al., 2007).

### DISC1 Knockout Mice

Since expression of dominant negative proteins frequently has been used successfully in animal models to achieve partial loss of function for relevant proteins (Oike et al., 1999), transgenic mice harboring a C-terminally truncated, dominant negative DISC1 (*DN-DISC1*), expressed under the control of a promoter for *αCaMKII*, were generated (Hikida et al., 2007). This model displays several abnormalities including hyperactivity, disturbance in sensorimotor gating, the dynamic modulation of reward value by effortful action, progressive ratio performance, social behavior, and an anhedonia/depression-like deficit (Hikida et al., 2007; Pletnikov et al., 2008; Johnson et al., 2013). In distinction from *DN-DISC1* mice, *N*-ethyl-*N*-nitrosourea (ENU) was used to induce mutations in exon 2 of mouse Disc1 gene, resulting in the occurrence of missense mutations such as Q31L (glutamine to leucine) or L100P (leucine to proline), causing an increase in depression-like behaviors in Q31L mice and schizophrenia-like behaviors including impaired prepulse inhibition (PPI) and latent inhibition in L100P mice (Clapcote et al., 2007; Shoji et al., 2012). Furthermore, the phenotypes of Q31L mutant mice were partly improved with administration of an antidepressant. Thus, DISC1 dysfunction, likely can exert its influence on neuropsychiatric disorders from its role in both neurons and glia.

### An Increase or Decrease of DISC1 Expression in Oligodendrocytes

Expression of *ΔhDISC1* could exert a significant influence on oligodendrocyte proliferation, differentiation, and function (Katsel et al., 2011). In fact, DISC1 is expressed in oligodendrocytes in the corpus callosum (Seshadri et al., 2010). In rat oligodendrocyte precursor cell cultures (Hattori et al., 2014), DISC1 expression decreases in the course of oligodendrocyte differentiation. Furthermore, the expression of CNPase and *myelin basic protein* (MBP) known to markers of myelin maturation were decreased following full length DISC1 overexpression. In contrast, the knockdown of endogenous DISC1 using RNA interference increased the expression of CNPase as well as the number of mature oligodendrocytes (Hattori et al., 2014). SRY box containing (Sox) family member, Sox10, the homeobox containing (Hox) transcription factor Nkx2.2, the basic helix-loop-helix (bHLH) family members Olig1 and Olig2 and the inhibitor of DNA binding (Id) family of proteins Id2 and Id4 have all been shown to be involved in the control of oligodendrocyte differentiation (Nicolay et al., 2007; Emery, 2010). Against this backdrop, it is perhaps not surprising that knockdown of DISC1 increased the expression of Sox10 and/or Nkx2.2, and DISC1 overexpression led to the reduced expression of these transcription factors. These findings are strongly supportive of a role for DISC1 in negatively regulating oligodendrocyte differentiation by acting upstream of Sox10 and/or Nkx2.2 to regulate their transcription (Hattori et al., 2014).

### A Decrease of DBZ Expression in Oligodendrocytes

DISC1 binding zinc finger protein (DBZ), also known as ZNF365 or Su48, is a CNS specific member of the DISC1 interactome and is a novel DISC1 binding protein with a predicted C2H2-type zinc-finger motif and coil domains (Hattori et al., 2007). DBZ regulates neurite outgrowth via the DISC1-DBZ interaction in primary neurons and cultured PC12 cells *in vitro* (Hattori et al., 2007). In DBZ knockout mice, oligodendrocytes displaying an immature structural morphology are more abundant than in control mice and the timing of myelination in the corpus callosum is delayed (Koyama et al., 2013). Although this model implicates DBZ function in oligodendrocyte development and myelination, further studies using more specific models such as oligodendrocyte-specific DBZ knockout mice are needed to elucidate the precise function of DBZ (Shimizu et al., 2014).

### DISC1-Deficiency in Astrocytes

Since the administration of the *N*-methyl-*D*-aspartic acid (NMDA) receptor antagonists phencyclidine and MK-801 induce behaviors that closely resemble those observed in schizophrenic patients, dysfunction of the NMDA receptor is regarded as a particularly strong candidate for being a component of the mechanism of schizophrenia (Javitt and Zukin, 1991; Goff and Coyle, 2001). The stereoisomer D-serine binds to the "glycine site" on the NR1 subunit and it is crucial for the activation of this receptor. D-serine acting as co-agonist at the NMDA receptor is involved in synaptic plasticity (Fossat et al., 2012; Rosenberg et al., 2013), and D-amino acid oxidase (DAAO) degrades the D-serine, modulating D-serine levels and thence NMDA receptor function (Duplantier et al., 2009; Strick et al., 2011). The biosynthesis of D-serine was clarified by the purification and molecular cloning of serine racemase (SR), which transforms L-serine to D-serine, and, interestingly, DISC1 binds to and stabilizes SR (Wolosker et al., 1999a,b; De Miranda et al., 2000). Furthermore, D-serine and SR have been predominantly localized to astrocytes ensheathing synapses, especially in brain regions with enriched NMDA receptors, suggesting that D-serine could be acting as a glial transmitter (Puyal et al., 2006; Williams et al., 2006). In this model of selective and inducible expression of mutant DISC1 in astrocytes, the expression of mutant DISC1 downregulates the level of endogenous DISC1 expression in astrocytes. The disruption of DISC1 binding to SR leads to increased ubiquitination and degradation of SR in astrocytes. The decrease of SR in astrocytes results in diminished production of D-serine in astrocytes. This mouse model displays abnormal behaviors like schizophrenia including sensitivity to an NMDA antagonist; MK-801, in an open field test and pre-pulse inhibition of acoustic startle test, and responds to the ameliorative effects of D-serine (Ma et al., 2013).

## Neuregulin-ErbB Signaling

Neuregulins comprise a large family of widely expressed, alternatively spliced epidermal growth factor (EGF)-like domain-containing proteins that have been strongly implicated in neural development (Corfas et al., 2004; Mei and Xiong, 2008). NRG proteins act by binding to and activating members of the ErbB receptor tyrosine kinase family. After the initial discovery of what came to be known as NRG1, five additional NRG1 homologs (NRG2, NRG3, NRG4, NRG5, and NRG6) have been identified. NRG1 proteins bind only to either ErbB3 or ErbB4 causing a conformational change that promotes receptor dimerization and auophosphorylation, and the subsequent activation of downstream signaling pathways. However, NRG1 does not bind to the ErbB2 receptor, which functions as a co-receptor that heterodimerizes with ErbB3 or ErbB4. Additionally, ErbB4 is known to be able to function as a homodimer. In adult brains, ErbB receptors are widely and differentially expressed. In general, ErbB2 is expressed in most cells, ErbB3 is mainly found in glial populations, and ErbB4 is enriched in neurons. NRG/ErbB signaling has been widely implicated in psychiatric disorders including schizophrenia, bipolar disorder, or depression (Corfas et al., 2004; Mei and Nave, 2014).

### Astrocyte Specific Disruption of synCAM1 Signaling

Synaptic cell adhesion molecule 1 (SynCAM1) is a member of the immunoglobulin (Ig) superfamily, a large group of proteins involved in cell surface recognition (Williams, 1992; Rougon and Hobert, 2003). SynCAM1 plays an important role in CNS developmental processes such as synaptic assembly (Biederer et al., 2002), enhancement of excitatory synaptic transmission (Sara et al., 2005; Fogel et al., 2007), functional presynaptic differentiation (Sara et al., 2005) and the regulation of synapse number and plasticity (Robbins et al., 2010). SynCAM1 is produced in astrocytes and plays a major role in facilitating astrocyte-to-astrocyte and astrocyte-to-neuron adhesive communication (Sandau et al., 2011). SynCAM1 is co-expressed with ErbB4 in astrocytes (Sandau et al., 2011) and is functionally related to ErbB4 receptors (Carpenter, 2003). Mice carrying a dominant-negative form of SynCAM1, specifically targeted to astrocytes, exhibited an attenuation of changes in diurnal rhythm activity. In addition, the locomotor activity in a dark field is increased and it is attenuated with the psychostimulant D, L-amphetamine, and anxiety is reduced in a zero maze test and an acoustic startle paradigm in these mice. These findings imply that these mice could be utilized as a model of neurodevelopmental disorder (Sandau et al., 2012).

### Neuregulin-ErbB4 Receptors Signaling-Deficiency in Oligodendrocytes

Neuregulin 1-ErbB receptor signaling appears to play a critical role in the ontogeny of psychiatric disorders and this hypothesis has been supported by the identification of altered expression levels and/or function of NRG1, ErbB3, and ErbB4 in patients with schizophrenia (Corfas et al., 2004; Silberberg et al., 2006). Moreover, mice with reduced levels of NRG1 or ErbB4 have exhibited behavioral alterations akin to those found in schizophrenia (Gerlai et al., 2000; Golub et al., 2004; Rimer et al., 2005).

Transgenic mice expressing a dominant-negative ErbB4 receptor in oligodendrocytes exhibit thinner myelin and less complex oligodendrocyte morphology and show schizophrenia-like behaviors including high anxiety and an enhanced sensitization to amphetamine. This abnormal response to amphetamine might be due to altered dopamine signaling as aberrant expressions of dopamine transporter (DAT) and dopamine1-like receptor in the cortex, nucleus accumbens, and striatum are evident (Roy et al., 2007).

### Neuregulin-ErbB3 Receptor Signaling-Deficiency in Oligodendrocytes

Neuregulin 1-ErbB signaling plays, at least in part, a critical role in oligodendrocyte development and CNS myelination (Michailov et al., 2004; Taveggia et al., 2005; Chen et al., 2006). In human prefrontal cortex, microarray analyses revealed that the level of ErbB3 was significantly reduced in schizophrenia subjects relative to a normal cohort (Hakak et al., 2001). This decrement was reproduced by another study (Tkachev et al., 2003). Consistent with the results of human studies, mice with selective ErbB3 receptor deletion in oligodendrocytes demonstrate deficits in social interaction and working memory (Makinodan et al., 2012), suggesting that NRG1-ErbB3 signaling in oligodendrocyte might contribute to the pathogenesis of schizophrenia (Makinodan et al., 2012).

## Other Studies

### Mice with Proteolipid Protein Overexpression

*Proteolipid protein* 1, a major protein in CNS myelin (Inoue et al., 1996; Mimault et al., 1999), is regarded as an "adhesive strut" that binds adjacent lamellae of the compacted myelin membrane (Boison et al., 1995).

Transgenic mice harboring extra copies of the myelin PLP1 gene have demonstrated that at the 2 months of age, the myelin was intact with a normally appearing ion channel distribution (Inoue et al., 1996), whereas the conduction velocity in all axonal tracts tested in the CNS was markedly reduced at this age (Tanaka et al., 2009). This observation was supported by subsequent analysis that these mice showed altered neuron–glia interaction with subtle changes in axonal diameters and paranodal structures, leading to schizophrenia-like behaviors including increased anxiety-related behaviors, reduced PPI, spatial learning deficits, and working memory deficits.

### Nogo-A Knockout Mice

Nogo signaling plays a crucial role in restricting axonal regeneration and compensatory fiber growth in the injured adult mammalian CNS (Schwab, 2004; Yiu and He, 2006). The membrane protein Nogo-A, which is predominantly expressed in oligodendrocytes in the adult brain and in neurons mainly during development, is well-known for its role as one of several currently known inhibitors of neurite outgrowth (Huber et al., 2002; Wang et al., 2002). Postmortem and genetic studies have implicated Nogo-A and its choromosomal location in schizophrenia and bipolar disorder (Coon et al., 1998; Novak et al., 2002).

These mice showed sensorimotor deficits, disrupted latent inhibition, and perseverative behaviors. Furthermore, they displayed an enhanced response to systemic amphetamine in an open field test. These behavioral phenotypes might be due to altered monoaminergic transmitter levels in the striatal and limbic regions and/or increased dopamine D2 receptor expression in the identical brain regions. In contrast, adult mice acutely treated with anti-Nogo-A antibodies did not exhibit abnormal behaviors, but showed increased dopamine D2 receptor expression (Willi et al., 2010).

### Selective Overexpression of Heme Oxygenase-1 (HO-1) in Astrocytes

The heme oxygenases (HOs), which are responsible for the degradation of heme to biliverdin/bilirubin, free iron and carbon monoxide (CO), has been strongly implicated in mammalian CNS aging and diseases (Schipper et al., 2009). Mammalian cells express two isoforms such as an inducible isoform, HO-1, and a constitutively active form, HO-2. Specifically, HO-1, encoded by the HMOX1 gene, is a 32-kDa stress protein, and the induction of the glial HMOX1 gene may lead to pathological brain iron deposition, intracellular oxidative damage, and bioenergetic failure in Alzheimer's disease and other human CNS disorders such as Parkinson's disease and schizophrenia (Schipper et al., 2009; Brown, 2011). This mice model displayed sensorimotor deficits, increased spontaneous horizontal movements, and stereotypy. Hyperdopaminergic signaling was identified in the striatum and substantia nigra and the associated neurochemical alterations may contribute to these behaviors (Song et al., 2012).

## Conclusion

In conclusion, studies leveraging different animal models for the enhanced biochemical and physiological understanding of mental disorders have moved from strictly targeting the biology of neurons to also include an examination of the glia, especially since glial cells such as oligodendrocytes, astrocytes, and microglia have emerged as critically important modifiers of both CNS development and function. Postmortem brain analyses have clearly indicated that glial cell abnormalities are present in the brains of patients with schizophrenia. However, it remains uncertain whether the dysregulation and symptoms seen are a primary result of alterations in glial cell biology or the deficits in glial function occur as a side product of neuronal dysfunction. Nonetheless, as we have described, continued use of cell-type specific conditional knockout mice will allow us to better dissect how glial cells are implicated in nervous system dysfunction and perhaps illuminate their role in the pathobiology of psychiatric diseases such as schizophrenia.

## Acknowledgment

This work was supported by the Naito Foundation.

## References

Alvarez-Saavedra, M., Saez, M. A., Kang, D., Zoghbi, H. Y., and Young, J. I. (2007). Cell-specific expression of wild-type MeCP2 in mouse models of Rett syndrome yields insight about pathogenesis. *Hum. Mol. Genet.* 16, 2315–2325. doi: 10.1093/hmg/ddm185

Amir, R. E., Van den Veyver, I. B., Wan, M., Tran, C. Q., Francke, U., and Zoghbi, H. Y. (1999). Rett syndrome is caused by mutations in X-linked MECP2, encoding methyl-CpG-binding protein 2. *Nat. Genet.* 23, 185–188. doi: 10.1038/13810

Armstrong, D. D. (2005). Neuropathology of Rett syndrome. *J. Child Neurol.* 20, 747–753. doi: 10.1177/08830738050200082401

Asaka, Y., Jugloff, D. G., Zhang, L., Eubanks, J. H., and Fitzsimonds, R. M. (2006). Hippocampal synaptic plasticity is impaired in the Mecp2-null mouse model of Rett syndrome. *Neurobiol. Dis.* 21, 217–227. doi: 10.1016/j.nbd.2005.07.005

Azevedo, F. A., Carvalho, L. R., Grinberg, L. T., Farfel, J. M., Ferretti, R. E., Leite, R. E., et al. (2009). Equal numbers of neuronal and nonneuronal cells make the human brain an isometrically scaled-up primate brain. *J. Comp. Neurol.* 513, 532–541. doi: 10.1002/cne.21974

Ballas, N., Lioy, D. T., Grunseich, C., and Mandel, G. (2009). Non-cell autonomous influence of MeCP2-deficient glia on neuronal dendritic morphology. *Nat. Neurosci.* 12, 311–317. doi: 10.1038/nn.2275

Bernstein, H. G., Steiner, J., Guest, P. C., Dobrowolny, H., and Bogerts, B. (2015). Glial cells as key players in schizophrenia pathology: recent insights and concepts of therapy. *Schizophr. Res.* 161, 4–18. doi: 10.1016/j.schres.2014.03.035

Bessis, A., Bechade, C., Bernard, D., and Roumier, A. (2007). Microglial control of neuronal death and synaptic properties. *Glia* 55, 233–238. doi: 10.1002/glia.20459

Biederer, T., Sara, Y., Mozhayeva, M., Atasoy, D., Liu, X., Kavalali, E. T., et al. (2002). SynCAM, a synaptic adhesion molecule that drives synapse assembly. *Science* 297, 1525–1531. doi: 10.1126/science.1072356

Blackwood, D. H., Fordyce, A., Walker, M. T., St Clair, D. M., Porteous, D. J., and Muir, W. J. (2001). Schizophrenia and affective disorders–cosegregation with a translocation at chromosome 1q42 that directly disrupts brain-expressed genes: clinical and P300 findings in a family. *Am. J. Hum. Genet.* 69, 428–433. doi: 10.1086/321969

Block, M. L., and Hong, J. S. (2005). Microglia and inflammation-mediated neurodegeneration: multiple triggers with a common mechanism. *Prog. Neurobiol.* 76, 77–98. doi: 10.1016/j.pneurobio.2005.06.004

Boison, D., Bussow, H., D'Urso, D., Muller, H. W., and Stoffel, W. (1995). Adhesive properties of proteolipid protein are responsible for the compaction of CNS myelin sheaths. *J. Neurosci.* 15, 5502–5513.

Brown, A. S. (2011). The environment and susceptibility to schizophrenia. *Prog. Neurobiol.* 93, 23–58. doi: 10.1016/j.pneurobio.2010.09.003

Camargo, L. M., Collura, V., Rain, J. C., Mizuguchi, K., Hermjakob, H., Kerrien, S., et al. (2007). Disrupted in Schizophrenia 1 Interactome: evidence for the close connectivity of risk genes and a potential synaptic basis for schizophrenia. *Mol. Psychiatry* 12, 74–86. doi: 10.1038/sj.mp.4001880

Carpenter, G. (2003). ErbB-4: mechanism of action and biology. *Exp. Cell Res.* 284, 66–77. doi: 10.1016/S0014-4827(02)00100-3

Chang, Q., Khare, G., Dani, V., Nelson, S., and Jaenisch, R. (2006). The disease progression of Mecp2 mutant mice is affected by the level of BDNF expression. *Neuron* 49, 341–348. doi: 10.1016/j.neuron.2005.12.027

Chao, H. T., Zoghbi, H. Y., and Rosenmund, C. (2007). MeCP2 controls excitatory synaptic strength by regulating glutamatergic synapse number. *Neuron* 56, 58–65. doi: 10.1016/j.neuron.2007.08.018

Chen, R. Z., Akbarian, S., Tudor, M., and Jaenisch, R. (2001). Deficiency of methyl-CpG binding protein-2 in CNS neurons results in a Rett-like phenotype in mice. *Nat. Genet.* 27, 327–331. doi: 10.1038/85906

Chen, S., Velardez, M. O., Warot, X., Yu, Z. X., Miller, S. J., Cros, D., et al. (2006). Neuregulin 1-erbB signaling is necessary for normal myelination and sensory function. *J. Neurosci.* 26, 3079–3086. doi: 10.1523/JNEUROSCI.3785-05.2006

Clapcote, S. J., Lipina, T. V., Millar, J. K., Mackie, S., Christie, S., Ogawa, F., et al. (2007). Behavioral phenotypes of Disc1 missense mutations in mice. *Neuron* 54, 387–402. doi: 10.1016/j.neuron.2007.04.015

Coon, H., Myles-Worsley, M., Tiobech, J., Hoff, M., Rosenthal, J., Bennett, P., et al. (1998). Evidence for a chromosome 2p13-14 schizophrenia susceptibility locus in families from Palau, Micronesia. *Mol. Psychiatry* 3, 521–527. doi: 10.1038/sj.mp.4000453

Corfas, G., Roy, K., and Buxbaum, J. D. (2004). Neuregulin 1-erbB signaling and the molecular/cellular basis of schizophrenia. *Nat. Neurosci.* 7, 575–580. doi: 10.1038/nn1258

Dani, V. S., Chang, Q., Maffei, A., Turrigiano, G. G., Jaenisch, R., and Nelson, S. B. (2005). Reduced cortical activity due to a shift in the balance between excitation and inhibition in a mouse model of Rett syndrome. *Proc. Natl. Acad. Sci. U.S.A.* 102, 12560–12565. doi: 10.1073/pnas.0506071102

Davalos, D., Grutzendler, J., Yang, G., Kim, J. V., Zuo, Y., Jung, S., et al. (2005). ATP mediates rapid microglial response to local brain injury in vivo. *Nat. Neurosci.* 8, 752–758. doi: 10.1038/nn1472

De Miranda, J., Santoro, A., Engelender, S., and Wolosker, H. (2000). Human serine racemase: moleular cloning, genomic organization and functional analysis. *Gene* 256, 183–188. doi: 10.1016/S0378-1119(00)00356-5

Derecki, N. C., Cronk, J. C., Lu, Z., Xu, E., Abbott, S. B., Guyenet, P. G., et al. (2012). Wild-type microglia arrest pathology in a mouse model of Rett syndrome. *Nature* 484, 105–109. doi: 10.1038/nature10907

Dracheva, S., Davis, K. L., Chin, B., Woo, D. A., Schmeidler, J., and Haroutunian, V. (2006). Myelin-associated mRNA and protein expression deficits in the anterior cingulate cortex and hippocampus in elderly schizophrenia patients. *Neurobiol. Dis.* 21, 531–540. doi: 10.1016/j.nbd.2005.08.012

Duan, X., Chang, J. H., Ge, S., Faulkner, R. L., Kim, J. Y., Kitabatake, Y., et al. (2007). Disrupted-In-Schizophrenia 1 regulates integration of newly generated neurons in the adult brain. *Cell* 130, 1146–1158. doi: 10.1016/j.cell.2007.07.010

Duplantier, A. J., Becker, S. L., Bohanon, M. J., Borzilleri, K. A., Chrunyk, B. A., Downs, J. T., et al. (2009). Discovery, SAR, and pharmacokinetics of a novel 3-hydroxyquinolin-2(1H)-one series of potent D-amino acid oxidase (DAAO) inhibitors. *J. Med. Chem.* 52, 3576–3585. doi: 10.1021/jm900128w

Dwork, A. J., Mancevski, B., and Rosoklija, G. (2007). White matter and cognitive function in schizophrenia. *Int. J. Neuropsychopharmacol.* 10, 513–536. doi: 10.1017/S1461145707007638

Emery, B. (2010). Regulation of oligodendrocyte differentiation and myelination. *Science* 330, 779–782. doi: 10.1126/science.1190927

Farina, C., Aloisi, F., and Meinl, E. (2007). Astrocytes are active players in cerebral innate immunity. *Trends Immunol.* 28, 138–145. doi: 10.1016/j.it.2007.01.005

Fogel, A. I., Akins, M. R., Krupp, A. J., Stagi, M., Stein, V., and Biederer, T. (2007). SynCAMs organize synapses through heterophilic adhesion. *J. Neurosci.* 27, 12516–12530. doi: 10.1523/JNEUROSCI.2739-07.2007

Fossat, P., Turpin, F. R., Sacchi, S., Dulong, J., Shi, T., Rivet, J. M., et al. (2012). Glial D-serine gates NMDA receptors at excitatory synapses in prefrontal cortex. *Cereb. Cortex* 22, 595–606. doi: 10.1093/cercor/bhr130

Gerlai, R., Pisacane, P., and Erickson, S. (2000). Heregulin, but not ErbB2 or ErbB3, heterozygous mutant mice exhibit hyperactivity in multiple behavioral tasks. *Behav. Brain Res.* 109, 219–227. doi: 10.1016/S0166-4328(99)00175-8

Goff, D. C., and Coyle, J. T. (2001). The emerging role of glutamate in the pathophysiology and treatment of schizophrenia. *Am. J. Psychiatry* 158, 1367–1377. doi: 10.1176/appi.ajp.158.9.1367

Golub, M. S., Germann, S. L., and Lloyd, K. C. (2004). Behavioral characteristics of a nervous system-specific erbB4 knock-out mouse. *Behav. Brain Res.* 153, 159–170. doi: 10.1016/j.bbr.2003.11.010

Greig, N. H., Mattson, M. P., Perry, T., Chan, S. L., Giordano, T., Sambamurti, K., et al. (2004). New therapeutic strategies and drug candidates for neurodegenerative diseases: p53 and TNF-alpha inhibitors, and GLP-1 receptor agonists. *Ann. N. Y. Acad. Sci.* 1035, 290–315. doi: 10.1196/annals.1332.018

Guy, J., Gan, J., Selfridge, J., Cobb, S., and Bird, A. (2007). Reversal of neurological defects in a mouse model of Rett syndrome. *Science* 315, 1143–1147. doi: 10.1126/science.1138389

Guy, J., Hendrich, B., Holmes, M., Martin, J. E., and Bird, A. (2001). A mouse Mecp2-null mutation causes neurological symptoms that mimic Rett syndrome. *Nat. Genet.* 27, 322–326. doi: 10.1038/85899

Hagberg, B. (2002). Clinical manifestations and stages of Rett syndrome. *Ment. Retard. Dev. Disabil. Res. Rev* 8, 61–65. doi: 10.1002/mrdd.10020

Hakak, Y., Walker, J. R., Li, C., Wong, W. H., Davis, K. L., Buxbaum, J. D., et al. (2001). Genome-wide expression analysis reveals dysregulation of myelination-related genes in chronic schizophrenia. *Proc. Natl. Acad. Sci. U.S.A.* 98, 4746–4751. doi: 10.1073/pnas.081071198

Harrison, P. J., and Weinberger, D. R. (2005). Schizophrenia genes, gene expression, and neuropathology: on the matter of their convergence. *Mol. Psychiatry* 10, 40–68. doi: 10.1038/sj.mp.4001558

Hattori, T., Baba, K., Matsuzaki, S., Honda, A., Miyoshi, K., Inoue, K., et al. (2007). A novel DISC1-interacting partner DISC1-Binding Zinc-finger protein: implication in the modulation of DISC1-dependent neurite outgrowth. *Mol. Psychiatry* 12, 398–407. doi: 10.1038/sj.mp.4001945

Hattori, T., Shimizu, S., Koyama, Y., Emoto, H., Matsumoto, Y., Kumamoto, N., et al. (2014). DISC1 (disrupted-in-schizophrenia-1) regulates differentiation of oligodendrocytes *PLoS ONE* 9:e88506. doi: 10.1371/journal.pone.0088506

Hikida, T., Jaaro-Peled, H., Seshadri, S., Oishi, K., Hookway, C., Kong, S., et al. (2007). Dominant-negative DISC1 transgenic mice display schizophrenia-associated phenotypes detected by measures translatable to humans. *Proc. Natl. Acad. Sci. U.S.A.* 104, 14501–14506. doi: 10.1073/pnas.0704774104

Huber, A. B., Weinmann, O., Brosamle, C., Oertle, T., and Schwab, M. E. (2002). Patterns of Nogo mRNA and protein expression in the developing and adult rat and after CNS lesions. *J. Neurosci.* 22, 3553–3567.

Inoue, K., Osaka, H., Sugiyama, N., Kawanishi, C., Onishi, H., Nezu, A., et al. (1996). A duplicated PLP gene causing Pelizaeus-Merzbacher disease detected by comparative multiplex PCR. *Am. J. Hum. Genet.* 59, 32–39.

Iwamoto, K., Bundo, M., and Kato, T. (2005). Altered expression of mitochondria-related genes in postmortem brains of patients with bipolar disorder or schizophrenia, as revealed by large-scale DNA microarray analysis. *Hum. Mol. Genet.* 14, 241–253. doi: 10.1093/hmg/ddi022

Javitt, D. C., and Zukin, S. R. (1991). Recent advances in the phencyclidine model of schizophrenia. *Am. J. Psychiatry* 148, 1301–1308. doi: 10.1176/ajp.148.10.1301

Johnson, A. W., Jaaro-Peled, H., Shahani, N., Sedlak, T. W., Zoubovsky, S., Burruss, D., et al. (2013). Cognitive and motivational deficits together with prefrontal oxidative stress in a mouse model for neuropsychiatric illness. *Proc. Natl. Acad. Sci. U.S.A.* 110, 12462–12467. doi: 10.1073/pnas.1307925110

Kamiya, A., Tomoda, T., Chang, J., Takaki, M., Zhan, C., Morita, M., et al. (2006). DISC1-NDEL1/NUDEL protein interaction, an essential component for neurite outgrowth, is modulated by genetic variations of DISC1. *Hum. Mol. Genet.* 15, 3313–3323. doi: 10.1093/hmg/ddl407

Katsel, P., Davis, K. L., Gorman, J. M., and Haroutunian, V. (2005). Variations in differential gene expression patterns across multiple brain regions in schizophrenia. *Schizophr. Res.* 77, 241–252. doi: 10.1016/j.schres.2005.03.020

Katsel, P., Tan, W., Abazyan, B., Davis, K. L., Ross, C., Pletnikov, M. V., et al. (2011). Expression of mutant human DISC1 in mice supports abnormalities in differentiation of oligodendrocytes. *Schizophr. Res.* 130, 238–249. doi: 10.1016/j.schres.2011.04.021

Kimelberg, H. K. (2007). Supportive or information-processing functions of the mature protoplasmic astrocyte in the mammalian CNS? A critical appraisal. *Neuron Glia Biol.* 3, 181–189. doi: 10.1017/S1740925X08000094

Koyama, Y., Hattori, T., Shimizu, S., Taniguchi, M., Yamada, K., Takamura, H., et al. (2013). DBZ (DISC1-binding zinc finger protein)-deficient mice display abnormalities in basket cells in the somatosensory cortices. *J. Chem. Neuroanat.* 53, 1–10. doi: 10.1016/j.jchemneu.2013.07.002

Kubicki, M., McCarley, R., Westin, C. F., Park, H. J., Maier, S., Kikinis, R., et al. (2007). A review of diffusion tensor imaging studies in schizophrenia. *J. Psychiatr. Res.* 41, 15–30. doi: 10.1016/j.jpsychires.2005.05.005

Lioy, D. T., Garg, S. K., Monaghan, C. E., Raber, J., Foust, K. D., Kaspar, B. K., et al. (2011). A role for glia in the progression of Rett's syndrome. *Nature* 475, 497–500. doi: 10.1038/nature10214

Lu, Z., Elliott, M. R., Chen, Y., Walsh, J. T., Klibanov, A. L., Ravichandran, K. S., et al. (2011). Phagocytic activity of neuronal progenitors regulates adult neurogenesis. *Nat. Cell Biol.* 13, 1076–1083. doi: 10.1038/ncb2299

Ma, T. M., Abazyan, S., Abazyan, B., Nomura, J., Yang, C., Seshadri, S., et al. (2013). Pathogenic disruption of DISC1-serine racemase binding elicits schizophrenia-like behavior via D-serine depletion. *Mol. Psychiatry* 18, 557–567. doi: 10.1038/mp.2012.97

Maezawa, I., and Jin, L. W. (2010). Rett syndrome microglia damage dendrites and synapses by the elevated release of glutamate. *J. Neurosci.* 30, 5346–5356. doi: 10.1523/JNEUROSCI.5966-09.2010

Maezawa, I., Swanberg, S., Harvey, D., LaSalle, J. M., and Jin, L. W. (2009). Rett syndrome astrocytes are abnormal and spread MeCP2 deficiency through gap junctions. *J. Neurosci.* 29, 5051–5061. doi: 10.1523/JNEUROSCI.0324-09.2009

Makinodan, M., Rosen, K. M., Ito, S., and Corfas, G. (2012). A critical period for social experience-dependent oligodendrocyte maturation and myelination. *Science* 337, 1357–1360. doi: 10.1126/science.1220845

Mao, Y., Ge, X., Frank, C. L., Madison, J. M., Koehler, A. N., Doud, M. K., et al. (2009). Disrupted in schizophrenia 1 regulates neuronal progenitor proliferation via modulation of GSK3beta/beta-catenin signaling. *Cell* 136, 1017–1031. doi: 10.1016/j.cell.2008.12.044

Mei, L., and Nave, K. A. (2014). Neuregulin-ERBB signaling in the nervous system and neuropsychiatric diseases. *Neuron* 83, 27–49. doi: 10.1016/j.neuron.2014.06.007

Mei, L., and Xiong, W. C. (2008). Neuregulin 1 in neural development, synaptic plasticity and schizophrenia. *Nat. Rev. Neurosci.* 9, 437–452. doi: 10.1038/nrn2392

Michailov, G. V., Sereda, M. W., Brinkmann, B. G., Fischer, T. M., Haug, B., Birchmeier, C., et al. (2004). Axonal neuregulin-1 regulates myelin sheath thickness. *Science* 304, 700–703. doi: 10.1126/science.1095862

Millar, J. K., Christie, S., Anderson, S., Lawson, D., Hsiao-Wei Loh, D., Devon, R. S., et al. (2001). Genomic structure and localisation within a linkage hotspot of Disrupted In Schizophrenia 1, a gene disrupted by a translocation segregating with schizophrenia. *Mol. Psychiatry* 6, 173–178. doi: 10.1038/sj.mp.4000784

Millar, J. K., Wilson-Annan, J. C., Anderson, S., Christie, S., Taylor, M. S., Semple, C. A., et al. (2000). Disruption of two novel genes by a translocation co-segregating with schizophrenia. *Hum. Mol. Genet.* 9, 1415–1423. doi: 10.1093/hmg/9.9.1415

Miller, R. H. (2002). Regulation of oligodendrocyte development in the vertebrate CNS. *Prog. Neurobiol.* 67, 451–467. doi: 10.1016/S0301-0082(02)00058-8

Mimault, C., Giraud, G., Courtois, V., Cailloux, F., Boire, J. Y., Dastugue, B., et al. (1999). Proteolipoprotein gene analysis in 82 patients with sporadic Pelizaeus-Merzbacher disease: duplications, the major cause of the disease, originate more frequently in male germ cells, but point mutations do not. The Clinical European Network on Brain Dysmyelinating Disease. *Am. J. Hum. Genet.* 65, 360–369. doi: 10.1086/302483

Mizuno, T., Kawanokuchi, J., Numata, K., and Suzumura, A. (2003). Production and neuroprotective functions of fractalkine in the central nervous system. *Brain Res.* 979, 65–70. doi: 10.1016/S0006-8993(03)02867-1

Mizuno, T., Sawada, M., Suzumura, A., and Marunouchi, T. (1994). Expression of cytokines during glial differentiation. *Brain Res.* 656, 141–146. doi: 10.1016/0006-8993(94)91375-7

Moretti, P., Levenson, J. M., Battaglia, F., Atkinson, R., Teague, R., Antalffy, B., et al. (2006). Learning and memory and synaptic plasticity are impaired in a mouse model of Rett syndrome. *J. Neurosci.* 26, 319–327. doi: 10.1523/JNEUROSCI.2623-05.2006

Muir, W. J., Pickard, B. S., and Blackwood, D. H. (2008). Disrupted-in-Schizophrenia-1. *Curr. Psychiatry Rep.* 10, 140–147. doi: 10.1007/s11920-008-0025-2

Nave, K. A. (2010). Myelination and the trophic support of long axons. *Nat. Rev. Neurosci.* 11, 275–283. doi: 10.1038/nrn2797

Newman, E. A. (2003). New roles for astrocytes: regulation of synaptic transmission. *Trends Neurosci.* 26, 536–542. doi: 10.1016/S0166-2236(03)00237-6

Nguyen, M. V., Du, F., Felice, C. A., Shan, X., Nigam, A., Mandel, G., et al. (2012). MeCP2 is critical for maintaining mature neuronal networks and global brain anatomy during late stages of postnatal brain development and in the mature adult brain. *J. Neurosci.* 32, 10021–10034. doi: 10.1523/JNEUROSCI.1316-12.2012

Nguyen, M. V., Felice, C. A., Du, F., Covey, M. V., Robinson, J. K., Mandel, G., et al. (2013). Oligodendrocyte lineage cells contribute unique features to Rett syndrome neuropathology. *J. Neurosci.* 33, 18764–18774. doi: 10.1523/JNEUROSCI.2657-13.2013

Nicolay, D. J., Doucette, J. R., and Nazarali, A. J. (2007). Transcriptional control of oligodendrogenesis. *Glia* 55, 1287–1299. doi: 10.1002/glia.20540

Nimmerjahn, A., Kirchhoff, F., and Helmchen, F. (2005). Resting microglial cells are highly dynamic surveillants of brain parenchyma in vivo. *Science* 308, 1314–1318. doi: 10.1126/science.1110647

Novak, G., Kim, D., Seeman, P., and Tallerico, T. (2002). Schizophrenia and Nogo: elevated mRNA in cortex, and high prevalence of a homozygous CAA insert. *Brain Res. Mol. Brain Res.* 107, 183–189. doi: 10.1016/S0169-328X(02)00492-8

Oike, Y., Hata, A., Mamiya, T., Kaname, T., Noda, Y., Suzuki, M., et al. (1999). Truncated CBP protein leads to classical Rubinstein-Taybi syndrome phenotypes in mice: implications for a dominant-negative mechanism. *Hum. Mol. Genet.* 8, 387–396. doi: 10.1093/hmg/8.3.387

Parpura, V., Heneka, M. T., Montana, V., Oliet, S. H., Schousboe, A., Haydon, P. G., et al. (2012). Glial cells in (patho)physiology. *J. Neurochem.* 121, 4–27. doi: 10.1111/j.1471-4159.2012.07664.x

Parpura, V., and Verkhratsky, A. (2012). Homeostatic function of astrocytes: Ca(2+) and Na(+) signalling. *Transl. Neurosci.* 3, 334–344. doi: 10.2478/s13380-012-0040-y

Pelvig, D. P., Pakkenberg, H., Stark, A. K., and Pakkenberg, B. (2008). Neocortical glial cell numbers in human brains. *Neurobiol. Aging* 29, 1754–1762. doi: 10.1016/j.neurobiolaging.2007.04.013

Perea, G., Navarrete, M., and Araque, A. (2009). Tripartite synapses: astrocytes process and control synaptic information. *Trends Neurosci.* 32, 421–431. doi: 10.1016/j.tins.2009.05.001

Pletnikov, M. V., Ayhan, Y., Nikolskaia, O., Xu, Y., Ovanesov, M. V., Huang, H., et al. (2008). Inducible expression of mutant human DISC1 in mice is associated with brain and behavioral abnormalities reminiscent of schizophrenia. *Mol. Psychiatry* 13, 173–186, 115. doi: 10.1038/sj.mp.4002079

Puyal, J., Martineau, M., Mothet, J. P., Nicolas, M. T., and Raymond, J. (2006). Changes in D-serine levels and localization during postnatal development of the rat vestibular nuclei. *J. Comp. Neurol.* 497, 610–621. doi: 10.1002/cne.21016

Rimer, M., Barrett, D. W., Maldonado, M. A., Vock, V. M., and Gonzalez-Lima, F. (2005). Neuregulin-1 immunoglobulin-like domain mutant mice: clozapine sensitivity and impaired latent inhibition. *Neuroreport* 16, 271–275. doi: 10.1097/00001756-200502280-00014

Robbins, E. M., Krupp, A. J., Perez de Arce, K., Ghosh, A. K., Fogel, A. I., Boucard, A., et al. (2010). SynCAM 1 adhesion dynamically regulates synapse number and impacts plasticity and learning. *Neuron* 68, 894–906. doi: 10.1016/j.neuron.2010.11.003

Rosenberg, D., Artoul, S., Segal, A. C., Kolodney, G., Radzishevsky, I., Dikopoltsev, E., et al. (2013). Neuronal D-serine and glycine release via the Asc-1 transporter regulates NMDA receptor-dependent synaptic activity. *J. Neurosci.* 33, 3533–3544. doi: 10.1523/JNEUROSCI.3836-12.2013

Rougon, G., and Hobert, O. (2003). New insights into the diversity and function of neuronal immunoglobulin superfamily molecules. *Annu. Rev. Neurosci.* 26, 207–238. doi: 10.1146/annurev.neuro.26.041002.131014

Roy, K., Murtie, J. C., El-Khodor, B. F., Edgar, N., Sardi, S. P., Hooks, B. M., et al. (2007). Loss of erbB signaling in oligodendrocytes alters myelin and dopaminergic function, a potential mechanism for neuropsychiatric disorders. *Proc. Natl. Acad. Sci. U.S.A.* 104, 8131–8136. doi: 10.1073/pnas.0702157104

Sandau, U. S., Alderman, Z., Corfas, G., Ojeda, S. R., and Raber, J. (2012). Astrocyte-specific disruption of SynCAM1 signaling results in ADHD-like behavioral manifestations. *PLoS ONE* 7:e36424. doi: 10.1371/journal.pone.0036424

Sandau, U. S., Mungenast, A. E., McCarthy, J., Biederer, T., Corfas, G., and Ojeda, S. R. (2011). The synaptic cell adhesion molecule, SynCAM1, mediates astrocyte-to-astrocyte and astrocyte-to-GnRH neuron adhesiveness in the mouse hypothalamus. *Endocrinology* 152, 2353–2363. doi: 10.1210/en.2010-1434

Sara, Y., Biederer, T., Atasoy, D., Chubykin, A., Mozhayeva, M. G., Sudhof, T. C., et al. (2005). Selective capability of SynCAM and neuroligin for functional synapse assembly. *J. Neurosci.* 25, 260–270. doi: 10.1523/JNEUROSCI.3165-04.2005

Sawada, M., Kondo, N., Suzumura, A., and Marunouchi, T. (1989). Production of tumor necrosis factor-alpha by microglia and astrocytes in culture. *Brain Res.* 491, 394–397. doi: 10.1016/0006-8993(89)90078-4

Schipper, H. M., Song, W., Zukor, H., Hascalovici, J. R., and Zeligman, D. (2009). Heme oxygenase-1 and neurodegeneration: expanding frontiers of engagement. *J. Neurochem.* 110, 469–485. doi: 10.1111/j.1471-4159.2009.06160.x

Schizophrenia Working Group of the Psychiatric Genomics, C. (2014). Biological insights from 108 schizophrenia-associated genetic loci. *Nature* 511, 421–427. doi: 10.1038/nature13595

Schurov, I. L., Handford, E. J., Brandon, N. J., and Whiting, P. J. (2004). Expression of disrupted in schizophrenia 1 (DISC1) protein in the adult and developing mouse brain indicates its role in neurodevelopment. *Mol. Psychiatry* 9, 1100–1110. doi: 10.1038/sj.mp.4001574

Schwab, M. E. (2004). Nogo and axon regeneration. *Curr. Opin. Neurobiol.* 14, 118–124. doi: 10.1016/j.conb.2004.01.004

Seshadri, S., Kamiya, A., Yokota, Y., Prikulis, I., Kano, S., Hayashi-Takagi, A., et al. (2010). Disrupted-in-Schizophrenia-1 expression is regulated by beta-site amyloid precursor protein cleaving enzyme-1-neuregulin cascade. *Proc. Natl. Acad. Sci. U.S.A.* 107, 5622–5627. doi: 10.1073/pnas.0909284107

Shimizu, S., Koyama, Y., Hattori, T., Tachibana, T., Yoshimi, T., Emoto, H., et al. (2014). DBZ, a CNS-specific DISC1 binding protein, positively regulates oligodendrocyte differentiation. *Glia* 62, 709–724. doi: 10.1002/glia.22636

Shoji, H., Toyama, K., Takamiya, Y., Wakana, S., Gondo, Y., and Miyakawa, T. (2012). Comprehensive behavioral analysis of ENU-induced Disc1-Q31L and -L100P mutant mice. *BMC Res. Notes* 5:108. doi: 10.1186/1756-0500-5-108

Silberberg, G., Darvasi, A., Pinkas-Kramarski, R., and Navon, R. (2006). The involvement of ErbB4 with schizophrenia: association and expression studies. *Am. J. Med. Genet. B Neuropsychiatr. Genet.* 141b, 142–148. doi: 10.1002/ajmg.b.30275

Song, W., Zukor, H., Lin, S. H., Hascalovici, J., Liberman, A., Tavitian, A., et al. (2012). Schizophrenia-like features in transgenic mice overexpressing human HO-1 in the astrocytic compartment. *J. Neurosci.* 32, 10841–10853. doi: 10.1523/JNEUROSCI.6469-11.2012

St Clair, D., Blackwood, D., Muir, W., Carothers, A., Walker, M., Spowart, G., et al. (1990). Association within a family of a balanced autosomal translocation with major mental illness. *Lancet* 336, 13–16. doi: 10.1016/0140-6736(90)91520-K

Strick, C. A., Li, C., Scott, L., Harvey, B., Hajos, M., Steyn, S. J., et al. (2011). Modulation of NMDA receptor function by inhibition of D-amino acid oxidase in rodent brain. *Neuropharmacology* 61, 1001–1015. doi: 10.1016/j.neuropharm.2011.06.029

Suzumura, A., Sawada, M., and Marunouchi, T. (1996). Selective induction of interleukin-6 in mouse microglia by granulocyte-macrophage colony-stimulating factor. *Brain Res.* 713, 192–198. doi: 10.1016/0006-8993(95)01535-3

Takeuchi, H., Mizuno, T., Zhang, G., Wang, J., Kawanokuchi, J., Kuno, R., et al. (2005). Neuritic beading induced by activated microglia is an early feature of neuronal dysfunction toward neuronal death by inhibition of mitochondrial respiration and axonal transport. *J. Biol. Chem.* 280, 10444–10454. doi: 10.1074/jbc.M413863200

Tanaka, H., Ma, J., Tanaka, K. F., Takao, K., Komada, M., Tanda, K., et al. (2009). Mice with altered myelin proteolipid protein gene expression display cognitive deficits accompanied by abnormal neuron-glia interactions and decreased conduction velocities. *J. Neurosci.* 29, 8363–8371. doi: 10.1523/JNEUROSCI.3216-08.2009

Taveggia, C., Zanazzi, G., Petrylak, A., Yano, H., Rosenbluth, J., Einheber, S., et al. (2005). Neuregulin-1 type III determines the ensheathment fate of axons. *Neuron* 47, 681–694. doi: 10 1016/j.neuron.2005.08.017

Tkachev, D., Mimmack, M. L., Ryan, M. M., Wayland, M., Freeman, T., Jones, P. B., et al. (2003). Oligodendrocyte dysfunction in schizophrenia and bipolar disorder. *Lancet* 362, 798–805. doi: 10.1016/S0140-6736(03)14289-4

Tomita, K., Kubo, K., Ishii, K., and Nakajima, K. (2011). Disrupted-in-Schizophrenia-1 (Disc1) is necessary for migration of the pyramidal neurons during mouse hippocampal development. *Hum. Mol. Genet.* 20, 2834–2845. doi: 10.1093/hmg/ddr194

Uranova, N. A., Vikhreva, O. V., Rachmanova, V. I., and Orlovskaya, D. D. (2011). Ultrastructural alterations of myelinated fibers and oligodendrocytes in the prefrontal cortex in schizophrenia: a postmortem morphometric study. *Schizophr. Res. Treatment* 2011:325789. doi: 10.1155/2011/325789

van den Pol, A. N., and Spencer, D. D. (2000). Differential neurite growth on astrocyte substrates: interspecies facilitation in green fluorescent protein-transfected rat and human neurons. *Neuroscience* 95, 603–616. doi: 10.1016/S0306-4522(99)00430-3

Wake, H., Moorhouse, A. J., Jinno, S., Kohsaka, S., and Nabekura, J. (2009). Resting microglia directly monitor the functional state of synapses in vivo and determine the fate of ischemic terminals. *J. Neurosci.* 29, 3974–3980. doi: 10.1523/JNEUROSCI.4363-08.2009

Wang, D. D., and Bordey, A. (2008). The astrocyte odyssey. *Prog. Neurobiol.* 86, 342–367. doi: 10.1016/j.pneurobio.2008.09.015

Wang, X., Chun, S. J., Treloar, H., Vartanian, T., Greer, C. A., and Strittmatter, S. M. (2002). Localization of Nogo-A and Nogo-66 receptor proteins at sites of axon-myelin and synaptic contact. *J. Neurosci.* 22, 5505–5515.

Weinberger, D. R. (1987). Implications of normal brain development for the pathogenesis of schizophrenia. *Arch. Gen. Psychiatry* 44, 660–669. doi: 10.1001/archpsyc.1987.01800190080012

Willi, R., Weinmann, O., Winter, C., Klein, J., Sohr, R., Schnell, L., et al. (2010). Constitutive genetic deletion of the growth regulator Nogo-A induces schizophrenia-related endophenotypes. *J. Neurosci.* 30, 556–567. doi: 10.1523/JNEUROSCI.4393-09.2010

Williams, A. F. (1992). The immunoglobulin superfamily in cell surface recognition. *C. R. Acad. Sci. III* 314, 27–29.

Williams, S. M., Diaz, C. M., Macnab, L. T., Sullivan, R. K., and Pow, D. V. (2006). Immunocytochemical analysis of D-serine distribution in the mammalian brain reveals novel anatomical compartmentalizations in glia and neurons. *Glia* 53, 401–411. doi: 10.1002/glia.20300

Wolosker, H., Blackshaw, S., and Snyder, S. H. (1999a). Serine racemase: a glial enzyme synthesizing D-serine to regulate glutamate-N-methyl-D-aspartate neurotransmission. *Proc. Natl. Acad. Sci. U.S.A.* 96, 13409–13414. doi: 10.1073/pnas.96.23.13409

Wolosker, H., Sheth, K. N., Takahashi, M., Mothet, J. P., Brady, R. O. Jr., et al. (1999b). Purification of serine racemase: biosynthesis of the neuromodulator D-serine. *Proc. Natl. Acad. Sci. U.S.A.* 96, 721–725. doi: 10.1073/pnas.96.2.721

Yiu, G., and He, Z. (2006). Glial inhibition of CNS axon regeneration. *Nat. Rev. Neurosci.* 7, 617–627. doi: 10.1038/nrn1956

Zoghbi, H. Y. (2003). Postnatal neurodevelopmental disorders: meeting at the synapse? *Science* 302, 826–830. doi: 10.1126/science.1089071

19

# Effect of MK-801 and Clozapine on the Proteome of Cultured Human Oligodendrocytes

*Juliana S. Cassoli[1], Keiko Iwata[2], Johann Steiner[3], Paul C. Guest[1], Christoph W. Turck[4]*, Juliana M. Nascimento[1,5] and Daniel Martins-de-Souza[1,6]**

*[1] Laboratory of Neuroproteomics, Department of Biochemistry and Tissue Biology, Institute of Biology, University of Campinas, Campinas, Brazil, [2] United Graduate School of Child Development, Department of Development of Functional Brain Activities, Research Center for Child Mental Development, Hamamatsu University School of Medicine, Osaka University and Kanazawa University and Chiba University and University of Fukui, Fukui, Japan, [3] Department of Psychiatry, University of Magdeburg, Magdeburg, Germany, [4] Department of Translational Research in Psychiatry, Max Planck Institute of Psychiatry, Munich, Germany, [5] D'Or Institute for Research and Education, Rio de Janeiro, Brazil, [6] UNICAMP Neurobiology Center, Campinas, Brazil*

***Correspondence:***
*Daniel Martins-de-Souza*
*dmsouza@unicamp.br;*
*Christoph W. Turck*
*turck@psych.mpg.de*

Separate lines of evidence have demonstrated the involvement of *N*-methyl-D-aspartate (NMDA) receptor and oligodendrocyte dysfunctions in schizophrenia. Here, we have carried out shotgun mass spectrometry proteome analysis of oligodendrocytes treated with the NMDA receptor antagonist MK-801 to gain potential insights into these effects at the molecular level. The MK-801 treatment led to alterations in the levels of 68 proteins, which are associated with seven distinct biological processes. Most of these proteins are involved in energy metabolism and many have been found to be dysregulated in previous proteomic studies of post-mortem brain tissues from schizophrenia patients. Finally, addition of the antipsychotic clozapine to MK-801-treated oligodendrocyte cultures resulted in changes in the levels of 45 proteins and treatment with clozapine alone altered 122 proteins and many of these showed opposite changes to the MK-801 effects. Therefore, these proteins and the associated energy metabolism pathways should be explored as potential biomarkers of antipsychotic efficacy. In conclusion, MK-801 treatment of oligodendrocytes may provide a useful model for testing the efficacy of novel treatment approaches.

**Keywords: glial cells, oligodendrocyte, proteomics, schizophrenia, pharmacology, clozapine, MK801**

## INTRODUCTION

The *N*-methyl-D-aspartate receptor (NMDAr) is an ionotropic receptor activated by glutamate, allowing the non-selective influx of calcium and sodium and outflow of potassium. The function of NMDAr in neurons is well-described as it participates actively on glutamatergic transmission, which is known to be defective in schizophrenia and related psychiatric disorders.

Schizophrenia presents with a variety of both positive and negative symptoms (Lewis, 2000). There are also disturbances in cognitive processes, such as attention and working memory, which can appear prior to the onset of the clinical condition. These cognitive problems represent core features of the illness and are associated to NMDAr dysfunction (Hahn et al., 2006). NMDAr antagonists exacerbate pre-existing symptoms in patients with schizophrenia and may drive schizophrenia-like symptoms in healthy mice and human volunteers (Gunduz-Bruce, 2009).

Moreover, these antagonists have been found to trigger sensory and motor disturbances in rats, similar to those displayed by patients with schizophrenia (Kovacic and Somanathan, 2010). At the cellular level, treatment with NMDAr antagonists have been shown to cause neuronal degeneration in retrosplenial, pyriform, and entorhinal cortices, as well as the *tenia tecti amygdalae* (Horváth et al., 1997).

While NMDAr function has been well-described in neurons, its function in glial cells such as astrocytes and oligodendrocytes still needs clarification despite intensive investigation over the past 10 years (Salter and Fern, 2005; Cao and Yao, 2013). This is likely to provide further insights into the pathways affected in schizophrenia, given the role of oligodendrocytes in the establishment and course of the disease (Cassoli et al., 2015). Cultured oligodendrocytes present glutamate-responsiveness to NMDAr, and may even release glutamate in certain conditions (Deng et al., 2003). This enables the study of the molecular mechanisms of oligodendrocytes *in vitro*.

One way of modulating NMDAr function in experimental settings is by employing pharmacological interventions. MK-801 (or [5R,10S]-[+]-5-methyl-10,11-dihydro-5*H*-dibenzo[*a,d*]cyclo hepten-5,10-imine or Dizocilpine) is a compound that belongs to the secondary bicyclic amine class and acts as non-competitive NMDAr antagonist, not only in neurons, but also in oligodendrocytes (Li et al., 2013). This compound binds to two sites on the NMDAr-ion channel complex in a manner similar to phencyclidine (PCP; Kornhuber et al., 1989) *in vivo* and *in vitro* (Murray et al., 2000). The NMDAr mediates glutamatergic transmission and plays a key role in neural plasticity of central nervous system (CNS; Harrison and Weinberger, 2004).

Besides the neuroprotective effects observed in stroke, trauma, Parkinson and organophosphate-induced seizure models, MK-801 also induces schizophrenia-like symptoms (Kovacic and Somanathan, 2010) such as alterations in prepulse inhibition (PPI; Zangrando et al., 2013). This has led researchers to employ MK-801 as a pharmacological model of schizophrenia (Paulson et al., 2007) for testing effects of antipsychotics such as clozapine (Paulson et al., 2007; Zuo et al., 2009; Vardigan et al., 2010; Brown et al., 2014).

Previous studies have shown that the NMDAr is also present in oligodendrocytes (Simon et al., 1984; Karadottir et al., 2005; Salter and Fern, 2005; Micu et al., 2006) and may be involved in regulation of myelination processes (Li et al., 2013). NMDA receptor signaling in oligodendrocytes also plays a crucial role in their energy metabolism and regulates differentiation and migration of these cells (for review see (Cao and Yao, 2013). Here, we have carried out a quantitative proteomic analysis to analyze protein expression changes in the human oligodendrocyte hybrid cell line (MO3.13) following treatment with MK-801 or the antipsychotic clozapine compared to control cells. The main objective was to shed light on the biochemical mechanisms involving NMDAr function in oligodendrocytes in order to determine whether these cells could be useful in future studies to model some aspects of schizophrenia.

# EXPERIMENTAL PROCEDURES

## Cell Cultures, Treatments, and Proteome Extraction

MO3.13 cells were maintained in DMEM medium supplemented with 2 mM L-glutamine, 1% penicillin/streptomicyn (Sigma-Aldrich, St. Louis, MO, USA) and 10% heat-inactivated fetal bovine serum (Life Technologies, Darmstadt, Germany), at 37°C in humidified atmosphere containing 5% $CO_2$, as described previously (Iwata et al., 2013). Cells were treated once and collected after 8 h as follows: Group 1 – 50 mM MK-801; Group 2 – 50 mM MK-801 plus 50 mM clozapine after 4 h; Group 3 – 50 mM clozapine; Group 4 – vehicle solution (0.01 M HCl; **Figure 1**). The glycine (0.4 mM) and glutamate (20 uM) contained in DMEM and FBS respectively are sufficiently high to activate NMDA receptors (Blanke and VanDongen, 2009; Cummings and Popescu, 2015).

MO3.13 cells were centrifuged at 1,000 *g* for 3 min and the pellets homogenized in 50 μL of 7 M urea, 2 M thiourea, 4% CHAPS, 2% ASB-14, and 70 mM DTT using a sample grinding kit (GE Healthcare, Uppsala, Sweden; Martins-de-Souza et al., 2007). Protein lysates were centrifuged for 10 min at 13,800 *g*, the supernatants collected and protein concentrations determined by Bradford assay (Bio-Rad, Munich, Germany).

## ICPL (Isotope-Coded Protein Labeling) Labeling

Cell lysate proteins were labeled with ICPL reagent from SERVA ICPL™ Quadruplex Kit (SERVA Electrophoresis, Heidelberg, Germany), as previously described (Maccarrone et al., 2014). Equal amounts of light and heavy labeled samples were combined and separated by 12% SDS gel electrophoresis before brilliant Coomassie staining. After staining, each gel lane was sliced in 10 pieces and the protein bands were digested in-gel using a 1:80 ratio of trypsin:ammonium bicarbonate. The resulting peptides were dried and stored at −80°C prior to shotgun mass spectrometry analyses.

## NanoLC-ESI MS/MS, Data Processing and Database Searching

Extracted peptides were dissolved in 0.1% formic acid aqueous solution and analyzed using a 2D-nano-LC system (Eksigent, Dublin, CA, USA) coupled online to an LTQ-Orbitrap XL mass spectrometer (Thermo Scientific, Bremen, Germany), as previously described (Maccarrone et al., 2013). The MS/MS fragmentation spectra were acquired in data dependent mode, and the five most intense signal ions (m/z) in each scan were selected for fragmentation. Nanoflow LC–MS/MS was performed in automatic mode via Xcalibur software (version 2.0.7, Thermo Scientific, San José, CA, USA). Each gel slice generated one MS raw data file, which was processed for generation of the.mgf file. The target and decoy (reverse sequence) databases were searched using the UniProt human protein database (release 2013 08, 20,266 sequences) through the Mascot server. The search parameters were (1) peptide and fragment ion mass accuracy 10 ppm and 0.5 Da, respectively, (2) protein and peptide FDRs

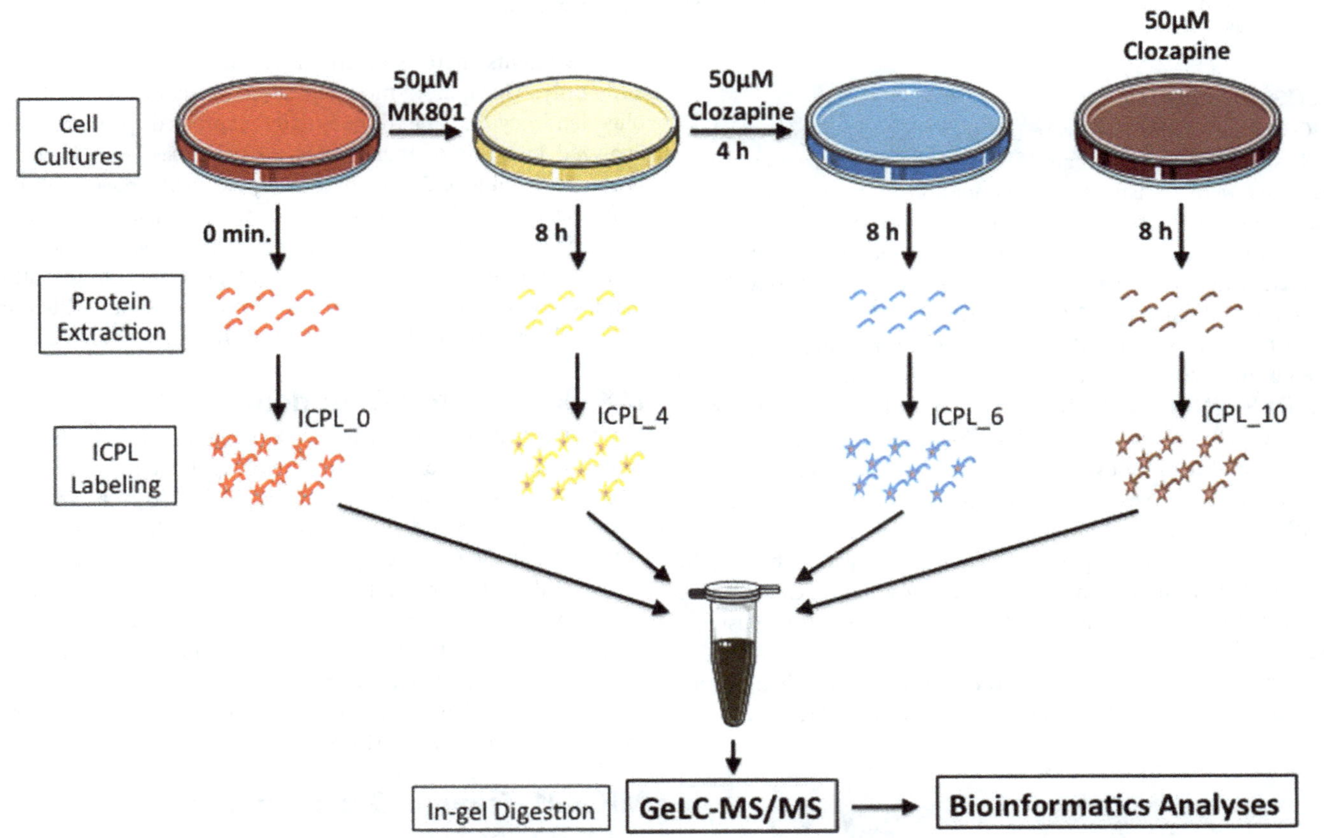


**FIGURE 1 | Experimental setup.** Briefly, MO3.13 cells were grown in the presence of MK-801 or clozapine or MK-801/clozapine. Proteins were extracted, labeled with ICPL and mixed with the same peptide amount. To reduce the proteome complexity, the samples were prior fractionated by SDS-PAGE, and protein bands were digested by trypsin at room temperature. In last step, the proteins from each gel slice were then subjected to LC-MS/MS analyses.

1%, (3) two missed cleavages, (4) trypsin as enzyme, (5) fixed modification = cysteine carbamidomethylation and variable modification = methionine oxidation and ICPL labeling.

## Proteome Quantification

Identified proteins had to fit the following criteria in all analyzed datasets to be considered for quantification as described previously (Maccarrone et al., 2014): (1) identification by at least 2 non-redundant peptides; (2) fold changes not greater than ±15; and (3) the standard deviation of quantified peptides not greater than 10. Determination of isotope-labeled peptide ratios was performed with MASCOT Distiller (Matrix Sciences). The software calculates the fold-changes of each identified peptide, considering the signal intensities of the same peptide across different samples. The fold changes of all peptides of a given protein were averaged, thereby determining the protein fold change. Based on our previous results (Maccarrone et al., 2014), we only considered proteins differentially expressed if they presented a fold-change greater than ±1.5 and proteins with fold changes between 1.5 and 2 were only considered if quantified by at least 5 peptides. In addition, all quantitated proteins were required to have a normal distribution at the peptide level, as determined by the Shapiro–Wilk *W*-test so an analysis of variance (ANOVA) could be employed to determine differentially expressed proteins. Only those with *p*-values lower than 0.05 were considered further.

## Pathway and Functional Correlation Analysis

The Uniprot accession codes of differentially expressed proteins were mapped to Gene Ontology (GO) categories (biological function and molecular process), using a script linked to the Human Protein Reference Database[1]. The same codes were also uploaded into the QIAGEN Ingenuity® Pathway Analysis software (IPA®, QIAGEN, Redwood City, CA, USA[2]), to the associated over-represented biological pathways and functions. IPA core analysis was performed using experimentally observed data from human and CNS cell lines, with canonical pathways, diseases and biological functions, and networks explored in detail. The refinement of the network generated by IPA was performed applying the following parameters: (1) direct/indirect interactions, (2) experimentally observed as confidence level,

[1]http://www.hprd.org/

[2]www.qiagen.com/ingenuity

(3) human as species, (4) tissues/cell lines, and (5) disease related to the CNS.

## Western Blot

MO3.13 protein lysates were (20 μg) were electrophoresed on 12% sodium dodecyl sulfate (SDS) minigels prepared in house. Proteins were transferred to Immobilon-FL polyvinyldiphenyl fluoride (PVDF) membranes (Millipore; Bedford, MA, USA) at 100 V for 1 h using a cooling system. PVDF membranes were then treated with 5% Carnation instant non-fat dry milk powder in Tris buffered saline (pH 7.4) containing 0.1% Tween -20 (TBS-T) for 4 h and rinsed in TBS-T three times for a total of 20 min. Membranes were incubated with Anti-Glutamate Receptor NMDAR1 (NR1) antibody produced in rabbit at a dilution of 1:000 in TBS-T overnight at 4°C (Sigma-Aldrich; Taufkirchen, Germany). Membranes were then washed twice with TBS-T for 15 min per wash. Next, the membranes were incubated with anti-c-MYC-peroxidase antibody (GE Healthcare; Uppsala, Sweden) for 40 min at room temperature, washed with water and TBS-T, and incubated with enhanced chemiluminescence (ECL) solution (GE Healthcare) for 1 min. The membranes were scanned using a Gel Doc™ XR+ System (Silk Scientific Incorporated; Orem, UT, USA) and the optical densities of the immunoreactive bands were measured using Quantity One software (Bio-Rad; **Figure 2**).

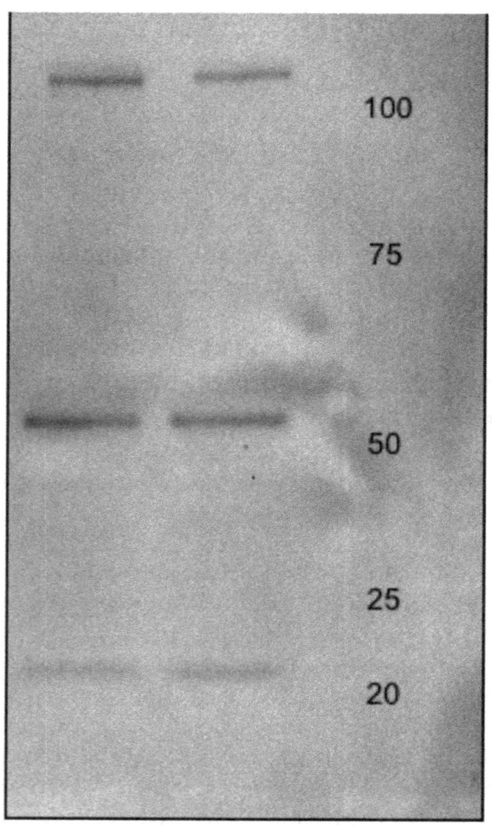


**FIGURE 2 | *N*-methyl-D-aspartate (NMDA) receptor Western Blot in MO3.13 protein lysates.**

## RESULTS

All treatments here studied (MK-801, MK-801+Clozapine and only clozapine) modified the proteome of cultured oligodendrocytes. The differentially expressed proteins were analyzed in terms of their biological processes, and the result is shown in **Figure 3**. All three analyzed proteomes presented differences in similar biological processes. For instance, proteins associated to protein metabolism were the most prevalent on all three different treatments in percentage terms. On the other hand, there are proteins and functional correlations, which are specifically modulated by each different treatment analyzed.

### MK-801-Treated Oligodendrocytes

MK-801 treatment for 8 h induced changes in the levels of 68 proteins in cultured oligodendrocytes (Supplementary Table S1). These proteins are mostly associated with energy metabolism functions and included aldolase A (ALDOA), aldolase C (ALDOC), malate dehydrogenase (MDH2), and transketolase (TKT; **Table 1**). In addition, proteins such as prohibitin (PHB) and annexin 5 (ANXA5), which are associated with communication and cell signaling, and the protein metabolism-related proteins nucleophosmin (NPM1), 40S ribosomal protein S16 (RPS16) and 60S ribosomal protein L7A (RPL7A), were specifically altered by the MK-801 treatment.

### MK-801-Treated Oligodendrocytes with Added Clozapine

The addition of clozapine after 4 h to the MK-801-treated cells affected the expression levels of 45 proteins, involved in six different biological processes. Most of these proteins are associated with energy metabolism, oxidative stress, and protein metabolism, and included changes in ALDOA, peroxiredoxin-6 (PRDX6), NPM1 and RPS16. In addition, profilin-1 (PFN1), a protein associated with cell growth and maintenance, showed the highest fold change of the proteins in this group (Supplementary Table S2).

### Clozapine-Treated Oligodendrocytes

Treatment with clozapine alone induced alterations in the levels of 122 proteins in cultured oligodendrocytes. Clozapine treatment mostly induced changes in proteins associated with regulation of nucleic acid metabolism, such as histone H2B (HIST1H2BJ), polyadenylate binding protein (PABPC1), and ribonucleoprotein (SNRPA1). In addition, ribosomal proteins as L32 (RPL32) and L8 (RPL8) were also affected (Supplementary Table S3). These effects are likely to represent early changes in the transcriptional and translational machinery as part of the clozapine response in oligodendrocyte cells.

### *In silico* Systems Biology

*In silico* analysis was performed using IPA, inputting the accession codes of the differentially proteins modulated in each treatment group. The results are shown in **Figure 4**. Essentially, the obtained proteomes were associated with some canonical pathways, biofunctions, disorders, and toxicities.

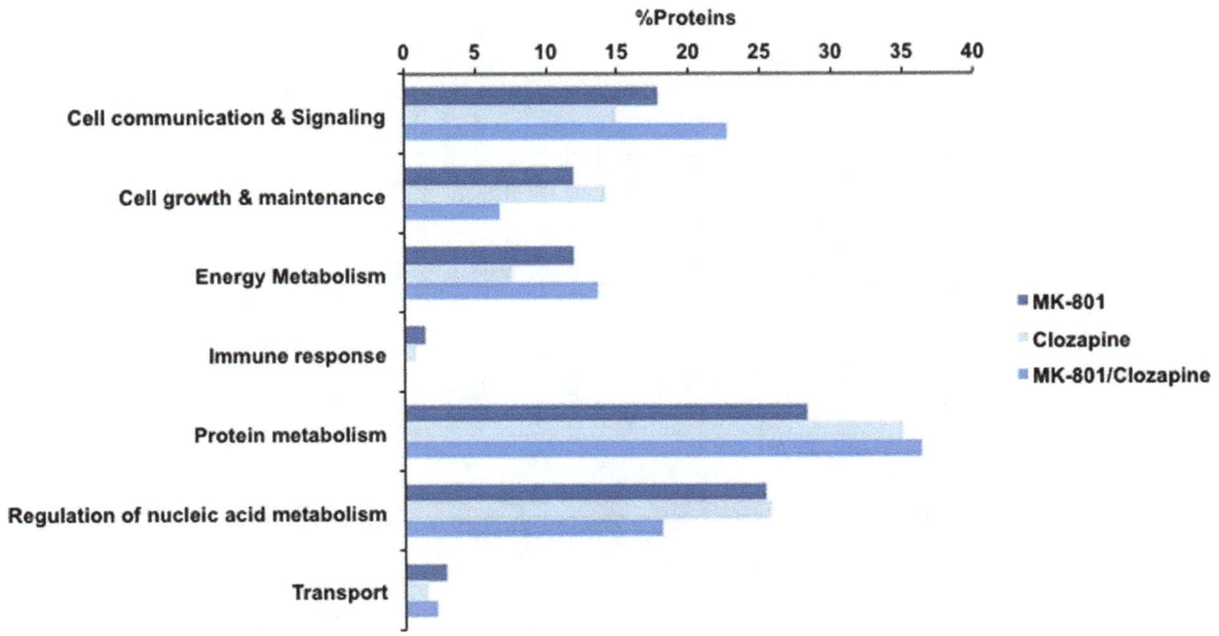


**FIGURE 3 | Biological processes involving the proteins identified with MK-801, Clozapine, and concomitant (MK-801 and Clozapine) treatment.** Bars in dark blue, blue, and light blue depict MK-801, Clozapine and MK-801/Clozapine treatments, respectively.

Among the canonical pathways, proteins altered in the MK-801-treated cells were related to cell signaling pathways mediated by 14-3-3 protein kinase, p70S6K and by the factor eIF2 at approximately equal levels. In contrast, the proteins altered by clozapine treatment showed a marked relationship to eIF2 signaling, followed by 14-3-3-mediated and p7056k signaling. The proteome changes in MK-801-treated oligodendrocytes with the addition of clozapine showed effects similar to the MK-801 treatment alone with additional changes in proteins involved in carbohydrate metabolism pathways (**Figure 4A**).

The MK-801 treatment resulted in similar values for all groups in the area of biofunctions and disorders, except for neurological disorder group, which showed the highest score. However, the altered proteins in the clozapine-treated cells were linked with neurological disease as well as psychological, and skeletal and muscular disorders (**Figure 4B**).

Toxicity pathways generated by the analysis were associated mainly with NRF2 oxidative stress and cell cycle G2/M DNA damage responses in the clozapine treatment group (**Figure 4C**). Furthermore, the proteome changes associated with the MK-801 treatment were mainly linked to reduction of mitochondrial membrane permeability, oxidative stress, and cell cycle G2/M DNA damage responses.

The list of altered proteins from the MK-801 treatment was also analyzed in terms of protein networks generated by the IPA software. This analysis can identify binding or interacting proteins which have not been detected by the proteomic approach (**Figure 5**). Hypoxia-inducing factor 1-α (HIF1-α), endothelial PAS domain-containing protein 1 (EPAS1), and MYC-proto-oncogene protein (MYCN), were the most associated transcription factors. In addition, proteins involved in energy metabolism, kinases, and heat shock proteins (HSPs) were the highly represented in the network generated (**Figure 5**).

## DISCUSSION

One of major challenges in neuropsychiatric research is the relatively limited knowledge of the molecular mechanisms of these diseases. The development of new preclinical models to improve such knowledge is also challenging for the same reasons. Biological assays using animals or cellular cultures as models are still emerging, with the aim to provide more information about the acute effects caused by administration of neuromodulators such as MK-801 and antipsychotic drugs (Paulson et al., 2004, 2007; Ji et al., 2009a,b; Ma et al., 2009; Martins-de-Souza et al., 2011b; Ahmed et al., 2012; Palmowski et al., 2014). Considering the known effects of oligodendrocyte dysfunction in schizophrenia, we have investigated the acute response of oligodendrocytic cells to the NMDA receptor antagonist MK-801 and clozapine treatment by identification of protein abundance changes using quantitative mass-spectrometry based proteomics. Analysis of quantitative data allowed the identification of proteins linked to a series of cellular processes and functions affected by MK-801 and showed how clozapine may block the effects of MK-801 in oligodendrocytic cells.

### Biological Process

Taken together, the different treatment groups resulted in changes in the levels of more than 200 proteins. Further studies are warranted to determine whether or not those proteins modulated by the MK-801 treatment are linked in any way

**TABLE 1 | Comparison of proteomic changes in oligodendrocytes (MO3.13 cells) after the indicated drug treatments.**

| Symbol | Description | Fold change CtrlxMK-801 | Fold change CtrlxCloz | Fold change CtrlxMK-801/Cloz | Location | Biological process |
|---|---|---|---|---|---|---|
| AKAP10 | A kinase (PRKA) anchor protein 10 | 1.77 | > −5 | > −5 | Cytoplasm | Cell communication and signaling |
| GDI2 | Rab GDP dissociation inhibitor beta | >5 | −4.76 | >5 | Cytoplasm | Cell communication and signaling |
| PHB | Prohibitin | >5 | 1.56 | >5 | Nucleus | Cell communication and signaling |
| LMNB1 | Lamin B1 | 2.65 | −4.35 | 1.71 | Nucleus | Cell growth and maintenance |
| ALDOC | Aldolase C. fructose-bisphosphate | >5 | −3.45 | 2.24 | Cytoplasm | Energy metabolism |
| PRDX6 | Peroxiredoxin 6 | 3.53 | 3.78 | >5 | Cytoplasm | Energy metabolism |
| CCT7 | Chaperonin containing TCP1. Subunit 7 (eta) | 2.28 | 3.96 | 1.58 | Cytoplasm | Protein metabolism |
| DNAJB11 | DnaJ (Hsp40) homolog. Subfamily B. Member 11 | −4.17 | −2.50 | −3.33 | Cytoplasm | Protein metabolism |
| EEF2 | Eukaryotic translation elongation factor 2 | >5 | > −5 | >5 | Cytoplasm | Protein metabolism |
| NPM1 | Nucleophosmin (nucleolar phosphoprotein B23. numatrin) | >5 | −3.03 | >5 | Nucleus | Protein metabolism |
| PDIA3 | Protein disulfide isomerase family A. member 3 | 3.00 | −4.54 | −3.45 | Cytoplasm | Protein metabolism |
| RPL17 | Ribosomal protein L17 | −3.03 | −3.85 | −2.13 | Cytoplasm | Protein metabolism |
| RPS16 | Ribosomal protein S16 | >5 | 3.59 | >5 | Cytoplasm | Protein metabolism |
| ANP32B | Acidic leucine-rich nuclear phosphoprotein 32 family member B | −2.22 | −2.86 | −2.13 | Nucleus | Regulation of nucleic acid metabolism |
| RALY | RNA-binding protein Raly | >5 | −2.44 | >5 | Nucleus | Regulation of nucleic acid metabolism |
| RBMX | RNA-binding motif protein, X chromosome | −2.63 | 2.41 | −2.222 | Nucleus | Regulation of nucleic acid metabolism |

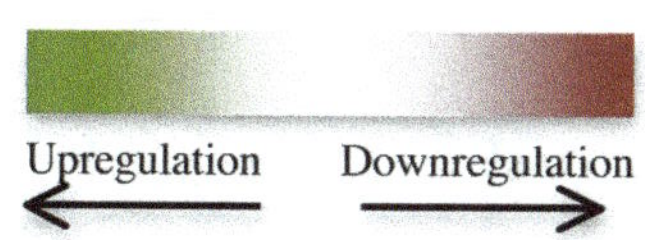

to schizophrenia. This would help to establish the validity of MK-801-treated oligodendrocytes as a potential model of some aspects of schizophrenia. On the other hand, some of the proteins modulated by the clozapine treatment may be biomarkers of drug response and some could provide links to novel therapeutic targets. The combined 200 proteins were mainly associated to "cell communication and signaling," "energy metabolism," "cell growth and maintenance," "protein metabolism," and "regulation of nucleic acid metabolism" in terms of biological processes (**Figure 3**). Several of these proteins have also been reported to be differentially expressed in brain tissue samples of schizophrenia patients (Nascimento and Martins-de-Souza, 2015) and in animals treated with such drugs (Paulson et al., 2004, 2007; Ji et al., 2009a,b; Ma et al., 2009; Palmowski et al., 2014). Similarly, a previous proteomic analysis was performed to understand the effects of MK-801 on cultured astrocytes (Martins-de-Souza et al., 2011b).

In the present study, proteins associated to energy metabolism were mostly upregulated in the MK-801 treated oligodendrocyte cell line (Supplementary Table S2). This effect is consistent with a number of studies which have used NMDAr antagonist treatment to investigate its effects on neuronal cell cultures (Guest et al., 2015) and rat brains (Paulson et al., 2004, 2007; Zhou et al., 2012). Similar effects have been also been reported in proteomic and transcriptomic studies using post-mortem samples from schizophrenia patients (Martins-de-Souza, 2010; Martins-de-Souza et al., 2011a; Cassoli et al., 2015). Taken together, these findings suggest that dysfunctions of NMDA activity can cause disruptions in energy metabolism pathways and vice-versa. However, further studies are necessary to extrapolate these findings to schizophrenia pathophysiology.

Effects of clozapine on cell cultures have already been reported. This drug induced oxidation of proteins involved in energy metabolism in SKNSH neuroblastoma cells, seen as effects on mitochondrial ribosomal protein S22 (MRPS22), mitochondrial malate dehydrogenase (MDH), calumenin (CALU), pyruvate kinase (PK1), and 3-oxoacid CoA transferase (OXCT1; Walss-Bass et al., 2008). Likewise, this antipsychotic provoked an increased oxidation of specific proteins, such as enolase (ENO), triosephosphate isomerase (TPI), glyceraldehyde-3-phosphate dehydrogenase (GAPD), Rho GDP dissociation inhibitor (GDI), cofilin (CFL), uridine monophosphate/cytidine monophosphate (UMP-CMP) kinase, and translation elongation factor, in lymphoblastoid cells obtained from patients with schizophrenia compared to those from healthy subjects (Baig et al., 2010). In this study, we also found that clozapine influenced the expression levels of proteins from the same biological processes in oligodendrocyte cells.

## Effects of Clozapine on MK-801-Treated Cells

Treatment with clozapine appeared to reverse some of the proteome changes caused by the MK-801 treatment, suggesting that such proteins might be associated with the medication response. Additionally, 16 proteins were affected in a similar manner in all three treatment groups (**Table 1**; **Figure 6**). Some

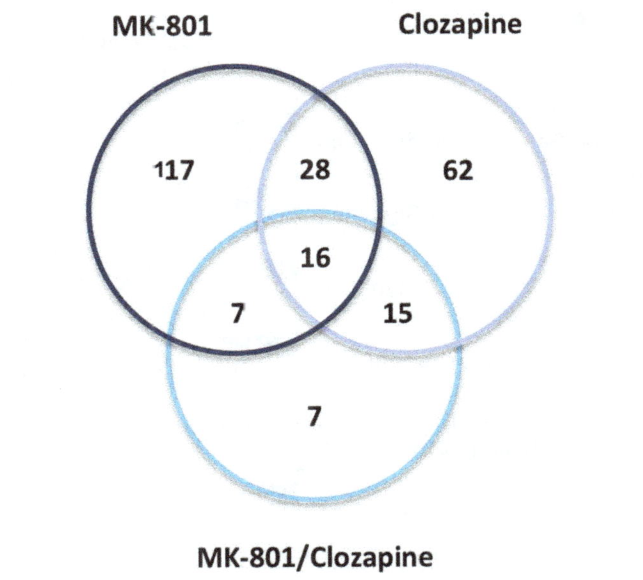


**FIGURE 6 | Venn diagram.** Protein overlap between the three drug treatments (MK-801, Clozapine, and MK-801, and Clozapine) applied to the characterization of oligodendrocyte proteomes.

of these proteins showed opposite directional changes depending on whether cells were treated with MK-801, clozapine or both. This suggests that these proteins may be involved in both the pathophysiology and the medication response. Such proteins included the AKAP10, ALDOC, protein disulfide isomerase family A member 3 (PDIA3), PHB, Rab GDP dissociation inhibitor beta (GDI2), and PRDX6 (**Table 1**), which are discussed below.

AKAP10 levels were increased by the MK-801 treatment and decreased by clozapine. The AKAP family of scaffold proteins are a diverse group of functionally related proteins that anchor the cAMP-dependent protein kinase (PKA) as well as other signaling proteins to coordinate signal transduction in different subcellular locations (Sanderson and Dell'Acqua, 2011). They have also been associated with synaptic plasticity, which is induced by activation of NMDA-type glutamate receptors. This suggests that clozapine may act on processes related to synaptic plasticity via effects on AKAP10. Moreover, this protein has been found to be differentially expressed in samples of corpus callosum from schizophrenia patients (Saia-Cereda et al., 2015).

Aldolase C has been previously reported to be upregulated in the frontal cortex (FC), insulate cortex (IC) and dorsolateral prefrontal cortex (DLPFC) and downregulated in the prefrontal cortex (PFC), Wernicke's area (WA), anterior temporal lobe (ATL) and anterior cingulate cortex (ACC) of schizophrenia patients compared to controls (Martins-de-Souza et al., 2011a). ALDOC is a glycolytic enzyme that catalyzes the reversible aldol cleavage of fructose-1,6-biphosphate and fructose 1-phosphate to produce dihydroxyacetone phosphate and either glyceraldehyde-3-phosphate or glyceraldehyde, respectively. In the present study, we found that the clozapine co-treatment resulted in a lowering of ALDOC levels in relation to increased levels induced by the

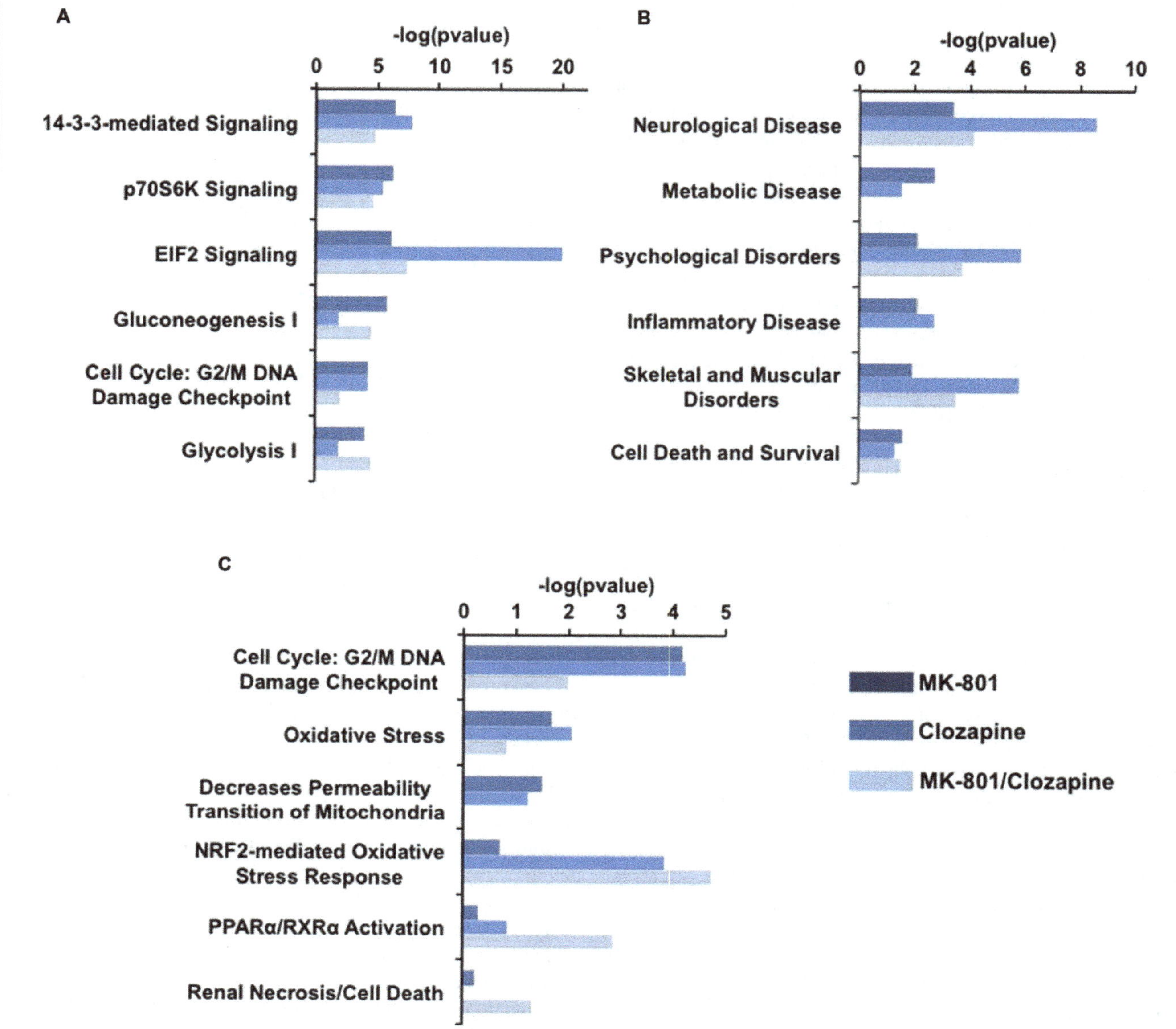


**FIGURE 4 | IPA analysis of proteomic data arisen each drug treatment. (A)** Canonical pathways, **(B)** related disorders and Biofunctions, and **(C)** toxicity pathways generated from IPA analysis. Bars in dark blue, blue, and light blue depict MK-801, Clozapine and MK-801/Clozapine treatments, respectively.

MK-801 treatment. Disturbances in ALDOC expression, and expression of the ALDOA isoform have also been reported by studies involving MK-801-treated animals and astrocyte cultures (Paulson et al., 2004; Martins-de-Souza et al., 2011b).

Clozapine treatment resulted in increased levels of PDIA3, a protein belonging to a family of enzymes that introduces disulfide bonds into proteins and catalyzes rearrangement of incorrect disulfide bonds (Wilkinson and Gilbert, 2004). Distinct from the present result, protein previous study showed that PDIA3 was downregulated after treatment of astrocytes with MK-801 (Martins-de-Souza et al., 2011b). This suggests that MK-801 and clozapine may have opposite effects on PDIA3 levels in oligodendrocytes and astrocytes. The MK-801 treatment promoted an upregulation of PHB in oligodendrocytes, which was similarly upregulated in the DLPFC and ACC, and decreased in the PFC of schizophrenia patient brain samples (Smalla et al., 2008; Martins-de-Souza et al., 2010). PHB is a multifunctional protein which acts as a chaperone for respiration chain proteins, a general structuring scaffold in mitochondrial morphology, and it is involved in cell proliferation and transcriptional modulation (Zhou and Qin, 2013; Peng et al., 2015). Rats treated with ketamine – another NMDAr antagonist – have also shown PHB upregulation in post-synaptic density preparations of DLPFC from chronic schizophrenia patients (Smalla et al., 2008). Oligodendrocytes isolated from the DLPFC have also been found to have increased levels of PHB (Bernstein et al., 2012). Likewise, a recent proteomic study showed PHB upregulation in the peripheral blood serum and brain tissue from rats acutely

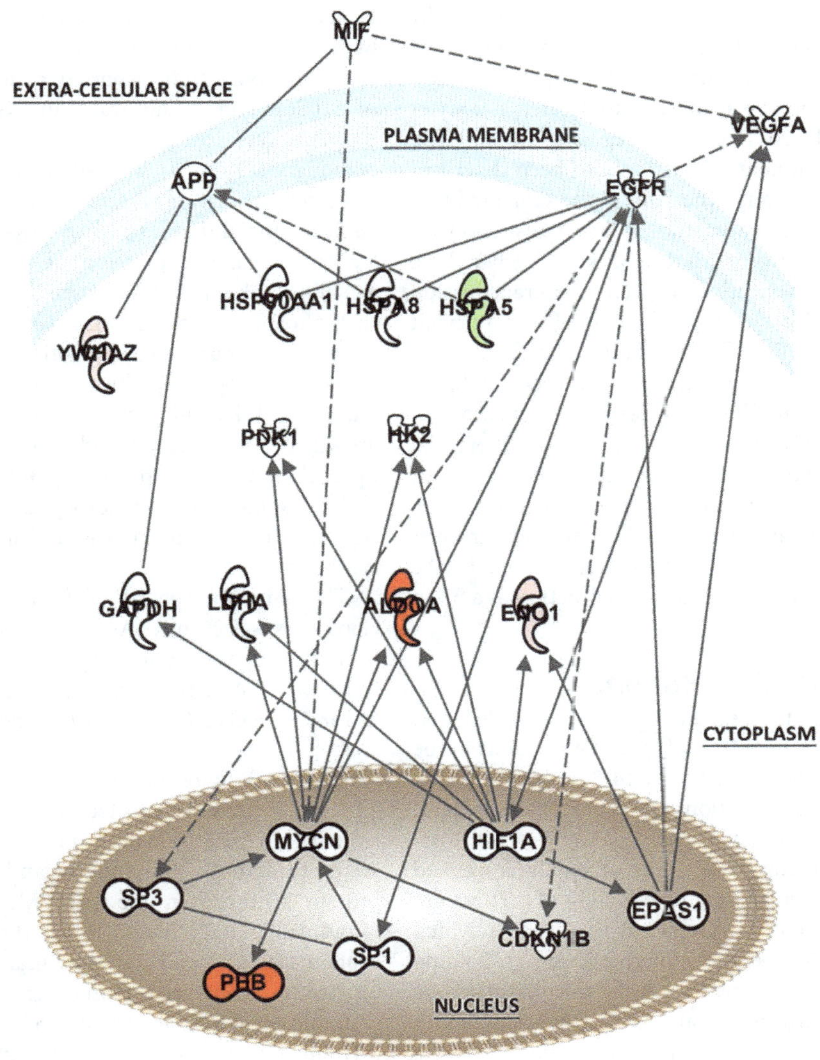


**FIGURE 5 | Potential network interactions, and their interactors, of differentially expressed proteins of MK-801-treated oligodendrocytes.** The network was generated from differentially expressed proteins by IPA (see "Pathway and Functional Correlation Analysis"). Colored interactors represent proteins previous found in the proteome. Full and dashed lines depict direct and indirect connections respectively.

treated with ketamine (Wesseling et al., 2015). Taken together, these findings indicate a relationship of PHB increased expression and hypofunction of NMDA receptor signaling.

Although, the Rab GDP dissociation inhibitor beta (GDI2) has not been found to be altered in schizophrenia proteomic studies, the Rab GDP dissociation inhibitor alpha (GDI1) isoform was previously found to be upregulated in samples of ACC and DLPFC of schizophrenia patients (English et al., 2009; Martins-de-Souza et al., 2010). The Rab proteins belong to the GDP dissociation inhibitor protein family, which regulates the GDP-GTP exchange reaction of members of small GTP-binding proteins. They are mainly involved in vesicular trafficking of molecules between cellular organelles (Shisheva et al., 1994). In our results, GDI2 was oppositely regulated by MK-801 and clozapine. However, addition of the antipsychotic to the MK-801-treated cultures was not sufficient to completely block GDI2 upregulation.

Another protein modulated by both MK-801 and clozapine in oligodendrocytes was peroxiredoxin 6 (PRDX6). The peroxiredoxins are a family of antioxidant enzymes that are ubiquitously distributed in the cell and can control cytokine-induced peroxide levels, which mediate signal transduction in mammalian cells. High abundance of peroxiredoxins in mammalian cells appears to protect the cellular components by removing accumulated peroxides produced as a result of normal cellular metabolism or as a response to oxidative stress (Rhee et al., 2005). In our study, PRDX6 was found to be upregulated by MK-801 and the clozapine single treatments. Interestingly, this effect was enhanced by the co-treatment resulting in markedly higher levels of this protein. PRDX6 has also been found to be altered in DLPFC and WA from schizophrenia patients (Martins-de-Souza et al., 2009a,b) as well as in MK-801-treated astrocytes (Martins-de-Souza et al., 2011b). An upregulation of PRDX6 following haloperidol treatment in rats has also been described (Andreazza et al., 2015), although the same study suggested that clozapine may also induce oxidative stress in liver, consistent with the documented adverse effects of this drug. Taken together, these findings show a potential connection between neurotransmission dysfunctions and oxidative damage, which might be relevant to disease pathogenesis (Ben-Shachar and Laifenfeld, 2004; Rajasekaran et al., 2015). Furthermore, the phospholipase A2 (PLA2) activity of PRDX6 is critical for regulation of phospholipid turnover (Chen et al., 2000) and differential regulation of PRDX6 may accelerate phospholipid turnover. Both of these PRDX6 activities may be related to schizophrenia pathogenesis since an enhancement of phospholipid turnover has been previously reported in schizophrenia frontal lobe (Gattaz et al., 1990). Therefore, PRDX6 could function as a brain marker for schizophrenia.

## *In silico* Functional Correlations

Functional correlation of the regulated proteins revealed that MK-801 and clozapine treatment could lead to alterations in the canonical signaling pathways mediated by 14-3-3 protein kinase, p70S6K and eIF2 factor. In addition, changes in carbohydrate metabolism pathways were also detected.

The 14-3-3 proteins compose a family of highly conserved acidic proteins, with molecular weights of 25–30 kD. There are seven mammalian 14-3-3 isoforms in eukaryotic cells which function as adaptor or "chaperone molecules" and scaffolding proteins that can translocate freely from the cytoplasm to the nucleus and vise-versa (Muslin et al., 1996). They are found as homo- or heterodimers and interact with cellular proteins representing a wide range of processes, such as neuronal development, mitogenic signal transduction, apoptotic cell death, cell cycle and cell growth controls (Mhawech, 2005). Several reports have shown disturbances in the expression of this protein family in schizophrenia brain tissue (Hayakawa et al., 1998; Wong et al., 2003; Middleton et al., 2005; Martins-de-Souza et al., 2012; Saia-Cereda et al., 2015; Schubert et al., 2015). Moreover, schizophrenia-related behavioral phenotypes have been described in 14-3-3 functional knockout mice (Cheah et al., 2012; Foote et al., 2015). Here, MK-801 and clozapine treatments resulted in increased levels of 14-3-3 proteins. Interestingly, when clozapine was administered to MK-801-treated cells, the levels of 14-3-3 protein theta (14-3-3ς) decreased and signaling mediated by the 14-3-3 family appeared to be abolished. Other studies have described changes in this protein family in the PFC of subjects with schizophrenia as a normalizing effect of antipsychotics, such as clozapine (Rivero et al., 2015). Furthermore, clozapine has been used to rescue the locomotor hyperactivity of 14-3-3ς knockout mice, which may indicate a novel role for 14-3-3ς in dopaminergic neurotransmission (Ramshaw et al., 2013). Considering these findings, further studies should be performed to determine whether or not dysregulation of 14-3-3 expression in oligodendrocytes is involved in schizophrenia, as suggested in by some post-mortem studies.

A previous study reported a decrease in phosphorylation of p70S6K and its substrates in frontal cortices of 7-days-old rats that were acutely treated with MK-801 (Yoon et al., 2008). Although, MK-801 is an NMDAr antagonist, the present results indicated that it may also antagonize p70S6K signaling. In contrast, the clozapine and co-MK-801/clozapine co-treatment led to increased expression of proteins involved in p70S6K signaling. The p70S6K protein is a serine/threonine kinase that phosphorylates the ribosomal S6 subunit, a component of the 40S subunit of eukaryotic ribosomes. It is activated by mTOR in mitogenic pathways downstream of phosphoinositide 3 kinase (PI3K) and plays a role in protein synthesis and in cell growth control (Fenton and Gout, 2011). Thus, the observed upregulation of the p70S6K pathway promoted by MK-801 and clozapine in oligodendrocytes might represent an adaptive response resulting in increased translation initiation in protein synthesis.

The initiation phase of protein synthesis, during which ribosomes select mRNAs to be translated, and identify the translational start site, requires a set of EIFs (eukaryotic translation initiation factors). EIF2 (eukaryotic initiation factor-2) is a GTP (guanosine triphosphate)-binding protein that enables transport of the initiation-specific form of Met-tRNA (Met-tRNAi) onto the ribosome. According to IPA analysis, all drug treatments affected the expression of many proteins related to EIF2 signaling in oligodendrocytes. This effect seems to activate the pathway and may reflect the increased protein synthesis in the cells. Members of EIFs have been found functionally linked to the disrupted in schizophrenia 1 protein (DISC1) and to stress granules (Ogawa et al., 2005). Moreover, many risk-promoting genes and a number of environmental risk factors are related to oligodendrocyte cell loss and hypomyelination via activation of EIF2-alpha kinases in schizophrenia (Carter, 2007). These can lead to an arrest of protein synthesis through the eventual inhibition of translation initiation factor EIF2-beta by phosphorylated eIF2-alpha (Carter, 2007).

## Toxicity Pathways

The toxicity pathways associated with the proteomic changes of all treatment groups were mainly cell cycle G2/M DNA damage and nuclear factor-erythroid 2-related factor 2 (NRF2)-mediated responses. The link to cell cycle G2/M DNA damage signaling was due to changes in the 14-3-3 family proteins (YWHAB, YWHAG, YWHAH, YWHAQ, and YWHAZ), in addition to the Wee1-like protein kinase (WEE1).

Other proteins predicted to be involved in drug treatment responses included alcohol dehydrogenase [NADP(+)] (AKR1A1), T-complex protein 1 subunit eta (CCT7), DnaJ homolog subfamily B member 11 (DNAJB11), dual specificity mitogen-activated protein kinase kinases 1 (MAP2K1) and 2 (MAP2K2), although this occurred most predominantly in the MK-801 and clozapine co-treatment condition. NRF2 is a reactive oxygen species-responsive transcription factor, which binds to the antioxidant response elements (AREs) within the promoter of antioxidant enzyme genes and activates their transcription. NRF2 signaling takes place upon exposure of cells to oxidative stress through phosphorylation of the protein in response to activation of protein kinase C, phosphatidylinositol 3-kinase and MAP kinase pathways (Petri et al., 2012). After phosphorylation, NRF2 translocates to the nucleus, binds AREs and transactivates detoxifying enzymes and antioxidant enzymes, such as glutathione S-transferase, NAD(P)H quinone oxidoreductase, sulfiredoxin 1 (SRXN1) and thioredoxin reductase 1 (TXNRD1). SRXN1 and TXNRD1 are involved in the reduction and recovery of peroxiredoxins (Neumann et al., 2009; Soriano et al., 2009). The current results suggest that differential expression of NRF2 signaling proteins can affect PRDXs expression, although additional analyses should be performed to confirm these findings.

### Potential Interactions

The analysis of potential protein interactions showed that MK-801 treatment of oligodendrocytes included changes in proteins linked to other proteins which were mostly associated with energy and protein metabolism. However, nuclear transcription factors also appeared as highly connected proteins such as hypoxia-inducing factor 1-α (HIF1-α), MYCN and endothelial PAS domain-containing protein 1 (EPAS1). This suggests that these factors may be upstream regulators of the energy metabolism proteins altered by the MK-801 treatment.

HIF1-α is a subunit of a heterodimeric transcription factor hypoxia-inducible factor 1 (HIF-1) encoded by the *HIF1A* gene. HIF1 is the main transcriptional factor regulating the effects of hypoxia in expression of genes for angiogenesis, glycolysis and protective responses (Semenza, 2001). This factor is important in embryonic development and neural fold formation (Maltepe and Simon, 1998). Moreover, HIF1 has been related to regulation of many risk genes of schizophrenia. A meta-analysis study revealed that more than 50% of schizophrenia candidate genes met the criteria for a link to ischemia, hypoxia and/or vascular factors (Schmidt-Kastner et al., 2012) and epidemiological studies have shown that, events that lead to development of fetal hypoxia and inflammation during pregnancy are associated with increased risk of schizophrenia later in life (Nicodemus et al., 2008; Khandaker et al., 2013).

### Final Remarks

Considering all findings discussed above, the current study supports the concept that dysfunctions in NMDAr signaling in oligoendrocytes may be a central process in schizophrenia. MK-801-treated oligodendrocytes exhibited differences on cellular processes that have been previously observed in schizophrenia samples and have also revealed new pathways that could be pivotal in the development of this disorder. Although, the MK-801 treated oligodendrocyte model cannot reflect the pathophysiology of a complex psychiatric disorder as schizophrenia in its entirety, employing this approach might provide insights about specific aspects of the disease and lead to a novel preclinical tool for drug target discovery

## AUTHOR CONTRIBUTIONS

JC helped in experimental design, analyzed and interpreted the data and wrote the original version of the manuscript. Also corrected the manuscript according to reviewers advice. KI performed cell cultures experiments and pharmacological treatments. Helped in data interpretation and manuscript revision. JS has interpreted the data and has revised the manuscript carefully. PG analyzed the data and rewrote the manuscript carefully. CT analyzed the data and has revised the manuscript carefully. JN analyzed and interpreted the data and revised the manuscript carefully. DM-d-S conceptualized the study and experimental design. Analyzed the data and revised critically the original version of the manuscript. Later, corrected the manuscript according to reviewers advice.

## ACKNOWLEDGMENTS

Authors thank Prof. Sabine Bahn (University of Cambridge, UK) for providing access to IPA®.

## FUNDING

DM-d-S, JN, and JC are supported by Sao Paulo Research Foundation (FAPESP), grants 13/08711-3, 14/21035-0, 14/14881-1, and 14/10068-4; by the Brazilian National Council for Scientific and Technological Development (CNPq) grant 460289/2014-4; and the Research Fund (FAEPEX) from University of Campinas, grant 0986/14.

## REFERENCES

Ahmed, E. U., Ahmed, S., Ukai, W., Matsumoto, I., Kemp, A., Mcgregor, I. S., et al. (2012). Antipsychotic induced alteration of growth and proteome of rat neural stem cells. *Neurochem. Res.* 37, 1649–1659. doi: 10.1007/s11064-012-0768-3

Andreazza, A. C., Barakauskas, V. E., Fazeli, S., Feresten, A., Shao, L., Wei, V., et al. (2015). Effects of haloperidol and clozapine administration on oxidative stress in rat brain, liver and serum. *Neurosci. Lett.* 591, 36–40. doi: 10.1016/j.neulet.2015.02.028

Baig, M. R., Navaira, E., Escamilla, M. A., Raventos, H., and Walss-Bass, C. (2010). Clozapine treatment causes oxidation of proteins involved in energy metabolism in lymphoblastoid cells: a possible mechanism for antipsychotic-induced metabolic alterations. *J. Psychiatr. Pract.* 16, 325–333. doi: 10.1097/01.pra.0000388627.36781.6a

Ben-Shachar, D., and Laifenfeld, D. (2004). Mitochondria, synaptic plasticity, and schizophrenia. *Int. Rev. Neurobiol.* 59, 273–296. doi: 10.1016/s0074-7742(04)59011-6

Bernstein, H. G., Smalla, K. H., Durrschmidt, D., Keilhoff, G., Dobrowolny, H., Steiner, J., et al. (2012). Increased density of prohibitin-immunoreactive oligodendrocytes in the dorsolateral prefrontal white matter of subjects with schizophrenia suggests extraneuronal roles for the protein in the disease. *Neuromolecular Med.* 14, 270–280. doi: 10.1007/s12017-012-8185-y

Blanke, M. L., and VanDongen, A. M. J. (2009). "Activation mechanisms of the NMDA receptor," in *Biology of the NMDA Receptor*, ed. A. M. Van Dongen (Boca Raton, FL: CRC Press/Taylor & Francis).

Brown, J. W., Rueter, L. E., and Zhang, M. (2014). Predictive validity of a MK-801-induced cognitive impairment model in mice: implications on the potential limitations and challenges of modeling cognitive impairment associated with schizophrenia preclinically. *Prog. Neuropsychopharmacol. Biol. Psychiatry* 49, 53–62. doi: 10.1016/j.pnpbp.2013.11.008

Cao, N., and Yao, Z. X. (2013). Oligodendrocyte N-methyl-D-aspartate receptor signaling: insights into its functions. *Mol. Neurobiol.* 47, 845–856. doi: 10.1007/s12035-013-8408-8

Carter, C. J. (2007). EIF2B and oligodendrocyte survival: where nature and nurture meet in bipolar disorder and Schizophrenia? *Schizophr. Bull.* 33, 1343–1353. doi: 10.1093/schbul/sbm007

Cassoli, J. S., Guest, P. C., Malchow, B., Schmitt, A., Falkai, P., and Martins-De-Souza, D. (2015). Disturbed macro-connectivity in schizophrenia linked to oligodendrocyte dysfunction: from structural findings to molecules. *NPJ Schizophr.* 1, 15034. doi: 10.1038/npjschz.2015.34

Cheah, P. S., Ramshaw, H. S., Thomas, P. Q., Toyo-Oka, K., Xu, X., Martin, S., et al. (2012). Neurodevelopmental and neuropsychiatric behaviour defects arise from 14-3-3zeta deficiency. *Mol. Psychiatry* 17, 451–466. doi: 10.1038/mp.2011.158

Chen, J. W., Dodia, C., Feinstein, S. I., Jain, M. K., and Fisher, A. B. (2000). 1-Cys peroxiredoxin, a bifunctional enzyme with glutathione peroxidase and phospholipase A2 activities. *J. Biol. Chem.* 275, 28421–28427. doi: 10.1074/jbc.M005073200

Cummings, K. A., and Popescu, G. K. (2015). Glycine-dependent activation of NMDA receptors. *J. Gen. Physiol.* 145, 513–527. doi: 10.1085/jgp.2014 11302

Deng, W., Rosenberg, P. A., Volpe, J. J., and Jensen, F. E. (2003). Calcium-permeable AMPA/kainate receptors mediate toxicity and preconditioning by oxygen-glucose deprivation in oligodendrocyte precursors. *Proc. Natl. Acad. Sci. U. S. A.* 100, 6801–6806. doi: 10.1073/pnas.11366 24100

English, J. A., Dicker, P., Föcking, M., Dunn, M. J., and Cotter, D. R. (2009). 2-D DIGE analysis implicates cytoskeletal abnormalities in psychiatric disease. *Proteomics* 9, 3368–3382. doi: 10.1002/pmic.200900015

Fenton, T. R., and Gout, I. T. (2011). Functions and regulation of the 70 kDa ribosomal S6 kinases. *Int. J. Biochem. Cell Biol.* 43, 47–59. doi: 10.1016/j.biocel.2010.09.018

Foote, M., Qiao, H., Graham, K., Wu, Y., and Zhou, Y. (2015). Inhibition of 14-3-3 proteins leads to schizophrenia-related behavioral phenotypes and synaptic defects in mice. *Biol. Psychiatry* 78, 386–395. doi: 10.1016/j.biopsych.2015.02.015

Gattaz, W. F., Hubner, C. V., Nevalainen, T. J., Thuren, T., and Kinnunen, P. K. (1990). Increased serum phospholipase A2 activity in schizophrenia: a replication study. *Biol. Psychiatry* 28, 495–501.

Guest, P. C., Iwata, K., Kato, T. A., Steiner, J., Schmitt, A., Turck, C. W., et al. (2015). MK-801 treatment affects glycolysis in oligodendrocytes more than in astrocytes and neuronal cells: insights for schizophrenia. *Front. Cell. Neurosci.* 9:180. doi: 10.3389/fncel.2015.00180

Gunduz-Bruce, H. (2009). The acute effects of NMDA antagonism: from the rodent to the human brain. *Brain Res. Rev.* 60, 279–286. doi: 10.1016/j.brainresrev.2008.07.006

Hahn, C.-G., Wang, H.-Y., Cho, D.-S., Talbot, K., Gur, R. E., Berrettini, W. H., et al. (2006). Altered neuregulin 1-erbB4 signaling contributes to NMDA > receptor hypofunction in schizophrenia. *Nat. Med.* 12, 824–828. doi: 10.1038/nm1418

Harrison, P. J., and Weinberger, D. R. (2004). Schizophrenia genes, gene expression, and neuropathology: on the matter of their convergence. *Mol. Psychiatry* 10, 40–68. doi: 10.1038/sj.mp.4001558

Hayakawa, T., Ishiguro, H., Toru, M., Hamaguchi, H., and Arinami, T. (1998). Systematic search for mutations in the 14-3-3 eta chain gene on chromosome 22 in schizophrenics. *Psychiatr. Genet.* 8, 33–36. doi: 10.1097/00041444-199800810-00006

Horváth, Z. C., Czopf, J., and Buzsáki, G. (1997). MK-801-induced neuronal damage in rats. *Brain Res.* 753, 181–195. doi: 10.1016/S0006-8993(96)01290-5

Iwata, K., Cafe-Mendes, C. C., Schmitt, A., Steiner, J., Manabe, T., Matsuzaki, H., et al. (2013). The human oligodendrocyte proteome. *Proteomics* 13, 3548–3553. doi: 10.1002/pmic.201300201

Ji, B., La, Y., Gao, L., Zhu, H., Tian, N., Zhang, M., et al. (2009a). A comparative proteomics analysis of rat mitochondria from the cerebral cortex and hippocampus in response to antipsychotic medications. *J. Proteome Res.* 8, 3633–3641. doi: 10.1021/pr800876z

Ji, B., Zhang, Z., Zhang, M., Zhu, H., Zhou, K., Yang, J., et al. (2009b). Differential expression profiling of the synaptosome proteome in a rat model of antipsychotic resistance. *Brain Res.* 1295, 170–178. doi: 10.1016/j.brainres.2009.07.097

Karadottir, R., Cavelier, P., Bergersen, L. H., and Attwell, D. (2005). NMDA receptors are expressed in oligodendrocytes and activated in ischaemia. *Nature* 438, 1162–1166. doi: 10.1038/nature04302

Khandaker, G. M., Zimbron, J., Lewis, G., and Jones, P. B. (2013). Prenatal maternal infection, neurodevelopment and adult schizophrenia: a systematic review of population-based studies. *Psychol. Med.* 43, 239–257. doi: 10.1017/s0033291712000736

Kornhuber, J., Mack-Burkhardt, F., Kornhuber, M. E., and Riederer, P. (1989). [3H]MK-801 binding sites in post-mortem human frontal cortex. *Eur. J. Pharmacol.* 162, 483–490. doi: 10.1016/0014-2999(89)90339-7

Kovacic, P., and Somanathan, R. (2010). Clinical physiology and mechanism of dizocilpine (MK-801): electron transfer, radicals, redox metabolites and bioactivity. *Oxid. Med. Cell. Longev.* 3, 13–22. doi: 10.4161/oxim.3.1.10028

Lewis, D. A. (2000). Is there a neuropathology of schizophrenia? Recent findings converge on altered thalamic-prefrontal cortical connectivity. *Neuroscientist* 6, 208–218. doi: 10.1177/107385840000600311

Li, C., Xiao, L., Liu, X., Yang, W., Shen, W., Hu, C., et al. (2013). A functional role of NMDA receptor in regulating the differentiation of oligodendrocyte precursor cells and remyelination. *Glia* 61, 732–749. doi: 10.1002/glia.22469

Ma, D., Chan, M. K., Lockstone, H. E., Pietsch, S. R., Jones, D. N., Cilia, J., et al. (2009). Antipsychotic treatment alters protein expression associated with presynaptic function and nervous system development in rat frontal cortex. *J. Proteome Res.* 8, 3284–3297. doi: 10.1021/pr800983p

Maccarrone, G., Lebar, M., and Martins-De-Souza, D. (2014). Brain quantitative proteomics combining GeLC-MS and isotope-coded protein labeling (ICPL). *Methods Mol. Biol.* 1156, 175–185. doi: 10.1007/978-1-4939-0685-7_11

Maccarrone, G., Rewerts, C., Lebar, M., Turck, C. W., and Martins-De-Souza, D. (2013). Proteome profiling of peripheral mononuclear cells from human blood. *Proteomics* 13, 893–897. doi: 10.1002/pmic.201200377

Maltepe, E., and Simon, M. C. (1998). Oxygen, genes, and development: an analysis of the role of hypoxic gene regulation during murine vascular development. *J. Mol. Med. (Berl.)* 76, 391–401. doi: 10.1007/s001090050231

Martins-de-Souza, D. (2010). Proteome and transcriptome analysis suggests oligodendrocyte dysfunction in schizophrenia. *J. Psychiatr. Res.* 44, 149–156. doi: 10.1016/j.jpsychires.2009.07.007

Martins-De-Souza, D., Dias-Neto, E., Schmitt, A., Falkai, P., Gormanns, P., Maccarrone, G., et al. (2010). Proteome analysis of schizophrenia brain tissue. *World J. Biol. Psychiatry* 11, 110–120. doi: 10.3109/15622970903490626

Martins-de-Souza, D., Gattaz, W. F., Schmitt, A., Novello, J. C., Marangoni, S., Turck, C. W., et al. (2009a). Proteome analysis of schizophrenia patients Wernicke's area reveals an energy metabolism dysregulation. *BMC Psychiatry* 9:17. doi: 10.1186/1471-244x-9-17

Martins-de-Souza, D., Gattaz, W. F., Schmitt, A., Rewerts, C., Maccarrone, G., Dias-Neto, E., et al. (2009b). Prefrontal cortex shotgun proteome analysis reveals altered calcium homeostasis and immune system imbalance in schizophrenia. *Eur. Arch. Psychiatry Clin. Neurosci.* 259, 151–163. doi: 10.1007/s00406-008-0847-2

Martins-de-Souza, D., Guest, P. C., Rahmoune, H., and Bahn, S. (2012). Proteomic approaches to unravel the complexity of schizophrenia. *Expert Rev. Proteomics* 9, 97–108. doi: 10.1586/epr.11.70

Martins-de-Souza, D., Harris, L. W., Guest, P. C., and Bahn, S. (2011a). The role of energy metabolism dysfunction and oxidative stress in schizophrenia revealed by proteomics. *Antioxid. Redox Signal.* 15, 2067–2079. doi: 10.1089/ars.2010.3459

Martins-de-Souza, D., Lebar, M., and Turck, C. W. (2011b). Proteome analyses of cultured astrocytes treated with MK-801 and clozapine: similarities with schizophrenia. *Eur. Arch. Psychiatry Clin. Neurosci.* 261, 217–228. doi: 10.1007/s00406-010-0166-2

Martins-de-Souza, D., Menezes De Oliveira, B., Dos Santos Farias, A., Horiuchi, R. S., Crepaldi Domingues, C., De Paula, E., et al. (2007). The use of ASB-14 in combination with CHAPS is the best for solubilization of human brain proteins for two-dimensional gel electrophoresis. *Brief. Funct. Genomics proteomics* 6, 70–75. doi: 10.1093/bfgp/elm009

Martins-de-Souza, D., Schmitt, A., Röder, R., Lebar, M., Schneider-Axmann, T., Falkai, P., et al. (2010). Sex-specific proteome differences in the anterior cingulate cortex of schizophrenia. *J. Psychiatr. Res.* 44, 989–991. doi: 10.1016/j.jpsychires.2010.03.003

Mhawech, P. (2005). 14-3-3 proteins – an update. *Cell Res.* 15, 228–236. doi: 10.1038/sj.cr.7290291

Micu, I., Jiang, Q., Coderre, E., Ridsdale, A., Zhang, L., Woulfe, J., et al. (2006). NMDA receptors mediate calcium accumulation in myelin during chemical ischaemia. *Nature* 439, 988–992. doi: 10.1038/nature04474

Middleton, F. A., Peng, L., Lewis, D. A., Levitt, P., and Mirnics, K. (2005). Altered expression of 14-3-3 genes in the prefrontal cortex of subjects with schizophrenia. *Neuropsychopharmacology* 30, 974–983. doi: 10.1038/sj.npp.1300674

Murray, F., Kennedy, J., Hutson, P. H., Elliot, J., Huscroft, I., Mohnen, K., et al. (2000). Modulation of [3H]MK-801 binding to NMDA receptors in vivo and in vitro. *Eur. J. Pharmacol.* 397, 263–270. doi: 10.1016/S0014-2999(00)00263-6

Muslin, A. J., Tanner, J. W., Allen, P. M., and Shaw, A. S. (1996). Interaction of 14-3-3 with signaling proteins is mediated by the recognition of phosphoserine. *Cell* 84, 889–897. doi: 10.1016/S0092-8674(00)81067-3

Nascimento, J. M., and Martins-de-Souza, D. (2015). The proteome of schizophrenia. *NPJ Schizophrenia* 1, 14003. doi: 10.1038/npjschz.2014.3

Neumann, C. A., Cao, J., and Manevich, Y. (2009). Peroxiredoxin 1 and its role in cell signaling. *Cell Cycle* 8, 4072–4078. doi: 10.4161/cc.8.24.10242

Nicodemus, K. K., Marenco, S., Batten, A. J., Vakkalanka, R., Egan, M. F., Straub, R. E., et al. (2008). Serious obstetric complications interact with hypoxia-regulated/vascular-expression genes to influence schizophrenia risk. *Mol. Psychiatry* 13, 873–877. doi: 10.1038/sj.mp.4002153

Ogawa, F., Kasai, M., and Akiyama, T. (2005). A functional link between Disrupted-In-Schizophrenia 1 and the eukaryotic translation initiation factor 3. *Biochem. Biophys. Res. Commun.* 338, 771–776. doi: 10.1016/j.bbrc.2005.10.013

Palmowski, P., Rogowska-Wrzesinska, A., Williamson, J., Beck, H. C., Mikkelsen, J. D., Hansen, H. H., et al. (2014). Acute phencyclidine treatment induces extensive and distinct protein phosphorylation in rat frontal cortex. *J. Proteome Res.* 13, 1578–1592. doi: 10.1021/pr4010794

Paulson, L., Martin, P., Ljung, E., Blennow, K., and Davidsson, P. (2007). Proteome analysis after co-administration of clozapine or haloperidol to MK-801-treated rats. *J. Neural Transm.* 114, 885–891. doi: 10.1007/s00702-007-0626-7

Paulson, L., Martin, P., Nilsson, C. L., Ljung, E., Westman-Brinkmalm, A., Blennow, K., et al. (2004). Comparative proteome analysis of thalamus in MK-801-treated rats. *Proteomics* 4, 819–825. doi: 10.1002/pmic.200300622

Peng, Y.-T., Chen, P., Ouyang, R.-Y., and Song, L. (2015). Multifaceted role of prohibitin in cell survival and apoptosis. *Apoptosis* 20, 1135–1149. doi: 10.1007/s10495-015-1143-z

Petri, S., Körner, S., and Kiaei, M. (2012). Nrf2/ARE signaling pathway: key mediator in oxidative stress and potential therapeutic target in ALS. *Neurol. Res. Int.* 2012, 7. doi: 10.1155/2012/878030

Rajasekaran, A., Venkatasubramanian, G., Berk, M., and Debnath, M. (2015). Mitochondrial dysfunction in schizophrenia: pathways, mechanisms and implications. *Neurosci. Biobehav. Rev.* 48, 10–21. doi: 10.1016/j.neubiorev.2014.11.005

Ramshaw, H., Xu, X., Jaehne, E. J., Mccarthy, P., Greenberg, Z., Saleh, E., et al. (2013). Locomotor hyperactivity in 14-3-3zeta KO mice is associated with dopamine transporter dysfunction. *Transl. Psychiatry* 3, e327. doi: 10.1038/tp.2013.99

Rhee, S. G., Chae, H. Z., and Kim, K. (2005). Peroxiredoxins: a historical overview and speculative preview of novel mechanisms and emerging concepts in cell signaling. *Free Radic. Biol. Med.* 38, 1543–1552. doi: 10.1016/j.freeradbiomed.2005.02.026

Rivero, G., Gabilondo, A. M., Garcia-Sevilla, J. A., La Harpe, R., Morentin, B., and Meana, J. J. (2015). Up-regulated 14-3-3beta and 14-3-3zeta proteins in prefrontal cortex of subjects with schizophrenia: effect of psychotropic treatment. *Schizophr. Res.* 161, 446–451. doi: 10.1016/j.schres.2014.12.014

Saia-Cereda, V. M., Cassoli, J. S., Schmitt, A., Falkai, P., Nascimento, J. M., and Martins-De-Souza, D. (2015). Proteomics of the corpus callosum unravel pivotal players in the dysfunction of cell signaling, structure, and myelination in schizophrenia brains. *Eur. Arch. Psychiatry Clin. Neurosci.* 265, 601–612. doi: 10.1007/s00406-015-0621-1

Salter, M. G., and Fern, R. (2005). NMDA receptors are expressed in developing oligodendrocyte processes and mediate injury. *Nature* 438, 1167–1171. doi: 10.1038/nature04301

Sanderson, J. L., and Dell'Acqua, M. L. (2011). AKAP signaling complexes in regulation of excitatory synaptic plasticity. *Neuroscientist* 17, 321–336. doi: 10.1177/1073858410384740

Schmidt-Kastner, R., Van Os, J., Esquivel, G., Steinbusch, H. W. M., and Rutten, B. P. F. (2012). An environmental analysis of genes associated with schizophrenia: hypoxia and vascular factors as interacting elements in the neurodevelopmental model. *Mol. Psychiatry* 17, 1194–1205. doi: 10.1038/mp.2011.183

Schubert, K. O., Focking, M., and Cotter, D. R. (2015). Proteomic pathway analysis of the hippocampus in schizophrenia and bipolar affective disorder implicates 14-3-3 signaling, aryl hydrocarbon receptor signaling, and glucose metabolism: potential roles in GABAergic interneuron pathology. *Schizophr. Res.* 167, 64–72. doi: 10.1016/j.schres.2015.02.002

Semenza, G. L. (2001). HIF-1 and mechanisms of hypoxia sensing. *Curr. Opin. Cell Biol.* 13, 167–171. doi: 10.1016/S0955-0674(00)00194-0

Shisheva, A., Südhof, T. C., and Czech, M. P. (1994). Cloning, characterization, and expression of a novel GDP dissociation inhibitor isoform from skeletal muscle. *Mol. Cell. Biol.* 14, 3459–3468. doi: 10.1128/MCB.14.5.3459

Simon, R. P., Swan, J. H., Griffiths, T., and Meldrum, B. S. (1984). Blockade of N-methyl-D-aspartate receptors may protect against ischemic damage in the brain. *Science* 226, 850–852. doi: 10.1126/science.6093256

Smalla, K. H., Mikhaylova, M., Sahin, J., Bernstein, H. G., Bogerts, B., Schmitt, A., et al. (2008). A comparison of the synaptic proteome in human chronic schizophrenia and rat ketamine psychosis suggest that prohibitin is involved in the synaptic pathology of schizophrenia. *Mol. Psychiatry* 13, 878–896. doi: 10.1038/mp.2008.60

Soriano, F. X., Baxter, P., Murray, L. M., Sporn, M. B., Gillingwater, T. H., and Hardingham, G. E. (2009). Transcriptional regulation of the AP-1 and Nrf2 target gene sulfiredoxin. *Mol. Cells* 27, 279–282. doi: 10.1007/s10059-009-0050-y

Vardigan, J. D., Huszar, S. L., Mcnaughton, C. H., Hutson, P. H., and Uslaner, J. M. (2010). MK-801 produces a deficit in sucrose preference that is reversed by clozapine, D-serine, and the metabotropic glutamate 5 receptor positive allosteric modulator CDPPB: relevance to negative symptoms associated with schizophrenia? *Pharmacol. Biochem. Behav.* 95, 223–229. doi: 10.1016/j.pbb.2010.01.010

Walss-Bass, C., Weintraub, S. T., Hatch, J., Mintz, J., and Chaudhuri, A. R. (2008). Clozapine causes oxidation of proteins involved in energy metabolism: a possible mechanism for antipsychotic-induced metabolic alterations. *Int. J. Neuropsychopharmacol.* 11, 1097–1104. doi: 10.1017/s1461145708008882

Wesseling, H., Rahmoune, H., Tricklebank, M., Guest, P. C., and Bahn, S. (2015). A targeted multiplexed proteomic investigation identifies ketamine-induced changes in immune markers in rat serum and expression changes in protein kinases/phosphatases in rat brain. *J. Proteome Res.* 14, 411–421. doi: 10.1021/pr5009493

Wilkinson, B., and Gilbert, H. F. (2004). Protein disulfide isomerase. *Biochim. Biophys. Acta* 1699, 35–44. doi: 10.1016/j.bbapap.2004.02.017

Wong, A. H., Macciardi, F., Klempan, T., Kawczynski, W., Barr, C. L., Lakatoo, S., et al. (2003). Identification of candidate genes for psychosis in rat models, and possible association between schizophrenia and the 14-3-3eta gene. *Mol. Psychiatry* 8, 156–166. doi: 10.1038/sj.mp.4001237

Yoon, S. C., Seo, M. S., Kim, S. H., Jeon, W. J., Ahn, Y. M., Kang, U. G., et al. (2008). The effect of MK-801 on mTOR/p70S6K and translation-related proteins in rat frontal cortex. *Neurosci. Lett.* 434, 23–28. doi: 10.1016/j.neulet.2008.01.020

Zangrando, J., Carvalheira, R., Labbate, G., Medeiros, P., Longo, B. M., Melo-Thomas, L., et al. (2013). Atypical antipsychotic olanzapine reversed deficit on prepulse inhibition of the acoustic startle reflex produced by microinjection of dizocilpine (MK-801) into the inferior colliculus in rats. *Behav. Brain Res.* 257, 77–82. doi: 10.1016/j.bbr.2013.09.018

Zhou, K., Yang, Y., Gao, L., He, G., Li, W., Tang, K., et al. (2012). NMDA receptor hypofunction induces dysfunctions of energy metabolism and semaphorin signaling in rats: a synaptic proteome study. *Schizophr. Bull.* 38, 579–591. doi: 10.1093/schbul/sbq132

Zhou, T. B., and Qin, Y. H. (2013). Signaling pathways of prohibitin and its role in diseases. *J. Recept. Signal Transduct. Res.* 33, 28–36. doi: 10.3109/10799893.2012.752006

Zuo, D. Y., Cao, Y., Zhang, L., Wang, H. F., and Wu, Y. L. (2009). Effects of acute and chronic administration of MK-801 on c-Fos protein expression in mice brain regions implicated in schizophrenia with or without clozapine. *Prog. Neuropsychopharmacol. Biol. Psychiatry* 33, 290–295. doi: 10.1016/j.pnpbp.2008.12.002

# 20

# Proteomics Research in Schizophrenia

*Katarina Davalieva*[1], *Ivana Maleva Kostovska*[1] *and Andrew J. Dwork*[2, 3, 4*]

[1] *Research Centre for Genetic Engineering and Biotechnology "Georgi D Efremov," Macedonian Academy of Sciences and Arts, Skopje, Republic of Macedonia,* [2] *Department of Molecular Imaging and Neuropathology, New York State Psychiatric Institute, New York, NY, USA,* [3] *Departments of Psychiatry and Pathology and Cell Biology, College of Physicians and Surgeons of Columbia University, New York, NY, USA,* [4] *Macedonian Academy of Sciences and Arts, Skopje, Republic of Macedonia*

***Correspondence:***
*Andrew J. Dwork*
*ajd6@columbia.edu*

Despite intense scientific efforts, the neuropathology and pathophysiology of schizophrenia are poorly understood. Proteomic studies, by testing large numbers of proteins for associations with disease, may contribute to the understanding of the molecular mechanisms of schizophrenia. They may also indicate the types and locations of cells most likely to harbor pathological alterations. Investigations using proteomic approaches have already provided much information on quantitative and qualitative protein patterns in postmortem brain tissue, peripheral tissues and body fluids. Different proteomic technologies such as 2-D PAGE 2-D DIGE, SELDI-TOF, shotgun proteomics with label-based (ICAT), and label-free ($MS^E$) quantification have been applied to the study of schizophrenia for the past 15 years. This review summarizes the results, mostly from brain but also from other tissues and bodily fluids, of proteomics studies in schizophrenia. Emphasis is given to proteomics platforms, varying sources of material, proposed candidate biomarkers emerging from comparative proteomics studies, and the specificity of the putative markers in terms of other mental illnesses. We also compare proteins altered in schizophrenia with reports of protein or mRNA sequences that are relatively enriched in specific cell types. While proteomic studies of schizophrenia find abnormalities in the expression of many proteins that are not cell type-specific, there appears to be a disproportionate representation of proteins whose synthesis and localization are highly enriched in one or more brain cell type compared with other types of brain cells. Two of the three proteins most commonly altered in schizophrenia are aldolase C and glial fibrillary acidic protein, astrocytic proteins with entirely different functions, but the studies are approximately evenly divided with regard to the direction of the differences and the concordance or discordance between the two proteins. Alterations of common myelin-associated proteins were also frequently observed, and in four studies that identified alterations in at least two, all differences were downwards in schizophrenia, consistent with earlier studies examining RNA or targeting myelin-associated proteins.

**Keywords: brain tissue, 2D-DIGE, shotgun proteomics, glia, oligodendrocytes, astrocytes, myelin**

## THE NEED FOR PROTEOMICS STUDIES AND BIOMARKERS FOR SCHIZOPHRENIA

Genomic studies of schizophrenia, using genome wide association studies (GWAS), copy number variations (CNVs), microarrays, and next-generation sequencing (RNAseq) have linked schizophrenia with rare genetic variations (Sullivan et al., 2012).There is strong evidence that there are no known Mendelian variants identified for this disease. Instead, variations of many genes with confirmed involvement of rare structural variations and common variations with subtle effects are considered to be involved in the etiology of the disease (Owen et al., 2010). Genomics studies on schizophrenia have not answered the main questions on the pathophysiology of the disease, nor have they resulted in identification of diagnostic, prognostic, or therapeutic biomarkers. In addition, current research suggests that schizophrenia can arise from an interaction between neurodevelopmental processes and environmental effects (Albus, 2012).

Understanding schizophrenia as a complex disease therefore requires determination of not only gene expression and DNA variations, but also determination of the abundance and modifications of various proteins, and their distribution at gross anatomical, cellular, and subcellular levels. Proteomics aims to unravel biological processes based on qualitative and quantitative comparison of proteomes. It gives a different level of understanding than genomics for several reasons. First, the expression or function of proteins is modulated at many diverse points, from transcription of DNA to post-translational modifications (PTMs), and very little of this can be predicted from analysis of nucleic acids alone. Second, there is generally poor correlation between abundance of mRNA, transcribed from DNA, and abundance of protein translated from that mRNA. Third, many transcripts give rise to more than one protein, through alternative splicing or alternative PTMs such as phosphorylation, glycosylation, and acetylation, which profoundly affect their activities and lead to multiple protein products from the same gene.

Proteomic investigations have largely improved our understanding of schizophrenia, based on quantitative and qualitative identification of protein patterns in postmortem brain tissue, peripheral tissues, and body fluids (Martins-de-Souza et al., 2012b; Guest et al., 2013, 2014; Nascimento and Martins-de-Souza, 2015). This has enhanced our knowledge of complex protein networks and signal transduction pathways affected in this disease, as discussed in detail below. In addition, emerging proteomic platforms have facilitated the identification of biomarker candidates by simultaneous measurement of hundreds or thousands of molecules in non-hypothesis-driven comparative proteomics studies. This approach established the first blood-based test to aid in the diagnosis of schizophrenia (Schwarz et al., 2010). The test encompassed 51 biomarkers with an overall sensitivity and specificity of 83%. The clinical utility of this test has been studied in terms of specificity compared with other psychiatric disorders (Schwarz et al., 2012a), the ability to identify the disease prior to clinical manifestation, (Schwarz et al., 2012b) and the ability to define the complex schizophrenia syndrome on the basis of molecular profiles (Schwarz et al., 2014).

However, there is still an urgent need for biomarkers that will help to improve the diagnosis and stratification of patients and facilitate more effective treatments and care. The field of proteomics is rapidly developing, with improvements in mass spectrometry, peptide identification algorithms, and bioinformatics. Larger studies, standardized sample collection and processing, and highly sophisticated proteomics platforms promise new diagnostic, prognostic, and therapeutic biomarkers for schizophrenia.

## PROTEOMICS STUDIES OF SCHIZOPHRENIA

The history of proteomic studies of schizophrenia largely recapitulates that of proteomics in general, driven over the past few decades by advances in the instrumentation and analysis of data for mass spectroscopy. We refer the reader to a recent publication (Doerr et al., 2015), in which these developments are reviewed for a general scientific audience.

The earliest proteomic investigations of schizophrenia employed two-dimensional polyacrylamide gel electrophoresis (2-D PAGE), combined with mass spectrometry (MS) identification, mainly based on matrix-assisted laser desorption/ionization-(MALDI)-time-of-flight (TOF)-TOF instruments. Moreover, 2-D PAGE/MS and later on, 2-D difference in-gel electrophoresis (DIGE)/MS are the most reported platforms in the study of postmortem brain tissues. As summarized in **Table 1**, 14 out of 25 proteomic studies on autopsy brain tissue from people with schizophrenia used 2-D PAGE/MS or 2-D DIGE/MS alone, and 2 studies employed combinations of these platforms with shotgun proteomics.

Since its introduction in 1975 (O'Farrell, 1975), 2-D PAGE, combined with MS, has been widely used in proteomics studies. The platform is based on several steps of protein separation, detection, quantification and identification. Proteins are separated in two steps: by isoelectric point (pl) through isoelectric focusing on immobilized pH gradient (IPG) strips, followed by separation by molecular weight (MW) using SDS–PAGE. Proteins are detected using different staining protocols, and differences in abundances are quantified by image analysis software. The protein identification is based on excision of the 2D-spots of interest, enzymatic digestion (usually with trypsin), and analysis of the masses of these peptides by mass spectrometry [MALDI-TOF-MS or liquid chromatography (LC)–MS/MS]. Each protein produces a specific combination of peptide masses, known as a peptide mass fingerprint, which allows identification by comparison with database of fingerprints derived from protein sequences. To minimize ambiguity from gel-to-gel differences in 2-D PAGE, DIGE was introduced in 1997 (Unlü et al., 1997). DIGE combines multiple samples and internal standards in one gel by the fluorescent labeling of different samples with different cyanine dyes. This eliminates the need for technical replicates heavily used in conventional 2-D PAGE and improves reproducibility and sensitivity.

The advantages and limitations of this platform are well-established (Rabilloud and Lelong, 2011). The key advantages are high reproducibility, robustness, separation of intact proteins, visualization, and detection of PTMs, and cost-effectiveness of the procedure. A major disadvantage of any gel-based system, as recognized throughout the years, is limitation in the analysis

**TABLE 1 | Proteins with altered abundance in schizophrenia obtained by comparative proteomics studies of several human brain regions.**

| Number of proteins with altered abundances | Brain region (BA)** | Some of the proteins with altered abundances in schizophrenia compared to controls* | Processes and pathways affected | Study design | Method | References |
|---|---|---|---|---|---|---|
| **FRONTAL CORTEX** | | | | | | |
| 8 proteins | 10 | **DPYSL2↓ ALDOC↑ GFAP↓** | Differentiation, neurogenesis, glycolysis, development and organization of the central nervous system | Individuals with schizophrenia (*n* = 24), bipolar disorder (*n* = 23), major depressive disorder without psychotic features (*n* = 19) and unaffected controls (*n* = 23) | 2-D PAGE/MS | Johnston-Wilson et al., 2000 |
| **PREFRONTAL CORTEX** | | | | | | |
| 50 proteins | 9 white and gray matter | **PKM**1↓; **PKM** 2↓; **ACO2**↓; **HK1**↓; **PRDX1**↓; **PRDX2**↓; **ALDOC**↓; **ALDOA**↓; **HSPA1**↓;**HSPA**2↓; **HSPA5**↓; **HSPA8**↓; **TUBA2**↓; **TUBA6**↓; **TUBB5**↓; **ENO1/2**↓; **GSN**↓; **GLUL↓; ACTA/B/C**↓; **MDH1**↓; **SPTAN1**↓; **CNP↓; DNM1**/2↓; **DPYSL2**↓; **DPYSL5**↓; **DPYSL**4↓; **SEPT**3↓; **TF↑; GSTM3↓, GSTTLp28↓;** | Mitochondrial function, oxidative stress responses, peroxisomal function, cytoskeletal dysfunction, protein trafficking | 10 schizophrenia and 10 well-matched control individuals | 2-D DIGE/MS | Prabakaran et al., 2004 |
| 15 proteins | 9 (dorsolateral) | **DPYSL3↑;** PHGDH↑; **SEPT**5↑; **TCP1**↑; PGLS↑; **DNM1**↑; ERP29↑; ALB↑; **ENO2**↓; **GFAP**↑; GDA↓; **NEFL**↓; PACSIN1↓; **TF**↓; **ATP6V1B2**↓ | Development of the central nervous system, energy metabolism, cytoskeletal dysfunction | 35 individuals with schizophrenia, 35 with bipolar disorder and 35 controls | 2-D PAGE/MS | Pennington et al., 2008 |
| 16 proteins | 9 (dorsolateral) gray matter | LAMP↑; STXBP1↑; BASP1↑; NCAM↑; PHB↓; CNTN1↓; **CKB**↑; HBB↓; GNAI1↑; **TUBB/A↑; ATP6V1B2**↑; **VDAC1**↓ | Synaptic function, metabolism, signaling, cytoskeletal dysfunction | Pooled samples from schizophrenia, bipolar disorder and control cases (*n* = 10 per group) | 2-D DIGE/MS 1-D/LC-MS/MS | Behan et al., 2009 |
| Targeted one protein expression | 9 (dorsolateral) | **APOA1**↓ | May have role in neuronal and glial metabolism | 16 schizophrenia and 16 well-matched controls | Western blot | Huang et al., 2008 |
| 24 proteins | 46 (left dorsolateral) | **MBP**↓; **TF**↓; **ALDOC**↑; **PGK1**↑; **ACO2**↑; **MDH1**↓; **ATP5H**↑; **ATP5A1**↑; UQCRC1↓; HSP90AA1 ↓; **HSPD1**↑; **INA**↑; **PCMT1**↑; **GFAP**↑; **NEFL**↓; **DNM1**↑; **CFL1**↓; **CRYM**↓; **GNB1**↑; **DPYSL2↑;ACTG1**↓ | Alterations in oligodendrocytes, energy metabolism, glycolysis, oxidative stress, cytoskeletal dysfunction, cell signaling | pool of 9 schizophrenia patients and pool of 7 paired controls | 2-D PAGE/MS | Martins-de-Souza et al., 2009a |
| 84 proteins | 46 (dorsolateral) | SIRPA↓; SIRPB1↓; **PRDX2**↑; **PRDX6**↑; PLEC↑; **VIM**↑; LMNB2↑; DES↑; **TUBB2B**↑; TBCB↑; KIF21A↑; **MAP1A**↑; MAP2↑; MAP6↑; EPB41L1↑; SH3GL2↑; **PEBP1**↑; BSN↑; HOMER1↑; STRN↑; **MOG**↓; CSNK2A1↑; MYO1D↓; **HK1**↑; PFKM↑; **GAPDH**↑; **CNP**↓ | Immune system, cytoskeleton assembly, calcium homeostasis, energy metabolism, glycolysis | 9 schizophrenia patients and 7 controls | ICPL /IEF/LC-MALDI | Martins-de-Souza et al., 2009c |

*(Continued)*

**TABLE 1 | Continued**

| Number of proteins with altered abundances | Brain region (BA)** | Some of the proteins with altered abundances in schizophrenia compared to controls* | Processes and pathways affected | Study design | Method | References |
|---|---|---|---|---|---|---|
| 32 proteins | 46 (dorsolateral-white matter) | **NEFL**↓; **NEFM**↑; **NEFH**↓; **VIM**↑; **TUBB**↓; **YWHAE**↑; **YWHAZ**↓; **DPYSL2**↑; **DPYSL3**↑; **DPYSL5**↑; **PCMT1**↑; **STMN1**↓; GDI1↑; **ENO1**↓; **ALDOC**↓; **IMPA1**↑; **TPI1**↓; PRDX4↓; PDE8B↓,PLP1↑ | Cytoskeletal dysfunction, signal transduction, energy metabolism | 35 schizophrenia, 35 bipolar disorder and 35 controls | 2-D DIGE/MS | English et al., 2009 |
| 41 protein spots | NS (left dorsolateral synapse enriched fractions) | **PKM**↓; **ATP6V1B2**↑; **ATP5B**↑; GDF2↓; GNAQ↑; **PEBP1**↑; ANXA10↑; **CKB**↑; GNB3↑; **PPA2**↑; **ALDOC**↑; AK4↑; **ANXA2**↓; HDGF↑; MLF2↑; **ATP5H**↑; **VDAC1**↑; PDYN↑; | Energy metabolism, neurotransmission/signaling | 8 schizophrenia patients and 7 controls | 2-D PAGE/MS | Smalla et al., 2008 |
| Targeted one protein expression | 46 (dorsolateral) | **HINT1**↓ | May have role in cellular stress and apoptosis | 9 schizophrenia patients and 7 controls | Western blot | Varadarajulu et al., 2012 |
| Biomarker panel of 10 peaks | NS (dorsolateral) | No protein identifications (sensitivity and specificity of the panel 70%) | | 34 schizophrenia patients and 35 matched controls | SELDI-TOF-MS | Mei et al., 2006 |
| Biomarker panel of 21 protein peaks | NS (dorsolateral) | CD58 ↓; CALM1↓; MAGOH↓; MAXb↓; RGS11↓; UCHL1↓; CEBPZ↓; **HSPD1**↓; **PGAM1**↓; **ENO2**↓; **GLUL**↓; **PPA2**↓; **YWHAE**↓; **ALDOC**↓; PNP↓; NKX2-4↓; DECR2↓; MTAP↓; BYSL↓; SMPD1↓; ANKRD12↓; | Cell metabolism, glycolysis, intracellular signaling, oxidative stress | 17 schizophrenia patients, 20 bipolar disorder patients and 20 normal controls | SELDI-TOF-MS | Novikova et al., 2006 |
| **ANTERIOR CINGULATE CORTEX** | | | | | | |
| 36 proteins | 24 (gray matter) | **DPYSL2**↑; **CRMP1**↑; **ALDOC**↓; **DNM1**↑; **GFAP**↓; PPP1CA↓; **CS**↓; CA1↑; **TF**↓; IDH3B↓; ACAT2↑; **SOD1**↑; DDAH1↓; ANXA1↑; **ANXA5**↑; **CKB**↑; EHD3↑; **STMN1**↑; PHB↑; | Energy metabolism, oxidative stress, cytoskeletal dysfunction, protein trafficking, development and organization of the central nervous system | 10 schizophrenia patients and 10 healthy controls | 2-D PAGE/MS | Clark et al., 2006 |
| 27 proteins | 24 (white matter) | **DPYSL2**↓; **ALDOC**↓; **CS**↑; CBR1↓; **ATP5A1**↑; **IMPA1**↑; GPD1↓; LDHA↓; **NEFL**↓; **ATP6V1A**↑; PSMB4↑; **PGAM1**↓ | Energy metabolism, oxidative stress response, cytoskeletal dysfunction, cellular signaling | 10 schizophrenia patients and 10 healthy controls | 2-D PAGE/MS | Clark et al., 2007 |
| 19 proteins | NS | **ACO2**↑; **ALDOA**↑; **CRMP1**↑; **DPYSL2**↑; SRI↓; **CKB**↓; | Energy metabolism, glycolysis, cytoskeletal dysfunction | 15 schizophrenia patients, 15 bipolar, 15 major depressive disorder and 15 healthy controls | 2-D PAGE/MS | Beasley et al., 2006 |
| 32 proteins | NS | **DPYSL2**↑; **CRYAB**↑; **PRDX6**↓; **ALDOC**↑; **GLUL**↑ | Energy metabolism, cell communication/ signal transduction, cytoskeletal dysfunction | 11 schizophrenia patients and 8 healthy controls | 2-D PAGE/MS | Martins-de-Souza et al., 2010b |

*(Continued)*

**TABLE 1 | Continued**

| Number of proteins with altered abundances | Brain region (BA)** | Some of the proteins with altered abundances in schizophrenia compared to controls* | Processes and pathways affected | Study design | Method | References |
|---|---|---|---|---|---|---|
| 143 proteins | 24 (enrichment of the postsynaptic density) | ARF6↑; ARFGAP1↑; AP2B1↑; RAB11FIP5↑; AP2M1↓; ADRBK1↓; **DNM1**↑; **HSPA6**↓; **HSPA8**↓; RAP1A↑; GRIA2↓; MAPK3↓; SHANK3↓; SYNPO↓; MYL6↓; CYFIP2↓; ATP6V0A1↓; **PRDX1**↓; ESYT↑; GNAS↓; CAMK2B, CAMK2D↓; CAMK2G↓; CALM2↓; **VDAC1**↓; VDAC2↓ | Endocytosis, long-term potentiation, calcium signaling pathway | 10 schizophrenia patients and 10 healthy controls | Label-free LC–MS/MS | Föcking et al., 2015 |
| **CORPUS CALLOSUM** | | | | | | |
| 34 proteins | NS | **NEFL**↓; **NEFM**↓; **GFAP**↑; **ACTG1** ↓; **ACTB** ↓; **TUBB**↓; **INA**↑; ACTR1A↑; COTL1↑; **ATP5B**↓; ARHGDIA↑; **STMN1**↑; **DPYSL2**↓; **YWHAH**↓; **HSPA8**↓; HSPA1L↓; **HSPA5**↑; **GSTP1**↑; **SOD1**↑; **CKB**↓; **PRDX2**↓; UCHL1↑; PARK7↑; FTH1↓; **LDHB**↓; **ENO2**↓; | Cytoskeletal dysfunction, oxidative stress, glycolysis, neuroprotective dysfunction | 10 schizophrenia patients and 10 healthy controls | 2-D PAGE/MS | Sivagnanasundaram et al., 2007 |
| 65 proteins | NS | **INA**↓; CLTC↓; VCAN↓; **FSCN1**↑; **GSN**↓; **NEFL**↓; HAPLN2↓; **NEFM**↓; **NEFH**↑; **TUBA1A**↓; **TUBA4A**↓; **TUBB2B**↓; **TUBB4B**↑; **TUBB3**↑; **TUBB6**↑;**STMN1**↑; **VIM**↑; **CNP**↓; **ENO1/2**↑; **ATP5A1**↓; **ALDOA**↓; GLUD1↑; **GAPDH**↓; PYGB↓; PYGM↓; CRYL1↓; **MDH1**↓; **PRDX1**↓; **PKM**↑; **SOD1**↓; **TPI1**↓; **HINT1**↑; **MOG**↓; **YWHAB/H/Z/G**↓; **CRYAB**↓; **HSPA6**↑; **UBE2N**↑; **MBP**↓; **ATP6V1B2**↑; | Cell growth and maintenance, energy metabolism, cell communication and signaling, protein metabolism, transport and myelination | 9 schizophrenia patients and 7 healthy controls | Label-free nano LC-MS/MS | Saia-Cereda et al., 2015 |
| Targeted one protein expression | NS | S100B↓ | Disturbed oligodendrocyte maturation | 9 schizophrenia patients and 7 healthy controls | 2-D nano LC/MS Western blot | Steiner et al., 2014 |
| **TEMPORAL LOBE** | | | | | | |
| 25 proteins | 22 (left posterior superior-Wernicke's area) | **CKB**↑; **ALDOC**↓; **TPI1**↑; **GAPDH**↓; **PGAM1**↑; **ENO2**↑; **ATP6V1A**↑; **ATP5A1**↓; **QDPR**↑; **PRDX6**↑; **GFAP**↑; **PEBP1**↑; **ACO2**↑; **TUBB**↓ | Energy metabolism, glycolysis | 9 schizophrenia patients and 6 healthy controls | 2-D PAGE/MS | Martins-de-Souza et al., 2009b |
| 37 proteins | 38 (left anterior) | **MOG**↓; **MBP**↓; **GFAP**↓; **UBE2N**↓; **CNP**↓; PPP3CA↓; **SPTAN1**↓, **YWHAH**↓; **YWHAZ**↓; **YWHAG**↓; **ALDOC**↓; HIST1H3A↓; CA2↓; RPS10↓; SLC9A3R1↑; **TUBB**↑; **NEFL**↓; **NEFM**↓ | Oligodendrocyte-myelin regulated proteins, regulation Ca2+ homeostasis, energy metabolism | 5 schizophrenia patients and 4 healthy controls | ICPL /IEF/LC-MALDI | Martins-de-Souza et al., 2009d |

*(Continued)*

**TABLE 1 | Continued**

| Number of proteins with altered abundances | Brain region (BA)** | Some of the proteins with altered abundances in schizophrenia compared to controls* | Processes and pathways affected | Study design | Method | References |
|---|---|---|---|---|---|---|
| **HIPPOCAMPUS** | | | | | | |
| 34 proteins | anterior and posterior | Anterior (**CKB**↓; **ATP5H**↑; **LDHB**↓; NME1↑; COX5A↑; COX6B1↓; **PRDX2**↓; **PRDX6**↓; **SOD1**↓; **UBE2N**↑; PHB↑; HSPA1B↓; HSPA9↓; **ACTB**↓; **VIM**↑; **NEFM**↓; **STMN1**↑; FABP7↓; **YWHAZ**↑; **YWHAG**↑; **YWHAE**↑; **ANXA5**↑; **ATP6V1A**↓) Posterior (**PGAM1**↑; **CKB**↑; TALDO1↑; **GSN**↑; **ACTB**↑; **TUBA1**↓; **TUBB4**↓; **STMN1**↑) | Energy metabolism, oxidative stress, altered neurotransmission, mitochondrial dysfunction, abnormal neuronal and glial cytoarchitecture | Anterior hippocampus (7 schizophrenia patients and 7 controls) Posterior hippocampus (9 schizophrenia patients and 9 controls) | 2-D PAGE/MS | Nesvaderani et al., 2009 |
| 108 proteins | mid | **GFAP**↓; **HSPA8**↓; CTSD↑; **STMN1**↑; **SOD1**↑; **DPYSL3**↓; **NEFL**↓; **FSCN1**↓; **ANXA6**↓; **TUB**↑; SEPT11↓; SNCA↓; **ATP6V1B2**↓; **ENO1**↓; **YWHAE**↓; PCMT1↓; **SPTAN1**↓; **PRDX1**↓; | cytoskeletal and metabolic changes, clathrin-mediated endocytosis | 20 subjects with schizophrenia, 20 subjects with bipolar disorder, and 20 control cases | 2-D DIGE/MS | Föcking et al., 2011 |
| **MEDIODORSAL THALAMUS** | | | | | | |
| 10 proteins (2-D) 41 proteins (shotgun) | NS | TKT↑; **GSTP1**↑; **PGAM1**↑; **GAPDH**↑; **QDPR**↑; **TPI1**↑; **YWHAZ**↓; **CFL1**↑; **MBP**↑; **MOG**↑; **NEFM**↓; PRKCG↑; **GFAP**↓; **HSPA8**↓; **VIM**↑; **HSPA1A**↑; **ACT**↑; **GLUL**↑; **MAP1A**↑; MAPT↓; SYT5↑; SYN3↑; SEPT2↓ | Energy metabolism, oligodendrocyte metabolism, cytoskeleton assembly | Samples from 11 schizophrenia patients and 8 controls | 2-D PAGE/MS ICPL/IEF/LC-MALDI | Martins-de-Souza et al., 2010a |
| Targeted one protein expression | NS | **HINT1**↑ | May have role in cellular stress and apoptosis | 11 schizophrenia patients and 8 controls | Western blot | Varadarajulu et al., 2012 |

*Proteins found in more than one independent study are highlighted in bold. The arrows indicate the increase (↑) or decrease (↓) of the protein level in the schizophrenia group compared to control group(s). **Brodmann area. NS, Brodmann area not specified or not applicable.*

of hydrophobic (membrane) proteins, high molecular weight proteins (Mw > 100 kDa), and highly acidic (pI < 3), or basic (pI > 9) proteins. Another important drawback is the limitation of the dynamic range of detection, as highly abundant proteins typically mask the identification of less abundant proteins with similar pI and MW. However, efforts to overcome these limitations are improving resolution (Butt and Coorssen, 2005) and increasing dynamic range (Wright et al., 2014a,b).

"Shotgun" proteomic techniques do not employ gels and are aimed to touch all possible targets at once. These are powerful tools for studying large-scale protein expression and characterization of complex biological systems. Shotgun methods begin with digestion of the whole proteome of interest, followed by high resolution separation of the resultant peptides by liquid chromatography (LC) and their identification based on tandem mass spectrometry (MS/MS) data; (Link et al., 1999). Increased resolution can be achieved by including pre-fractionation steps prior to LC-MS/MS. Pre-fractionation methods can include other types of chromatography (e.g., affinity chromatography), initial separation by isoelectric focusing (IEF), or one dimensional sodium dodecyl sulfate PAGE (1-D SDS PAGE). In the case of IEF and 1-D SDS PAGE, gels are divided into a number of pieces, and each piece is subjected to digestion and subsequent LC-MS/MS. IEF pre-fractionation has been used in 3 published studies of schizophrenia, and 1-D SDS PAGE pre-fractionation in one (Behan et al., 2009; Martins-de-Souza et al., 2009c,d, 2010b). In addition, the number of protein identifications can be increased by using two-dimensional liquid chromatography (2-D nano-LC), which has been done on postmortem brain tissue (Steiner et al., 2014). In shotgun proteomics, protein identification relies strongly on computational resources that combine and interpret data generated by MS/MS (Haas et al., 2006). The quantification of proteins in a shotgun-MS comparative analysis can be based on labeled or unlabeled peptides. Labeling methods used in schizophrenia proteomics studies include stable isotope labeling methods, such as isobaric tags for relative and absolute concentration (iTRAQ) and isotope-coded protein labeling (ICPL). However, most labeling-based quantification approaches have potential limitations, such as increased time and complexity of sample preparation, requirement for higher sample concentration, high cost of the reagents, incomplete labeling, requirement for specific quantification software, and a limited number of samples (2–8) per analysis. Most of these limitations, especially limits on number of samples, are eliminated in label-free approaches (Patel et al., 2009). The quantification in label-free proteomics is based on the theoretical assumption that the chromatographic peak areas of peptides correlate with their concentrations. Label-free proteomics analysis can be data-dependent (DDA; Stahl et al., 1996) or data-independent ($MS^E$; Li et al., 2009), based on the selection of the peptide peaks for identification. In schizophrenia studies, $MS^E$ has been used in several studies of peripheral tissues and body fluids (reviewed below) and is preferred over DDA because of the higher percentage of protein identifications and higher coverage of the proteome (Geromanos et al., 2009). $MS^E$ was used to identify a serum biomarker panel capable of distinguishing first-onset drug-naive schizophrenia subjects from healthy subjects. This final panel was validated by immunoassay and later adapted into the multiplex immunoassay platform (MAP) leading to the first blood-based laboratory test for schizophrenia (Schwarz et al., 2010).

The strengths of the shotgun approach are experimental simplicity, greater proteomic coverage than gel-based platforms, and accurate quantification. Its weaknesses involve technical reproducibility, limited dynamic range, and informatics challenges related to the enormous complexity of the generated peptide samples (Domon and Aebersold, 2006). In addition, this approach cannot identify proteins with multiple modifications because the connection between the peptides that are analyzed in the mass spectrometer and the protein(s) from which the peptides originate is lost during proteolysis.

Surface-enhanced laser desorption/ionization time-of-flight mass spectrometry (SELDI-TOF-MS) has also been applied in the study of schizophrenia. SELDI-TOF is a variant MALDI-TOF that makes use of chemically-modified surfaces to reduce the complexity of biological samples prior to separation in the mass analyzer. Its invention increased interest in using patterns from mass spectra to differentiate samples with and without disease (Wright, 2002). SELDI provided several important advantages, such as ability to analyze complex biological samples with minimal pre-processing, ease of handling, and high throughput. However, over time, its lack of definitive protein identification and low reproducibility, influenced mainly by sample processing (Baggerly et al., 2004), became evident, and it is now used only rarely. There are several SELDI-TOF-MS schizophrenia studies of brain tissue and body fluids that appeared a decade ago, with and without identification of the affected proteins (Huang et al., 2006, 2008; Mei et al., 2006; Novikova et al., 2006; Craddock et al., 2008).

While all the proteomics platforms discussed have their strengths and weaknesses, it is becoming more widely accepted that combinations of different proteomics methods can take advantage of each method to increase the number of identified and quantified proteins, to detect and characterize PTMs and to increase statistical significance of the results. So far, schizophrenia studies combining 2-D PAGE or 2-D DIGE with shotgun proteomics are limited to one study of brain tissue (Behan et al., 2009), one study of both brain tissue and cerebrospinal fluid (Martins-de-Souza et al., 2010a) and one study of post-mortem pituitary glands (Krishnamurthy et al., 2013). However, as the growing number of studies demonstrate the power of combining these two platforms, it seems that a combination of gel-based and shotgun proteomics will be the best route to an understanding of the biological pathways of schizophrenia and to the discovery of reliable biomarkers for diagnosis, stratification and therapy.

Combinations of proteomics techniques other than gel-based and shotgun proteomics reportedly result in high confidence biomarker discovery. MALDI mass spectrometric imaging (MSI), combined with high resolution top-down tandem MS identification, has been used for the discovery of biomarkers for neurodevelopment disorders (Ye et al., 2014) but has not yet been used to study schizophrenia. MALDI MSI is a relatively new imagining technique that is label-free and enables simultaneous mapping of proteins and numerous molecules in tissue samples with great sensitivity and chemical specificity (Seeley and Caprioli, 2008). It has enabled discovery of tissue biomarkers for various cancers. The top-down tandem MS approach differs from the shotgun approach by directly analyzing intact proteins and allowing assessment of protein modifications, such as PTMs and sequence variants, with no prior knowledge (Kelleher, 2004; Michalski et al., 2012). This combination is reported to be fast and robust, and it has provided highly reproducible proteome "snapshots" of anatomical regions in sections of infant rat brain. It has high potential for future studies in schizophrenia.

## CANDIDATE PROTEINS IMPLICATED IN SCHIZOPHRENIA

### Tissue Biomarkers

As schizophrenia is presumably a brain disease, the comparative proteomic analysis of human postmortem brain tissue is of highest interest as it may reveal the disease-related proteins. This may help in the understanding the molecular mechanisms of the disease and in addition indicate potential biomarkers as candidates for diagnosis, prognosis, and therapy.

We have found 25 published articles on the proteomics of human brain tissue in schizophrenia. These studies investigated the relationship between schizophrenia and the protein profiles of six distinct brain regions: frontal or prefrontal cortex, anterior cingulate cortex, corpus callosum, temporal lobe neocortex, hippocampus, and mediodorsal thalamus. Detailed review of these studies regarding the study design, brain regions, number of identified proteins with altered abundancies, some of the candidate biomarker proteins, affected pathways in relation to schizophrenia and proteomics platforms used, are given in **Table 1**.

The most extensively studied brain region by proteomics studies is prefrontal cortex (PFC). The primary functions of PFC include the organization of thoughts and actions (cognitive control) such as willed action, decision making, and working memory (Frith and Dolan, 1996; Miller and Cohen, 2001). Individuals with schizophrenia exhibit poor working memory (Park and Holzman, 1992), abnormal eye movements (Park and Holzman, 1993), and abnormal executive functioning (Velligan and Bow-Thomas, 1999). Well-known abnormalities of dorsolateral (DL) PFC reported in schizophrenia include failure to activate during the Wisconsin card-sorting test (Daniel et al., 1991), decreased expression of calcium-binding proteins and glutamic acid decarboxylase in interneurons (Hashimoto et al., 2003), decreased density of spines on pyramidal cell dendrites (Glantz and Lewis, 2000), and decreased cortical volume without loss of neurons (Selemon et al., 1995).

The first proteomics study of schizophrenia (Johnston-Wilson et al., 2000) used 2-D PAGE/MS to compare PFC, specifically Brodmann area (BA) 10, of *post mortem* human brains from individuals with schizophrenia, individuals with other psychiatric disorders, and "controls" (i.e., individuals who died without history of psychiatric disorder). Half of the published proteomics studies on schizophrenia so far have investigated the PFC, mostly dorsolateral PFC (Brodmann areas 9 and 46; Prabakaran et al., 2004; Mei et al., 2006; Novikova et al., 2006; Huang et al., 2008; Pennington et al., 2008; Smalla et al., 2008; Behan et al., 2009; English et al., 2009; Martins-de-Souza et al., 2009a,c; Varadarajulu et al., 2012). Different proteomics platforms were used, mostly gel-based platforms (2-D PAGE/2-D DIGE) followed by shotgun proteomics or SELDI-TOF-MS. Western blot was used for targeted analysis of particular proteins of interest or validation of selected candidates.

The anterior cingulate cortex (ACC) is involved in emotion and behavior (Luu and Posner, 2003). The association between ACC and schizophrenia was based on abnormal activation of the ACC during hallucinations (Cleghorn et al., 1990) and task performances (Carter et al., 1997; Quintana et al., 2004) and on histological abnormalities (Benes et al., 2001; Bouras et al., 2001; Chana et al., 2003; Salgado-Pineda et al., 2003). The differential protein expression between schizophrenia and non-psychiatric groups was investigated in 4 studies using 2-D PAGE/MS (Beasley et al., 2006; Clark et al., 2006, 2007; Martins-de-Souza et al., 2010b) and one recent study using LC-MS/MS to study expression of proteins in postsynaptic densities (Föcking et al., 2015).

Neuropathological and neuroimaging studies have repeatedly reported structural abnormalities of the corpus callosum (CC) in schizophrenia, such as smaller volume, poor structural integrity of the axonal fiber tracts, and decrease in density of axons (Shenton et al., 2001; Mehler and Warnke, 2002; Innocenti et al., 2003). CC has been investigated by two comparative proteomics studies using 2-D PAGE/MS (Sivagnanasundaram et al., 2007), and LC-MS (Saia-Cereda et al., 2015), respectively. There is one more proteomics study of corpus callosum (Steiner et al., 2014), which used targeted 2-D nano LC/MS and western blot, to analyze S100B protein. In temporal lobe (TL) neocortex, Wernicke's area (posterior region of Brodmann area 22) and left temporal pole (Brodmann area 38) have been implicated in the pathophysiology of schizophrenia because of their roles in speech, language, and communication. There are two comparative proteome analyses of these brain regions, performed by 2-D PAGE/MS and shotgun proteomics (Martins-de-Souza et al., 2009b,d).

Hippocampus and mediodorsal thalamus (MDT) are both areas of interest in schizophrenia where early studies reported structural abnormalities that were later called into question (Dwork, 1997; Romanski et al., 1997; Harrison and Eastwood, 2001) and were subsequently subjected to proteomics investigation. There are 2 comparative studies of hippocampus using gel-based proteomics (Nesvaderani et al., 2009; Föcking et al., 2011), 1 comparative study of MDT using combination of 2-D PAGE/MS and shotgun proteomics (Martins-de-Souza et al., 2010a), and one targeted analysis of specific protein expression in mediodorsal thalamus by Western blot (Varadarajulu et al., 2012).

What is common to all of the proteomics studies of brain tissue is that, regardless of the platform and brain region analyzed, there has been constantly observed alteration of energy metabolism expressed as disturbed levels of proteins included in glycolysis, Krebs cycle, mitochondrial function, oxidative stress, and various other energy pathways. Abnormalities of proteins mediating synaptic function and signal transduction were also observed.

The central pathway for energy metabolism is glycolysis. Proteome analyses of different brain regions from individuals with schizophrenia have consistently revealed a number of differentially expressed glycolytic enzymes, as shown in **Table 1**. Aldolase C and A (ALDOC/A), have been found with differential abundance in 13 proteomics studies investigating FC, PFC, ACC, CC, and TL. Alpha and gamma enolase (ENO1/2) were found with differential abundance in 8 studies of PFC, CC, TL, and hippocampus. Glyceraldehyde-3-phosphate dehydrogenase (GAPDH), triosephosphate isomerase (TPI1), and phosphoglycerate mutase 1 (PGAM1) were also found with differential abundance in all of the investigated brain regions except FC, while dysregulation of hexokinase (HK1) was observed in two studies of PFC. Dysregulation of lactate dehydrogenase complex (LDHA/B), which reduces pyruvate into lactate and represents the intersection of key pathways of energy metabolism, was observed in 3 studies analyzing ACC, CC, and hippocampus.

Dysregulation of the Krebs cycle has also been implicated in schizophrenia as a result of differential abundance of several involved enzymes: such as aconitase 2 (ACO2), malate dehydrogenase 1 (MDH1), and citrate synthase (CS). The dysregulation of these enzymes was mainly observed in the ACC, 2 studies of PFC, and 2 studies of CC and TL.

Dysregulation of different ATP synthase subunits, such as ATP5A1, ATP5B, and ATP5H in PFC, ACC, CC, TL, and hippocampus suggests abnormalities of mitochondrial function. Overall dysregulation of energy metabolism leads, among other consequences, to overproduction of reactive oxygen species (ROS) and oxidative stress. Oxidative stress events present in schizophrenia and have been identified on a proteomic level through dysregulation of several groups of enzymes, mainly peroxiredoxins (PRDXs), glutathione transferases (GST), NADPH-dependent oxidoreductases, and antioxidant enzymes.

The most prominent dysregulation was observed at peroxiredoxins (PRDX1, 2, 3, 6) found with differential abundancies in 11 proteomics studies and in all investigated brain regions except MDT. Glutathione S-transferase P (GSTP1), carbonyl reductase 1 (CBR1), quinoid dihydropteridine reductase (QDPR), and antioxidant enzyme superoxide dismutase (SOD1) were also found with differential abundances in several studies and various brain regions, but not in FC and PFC. From the proteins involved in other energy pathways, vacuolar ATP synthases (ATP6V1A, ATP6V1B2, ATP6V0A1) and creatine kinase (CKB) were consistently found with differential abundance in all of the investigated brain regions of schizophrenia patients. The rest of the proteins from this group (glutamine synthase [GLUL], transketolase [TKT], and carbonic anhydrase 1 and 2 [CA1/2]) were found with differential abundance in some brain regions, as presented in **Table 1**.

As with the proteins involved in energy metabolism, proteomics studies of the brain tissue consistently revealed changes in the abundance of some of the cytoskeletal components of the cell. These encompassed 4 major components: (1) microfilaments composed of actin, (2) microtubules composed of tubulin, (3) intermediate filaments, which are a family of about 70 different proteins, and (4) microtubule associated proteins. Differential abundance of beta and gamma actin isoforms was observed in 8 studies, including three studies of dorsolateral PFC, while the others included all other investigated brain areas. Alpha and beta tubulins were also found with differential abundance in 12 independent studies, mainly in PFC, ACC, CC, and hippocampus. There were 5 intermediate filament proteins with disturbed abundance in schizophrenia: desmin (DES), vimentin (VIM), glial fibrillary acidic protein (GFAP), and neurofilament medium and light chains (NEFM and NEFL). The most prominent change inivolved neurofilament proteins, observed in 11 studies, followed by GAFP in 9 studies, and in all investigated brain regions. Disturbed levels of VIM and DES were observed less frequently, in 5 (English et al., 2009; Martins-de-Souza et al., 2009c, 2010b; Nesvaderani et al., 2009; Saia-Cereda et al., 2015) and 1 study (Martins-de-Souza et al., 2009c), respectively. Microtubule-associated proteins (MAPs) with differential abundance in schizophrenia encompassed microtubule-associated proteins 1A (MAP1A), 2 (MAP2), and tau (MAPT), and dynamin 1 (DNM1). The differential abundance of these proteins was observed at lower rates than were other cytoskeletal proteins. Changed levels of DNM1 were found in 5 studies of which 3 assayed PFC (Prabakaran et al., 2004; Pennington et al., 2008; Martins-de-Souza et al., 2009a) and 2 assayed ACC (Clark et al., 2006; Föcking et al., 2015), while MAP1A and MAPT were found in only 2 studies, 1 of PFC (also including MAP2) and 1 of MDT (Martins-de-Souza et al., 2009c, 2010b).

Cytoskeleton associated proteins dihydropyrimidinase-related protein 2 (DPYSL2), 14-3-3 protein family (YWHAE, YWHAZ, YWHAG, YWHAH, YWHAB), spectrin (SPTAN1), stathmin (STMN1), and various representatives from the heat shock proteins (HSPD1, HSPA5, HSPA8, HSPA1L, HSPA1A, HSPA1B) were detected with abnormal abundance in more than 5 independent studies, providing further support for cytoskeletal dysfunction in schizophrenia.

Oligodendrocyte dysfunction in schizophrenia has been suggested by brain imaging, epigenetic and transcriptomics studies, discussed in detail elsewhere (Dwork et al., 2007; Martins-de-Souza, 2010; Haroutunian et al., 2014). Six proteomics studies from 2 independent groups so far have found altered expression of some of the oligodendrocyte-related proteins in schizoprenia brain tissues such as 2′,3′-cyclic nucleotide 3′-phosphodiesterase (CNP), myelin basic protein (MBP), myelin oligodendrocyte glycoprotein (MOG), and gelsolin (GSN; Prabakaran et al., 2004; Martins-de-Souza et al., 2009a,c,d, 2010b; Saia-Cereda et al., 2015). We found 5 proteomics studies focused on white matter. Three (Sivagnanasundaram et al., 2007; Steiner et al., 2014; Saia-Cereda et al., 2015) examined corpus callosum. One (Steiner et al., 2014) was focused on S100B, reportedly elevated in blood and CSF of individuals with schizophrenia, and found a decrease of 50–70% by mass spectroscopy and western blot. The more recent (Saia-Cereda et al., 2015) of the other two studies, employing label-free nano LC/MS/MS, identified downregulation of CNP, MBP, MOG, and GSN, while they were not found to be abnormal in the older study (Sivagnanasundaram et al., 2007), which employed 2-D PAGE/MS. Proteins involved in filaments and microtubules were abundantly represented in the results from both studies, although fiber densities in the corpus callosum have mostly been found unaffected by schizophrenia (reviewed in Dwork et al., 2007). The other two proteomics studies analyzed post mortem white matter from PFC (English et al., 2009) and ACC (Clark et al., 2007). Both found reduced levels of ALDOC in schizophrenia. Among myelin-related proteins, the only change in schizophrenia was upregulation of PLP1 in prefrontal white matter. In contrast, *in situ* hybridization of ACC white matter showed downregulation of mRNA for CNP and MAG in schizophrenia (McCullumsmith et al., 2007). In a targeted study (Dracheva et al., 2006), western blot for CNP showed decreased levels in the hippocampus but not the putamen from individuals with schizophrenia.

One study (Krishnamurthy et al., 2013; included in **Table 2**) employed several platforms to study pituitary gland from autopsies of individuals with schizophrenia or without psychiatric illness. The pituitary glands from subjects with schizophrenia showed disturbance in hypothalamic- pituitary-adrenal axis, immune system, lipid transport, and metabolism. By LC-$MS^E$, prolactin was significantly lower, by approximately 35% in pituitary from chronically medicated individuals with schizophrenia, suggesting that despite antipsychotic medication, prolactin production was suppressed by elevated dopamine. While the same average difference was found by western blot, for schizophrenia and bipolar disorder as well, the differences from normal were not significant. By contrast, western blot gave virtually identical levels for follicle stimulating hormone across all diagnostic groups.

## Body Fluids Biomarkers

The comparative proteomics analysis of body fluids is of highest clinical interest as it may reveal biomarkers for diagnosis,

**TABLE 2 | Candidate protein biomarkers for schizophrenia obtained by proteomics studies using human body fluids and tissues other than brain.**

| Number of proteins with altered abundances | Body fluid | Candidate biomarkers | Processes and pathways affected | Study design | Method | References |
|---|---|---|---|---|---|---|
| 1 | CSF | **APOA4**↓ | Reverse cholesterol transport | 10 controls and 10 schizophrenia patients were pooled to form four pools for each group | 2-D PAGE/MS | Jiang et al., 2003 |
| 2 | CSF | VGF 23-62 peptide↑; **TTR**↓ | Synaptic plasticity, penile erection, circadian clock, thyroid hormone binding | 58 schizophrenia, 16 with depression, 5 with obsessive-compulsive disorder, 10 with Alzheimer disease and 90 controls | SELDI-TOF-MS | Huang et al., 2006 |
| 1 | CSF | **APOA1**↓ | Plasma cholesterol esters formation | CSF: 41 vs. 40; liver:15 vs. 15; RBC: 20 vs. 20; serum: 35 vs. 63; brain 1st exp: 8 vs. 8; brain 2nd exp: 9 vs. 9 | SELDI-TOF-MS | Huang et al., 2008 |
| 6 | CSF | **APOE**↑; **APOA1**↑; **TTR**↓; TGFBR1↓; CCDC3↓; PTGDS↑ | Molecular transport, signal transduction receptors | 17 first episode schizophrenia and 10 controls | Western blot | Martins-De-Souza et al., 2010c |
| 7 | plasma | **HP**↑; **SERPINA1**↑; **CFB**↑; **APOA1**↓; **APOA4**↑; **TTR**↓ | Acute phase proteins, molecular transport | 22 schizophrenia patients and 20 controls | 2-D PAGE/MS | Yang et al., 2006 |
| 6 | plasma | **HP**↑; **SERPINA1**↑; **APCS**↑; **AMBP**↑; SERPINC1↑; GC↑ | Acute phase, coagulation and transport | 42 schizophrenia patients and 46 healthy controls | 2-D PAGE/MS | Wan et al., 2007 |
| 1 | plasma | α-defensins (**DEFA**) ↑ | Dysregulation of immune pathway of peripheral white blood cells | T cell lysates from 15 schizophrenia and 15 controls | SELDI-TOF-MS | Craddock et al., 2008 |
| 79 | plasma | BDNF↑; EGF↑; CXCL5↑; TIMP1↑; **MMP9**↑; **Insulin**↑ | Synaptic transmission, growth factors, chemo-attractants, proteolytic system | 245 major depressive disorder, 229 schizophrenia and 254 controls | Multiplexed immunoassay | Domenici et al., 2010 |
| 10 | serum | **CD5L**↓; **IGHM**↓; F13B↓; TF↓; **AHSG**↓; APOD↓; **APOA1**↓; **APOA4**↓; **APOA2**↓; **APOC1**↓ | Lipid metabolism, cholesterol transport pathway, immune response | 22 first onset schizophrenia patients and 33 matched controls | Label-free nano LC-MS/MS ($MS^E$) | Levin et al., 2010 |
| 181 tested | serum | 51 biomarker panel | Diverse protein functions | 577 schizophrenia patients and 229 controls | Multiplexed immunoassay | Schwarz et al., 2010 |
| 21 tested (7 selected) | serum | **Insulin** ↑; **CHGA**↑; PPY↑; PRL↑; Cortisol↑; GH1↓; Progesterone↑;**prolactin**↑ growth hormone↓ | Dysregulation of glucose metabolism, hypothalamic-pituitary-adrenalgonadal axis hormones | 236 first and recent onset schizophrenia patients and 230 matched controls | Multiplex immunoassay; 2D-DIGE | Guest et al., 2011 |
| 181 tested | serum | 34 biomarker panel | Diverse protein functions | 250 first and recent onset schizophrenia, 35 major depressive disorder, 32 bipolar disorder, 45 Asperger syndrome and 280 control subjects | Multiplexed immunoassay | Schwarz et al., 2012a |

*(Continued)*

**TABLE 2 | Continued**

| Number of proteins with altered abundances | Body fluid | Candidate biomarkers | Processes and pathways affected | Study design | Method | References |
|---|---|---|---|---|---|---|
| 20 | serum | SPP1↓; CALB1↑; CTGF↑; TBG↑; **APOA1**↑; APOB↑; **CHGA**↑; **AMBP**↓; IL6R↓; IL17↓; **CD5L**↑; **PROS1**↑; **APCS**↑; CA125↓; TFF3↓; GOT1↓; **HGF**↓ | Inflammation and immune response | 75 schizophrenia, 110 bipolar disorder patients and their matched controls (75+110) | Multiplexed immunoassay | Schwarz et al., 2012b |
| 191 tested | serum | Symptom severity (FABP5; **CKB**; MB; CRP; MMP9; **HGF**) Response prediction (**insulin**) Time to relapse (LEP↓; **proinsulin** ↓; TGFA↑; **CD5L**↓; B2M↓; **MMP9**↑; CD40↓; **APOC1**↓) | Acute phase response pathway, transport, immune response, glucose metabolic pathways | 77 schizophrenia patients were analyzed to identify molecules associated with symptom severity, predict response over a 6-week treatment period and predict the time to relapse | Multiplexed immunoassay | Schwarz et al., 2012c |
| 35 (additional 59 with only phosporilation pattern changes) | serum | Altered abundance and phosphorylation: ALS2↑; MAST1↑; **CFB**↑; C4BPA↑; CFHR3↑; C6↑; ITIH3↑; **APOA1**↓; MYOF↓; **APOA2**↓; CCDC57↓; SMC1A↓; GPLD1↓ | Acute phase response signaling pathway, Complement system, LXR/RXR activation, Coagulation system, Intristic prothrombin activation pathway | 20 antipsychotic-naïve schizophrenia patients and 20 matched healthy controls | IMAC/LC-MS/MS ($MS^E$) | Jaros et al., 2012 |
| 27 | serum | ANPEP↓; APOC2↓;APOF↓; APOL1↓; C4BPB↓; C8B↑; **CD5L**↑; DBH↑; F7↓; GGH↓; ICAM2↓; IGFALS↓; IGHG4↑; SERPINA5↑; **IGHM**↑; ITIH4↑; KNG1↑; LBP↓; PGLYRP2↑; PI16↑; PLTP↑; **PROS1**↓; ZNF57↓ | Complement system, coagulation cascades | 10 antipsychotic drug- naïve schizophrenia patients and 10 healthy volunteers | LC-MS/MS | Li et al., 2012 |
| 23 immune molecules and 30 growth factors and hormones | serum | group 1 (MIF, CXCL8, IL1RN, IL18, and IL16) group 2 (**prolactin**, resistin, testosterone, **insulin**, PDGFRA, LEPROT, and AGT) | Identified 2 subgroups of schizophrenia patients based on molecular serum profiles. Group 1 had changes in immune molecules, and group 2 changes in growth factors and hormones | 180 antipsychotic-naive schizophrenia patients and 398 matched controls | Multiplexed immunoassay | Schwarz et al., 2014 |
| 5 | blood | **Insulin**↑; **proinsulin**↑; des-31,32-proinsulin↑; C-peptide↑; **CHGA**↑ | Dysregulation of glucose metabolic pathways | 66 schizophrenia, 10 bipolar and 78 matched controls | Fluorescence assays and immunoassays | Guest et al., 2010 |
| 17 validated by MRM/MS | sweat | AZGP1↑; ANXA5↑; TXN↑; ARG2↑; BLMH↑; CDSN↑; CALML5↑; CASP14↑; **CSTA**↑; DSG↑; PARK7↑; G3PDH↑; KLK11↑; PSBP1↑; S100A7↑; **PRDX1**↑; PIP↓ | Oxidative stress, lipid metabolism, Ca and others binding proteins, epidermal differentiation and integrity, proteinase inhibitors, cell-cell adhesion, glycolysis | The first set was made by pooling of 8 patients samples and 8 controls. The second set was made by pooling of 4 patients and 4 controls | LC–MS/MS; MRM/MS | Raiszadeh et al., 2012 |

(Continued)

**TABLE 2 | Continued**

| Number of proteins with altered abundances | Body fluid | Candidate biomarkers | Processes and pathways affected | Study design | Method | References |
|---|---|---|---|---|---|---|
| 8 | saliva | **DEFA1-4**↑; S100A12↑; **CSTA**↑; S-derivatives of CSTB↑ | Dysregulation of immune pathway of peripheral white blood cells | 32 schizophrenia, 17 bipolar and 31 healthy controls | RP-HPLC–ESI-MS (top-down) | Iavarone et al., 2014 |
| 18 | peripheral blood mononuclear cells (PBMCs) | Unstimulated PBMCs (CNDP2↑; COTL1↓; GPI↓; **HSPA2**↓; **LDHB**↑) Stimulated PBMCs (**ALDOC**↑; **HSPD1**↓; **GAPDH**↑; HNRPK↑; **LDHB**↑; NAMPT↑; MYH14/15↑; **PGK1**↑; PPIA↑; **TPI1**↑; PKLR↑; PGAM4↑) | Dysregulation of glucolytic pathway | 12 first onset schizophrenia patients, 7 chronically ill antipsychotic treated schizophrenia patients and 19 healthy controls | Label-free nano LC-MS/MS ($MS^E$) | Herberth et al., 2011 |
| 29 (LC-$MS^E$) 13 (2-D DIGE) | pituitary gland | LC-$MS^E$ (SIPA1↑; CEMIP↑; FGB↑; CFAP43↑; MYH9↑; HNRNPA2B↓TTC28↓; PIWIL3↓; **APOA1**↓; **APOA2**↓; **CKB**↓; **TUBA1A**↓; **TUBB1B**↓; **TUBB2C**↓; **AHSG**↓; TGM2↓; TUBB4B↓; LMX1B↓; CTNND2↓; YWHAQ↓; **HP**↓; **CRYM**↓; HSPB1↓; SCGN↓; SETD5↓; TIAM2↓; | Disturbance in hypothalamic–pituitary–adrenal axis, immune system, lipid transport and metabolism | 14 schizophrenia and 15 control subjects were analyzed by comparative proteomics. Additional 13 bipolar disorder and 14 major depression patients were included in Western validation | LC-MS/MS ($MS^E$) Multiplexed immunoassay, 2-D DIGE, Western blot | Krishnamurthy et al., 2013 |

*Candidate biomarkers found in more than one independent study are highlighted in bold. The arrows indicate the increase (↑) or decrease (↓) of the protein level in schizophrenia group compared to control group(s).*

choice of therapy and future course of schizophrenia. We found 20 proteomics studies investigating potential schizophrenia biomarkers in cerebrospinal fluid, blood, sweat, and saliva, and 2 additional studies investigating protein alterations in peripheral blood mononuclear cells (PBMCs) and the aforementioned study of pituitary gland (**Table 2**).

Cerebrospinal fluid (CSF) and blood are the main body fluids used in proteomic studies of neurological or psychiatric disorders, including schizophrenia. CSF is presumed to be representative of the extracellular space in the CNS. Consequently, pathological abnormalities of the brain might be directly reflected in CSF. Normal CSF protein concentrations are ~0.5% those of normal serum or plasma, requiring highly sensitive analytical techniques. Fewer proteins can normally be detected. CSF sampling is moderately invasive, so it is difficult to perform longitudinal studies. The first 2-D map of human CSF proteome was presented by Goldman and collaborators in 1980 (Goldman et al., 1980). With the development of proteomics technologies, different approaches were used for discovering CSF biomarkers for schizophrenia: 2-D PAGE and 2-D DIGE followed by MALDI-MS identification (Jiang et al., 2003; Martins-De-Souza et al., 2010c) and SELDI-MS (Huang et al., 2006, 2008). These studies revealed altered levels of proteins involved in molecular transport of cholesterol and of proteins involved in phospholipid metabolism [apolipoprotein A-I (APOA1), apolipoprotein A-IV (APOA4), and apolipoprotein E (APOE), 23-62 VGF peptide], transthyretin (TTR), arachidonic acid metabolism enzyme-prostaglandin-H2 D-isomerase (PTGDS), coiled-coil domain-containing protein 3 precursor (CCDC3), and transforming growth factor-β receptor type-1 (TGFBR1).

The major advantage of using blood for biomarker discovery arises from two main blood characteristics. With the exception of the urine, which usually contains no protein, blood is the most easily and least invasively sampled body fluid for clinical studies. This accessibility allows multiple samplings at various stages of the disease and treatment. Second, blood interacts with all tissues, and therefore can indicate changes anywhere in the body.

We found 14 proteomic studies investigating potential biomarkers in plasma and serum. The first 2 studies investigated the plasma proteome by 2-D PAGE coupled with MS. They revealed altered levels of acute phase response proteins (Yang et al., 2006; Wan et al., 2007), suggesting a link between inflammatory response systems and pathophysiology of schizophrenia. The affected proteins included haptoglobin (HP), α-1-antitrypsin (SERPINA1), complement factor B precursor (CFB), apolipoprotein A1 (APOA1), apolipoprotein A4 (APOA4), transthyretin (TTR), serum amyloid P-component (APCS), alpha-1-microglobulin (AMBP), and antithrombin III (SERPINC1). A study using a SELDI-TOF platform to analyze lysates of stimulated T lymphocytes found alterations of α-defensin (DEFA) in minimally medicated subjects with schizophrenia, and also in their monozygotic twins without schizophrenia (Craddock et al., 2008), suggesting a marker for susceptibility.

There are 3 studies of serum proteome so far using label-free LC-MS/MS. The first study of serum proteome found that the most significantly changed proteins belong to the apolipoprotein family (apolipoprotein D [APOD], apolipoprotein A1 [APOA1], apolipoprotein A4 [APOA4], apolipoprotein A2 [APOA2], and apolipoprotein C1 [APOC1]), involved in the metabolism of high-density lipoprotein and triglyceride-rich lipoproteins, and in the reverse cholesterol transport pathway. These were followed by proteins involved in immune response (CD5 molecule-like [CD5L], IgM [IGHM], transferrin [TF]) and in insulin resistance (α-2-HS glycoprotein [AHSG]; Levin et al., 2010). Subsequent studies (Jaros et al., 2012; Li et al., 2012) confirmed that subjects with schizophrenia feature serum abnormalities in levels and phosphorylation of proteins involved in immune response. These studies also implicated the complement and coagulation cascades as the most significant pathways disturbed in schizophrenia.

However, the majority of the studies on plasma and serum have used multiplexed immunoassays containing selected subsets of biomarkers, constructed based on the findings from previous discovery proteomics studies. The first attempt to develop a molecular test with clinical utility for diagnosis of schizophrenia resulted in formation of a 51-plex biomarker panel with sensitivity and specificity of 83% (Schwarz et al., 2010). The study of specificity of this panel for schizophrenia compared with other psychiatric disorders led to establishment of a reduced, 34-biomarker panel that gave a separation of 60–75% of schizophrenia subjects from controls across 5 independent cohorts (Schwarz et al., 2012a). In the most recent studies, the multiplexed immunoassay test was also investigated for the ability to identify the disease prior to clinical manifestation (Schwarz et al., 2012b) and to characterize subgroups of individuals with schizophrenia on the basis of the molecular pathways affected (Schwarz et al., 2014).

Several multiplex immunoassay studies identified elevated insulin-related peptides in untreated first-onset schizophrenia subjects, suggesting that dysregulation of glucose metabolic pathways may have a role in the development of schizophrenia (Guest et al., 2010, 2011; Schwarz et al., 2012c). Immune response alterations have also been observed by several studies (Schwarz et al., 2012b,c). Also, altered levels of hormones (prolactin, cortisol, progesterone, and growth hormone) in blood have been observed in people with schizophrenia, indicating that functions of multiple components of the hypothalamic-pituitary-adrenal-gonadal axis may be affected (Domenici et al., 2010; Guest et al., 2011).

There is only one report describing sweat proteome alteration in schizophrenia (Raiszadeh et al., 2012). The eccrine sweat glands, controlled by the sympathetic nervous system, are responsible for thermoregulation. Distributed over the entire body, they produce a fluid that is composed of inorganic ions, lactate, urea, ammonia, amino acids, and proteins, including plasma and epidermal proteins. The study of Raiszadeh et al. (2012) revealed 17 proteins with differential abundance of approximately two-fold or greater between schizophrenia and healthy subjects (listed in **Table 2**). These proteins involve diverse biological functions: oxidative stress, lipid metabolism, calcium-binding and other binding proteins, epidermal differentiation and integrity, protease inhibition, cell-cell adhesion, and glycolysis. The potential of sweat as a source for new schizophrenia biomarkers was highlighted, since only 5 proteins [albumin (ALB), alpha-2-glycoprotein 1 (AZGP1), clusterin isoform 1 (CLU), apolipoprotein D precursor (APOD), and gelsolin isoform b (GSN)] were found in common between sweat and serum.

Saliva allows non-invasive specimen collection, and it can sometimes be a good substitute for plasma or blood. Until now, only one study has investigated saliva as a potential source for schizophrenia and bipolar disease biomarkers using top down proteomics platform (RP-HPLC–ESI-MS; Iavarone et al., 2014). All significantly altered proteins and peptides were involved in innate immunity (α-defensins 1–4, S100A12, cystatin A and S-derivatives of cystatin B). However, as increased levels of these proteins were also found in association with neoplasms and infectious diseases, the authors concluded that this set of proteins has low diagnostic potential for schizophrenia.

One small study (Herberth et al., 2011) used LC-$MS^E$ to investigate the proteomes of PBMCs, at baseline and after 72 h of stimulation by staphylococcal enterotoxin and CD28. Cells from antipsychotic-naïve subjects in the first episode of schizophrenia, compared with cells from healthy subjects, showed altered levels of some glycolytic enzymes at rest, and more after stimulation, while these alterations were not seen in PBMC from individuals with chronic schizophrenia and antipsychotic treatment. Curiously, the post-stimulation levels of ALDOC were greater in the cells from anti-psychotic-naïve schizophrenia subjects than in the cells from healthy subjects, while there was no reported abnormality of ALDOA, which in PBMC is an order of magnitude more abundant than ALDOC, and two orders of magnitude more abundant than ALDOB (see: http://moped.proteinspire.org/; Kim et al., 2014; Montague et al., 2015). As discussed elsewhere in this review, in schizophrenia, ALDOC is the most frequently abnormally-expressed protein identified in proteomic studies of the brain, where its expression is predominantly astrocytic, but some studies of schizophrenia find elevated levels and others find depressed levels (see below and **Tables 1, 5**). An abnormal response of the C isoform in a cell that normally expresses predominantly the A isoform could point to a specific dysregulation of the C isoform in schizophrenia, but it could also indicate a general lability of the C isoform in the presence of independent abnormalities of glycolysis.

## THE SPECIFICITY OF THE CANDIDATE BIOMARKERS FOR SCHIZOPHRENIA

To evaluate the overlap of the schizophrenia-associated candidate biomarkers with candidate biomarkers for other neurological diseases, we reviewed proteomic studies and reviews of several diseases such as bipolar disorder, major depressive disorder, Alzheimer's disease and Parkinson's disease.

We found 5 proteomics studies where both schizophrenia and bipolar disorder were compared with a non-psychiatric group (Novikova et al., 2006; Pennington et al., 2008; Behan et al., 2009; English et al., 2009; Föcking et al., 2011). Pennington et al. (2008) found 6 out of 66 proteins to be altered in both diseases, with cytoskeleton and synaptic-associated function (two

**TABLE 3 | Proteins with differential abundance in schizophrenia reported as characteristic of individual cell types by transcriptional studies of mouse brain cells and mononuclear cells.**

| Gene | Cell type | Descriptive Group* | Citations** | | | | | | | | | | |
|---|---|---|---|---|---|---|---|---|---|---|---|---|---|
| ALDOC | astrocytes | C: 13/40; C: well-described; C: astrocyte-enriched | Martins-de-Souza et al., 2009d | Novikova et al., 2006 | Johnston-Wilson et al., 2000 | English et al., 2009 | Martins-de-Souza et al., 2009a | Prabakaran et al., 2004 | Smalla et al., 2008 | Clark et al., 2006 | Clark et al., 2007 | Martins-de-Souza et al., 2009b | Martins-De-Souza et al., 2010c |
| GFAP | astrocytes | C: 13/40; C: well-described; C: astrocyte-enriched | Martins-de-Souza et al., 2009d | Martins-de-Souza et al., 2010a | Johnston-Wilson et al., 2000 | Martins-de-Souza et al., 2009a | Pennington et al., 2008 | Clark et al., 2006 | Sivagnanasundaram et al., 2007 | Martins-de-Souza et al., 2009b | Föcking et al., 2011 | | |
| HIST1H3G | astrocytes | C: developmental | Martins-de-Souza et al., 2009d | | | | | | | | | | |
| HSPA1B | astrocytes | C: developmental | Nesvaderani et al., 2009 | | | | | | | | | | |
| PDE8B | astrocytes | C: developmental | English et al., 2009 | | | | | | | | | | |
| PYGM | astrocytes | C: developmental | Saia-Cereda et al., 2015 | | | | | | | | | | |
| SLC9A3R1 | astrocytes | C: astrocyte-enriched | Martins-de-Souza et al., 2009d | | | | | | | | | | |
| GNAQ | microglia | Y: MG-enriched | Smalla et al., 2008 | | | | | | | | | | |
| MAPK3 | microglia | Y: MG-enriched | Martins-de-Souza et al., 2010b | | | | | | | | | | |
| GAPDH | monocytes | Y: monocyte-enriched | Martins-de-Souza et al., 2009c | Martins-de-Souza et al., 2010a | Saia-Cereda et al., 2015 | Martins-de-Souza et al., 2009b | | | | | | | |
| PGK1 | monocytes | Y: monocyte-enriched | Martins-de-Souza et al., 2009a | | | | | | | | | | |
| NEFL | neurons | C: well-described; C: neuron-enriched | Martins-de-Souza et al., 2009d | English et al., 2009 | Martins-de-Souza et al., 2009a | Pennington et al., 2008 | Clark et al., 2007 | Saia-Cereda et al., 2015 | Sivagnanasundaram et al., 2007 | Föcking et al., 2011 | | | |
| NEFM | neurons | C: neuron-enriched | Martins-de-Souza et al., 2009d | Martins-de-Souza et al., 2010a | English et al., 2009 | Saia-Cereda et al., 2015 | Sivagnanasundaram et al., 2007 | Nesvaderani et al., 2009 | | | | | |
| CAMK2B | neurons | C: neuron-enriched | Martins-de-Souza et al., 2010b | | | | | | | | | | |
| GDA | neurons | C: 29/40; C: neuron-enriched | Pennington et al., 2008 | | | | | | | | | | |
| CNP | oligodendrocytes | C: oligodendrocyte-enriched | Martins-de-Souza et al., 2009c | Martins-de-Souza et al., 2009d | Prabakaran et al., 2004 | Saia-Cereda et al., 2015 | | | | | | | |
| MBP | oligodendrocytes | C: 27/40; C: well-described; C: oligodendrocyte-enriched C:developmental | Martins-de-Souza et al., 2009d | Martins-de-Souza et al., 2010a | Martins-de-Souza et al., 2009a | Saia-Cereda et al., 2015 | | | | | | | |
| MOG | oligodendrocytes | C: 2/40; C: well-described; C: oligodendrocyte-enriched; C: developmental | Martins-de-Souza et al., 2009c | Martins-de-Souza et al., 2009d | Martins-de-Souza et al., 2010a | Saia-Cereda et al., 2015 | | | | | | | |
| GSN | oligodendrocytes | C: 10/40; C: oligodendrocyte-enriched | Prabakaran et al., 2004 | Saia-Cereda et al., 2015 | Nesvaderani et al., 2009 | | | | | | | | |

*(Continued)*

**TABLE 3 | Continued**

| Gene | Cell type | Descriptive Group* | Citations** |
|---|---|---|---|
| HAPLN2 | oligodendrocytes | C: oligodendrocyte-enriched; C:developmental | Saia-Cereda et al., 2015 |
| MYO1D | oligodendrocytes | C: oligodendrocyte-enriched; C:developmental | Martins-de-Souza et al., 2009c |
| PLP1 | oligodendrocytes | C: 17/40; C: oligodendrocyte-enriched; C:developmental | English et al., 2009 |

*Descriptive Group refers to the heading of the table(s) from Cahoy et al. (2008) (C) or Yamasaki et al. (2014) (Y) in which the gene was listed.
[Number]/40 refers to the rank on the list of "Top 40" genes for that cell type. **Citations are the references for proteomic studies reporting that the protein is altered in schizophrenia.

forms of SEPT5, SEPT11, DPYSL3, TCP1), metabolism and CNS development (PHGDH). However, half of the proteins with altered abundance in bipolar disorder were cytoskeletal, metabolic or mitochondrial-associated proteins and some, such as TUBA, TUBB, NEFM, ATP5B, ENO2, PRDX2, PRDX6, ATP6V1A have been frequently found in schizophrenia studies (**Table 1**). Behan et al. (2009) identified three proteins involved in synapse-associated functions (LSAMP, BASP1, and STXBP1) while in a subsequent study from the same group (English et al., 2009), some intermediate filaments (NEFH, vimentin) and cytoskeleton-associated proteins (DPYSL2, DPYSL3, YWHAE) showed the same change in abundance in bipolar disorder as in schizophrenia. Novikova et al. (2006) found 5 proteins that were altered in both schizophrenia and bipolar disorder (CEBPZ, DECR2, BYSL, ANKARD, and ALDOC), associated with cell signaling, lipid and glucose metabolism, and other intracellular processes. The comparative proteomic analysis of hippocampus reported similar protein changes in schizophrenia and bipolar disorder with two-thirds of the proteins with altered abundances in schizophrenia showing the same trend in bipolar disorder as well (Föcking et al., 2011). These proteins were mostly involved in cytoskeletal and metabolic cellular mechanisms.

Two proteomic studies included major depressive disorder (MDD) in addition to schizophrenia and bipolar disorder. In one of the first proteomics studies of the brain, abundance of 3 proteins (DPYSL2, ALDOC, and GFAP) were altered in the frontal cortex in all three disorders (Johnston-Wilson et al., 2000). Altered levels of these proteins, associated with synaptic function, glycolysis, and cytoskeletal structure, respectively, were subsequently confirmed by most other proteomic studies of the brain in schizophrenia. A study of the protein changes in ACC in schizophrenia, MDD and bipolar disorder found that cytoskeletal and mitochondrial proteins are the most prominently altered in all of these disorders, but only 2 identified proteins (SRI, ALDOC) were found with changed levels in both schizophrenia and MDD (Beasley et al., 2006). The rest of the MDD - focused studies identified candidate biomarkers that to some extent overlap with those for schizophrenia (Martins-de-Souza, 2014). The biological functions implicated in MDD, such as energy metabolism, cellular transport, and cell communication and signaling are also the main pathways implicated in schizophrenia. However, several important differences that help in differentiation of these diseases on a protein level were observed: The disorders were associated with different pathways of energy metabolism (glycolysis is the main affected pathway in schizophrenia, while oxidative phosphorylation is more affected in MDD) and opposite changes of the same proteins were identified in both diseases (Martins-de-Souza et al., 2012a).

From the 93 proteins that have shown quantitative changes or modifications in 43 2-D based proteomic studies in 13 different brain regions in Alzheimer's disease between 1999 and 2010 (Korolainen et al., 2010), 34 proteins have been reported in schizophrenia brain proteomics studies as well. These 34 proteins point to the same disturbances in two major pathways: One is energy metabolism, especially glycolysis (ALDOA/C, ENO1/2, GAPDH, LDHB, PGAM1, PKM2, TPI1), Krebs cycle (ACO2, MDH1), mitochondrial function (ATP5A1, ATP5B), and oxidative stress (Piredoxins [PRDX2, 3, 6], SOD, CKB). The other pathway is cytoskeletal, through tubulins (TUBA1B, TUBA1C, TUBB), intermediate filaments (GFAP, NEFL,) cytoskeleton associated proteins (DPYSL2, YWHAE, YWHAG, STMN1,) and heat shock proteins (HSPA9, HSPA5, HSPD1, HSPA1A, HSPA2, HSPA8). Although the comparative proteomics studies of postmortem human brains from Parkinson's disease are quite limited, the reported proteins showed some overlap with schizophrenia in neurofilaments (NEFL, NEFM), peroxiredoxins, and proteins involved in ATP synthesis (Srivastava et al., 2010).

The majority of the blood-based candidate proteins for schizophrenia are also involved in Parkinson's disease, Alzheimer's disease, and MDD. Several acute phase proteins (A2M, C3, SERPINA1, and ALB), proposed as candidate biomarkers for schizophrenia, were also found to be associated with Parkinson's disease, Alzheimer's disease, and MDD (Chiam et al., 2015). In addition, APOE and APCS were associated with both Parkinson's disease and Alzheimer's disease.

From the proposed candidate cerebrospinal fluid biomarkers for schizophrenia (**Table 2**), APOA1, APOA4, APOE, and PTGDS have been also proposed as candidate biomarkers for Alzheimer's disease and TTR (synthesized in the brain uniquely by choroid plexus, Herbert et al., 1986) as a candidate biomarker for Parkinson's and Alzheimer's diseases (Korolainen et al., 2010; Kroksveen et al., 2011).

## CELL-SPECIFIC PROTEINS

Since different cells produce different proteins, one could look to proteomics for evidence of specific cell types affected in schizophrenia. We therefore compared the proteins in **Table 1** with lists of genes identified in a large study of transcriptional signatures of cell type in mouse CNS (Cahoy et al., 2008) and a comparison of microglia with circulating monocytes (Yamasaki et al., 2014). From the former report, we extracted 240 genes, of which 106 were preferentially expressed in astrocytes, 83 in oligodendrocytes, 43 in neurons, 5 in endothelial cells, and 3 in microglia. From the latter, we extracted 76 genes, of which 48 were preferentially expressed in microglia and 28 in monocytes. Of the 221 proteins reported as differentially expressed in schizophrenia (**Table 1**), mRNA sequences for 22 were also reported as characteristic of individual cell types (**Table 3**). These include the 2 proteins most frequently reported altered in schizophrenia, ALDOC (11 reports) and GFAP (9 reports), both expressed predominantly in astrocytes.

For a more inclusive analysis, we made use of a published dataset (http://jiaqianwulab.org/resource.htm) from mouse RNA sequencing (RNAseq) expriments (Zhang et al., 2014; Dong et al., 2015). This dataset includes expression levels of 22,462 genes from neurons (NEU), astrocytes (ASTRO), endothelial cells (ENDO), microglia (MGL), myelinating oligodendrocytes (MO), newly formed oligodendrocytes (NFO), and oligodendrocyte precursor cells (OPC). Expression levels in different cell types were highly correlated (**Figure 1A**), so gene expression in two cell types can be compared, and genes enriched in either cell type, relative to the other, can be determined by linear regression (e.g., **Figure 1B**). Similarly, one cell type can be compared with

**TABLE 4 | Oligodendroglial proteins most commonly cited.**

| Region | MBP | CNP | MOG | GSN | References |
|---|---|---|---|---|---|
| BA9 gray and white matter | | ↓ | | ↓ | Prabakaran et al., 2004 |
| BA46 | | ↓ | ↓ | | Martins-de-Souza et al., 2009c |
| Corpus callosum | ↓ | ↓ | ↓ | ↓ | Saia-Cereda et al., 2015 |
| BA38, left | ↓ | ↓ | ↓ | | Martins-de-Souza et al., 2009d |
| BA46, left | ↓ | | | | Martins-de-Souza et al., 2009a |
| Hippocampus | | | | ↑ | Nesvaderani et al., 2009 |
| Mediodorsal thalamus | | | ↑ | | Martins-de-Souza et al., 2010a |

*Proteomics studies of brain reporting altered levels of myelin-associated proteins MBP, CNP, MOG, or GSN. Arrows as in* ***Table 1****.*

**TABLE 5 | Astrocytic proteins most commonly cited.**

| Schizophrenia relative to nonpsychiatric | | GFAP | | | |
|---|---|---|---|---|---|
| | | Higher | Lower | Neither | Total |
| ALDOC | Higher | 1 | 1 | 2 | 4 |
| | Lower | 1 | 2 | 4 | 7 |
| | Neither | 2 | 2 | | 4 |
| | Total | 4 | 5 | 6 | 15 |

*Numbers of studies from* ***Table 1*** *reporting differences between schizophrenia and non-psychiatric cases in GFAP, ALDOC, or both. Since most reports do not include tabulations of all identified proteins, the category of "Neither" higher nor lower does not distinguish failure to identify the protein and a failure to find a significant difference between schizophrenia and non-psychiatric cases.*

several others simultaneously by performing multiple linear regression and identifying the genes with standardized residuals greater than 2 (**Figure 1C**). By regression of each of 6 brain cell types against the others we found 714 such genes, of which 78 code for proteins that proteomic studies have identified as affected in schizophrenia. These include 7 of 14 genes expressed preferentially in MO, 13/174 in ASTRO, 9/108 in OPC, 54/362 in NEU, 2/129 in ENDO, and 6/46 in MGL (**Figure 2**). These regressions are restricted to comparisons amongst different types of brain cells; they do not imply any comparison with expression of transcripts in other organs.

The comparisons among cell types are based on RNA, which does not necessarily correlate with levels of the encoded protein. Furthermore, they are based on cells from mice, not humans. However, the specificities (at least within the brain) of the most commonly cited astrocytic proteins, ALDOC and GFAP are well-established by immunohistochemistry on the human brain [except for the presence of ALDOC in cerebellar Purkinje cells (Thompson et al., 1982; Kumanishi et al., 1985), which were not included in any of the proteomic studies]. Similarly, the specificities of the most commonly cited oligodendroglial proteins, MBP, CNP, MOG, and GSN (Tanaka and Sobue, 1994), all associated with myelin, are also well-established by immunohistochemistry.

A

| Pearson's r | nfo | opc | neu | endo | astro | mgl |
|---|---|---|---|---|---|---|
| mo | 0.958 | 0.060 | 0.034 | 0.031 | 0.016 | 0.018 |
| nfo | | 0.112 | 0.111 | 0.058 | 0.056 | 0.032 |
| opc | | | 0.578 | 0.524 | 0.392 | 0.342 |
| neu | | | | 0.417 | 0.366 | 0.167 |
| endo | | | | | 0.176 | 0.159 |
| astro | | | | | | 0.451 |

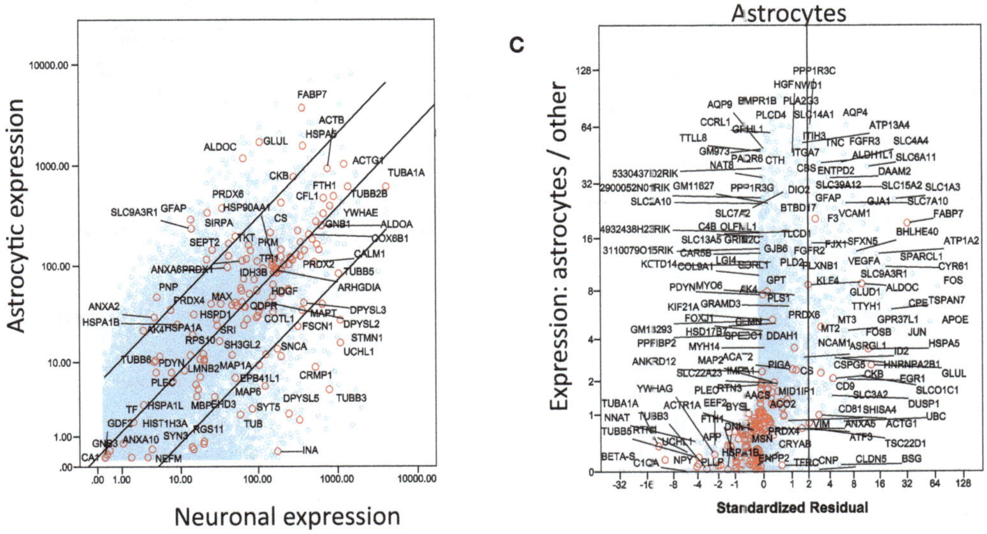


**FIGURE 1 | Analysis of mouse RNAseq data from http://jiaqianwulab.org/resource.htm (Zhang et al., 2014; Dong et al., 2015). (A)** Correlation coefficients between cell types for all genes. **(B)** Linear regression of gene expression in ASTRO and NEU. Genes for proteins included in **Table 1** are represented by red circles and labeled where space permits. Other genes are represented by blue circles. Center line represents best fit and outer lines 95% confidence limits after log transformation of data. **(C)** Multiple regression of ASTRO against other cell types. Linear regression of untransformed expression data for ASTRO against data for MO, OPC, NEU, and ENDO, was performed, and standardized residuals were computed. NFO were omitted from all multiple correlations because of their very high correlation with MO. Standardized residuals are potted on X-axis. The Y axis represents the ratio between expression level in ASTRO and the average expression levels in the other five cell types. Genes with standardized residual values above two (i.e., to the right of the vertical line) were considered enriched in astrocytes. Colors are as in **(B)**; both red and blue circles are labeled where space permits.

## CONCLUSION AND FUTURE PERSPECTIVES IN SCHIZOPHRENIA PROTEOMICS RESEARCH

We have attempted to review all studies of schizophrenia by proteomics, including studies of autopsy brain tissues and bodily fluids. The data lead us to conclude that there are important issues regarding the proteomics platforms and samples that make comparisons across studies quite difficult, especially when different platforms are used. More comparisons with other psychiatric illnesses are needed to address specificity. Proteomic studies have been confined to a small number of brain regions, with little attention to white matter.

Overall, however, the data from brain tissue point to prominent changes in metabolic pathways and cytoskeleton. The majority of studies of bodily fluids point toward immune response, lipid metabolism and to a lesser extent, dysregulation of glucose metabolic pathways. The discrepancy between findings in tissue and body fluids has been observed generally in biomarker studies, particularly in studies of cancer (Hanash et al., 2008). This lack of tissue biomarker detection in the circulation may be caused by low levels of release of disease-associated proteins from tissues to body fluids, where they are susceptible to masking by highly abundant blood proteins. Alternatively, circulating proteins associated with a particular disease may be too dilute for detection by the methods used for proteomics.

The comparison of the candidate biomarkers for schizophrenia with candidate biomarkers for other neurological diseases, such as bipolar disorder, MDD, Alzheimer's disease, and Parkinson's disease reveal overlap. This could be due to common disturbances in energy pathways and cytoskeletal function, or to bias associated with the proteomics method used. Most of the proteomics studies of brain tissues reviewed here and most of the proteomics studies of common neurological disorders, reviewed extensively elsewhere (Korolainen et al., 2010; Srivastava et al., 2010), have been based on2-D gel-based platforms. This approach is known to resolve only a limited collection of highly abundant and soluble proteins (Petrak et al., 2008; Wang et al., 2009). These proteins are mainly involved in central metabolism, protein production (e.g., ribosomal proteins, some RNA binding proteins, translation factors), protein conformational control and degradation (chaperones, disulfide isomerases, proline isomerases, proteasome subunits), cytoskeleton (including some cytoskeleton modifying proteins), adaptor proteins (14-3-3,

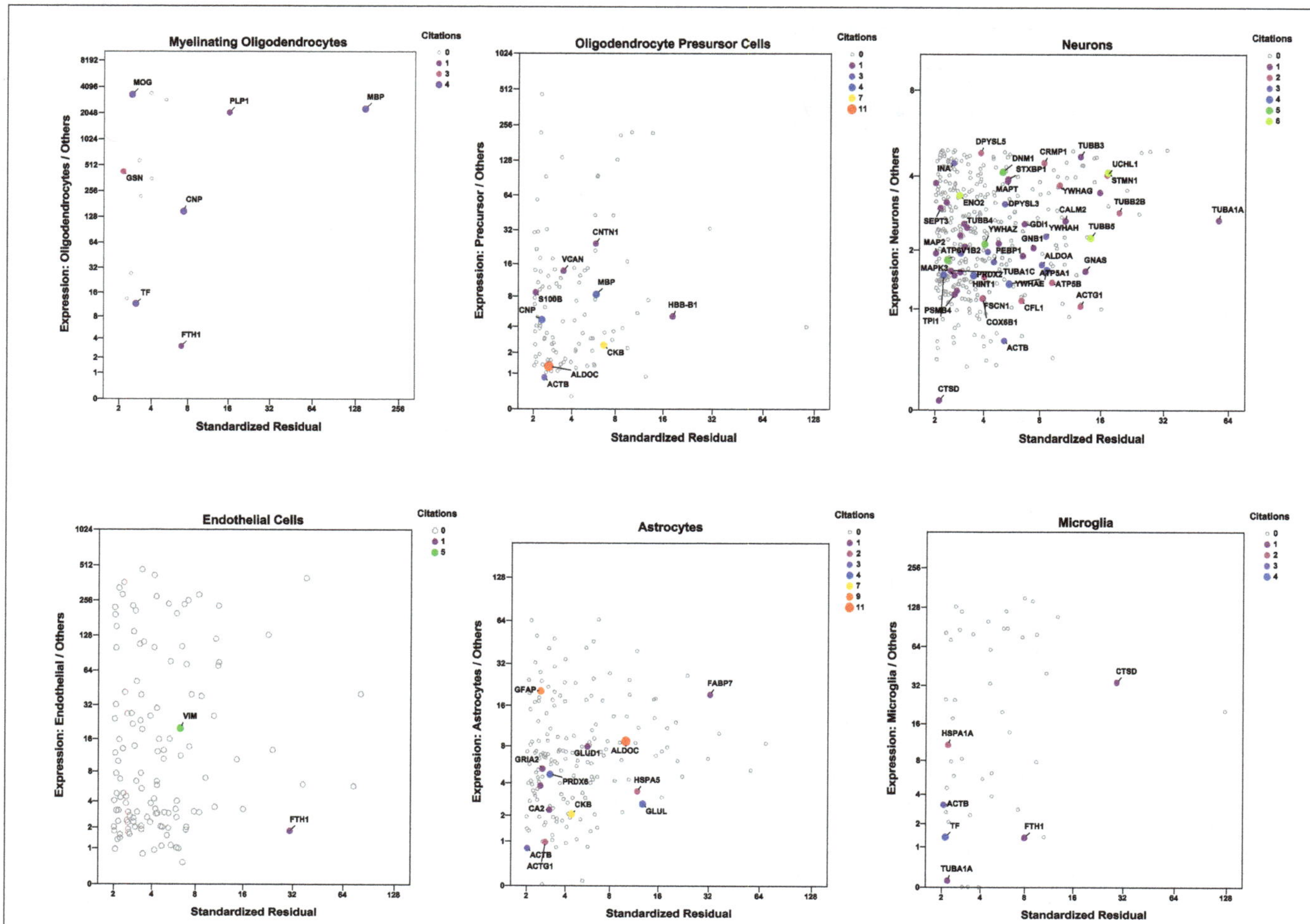


**FIGURE 2 | Multiple regression was performed and plotted as in Figure 1C, except that only data points with standardized residuals >2 are shown.** The color of the symbols represents the number of proteomic studies in which the level of each protein was found differentially expressed in brain tissue from individuals with schizophrenia (**Table 1**). Only genes for proteins cited at least once are labeled. Because of their biological relationship, MO expression was not included as an independent variable in the regression of OPC, and OPC was not included in the regression of MO.

annexins), and oxidative stress response (catalase, superoxide dismutases, peroxiredoxins, glutathione transferases). This limited scope of 2-D gels might explain why so many so called "specific" markers of various neurological diseases belong to the same classes. However, the research using shotgun label-free approaches, in comparative brain studies with MDD, provides a more detailed and specific overview of the energy metabolism pathways involved in the disease, with clues that these pathways are different from those implicated in schizophrenia (Martins-de-Souza et al., 2012a). Quantitative shotgun proteomics with data-independent acquisition ($MS^E$) coupled with wave ion mobility has been applied to a wide variety of samples including cells, tissues, clinical samples, and affinity pull downs, with power and effectiveness firmly established and extensively validated by many independent groups (Brown, 2014). Therefore, future extensive studies using proteomics platforms with wider dynamic range, such as label-free data-independent ($MS^E$) shotgun approach or MALDI MSI combined with high resolution top-down tandem MS identification could provide a more specific picture of the affected pathways in schizophrenia.

Assessment of the cell specificity of candidate biomarkers for schizophrenia did not point to exclusive dysfunction of one specific brain cell type. However, transcripts for 35% (78/221) of the proteins reported as affected in schizophrenia are enriched in one or more cell types in mouse brain. Since the vast majority (>95%) of mouse genes are not selectively expressed in any one type of brain cell compared with the others, there is clearly a preferential involvement of genes selectively expressed by specific types of brain cells. Among these 78 proteins, twice as many are highly expressed in neurons as in glia, but the glial proteins are found more consistently. Overall, ~50% of citations are to proteins not specifically expressed by individual types of brain cells, 30% to proteins preferentially expressed by neurons, and 20% to proteins predominantly expressed by glia. The most frequently referenced proteins are ALDOC (astrocytic), followed by GFAP (astrocytic) and DPYSL2 (nonspecific), followed by NEFL (nonspecific) and then CKB (oligodendroglial precursor and astrocytic). It is important to remember that the expression profiles on which this analysis relies are based solely on mRNA in mouse brain cells, since quantitative data on proteins in individual cell types from human brain are not available.

Studies of white matter, which is nearly devoid of neuronal cell bodies but abundantly, populated with oligodendroglia, oligodendroglial precursor (NG2) cells, astrocytes, and microglia showed some abnormalities of oligiodendroglial protein levels, with considerable variation across studies, and little or no replication of more consistent deficits in oligodendroglial mRNA. Abnormal content of astrocytic proteins in white matter was somewhat more consistent, with two studies reporting altered levels of ALDOC, and one reporting abnormal levels of GFAP. However, the picture changes somewhat when one looks beyond the handful of studies restricted to white matter. Gray matter includes myelin and all types of glia, and cortical samples cut macroscopically from frozen brain slices will almost inevitably include some white matter, intentionally or otherwise, since the cortex curves in 3 dimensions. The 7 studies reporting alterations in MBP, MOG, CNP, or GSN are listed in **Table 4**. In schizophrenia, levels of all 4 were depressed in 1 study of corpus callosum, while the 4 studies of neocortex found depressions of 1, 2, 2, and 3 of the proteins, respectively, with none elevated. Two studies, one of hippocampus and one of thalamus, reported elevation of GSN and MOG, respectively. Overall, these results corroborate the numerous reports from RNA and targeted protein studies of myelin-related deficits in schizophrenia. By contrast, while abnormalities of the astrocytic proteins ALDOC and GFAP are the most frequently reported, both are up in some studies and down in others, concordantly in some studies and discordantly in others (**Table 5**). There are many possible explanations, which must include the very varied functions of astrocytes in healthy and diseased brains.

At this time, exhaustive proteomic studies are new, and their interpretation is far from straightforward. This difficulty would be alleviated if researchers published entire datasets, rather than just positive findings. This is especially important for proteomics because, in contrast to mRNA expression studies, the total set of identified proteins varies dramatically between studies, so that proteins that are affected by disease in one study may not be detected at all in another. The potentially confounding influence of pre- and postmortem factors such as tissue pH, postmortem interval, medication exposure, and in particular, agonal state must always be reported and considered. Detailed and complete clinical and demographic data should also be included. Discovery proteomic studies, using well-matched sub-pools of disease and control subjects, should be followed by validation of important findings with other methods *in larger samples*, not just in those employed for discovery. Overall, the proteomics studies of schizophrenia so far have paved the way for future research that should contribute to greater understanding of the molecular mechanisms of the disease and identify biomarkers for clear and effective diagnosis, nosology, prognosis, and therapy. This is possible by using well-defined samples, larger cohorts, combinations of proteomics techniques to overcome limitations associated with individual techniques, and extensive validation.

## AUTHOR CONTRIBUTIONS

KD collected literature, assembled **Tables 1** and **2**, wrote the first draft of the manuscript, and edited subsequent drafts. IM collected literature, assembled **Tables 1** and **2**, and edited the manuscript. AJD outlined the project, compared the human and mouse data, prepared the figures and **Tables 3–5**, and revised and edited the manuscript.

## FUNDING

This study was supported by NIH Research Grants R01 MH098786, funded by the Fogarty International Center and the National Institute of Mental Health, and R01 MH064168, funded by the National Institute of Mental Health.

## REFERENCES


Albus, M. (2012). Clinical courses of schizophrenia. *Pharmacopsychiatry* 45(Suppl. 1), S31–S35. doi: 10.1055/s-0032-1308968

Baggerly, K. A., Morris, J. S., and Coombes, K. R. (2004). Reproducibility of SELDI-TOF protein patterns in serum: comparing datasets from different experiments. *Bioinformatics* 20, 777–785. doi: 10.1093/bioinformatics/btg484

Beasley, C. L., Pennington, K., Behan, A., Wait, R., Dunn, M. J., and Cotter, D. (2006). Proteomic analysis of the anterior cingulate cortex in the major psychiatric disorders: evidence for disease-associated changes. *Proteomics* 6, 3414–3425. doi: 10.1002/pmic.200500069

Behan, A. T., Byrne, C., Dunn, M. J., Cagney, G., and Cotter, D. R. (2009). Proteomic analysis of membrane microdomain-associated proteins in the dorsolateral prefrontal cortex in schizophrenia and bipolar disorder reveals alterations in LAMP, STXBP1 and BASP1 protein expression. *Mol. Psychiatry* 14, 601–613. doi: 10.1038/mp.2008.7

Benes, F. M., Vincent, S. L., and Todtenkopf, M. (2001). The density of pyramidal and nonpyramidal neurons in anterior cingulate cortex of schizophrenic and bipolar subjects. *Biol. Psychiatry* 50, 395–406. doi: 10.1016/S0006-3223(01)01084-8

Bouras, C., Kövari, E., Hof, P. R., Riederer, B. M., and Giannakopoulos, P. (2001). Anterior cingulate cortex pathology in schizophrenia and bipolar disorder. *Acta Neuropathol.* 102, 373–379. doi: 10.1007/s004010100392

Brown, L. M. (2014). Quantitative shotgun proteomics with data-independent acquisition and traveling wave ion mobility spectrometry: a versatile tool in the life sciences. *Adv. Exp. Med. Biol.* 806, 79–91. doi: 10.1007/978-3-319-06068-2_4

Butt, R. H., and Coorssen, J. R. (2005). Postfractionation for enhanced proteomic analyses: routine electrophoretic methods increase the resolution of standard 2D-PAGE. *J. Proteome Res.* 4, 982–991. doi: 10.1021/pr050054d

Cahoy, J. D., Emery, B., Kaushal, A., Foo, L. C., Zamanian, J. L., Christopherson, K. S., et al. (2008). A transcriptome database for astrocytes, neurons, and oligodendrocytes: a new resource for understanding brain development and function. *J. Neurosci.* 28, 264–278. doi: 10.1523/JNEUROSCI.4178-07.2008

Carter, C. S., Mintun, M., Nichols, T., and Cohen, J. D. (1997). Anterior cingulate gyrus dysfunction and selective attention deficits in schizophrenia: [15O]H2O PET study during single-trial Stroop task performance. *Am. J. Psychiatry* 154, 1670–1675. doi: 10.1176/ajp.154.12.1670

Chana, G., Landau, S., Beasley, C., Everall, I. P., and Cotter, D. (2003). Two-dimensional assessment of cytoarchitecture in the anterior cingulate cortex in major depressive disorder, bipolar disorder, and schizophrenia: evidence for decreased neuronal somal size and increased neuronal density. *Biol. Psychiatry* 53, 1086–1098. doi: 10.1016/s0006-3223(03)00114-8

Chiam, J. T., Dobson, R. J., Kiddle, S. J., and Sattlecker, M. (2015). Are blood-based protein biomarkers for Alzheimer's disease also involved in other brain disorders? A systematic review. *J. Alzheimers. Dis.* 43, 303–314. doi: 10.3233/JAD-140816

Clark, D., Dedova, I., Cordwell, S., and Matsumoto, I. (2006). A proteome analysis of the anterior cingulate cortex gray matter in schizophrenia. *Mol. Psychiatry* 11, 459–470. doi: 10.1038/sj.mp.4001806

Clark, D., Dedova, I., Cordwell, S., and Matsumoto, I. (2007). Altered proteins of the anterior cingulate cortex white matter proteome in schizophrenia. *Proteomics Clin. Appl.* 1, 157–166. doi: 10.1002/prca.200600541

Cleghorn, J. M., Garnett, E. S., Nahmias, C., Brown, G. M., Kaplan, R. D., Szechtman, H., et al. (1990). Regional brain metabolism during auditory hallucinations in chronic schizophrenia. *Br. J. Psychiatry* 157, 562–570. doi: 10.1192/bjp.157.4.562

Craddock, R. M., Huang, J. T., Jackson, E., Harris, N., Torrey, E. F., Herberth, M., et al. (2008). Increased alpha-defensins as a blood marker for schizophrenia susceptibility. *Mol. Cell. Proteomics* 7, 1204–1213. doi: 10.1074/mcp.M700459-MCP200

Daniel, D. G., Weinberger, D. R., Jones, D. W., Zigun, J. R., Coppola, R., Handel, S., et al. (1991). The effect of amphetamine on regional cerebral blood flow during cognitive activation in schizophrenia. *J. Neurosci.* 11, 1907–1917.

Doerr, A., Finkelstein, J., Jarchum, I., Goodman, C., and Dekker, B. (2015). Nature milestones: mass spectrometry. *Nat. Methods* 12, S1–S46.

Domenici, E., Wille, D. R., Tozzi, F., Prokopenko, I., Miller, S., McKeown, A., et al. (2010). Plasma protein biomarkers for depression and schizophrenia by multi analyte profiling of case-control collections. *PLoS ONE* 5:e9166. doi: 10.1371/journal.pone.0009166

Domon, B., and Aebersold, R. (2006). Mass spectrometry and protein analysis. *Science* 312, 212–217. doi: 10.1126/science.1124619

Dong, X., You, Y., and Wu, J. Q. (2015). Building an RNA sequencing transcriptome of the central nervous system. *Neuroscientist.* doi: 10.1177/1073858415610541. [Epub ahead of print].

Dracheva, S., Davis, K. L., Chin, B., Woo, D. A., Schmeidler, J., and Haroutunian, V. (2006). Myelin-associated mRNA and protein expression deficits in the anterior cingulate cortex and hippocampus in elderly schizophrenia patients. *Neurobiol. Dis.* 21, 531–540. doi: 10.1016/j.nbd.2005.08.012

Dwork, A. J. (1997). Postmortem studies of the hippocampal formation in schizophrenia. *Schizophr. Bull.* 23, 385–402. doi: 10.1093/schbul/23.3.385

Dwork, A. J., Mancevski, B., and Rosoklija, G. (2007). White matter and cognitive function in schizophrenia. *Int. J. Neuropsychopharmacol.* 10, 513–536. doi: 10.1017/S1461145707007638

English, J. A., Dicker, P., Föcking, M., Dunn, M. J., and Cotter, D. R. (2009). 2-D DIGE analysis implicates cytoskeletal abnormalities in psychiatric disease. *Proteomics* 9, 3368–3382. doi: 10.1002/pmic.200900015

Föcking, M., Dicker, P., English, J. A., Schubert, K. O., Dunn, M. J., and Cotter, D. R. (2011). Common proteomic changes in the hippocampus in schizophrenia and bipolar disorder and particular evidence for involvement of cornu ammonis regions 2 and 3. *Arch. Gen. Psychiatry* 68, 477–488. doi: 10.1001/archgenpsychiatry.2011.43

Föcking, M., Lopez, L. M., English, J. A., Dicker, P., Wolff, A., Brindley, E., et al. (2015). Proteomic and genomic evidence implicates the postsynaptic density in schizophrenia. *Mol. Psychiatry* 20, 424–432. doi: 10.1038/mp.2014.63

Frith, C., and Dolan, R. (1996). The role of the prefrontal cortex in higher cognitive functions. *Brain Res. Cogn. Brain Res.* 5, 175–181. doi: 10.1016/S0926-6410(96)00054-7

Geromanos, S. J., Vissers, J. P., Silva, J. C., Dorschel, C. A., Li, G. Z., Gorenstein, M. V., et al. (2009). The detection, correlation, and comparison of peptide precursor and product ions from data independent LC-MS with data dependant LC-MS/MS. *Proteomics* 9, 1683–1695. doi: 10.1002/pmic.200800562

Glantz, L. A., and Lewis, D. A. (2000). Decreased dendritic spine density on prefrontal cortical pyramidal neurons in schizophrenia. *Arch. Gen. Psychiatry* 57, 65–73. doi: 10.1001/archpsyc.57.1.65

Goldman, D., Merril, C. R., and Ebert, M. H. (1980). Two-dimensional gel electrophoresis of cerebrospinal fluid proteins. *Clin. Chem.* 26, 1317–1322.

Guest, P. C., Chan, M. K., Gottschalk, M. G., and Bahn, S. (2014). The use of proteomic biomarkers for improved diagnosis and stratification of schizophrenia patients. *Biomark. Med.* 8, 15–27. doi: 10.2217/bmm.13.83

Guest, P. C., Martins-de-Souza, D., Schwarz, E., Rahmoune, H., Alsaif, M., Tomasik, J., et al. (2013). Proteomic profiling in schizophrenia: enabling stratification for more effective treatment. *Genome Med.* 5, 25. doi: 10.1186/gm429

Guest, P. C., Schwarz, E., Krishnamurthy, D., Harris, L. W., Leweke, F. M., Rothermundt, M., et al. (2011). Altered levels of circulating insulin and other neuroendocrine hormones associated with the onset of schizophrenia. *Psychoneuroendocrinology* 36, 1092–1096. doi: 10.1016/j.psyneuen.2010.12.018

Guest, P. C., Wang, L., Harris, L. W., Burling, K., Levin, Y., Ernst, A., et al. (2010). Increased levels of circulating insulin-related peptides in first-onset, antipsychotic naive schizophrenia patients. *Mol. Psychiatry* 15, 118–119. doi: 10.1038/mp.2009.81

Haas, W., Faherty, B. K., Gerber, S. A., Elias, J. E., Beausoleil, S. A., Bakalarski, C. E., et al. (2006). Optimization and use of peptide mass measurement accuracy in shotgun proteomics. *Mol. Cell. Proteomics* 5, 1326–1337. doi: 10.1074/mcp.M500339-MCP200

Hanash, S. M., Pitteri, S. J., and Faca, V. M. (2008). Mining the plasma proteome for cancer biomarkers. *Nature* 452, 571–579. doi: 10.1038/nature06916

Haroutunian, V., Katsel, P., Roussos, P., Davis, K. L., Altshuler, L. L., and Bartzokis, G. (2014). Myelination, oligodendrocytes, and serious mental illness. *Glia* 62, 1856–1877. doi: 10.1002/glia.22716

Harrison, P. J., and Eastwood, S. L. (2001). Neuropathological studies of synaptic connectivity in the hippocampal formation in schizophrenia. *Hippocampus* 11, 508–519. doi: 10.1002/hipo.1067

Hashimoto, T., Volk, D. W., Eggan, S. M., Mirnics, K., Pierri, J. N., Sun, Z., et al. (2003). Gene expression deficits in a subclass of GABA neurons in the prefrontal cortex of subjects with schizophrenia. *J. Neurosci.* 23, 6315–6326.

Herbert, J., Wilcox, J. N., Pham, K. T., Fremeau, R. T. Jr., Zeviani, M., Dwork, A., et al. (1986). Transthyretin: a choroid plexus-specific transport protein in human brain. The 1986 S. Weir Mitchell award. *Neurology* 36, 900–911. doi: 10.1212/WNL.36.7.900

Herberth, M., Koethe, D., Cheng, T. M., Krzyszton, N. D., Schoeffmann, S., Guest, P. C., et al. (2011). Impaired glycolytic response in peripheral blood mononuclear cells of first-onset antipsychotic-naive schizophrenia patients. *Mol. Psychiatry* 16, 848–859. doi: 10.1038/mp.2010.71

Huang, J. T., Leweke, F. M., Oxley, D., Wang, L., Harris, N., Koethe, D., et al. (2006). Disease biomarkers in cerebrospinal fluid of patients with first-onset psychosis. *PLoS Med.* 3:e428. doi: 10.1371/journal.pmed.0030428

Huang, T. J., Wang, L., Prabakaran, S., Wengenroth, M., Lockstone, H. E., Bahn, S. et al. (2008). Independent protein-profiling studies show a decrease in apolipoprotein A1 levels in schizophrenia CSF, brain and peripheral tissues. *Mol. Psychiatry* 13, 1118–1128. doi: 10.1038/sj.mp.4002108

Iavarone, F., Melis, M., Platania, G., Cabras, T., Manconi, B., Petruzzelli, R., et al. (2014). Characterization of salivary proteins of schizophrenic and bipolar disorder patients by top-down proteomics. *J. Proteomics* 103, 15–22. doi: 10.1016/j.jprot.2014.03.020

Innocenti, G. M., Ansermet, F., and Parnas, J. (2003). Schizophrenia, neurodevelopment and corpus callosum. *Mol. Psychiatry* 8, 261–274. doi: 10.1038/sj.mp.4001205

Jaros, J. A., Martins-de-Souza, D., Rahmoune, H., Rothermundt, M., Leweke, F. M., Guest, P. C., et al. (2012). Protein phosphorylation patterns in serum from schizophrenia patients and healthy controls. *J. Proteomics 76*, 43–55. doi: 10.1016/j.jprot.2012.05.027

Jiang, L., Lindpaintner, K., Li, H. F., Gu, N. F., Langen, H., He, L., et al. (2003). Proteomic analysis of the cerebrospinal fluid of patients with schizophrenia. *Amino Acids* 25, 49–57. doi: 10.1007/s00726-003-0356-6

Johnston-Wilson, N. L., Sims, C. D., Hofmann, J. P., Anderson, L., Shore, A. D., Torrey, E. F., et al. (2000). Disease-specific alterations in frontal cortex brain proteins in schizophrenia, bipolar disorder, and major depressive disorder. *Mol. Psychiatry* 5, 142–149. doi: 10.1038/sj.mp.4000696

Kelleher, N. L. (2004). Top-down proteomics. *Anal, Chem. 76*, 197A–203A. doi: 10.1021/ac0415657

Kim, M. S., Pinto, S. M., Getnet, D., Nirujogi, R. S., Manda, S. S., Pandey, A., et al. (2014). A draft map of the human proteome. *Nature* 509, 575–581. doi: 10.1038/nature13302

Korolainen, M. A., Nyman, T. A., Aittokallio, T., and Pirttilä, T. (2010). An update on clinical proteomics in Alzheimer's research. *J. Neurochem.* 112, 1386–1414. doi: 10.1111/j.1471-4159.2009.06558.x

Krishnamurthy, D., Harris, L. W., Levin, Y., Koutroukides, T. A., Rahmoune, H., Pietsch, S., et al. (2013). Metabolic, hormonal and stress-related molecular changes in post-mortem pituitary glands from schizophrenia subjects. *World J. Biol. Psychiatry* 14, 478–489. doi: 10.3109/15622975.2011.601759

Kroksveen, A. C., Opsahl, J. A., Aye, T. T., Ulvik, R. J., and Berven, F. S. (2011). Proteomics of human cerebrospinal fluid: discovery and verification of biomarker candidates in neurodegenerative diseases using quantitative proteomics. *J. Proteomics* 74, 371–388. doi: 10.1016/j.jprot.2010.11.010

Kumanishi, T., Watabe, K., and Washiyama, K. (1985). An immunohistochemical study of aldolase C in normal and neoplastic nervous tissues. *Acta Neuropathol.* 67, 309–314. doi: 10.1007/BF00687817

Levin, Y., Wang, L., Schwarz, E., Koethe, D., Leweke, F. M., and Bahn, S. (2010). Global proteomic profiling reveals altered proteomic signature in schizophrenia serum. *Mol. Psychiatry* 15, 1088–1100. doi: 10.1038/mp.2009.54

Li, G. Z., Vissers, J. P., Silva, J. C., Golick, D., Gorenstein, M. V., and Geromanos, S. J. (2009). Database searching and accounting of multiplexed precursor and product ion spectra from the data independent analysis of simple and complex peptide mixtures. *Proteomics* 9, 1696–1719. doi: 10.1002/pmic.200800564

Li, Y., Zhou, K., Zhang, Z., Sun, L., Yang, J., Zhang, M., et al. (2012). Label-free quantitative proteomic analysis reveals dysfunction of complement pathway in peripheral blood of schizophrenia patients: evidence for the immune hypothesis of schizophrenia. *Mol. Biosyst.* 8, 2664–2671. doi: 10.1039/c2mb25158b

Link, A. J., Eng, J., Schieltz, D. M., Carmack, E., Mize, G. J., Morris, D. R. III. et al. (1999). Direct analysis of protein complexes using mass spectrometry. *Nat. Biotechnol.* 17, 676–682. doi: 10.1038/10890

Luu, P., and Posner, M. I. (2003). Anterior cingulate cortex regulation of sympathetic activity. *Brain* 126, 2119–2120. doi: 10.1093/brain/awg257

Martins-de-Souza, D. (2010). Proteome and transcriptome analysis suggests oligodendrocyte dysfunction in schizophrenia. *J. Psychiatr. Res.* 44, 149–156. doi: 10.1016/j.jpsychires.2009.07.007

Martins-de-Souza, D. (2014). Proteomics, metabolomics, and protein interactomics in the characterization of the molecular features of major depressive disorder. *Dialogues Clin. Neurosci.* 16, 63–73.

Martins-de-Souza, D., Gattaz, W. F., Schmitt, A., MacCarrone, G., Hunyadi-Gulyas, E., Eberlin, M. N., et al. (2009a). Proteomic analysis of dorsolateral prefrontal cortex indicates the involvement of cytoskeleton, oligodendrocyte, energy metabolism and new potential markers in schizophrenia. *J. Psychiatr. Res.* 43, 978–986. doi: 10.1016/j.jpsychires.2008.11.006

Martins-de-Souza, D., Gattaz, W. F., Schmitt, A., Novello, J. C., Marangoni, S., Turck, C. W., et al. (2009b). Proteome analysis of schizophrenia patients Wernicke's area reveals an energy metabolism dysregulation. *BMC Psychiatry* 9:17. doi: 10.1186/1471-244X-9-17

Martins-de-Souza, D., Gattaz, W. F., Schmitt, A., Rewerts, C., MacCarrone, G., Dias-Neto, E., et al. (2009c). Prefrontal cortex shotgun proteome analysis reveals altered calcium homeostasis and immune system imbalance in schizophrenia. *Eur. Arch. Psychiatry Clin. Neurosci.* 259, 151–163. doi: 10.1007/s00406-008-0847-2

Martins-de-Souza, D., Gattaz, W. F., Schmitt, A., Rewerts, C., Marangoni, S., Novello, J. C., et al. (2009d). Alterations in oligodendrocyte proteins, calcium homeostasis and new potential markers in schizophrenia anterior temporal lobe are revealed by shotgun proteome analysis. *J. Neural Transm.* 116, 275–289. doi: 10.1007/s00702-008-0156-y

Martins-de-Souza, D., Guest, P. C., Harris, L. W., Vanattou-Saifoudine, N., Webster, M. J., Rahmoune, H., et al. (2012a). Identification of proteomic signatures associated with depression and psychotic depression in post-mortem brains from major depression patients. *Transl. Psychiatry* 2, e87. doi: 10.1038/tp.2012.13

Martins-de-Souza, D., Guest, P. C., Rahmoune, H., and Bahn, S. (2012b). Proteomic approaches to unravel the complexity of schizophrenia. *Expert Rev. Proteomics* 9, 97–108. doi: 10.1586/epr.11.70

Martins-de-Souza, D., Maccarrone, G., Wobrock, T., Zerr, I., Gormanns, P., Reckow, S., et al. (2010a). Proteome analysis of the thalamus and cerebrospinal fluid reveals glycolysis dysfunction and potential biomarkers candidates for schizophrenia. *J. Psychiatr. Res.* 44, 1176–1189. doi: 10.1016/j.jpsychires.2010.04.014

Martins-de-Souza, D., Schmitt, A., Roder, R., Lebar, M., Schneider-Axmann, T., Falkai, P., et al. (2010b). Sex-specific proteome differences in the anterior cingulate cortex of schizophrenia. *J. Psychiatr. Res.* 44, 989–991. doi: 10.1016/j.jpsychires.2010.03.003

Martins-De-Souza, D., Wobrock, T., Zerr, I., Schmitt, A., Gawinecka, J., Schneider-Axmann, T., et al. (2010c). Different apolipoprotein E, apolipoprotein A1 and prostaglandin-H2 D-isomerase levels in cerebrospinal fluid of schizophrenia patients and healthy controls. *World J. Biol. Psychiatry* 11, 719–728. doi: 10.3109/15622971003758748

McCullumsmith, R E., Gupta, D., Beneyto, M., Kreger, E., Haroutunian, V., Davis, K. L., et al. (2007). Expression of transcripts for myelination-related genes in the anterior cingulate cortex in schizophrenia. *Schizophr. Res.* 90, 15–27. doi: 10.1016/j.schres.2006.11.017

Mehler, C., and Warnke, A. (2002). Structural brain abnormalities specific to childhood-onset schizophrenia identified by neuroimaging techniques. *J. Neural Transm.* 109, 219–234. doi: 10.1007/s007020200019

Mei, J. F., Kolbin, D., Kao, H. T., and Porton, B. (2006). Protein expression profiling of postmortem brain in schizophrenia. *Schizophr. Res.* 84, 204–213. doi: 10.1016/j.schres.2006.02.016

Michalski, A., Damoc, E., Lange, O., Denisov, E., Nolting, D., Müller, M., et al. (2012). Ultra high resolution linear ion trap Orbitrap mass spectrometer (Orbitrap Elite) facilitates top down LC MS/MS and versatile peptide fragmentation modes. *Mol. Cell. Proteomics* 11, O111.013698. doi: 10.1074/mcp.O111.013698

Miller, E. K., and Cohen, J. D. (2001). An integrative theory of prefrontal cortex function. *Annu. Rev. Neurosci.* 24, 167–202. doi: 10.1146/annurev.neuro.24.1.167

Montague, E., Janko, I., Stanberry, L., Lee, E., Choiniere, J., Anderson, N., et al. (2015). Beyond protein expression, MOPED goes multi-omics. *Nucleic Acids Res.* 43, D1145–D1151. doi 10.1093/nar/gku1175

Nascimento, J. M., and Martins-de-Souza, D. (2015). The proteome of schizophrenia. *Npj Schizophrenia* 1, 14003. doi: 10.1038/npjschz.2014.3

Nesvaderani, M., Matsumoto, I., and Sivagnanasundaram, S. (2009). Anterior hippocampus in schizophrenia pathogenesis: molecular evidence from a proteome study. *Aus. N.Z. J. Psychiatry* 43, 310–322. doi: 10.1080/00048670902721103

Novikova, S. I., He, F., Cutrufello, N. J., and Lidow, M. S. (2006). Identification of protein biomarkers for schizophrenia and bipolar disorder in the postmortem prefrontal cortex using SELDI-TOF-MS ProteinChip profiling combined with MALDI-TOF-PSD-MS analysis. *Neurobiol. Dis.* 23, 61–76. doi: 10.1016/j.nbd.2006.02.002

O'Farrell, P. H. (1975). High resolution two-dimensional electrophoresis of proteins. *J. Biol. Chem.* 250, 4007–4021.

Owen, M. J., Craddock, N., and O'Donovan, M. C. (2010). Suggestion of roles for both common and rare risk variants in genome-wide studies of schizophrenia. *Arch. Gen. Psychiatry* 67, 667–673. doi: 10.1001/archgenpsychiatry.2010.69

Park, S., and Holzman, P. S. (1992). Schizophrenics show spatial working memory deficits. *Arch. Gen. Psychiatry* 49, 975–982. doi: 10.1001/archpsyc.1992.01820120063009

Park, S., and Holzman, P. S. (1993). Association of working memory deficit and eye tracking dysfunction in schizophrenia. *Schizophr. Res.* 11, 55–61. doi: 10.1016/0920-9964(93)90038-K

Patel, V. J., Thalassinos, K., Slade, S. E., Connolly, J. B., Crombie, A., Murrell, J. C., et al. (2009). A comparison of labeling and label-free mass spectrometry-based proteomics approaches. *J. Proteome Res.* 8, 3752–3759. doi: 10.1021/pr900080y

Pennington, K., Beasley, C. L., Dicker, P., Fagan, A., English, J., Pariante, C. M., et al. (2008). Prominent synaptic and metabolic abnormalities revealed by proteomic analysis of the dorsolateral prefrontal cortex in schizophrenia and bipolar disorder. *Mol. Psychiatry* 13, 1102–1117. doi: 10.1038/sj.mp.4002098

Petrak, J., Ivanek, R., Toman, O., Cmejla, R., Cmejlova, J., Vyoral, D., et al. (2008). Deja vu in proteomics. A hit parade of repeatedly identified differentially expressed proteins. *Proteomics* 8, 1744–1749. doi: 10.1002/pmic.200700919

Prabakaran, S., Swatton, J. E., Ryan, M. M., Huffaker, S. J., Huang, T. J., Bahn, S., et al. (2004). Mitochondrial dysfunction in schizophrenia: evidence for compromised brain metabolism and oxidative stress. *Mol. Psychiatry* 9, 684–697. doi: 10.1038/sj.mp.4001532

Quintana, J., Wong, T., Ortiz-Portillo, E., Marder, S. R., and Mazziotta, J. C. (2004). Anterior cingulate dysfunction during choice anticipation in schizophrenia. *Psychiatry Res.* 132, 117–130. doi: 10.1016/j.pscychresns.2004.06.005

Rabilloud, T., and Lelong, C. (2011). Two-dimensional gel electrophoresis in proteomics: a tutorial. *J. Proteomics* 74, 1829–1841. doi: 10.1016/j.jprot.2011.05.040

Raiszadeh, M. M., Ross, M. M., Russo, P. S., Schaepper, M. A., Zhou, W., Deng, J., et al. (2012). Proteomic analysis of eccrine sweat: implications for the discovery of schizophrenia biomarker proteins. *J. Proteome Res.* 11, 2127–2139. doi: 10.1021/pr2007957

Romanski, L. M., Giguere, M., Bates, J. F., and Goldman-Rakic, P. S. (1997). Topographic organization of medial pulvinar connections with the prefrontal cortex in the rhesus monkey. *J. Comp. Neurol.* 379, 313–332.

Saia-Cereda, V. M., Cassoli, J. S., Schmitt, A., Falkai, P., Nascimento, J. M., and Martins-de-Souza, D. (2015). Proteomics of the corpus callosum unravel pivotal players in the dysfunction of cell signaling, structure, and myelination in schizophrenia brains. *Eur. Arch. Psychiatry Clin. Neurosci.* 265, 601–612. doi: 10.1007/s00406-015-0621-1

Salgado-Pineda, P., Baeza, I., Pérez-Gómez, M., Vendrell, P., Junqué, C., Bargalló, N., et al. (2003). Sustained attention impairment correlates to gray matter decreases in first episode neuroleptic-naive schizophrenic patients. *Neuroimage* 19, 365–375. doi: 10.1016/S1053-8119(03)00094-6

Schwarz, E., Guest, P. C., Rahmoune, H., Harris, L. W., Wang, L., Leweke, F. M., et al. (2012a). Identification of a biological signature for schizophrenia in serum. *Mol. Psychiatry* 17, 494–502. doi: 10.1038/mp.2011.42

Schwarz, E., Guest, P. C., Rahmoune, H., Martins-de-Souza, D., Niebuhr, D. W., Weber, N. S., et al. (2012b). Identification of a blood-based biological signature in subjects with psychiatric disorders prior to clinical manifestation. *World J. Biol. Psychiatry* 13, 627–632. doi: 10.3109/15622975.2011.599861

Schwarz, E., Guest, P. C., Steiner, J., Bogerts, B., and Bahn, S. (2012c). Identification of blood-based molecular signatures for prediction of response and relapse in schizophrenia patients. *Transl. Psychiatry* 2, e82. doi: 10.1038/tp.2012.3

Schwarz, E., Izmailov, R., Spain, M., Barnes, A., Mapes, J. P., Guest, P. C., et al. (2010). Validation of a blood-based laboratory test to aid in the confirmation of a diagnosis of schizophrenia. *Biomark. Insights* 5, 39–47.

Schwarz, E., van Beveren, N. J., Ramsey, J., Leweke, F. M., Rothermundt, M., Bogerts, B., et al. (2014). Identification of subgroups of schizophrenia patients with changes in either immune or growth factor and hormonal pathways. *Schizophr. Bull.* 40, 787–795. doi: 10.1093/schbul/sbt105

Seeley, E. H., and Caprioli, R. M. (2008). Molecular imaging of proteins in tissues by mass spectrometry. *Proc. Natl. Acad. Sci. U.S.A.* 105, 18126–18131. doi: 10.1073/pnas.0801374105

Selemon, L. D., Rajkowska, G., and Goldman-Rakic, P. S. (1995). Abnormally high neuronal density in the schizophrenic cortex. A morphometric analysis of prefrontal area 9 and occipital area 17. *Arch. Gen. Psychiatry* 52, 805–818. doi: 10.1001/archpsyc.1995.03950220015005

Shenton, M. E., Dickey, C. C., Frumin, M., and McCarley, R. W. (2001). A review of MRI findings in schizophrenia. *Schizophr. Res.* 49, 1–52. doi: 10.1016/S0920-9964(01)00163-3

Sivagnanasundaram, S., Crossett, B., Dedova, I., Cordwell, S., and Matsumoto, I. (2007). Abnormal pathways in the genu of the corpus callosum in schizophrenia pathogenesis: a proteome study. *Proteomics Clin. Appl.* 1, 1291–1305. doi: 10.1002/prca.200700230

Smalla, K. H., Mikhaylova, M., Sahin, J., Bernstein, H. G., Bogerts, B., Schmitt, A., et al. (2008). A comparison of the synaptic proteome in human chronic schizophrenia and rat ketamine psychosis suggest that prohibitin is involved in the synaptic pathology of schizophrenia. *Mol. Psychiatry* 13, 878–896. doi: 10.1038/mp.2008.60

Srivastava, G., Singh, K., Tiwari, M. N., and Singh, M. P. (2010). Proteomics in Parkinson's disease: current trends, translational snags and future possibilities. *Expert Rev. Proteomics* 7, 127–139. doi: 10.1586/epr.09.91

Stahl, D. C., Swiderek, K. M., Davis, M. T., and Lee, T. D. (1996). Data-controlled automation of liquid chromatography/tandem mass spectrometry analysis of peptide mixtures. *J. Am. Soc. Mass Spectrom.* 7, 532–540. doi: 10.1016/1044-0305(96)00057-8

Steiner, J., Schmitt, A., Schroeter, M. L., Bogerts, B., Falkai, P., Turck, C. W., et al. (2014). S100B is downregulated in the nuclear proteome of schizophrenia corpus callosum. *Eur. Arch. Psychiatry Clin. Neurosci.* 264, 311–316. doi: 10.1007/s00406-014-0490-z

Sullivan, P. F., Daly, M. J., and O'Donovan, M. (2012). Genetic architectures of psychiatric disorders: the emerging picture and its implications. *Nat. Rev. Genet.* 13, 537–551. doi: 10.1038/nrg3240

Tanaka, J., and Sobue, K. (1994). Localization and characterization of gelsolin in nervous tissues: gelsolin is specifically enriched in myelin-forming cells. *J. Neurosci.* 14, 1038–1052.

Thompson, R. J., Kynoch, P. A., and Willson, V. J. (1982). Cellular localization of aldolase C subunits in human brain. *Brain Res.* 232, 489–493. doi: 10.1016/0006-8993(82)90294-3

Unlü, M., Morgan, M. E., and Minden, J. S. (1997). Difference gel electrophoresis: a single gel method for detecting changes in protein extracts. *Electrophoresis* 18, 2071–2077. doi: 10.1002/elps.1150181133

Varadarajulu, J., Schmitt, A., Falkai, P., Alsaif, M., Turck, C. W., and Martins-de-Souza, D. (2012). Differential expression of HINT1 in schizophrenia brain tissue. *Eur. Arch. Psychiatry Clin. Neurosci.* 262, 167–172. doi: 10.1007/s00406-011-0216-4

Velligan, D. I., and Bow-Thomas, C. C. (1999). Executive function in schizophrenia. *Semin. Clin. Neuropsychiatry* 4, 24–33.

Wan, C., La, Y., Zhu, H., Yang, Y., Jiang, L., Chen, Y., et al. (2007). Abnormal changes of plasma acute phase proteins in schizophrenia and the relation between schizophrenia and haptoglobin (Hp) gene. *Amino Acids* 32, 101–108. doi: 10.1007/s00726-005-0292-8

Wang, P., Bouwman, F. G., and Mariman, E. C. (2009). Generally detected proteins in comparative proteomics–a matter of cellular stress response? *Proteomics* 9, 2955–2966. doi: 10.1002/pmic.200800826

Wright, E. P., Partridge, M. A., Padula, M. P., Gauci, V. J., Malladi, C. S., and Coorssen, J. R. (2014a). Top-down proteomics: enhancing 2D gel electrophoresis from tissue processing to high-sensitivity protein detection. *Proteomics* 14, 872–889. doi: 10.1002/pmic.201300424

Wright, E. P., Prasad, K. A., Padula, M. P., and Coorssen, J. R. (2014b). Deep imaging: how much of the proteome does current top-down technology already resolve? *PLoS ONE* 9:e86058. doi: 10.1371/journal.pone.0086058

Wright, G. L. Jr. (2002). SELDI proteinchip MS: a platform for biomarker discovery and cancer diagnosis. *Expert Rev. Mol. Diagn.* 2, 549–563. doi: 10.1586/14737159.2.6.549

Yamasaki, R., Lu, H., Butovsky, O., Ohno, N., Rietsch, A. M., Cialic, R., et al. (2014). Differential roles of microglia and monocytes in the inflamed central nervous system. *J. Exp. Med.* 211, 1533–1549. doi: 10.1084/jem.20132477

Yang, Y., Wan, C., Li, H., Zhu, H., La, Y., Xi, Z., et al. (2006). Altered levels of acute phase proteins in the plasma of patients with schizophrenia. *Anal. Chem.* 78, 3571–3576. doi: 10.1021/ac051916x

Ye, H., Mandal, R., Catherman, A., Thomas, P. M., Kelleher, N. L., Ikonomidou, C., et al. (2014). Top-down proteomics with mass spectrometry imaging: a pilot study towards discovery of biomarkers for neurodevelopmental disorders. *PLoS ONE* 9:e92831. doi: 10.1371/journal.pone.0092831

Zhang, Y., Chen, K., Sloan, S. A., Bennett, M. L., Scholze, A. R., O'Keeffe, S., et al. (2014). An RNA-sequencing transcriptome and splicing database of glia, neurons, and vascular cells of the cerebral cortex. *J. Neurosci.* 34, 11929–11947. doi: 10.1523/JNEUROSCI.1860-14.2014

# Permissions

All chapters in this book were first published by Frontiers; hereby published with permission under the Creative Commons Attribution License or equivalent. Every chapter published in this book has been scrutinized by our experts. Their significance has been extensively debated. The topics covered herein carry significant findings which will fuel the growth of the discipline. They may even be implemented as practical applications or may be referred to as a beginning point for another development.

The contributors of this book come from diverse backgrounds, making this book a truly international effort. This book will bring forth new frontiers with its revolutionizing research information and detailed analysis of the nascent developments around the world.

We would like to thank all the contributing authors for lending their expertise to make the book truly unique. They have played a crucial role in the development of this book. Without their invaluable contributions this book wouldn't have been possible. They have made vital efforts to compile up to date information on the varied aspects of this subject to make this book a valuable addition to the collection of many professionals and students.

This book was conceptualized with the vision of imparting up-to-date information and advanced data in this field. To ensure the same, a matchless editorial board was set up. Every individual on the board went through rigorous rounds of assessment to prove their worth. After which they invested a large part of their time researching and compiling the most relevant data for our readers.

The editorial board has been involved in producing this book since its inception. They have spent rigorous hours researching and exploring the diverse topics which have resulted in the successful publishing of this book. They have passed on their knowledge of decades through this book. To expedite this challenging task, the publisher supported the team at every step. A small team of assistant editors was also appointed to further simplify the editing procedure and attain best results for the readers.

Apart from the editorial board, the designing team has also invested a significant amount of their time in understanding the subject and creating the most relevant covers. They scrutinized every image to scout for the most suitable representation of the subject and create an appropriate cover for the book.

The publishing team has been an ardent support to the editorial, designing and production team. Their endless efforts to recruit the best for this project, has resulted in the accomplishment of this book. They are a veteran in the field of academics and their pool of knowledge is as vast as their experience in printing. Their expertise and guidance has proved useful at every step. Their uncompromising quality standards have made this book an exceptional effort. Their encouragement from time to time has been an inspiration for everyone.

The publisher and the editorial board hope that this book will prove to be a valuable piece of knowledge for researchers, students, practitioners and scholars across the globe.

# List of Contributors

**Berko Milleit**
Department of Psychiatry, Jena University Hospital, Jena, Germany
St. Joseph-Krankenhaus, Dessau-Roßlau, Germany

**Stefan Smesny and Heinrich Sauer**
Department of Psychiatry, Jena University Hospital, Jena, Germany

**Matthias Rothermundt**
Department of Psychiatry, University of Muenster, Muenster, Germany
Department of Psychiatry, St. Rochus Hospital, Telgte, Germany

**Christoph Preul**
Department of Neurology, Jena University Hospital, Jena, Germany

**Matthias L. Schroeter**
Max Planck Institute for Human Cognitive and Brain Sciences and Clinic for Cognitive Neurology, Leipzig, Germany

**Christof von Eiff**
Institute of Medical Microbiology, University of Muenster, Muenster, Germany

**Gerald Ponath**
Department of Psychiatry, University of Muenster, Muenster, Germany
Department of Neurology, School of Medicine, Yale University, New Haven, CT, USA

**Christine Milleit**
Department of Psychiatry, Jena University Hospital, Jena, Germany
Department of Psychiatry, Sophien- und Hufeland-Klinikum, Weimar, Germany

**Christian Gaser**
Department of Psychiatry, Jena University Hospital, Jena, Germany
Department of Neurology, Jena University Hospital, Jena, Germany

**Masahiro Ohgidani and Shigenobu Kanba**
Department of Neuropsychiatry, Graduate School of Medical Sciences, Kyushu University, Fukuoka, Japan

**Jawid Shariati and Andreas Knaus**
Department of Psychiatry and Psychotherapy, University of Göttingen, Göttingen, Germany

**Takahiro A. Kato**
Department of Neuropsychiatry, Graduate School of Medical Sciences, Kyushu University, Fukuoka, Japan
Brain Research Unit, Innovation Center for Medical Redox Navigation, Kyushu University, Fukuoka, Japan

**Silke Smolders**
BIOMED – Hasselt University, Hasselt, Belgium
Laboratory of Neuronal Differentiation, VIB Center for the Biology of Disease, Leuven and Center for Human Genetics, KU Leuven, Leuven, Belgium

**Sophie M. T. Smolders**
BIOMED – Hasselt University, Hasselt, Belgium
INSERM, UMR S 1130, Université Pierre et Marie Curie, Paris, France
CNRS, UMR 8246, Université Pierre et Marie Curie, Paris, France
UM 119 NPS, Université Pierre et Marie Curie, Paris, France

**Nina Swinnen, Jean-Michel Rigo and Bert Brône**
BIOMED – Hasselt University, Hasselt, Belgium

**Annette Gärtner**
Laboratory of Neuronal Differentiation, VIB Center for the Biology of Disease, Leuven and Center for Human Genetics, KU Leuven, Leuven, Belgium

**Pascal Legendre**
INSERM, UMR S 1130, Université Pierre et Marie Curie, Paris, France
CNRS, UMR 8246, Université Pierre et Marie Curie, Paris, France
UM 119 NPS, Université Pierre et Marie Curie, Paris, France

**Peter Falkai, Berend Malchow and Thomas Schneider-Axmann**
Department of Psychiatry and Psychotherapy, Ludwig Maximilians-University Munich, Munich, Germany

**Johann Steiner, Hans-Gert Bernstein and Bernhard Bogerts**
Department of Psychiatry and Psychotherapy, University of Magdeburg, Magdeburg, Germany

**Theo Kraus**
Center for Neuropathology and Prion Research (ZNP), Ludwig Maximilians-University Munich, Munich, Germany

**Andrea Schmitt**
Department of Psychiatry and Psychotherapy, Ludwig Maximilians-University Munich, Munich, Germany
Laboratory of Neuroscience (LIM27), Institute of Psychiatry, University of São Paulo, São Paulo, Brazil

**Hanzhi Wang, Shubao Liu, Yanping Tian, Xiyan Wu, Yangtao He, Chengren Li, Hongli Li and Lan Xiao**
Chongqing Key Laboratory of Neurobiology, Department of Histology and Embryology, Third Military Medical University, Chongqing, China

**Michael Namaka**
College of Pharmacy and Medicine, Joint Laboratory of Biological Psychiatry Between Shantou University Medical College and College of Medicine, University of Manitoba, Winnipeg, MB, Canada
Department of Human Anatomy and Cell Science, College of Medicine, University of Manitoba, Winnipeg, MB, Canada
Department of Rehabilitation Medicine, Health Sciences Centre (HSC), Winnipeg, MB, Canada

**Jiming Kong**
College of Pharmacy and Medicine, Joint Laboratory of Biological Psychiatry Between Shantou University Medical College and College of Medicine, University of Manitoba, Winnipeg, MB, Canada
Department of Human Anatomy and Cell Science, College of Medicine, University of Manitoba, Winnipeg, MB, Canada

**Hans-Gert Bernstein, Gabriela Meyer-Lotz, Henrik Dobrowolny, Jana Bannier, Johann Steiner and Bernhard Bogerts**
Department of Psychiatry, University of Magdeburg, Magdeburg, Germany

**Martin Walter**
Department of Psychiatry, University of Magdeburg, Magdeburg, Germany
Clinical Affective Neuroimaging Laboratory, University of Magdeburg, Magdeburg, Germany

**Katharina Schümberg and Maryna Polyakova**
Department of Cognitive Neurology, Max Planck Institute for Human Cognitive and Brain Sciences, Leipzig, Germany

**Yuta Takahashi**
Department of Disaster Psychiatry, International Research Institute of Disaster Science, Tohoku University, Sendai, Japan
Department of Disaster Psychiatry, Graduate School of Medicine, Tohoku University, Sendai, Japan
Department of Psychiatry, Graduate School of Medicine, Tohoku University, Sendai, Japan

**Johann Steiner**
Department of Psychiatry, University of Magdeburg, Magdeburg, Germany

**Matthias L. Schroeter**
Department of Cognitive Neurology, Max Planck Institute for Human Cognitive and Brain Sciences, Leipzig, Germany
Clinic for Cognitive Neurology, University of Leipzig, Leipzig, Germany
LIFE—Leipzig Research Center for Civilization Diseases, University of Leipzig, Leipzig, Germany
German Consortium for Frontotemporal Lobar Degeneration, Ulm, Germany

**Zhiqian Yu and Hiroaki Tomita**
Department of Disaster Psychiatry, International Research Institute of Disaster Science, Tohoku University, Sendai, Japan
Department of Disaster Psychiatry, Graduate School of Medicine, Tohoku University, Sendai, Japan
Group of Mental Health Promotion, Tohoku Medical Megabank Organization, Tohoku University, Sendai, Japan

**Mai Sakai**
Department of Disaster Psychiatry, International Research Institute of Disaster Science, Tohoku University, Sendai, Japan
Department of Disaster Psychiatry, Graduate School of Medicine, Tohoku University, Sendai, Japan

**Xianjun Chen, Tao Li, Yanping Tian, Fei Wang, Shubao Liu and Lan Xiao**
Department of Histology and Embryology, Chongqing Key Laboratory of Neurobiology, Third Military Medical University, Chongqing, China

**Weiguo Zhang and Yu Guo**
Department of Radiology, Institute of Surgery Research, Daping Hospital, Third Military Medical University, Chongqing, China

**Hai-Ying Shen**
Robert Stone Dow Neurobiology Laboratories, Legacy Research Institute, Portland, OR, USA

**Yue Feng**
Department of Pharmacology, Emory University School of Medicine, Atlanta, GA, USA

**Alexandre P. Muller**
Department of Biochemistry, Universidade Federal do Rio Grande do Sul, Porto Alegre, Brazil
Laboratory of Exercise, Biochemistry and Physiology, Universidade do Extremo Sul Catarinense, Criciúma, Brazil

**Eduardo R. Zimmer, Vitor R. Torrez, Marina C. Augustin, Kamila C. Zenki, Roberto F. Almeida, Gisele Hansel, Diogo O. Souza and Luis V. Portela**
Department of Biochemistry, Universidade Federal do Rio Grande do Sul, Porto Alegre, Brazil

**Eduardo Kalinine**
Department of Biochemistry, Universidade Federal do Rio Grande do Sul, Porto Alegre, Brazil
Department of Physiology, Universidade Federal de Sergipe, São Cristovão, Brazil

**Rodrigo Machado-Vieira**
Laboratory of Neuroscience, LIM-27, Institute and Department of Psychiatry, Universidade de São Paulo, São Paulo, Brazil
Center for Interdisciplinary Research on Applied Neurosciences (NAPNA), Universidade de São Paulo, São Paulo, Brazil
Experimental Therapeutics and Pathophysiology Branch, National Institute of Mental Health, National Institutes of Health, Bethesda, MD, USA

**Mami Noda**
Laboratory of Pathophysiology, Graduate School of Pharmaceutical Sciences, Kyushu University, 3-1-1 Maidashi, Higashi-ku, Fukuoka, Japan

**Daniela F. de Souza, Krista M. Wartchow, Paula S. Lunardi, Giovana Brolese, Lucas S. Tortorelli, Cristiane Batassini, Regina Biasibetti and Carlos-Alberto Gonçalves**
Departamento de Bioquímica, Instituto de Ciências Básicas da Saúde, Universidade Federal do Rio Grande do Sul, Porto Alegre, Brazil

**Maha Elsayed**
Laboratory of Neuroenergetics and Cellular Dynamics, Brain Mind Institute, Ecole Polytechnique Fédérale de Lausanne, Lausanne, Switzerland

**Pierre J. Magistretti**
Laboratory of Neuroenergetics and Cellular Dynamics, Brain Mind Institute, Ecole Polytechnique Fédérale de Lausanne, Lausanne, Switzerland
Division of Biological and Environmental Sciences and Engineering, King Abdullah University of Science and Technology, Thuwal, Saudi Arabia
Department of Psychiatry, Center for Psychiatric Neurosciences, University of Lausanne, Lausanne, Switzerland

**Takahiro A. Kato**
Department of Neuropsychiatry, Graduate School of Medical Sciences, Kyushu University, Fukuoka, Japan
Innovation Center for Medical Redox Navigation, Kyushu University, Fukuoka, Japan

**Francesco Petrelli, Luca Pucci and Paola Bezzi**
Department of Fundamental Neurosciences, University of Lausanne, Lausanne, Switzerland

**Paul C. Guest**
Laboratory of Neuroproteomics, Department of Biochemistry and Tissue Biology, Institute of Biology, University of Campinas, Campinas, Brazil

**Keiko Iwata**
Research Center for Child Mental Development, University of Fukui, Fukui, Japan
Department of Development of Functional Brain Activities, United Graduate School of Child Development, Osaka University-Kanazawa University-Hamamatsu University School of Medicine-Chiba University-University of Fukui, Fukui, Japan

**Johann Steiner**
Department of Psychiatry and Psychotherapy-Center for Behavioral Brain Sciences, University of Magdeburg, Magdeburg, Germany

**Andrea Schmitt**
Department of Psychiatry and Psychotherapy, Ludwig-Maximilians University, Munich, Germany
Laboratory of Neurosciences (LIM-27), Institute of Psychiatry, University of São Paulo, São Paulo, Brazil

**Christoph W. Turck**
Department of Translational Research in Psychiatry Proteomics and Biomarkers, Max Planck Institute of Psychiatry, Munich, Germany

**Daniel Martins-de-Souza**
Laboratory of Neuroproteomics, Department of Biochemistry and Tissue Biology, Institute of Biology, University of Campinas, Campinas, Brazil
Laboratory of Neurosciences (LIM-27), Institute of Psychiatry, University of São Paulo, São Paulo, Brazil
UNICAMP's Neurobiology Center, Campinas, Brazil

**Antonietta Gentile, Francesca De Vito and Diego Fresegna**
Fondazione Santa Lucia/Centro Europeo per la Ricerca sul Cervello (CERC), Rome, Italy
Clinica Neurologica, Dipartimento di Medicina dei Sistemi, Università Tor Vergata, Rome, Italy

**Alessandra Musella, Silvia Bullitta and Georgia Mandolesi**
Fondazione Santa Lucia/Centro Europeo per la Ricerca sul Cervello (CERC), Rome, Italy

**Fabio Buttari and Diego Centonze**
Clinica Neurologica, Dipartimento di Medicina dei Sistemi, Università Tor Vergata, Rome, Italy
IRCCS Istituto Neurologico Mediterraneo (INM) Neuromed, Pozzilli, Italy

**Leanne Stokes**
School of Medical Sciences, Health Innovations Research Institute, RMIT University, Melbourne, VIC, Australia
School of Pharmacy, University of East Anglia, Norwich, UK

**Sarah J. Spencer**
School of Health Sciences, Health Innovations Research Institute, RMIT University, Melbourne, VIC, Australia

**Trisha A. Jenkins**
School of Medical Sciences, Health Innovations Research Institute, RMIT University, Melbourne, VIC, Australia

**Kazuhiko Yamamuro, Sohei Kimoto, Toshifumi Kishimoto and Manabu Makinodan**
Department of Psychiatry, Faculty of Medicine, Nara Medical University, Kashihara, Japan

**Kenneth M. Rosen**
BioAxone BioSciences Inc., Cambridge, MA, USA

**Juliana S. Cassoli and Paul C. Guest**
Laboratory of Neuroproteomics, Department of Biochemistry and Tissue Biology, Institute of Biology, University of Campinas, Campinas, Brazil

**Keiko Iwata**
United Graduate School of Child Development, Department of Development of Functional Brain Activities, Research Center for Child Mental Development, Hamamatsu University School of Medicine, Osaka University and Kanazawa University and Chiba University and University of Fukui, Fukui, Japan

**Johann Steiner**
Department of Psychiatry, University of Magdeburg, Magdeburg, Germany

**Juliana M. Nascimento**
Laboratory of Neuroproteomics, Department of Biochemistry and Tissue Biology, Institute of Biology, University of Campinas, Campinas, Brazil
D'Or Institute for Research and Education, Rio de Janeiro, Brazil

**Daniel Martins-de-Souza**
Laboratory of Neuroproteomics, Department of Biochemistry and Tissue Biology, Institute of Biology, University of Campinas, Campinas, Brazil
UNICAMP Neurobiology Center, Campinas, Brazil

**Katarina Davalieva and Ivana Maleva Kostovska**
Research Centre for Genetic Engineering and Biotechnology "Georgi D Efremov," Macedonian Academy of Sciences and Arts, Skopje, Republic of Macedonia

**Andrew J. Dwork**
Department of Molecular Imaging and Neuropathology, New York State Psychiatric Institute, New York, NY, USA
Departments of Psychiatry and Pathology and Cell Biology, College of Physicians and Surgeons of Columbia University, New York, NY, USA
Macedonian Academy of Sciences and Arts, Skopje, Republic of Macedonia

# Index